Transplantation Immunology:
Methods and Protocols

Transplantation Immunology: Methods and Protocols

Edited by Kayla Streep

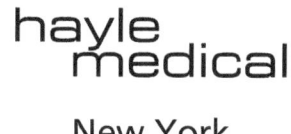

New York

Hayle Medical,
750 Third Avenue, 9th Floor,
New York, NY 10017, USA

Visit us on the World Wide Web at:
www.haylemedical.com

ISBN: 978-1-63241-869-2

Cataloging-in-Publication Data

Transplantation immunology : methods and protocols / edited by Kayla Streep.
    p. cm.
Includes bibliographical references and index.
ISBN 978-1-63241-869-2
1. Transplantation immunology. 2. Immunology. 3. Immunological tolerance. I. Streep, Kayla.
QR188.8 .T73 2020
617.95--dc23

Table of Contents

Preface

The world is advancing at a fast pace like never before. Therefore, the need is to keep up with the latest developments. This book was an idea that came to fruition when the specialists in the area realized the need to coordinate together and document essential themes in the subject. That's when I was requested to be the editor. Editing this book has been an honour as it brings together diverse authors researching on different streams of the field. The book collates essential materials contributed by veterans in the area which can be utilized by students and researchers alike.

Transplantation refers to the process of moving cells, tissues or organs from one part of the body to another, whether within the same person, or between a donor and a recipient. It is usually a life-saving intervention and is a major operation. However, the transplanted tissue or organ may be rejected by the immune system. Rejection is an adaptive immune response of the body that can occur due to the mechanisms of cellular immunity or humoral immunity. Different transplanted tissues favor different rejection mechanisms. Acute rejection occurs in all transplants unless immunosuppression has been achieved. An exception to this is transplantation between identical twins. Hyperacute rejection response sets in within minutes after a transplant, which if unattended may trigger a systemic inflammatory response syndrome. Rapid clumping, particularly the agglutination of red blood cells, is a common risk in kidney transplants. Chronic rejection can arise when there is a long-term loss of function in the transplanted organ. This loss in function arises due to fibrosis of the blood vessels of the transplanted tissues. This is responsible for the long-term morbidity witnessed in lung-transplant recipients. Transplant rejection can be lowered by using immunosuppressant drugs after transplantation and by prior determination of the molecular similitude between donor and recipient. This book provides comprehensive insights into the field of transplantation immunology. It presents researches and studies performed by experts across the globe on the methods and protocols of transplantation. It is a vital tool for all researching and studying this field.

Each chapter is a sole-standing publication that reflects each author's interpretation. Thus, the book displays a multi-facetted picture of our current understanding of application, resources and aspects of the field. I would like to thank the contributors of this book and my family for their endless support.

Editor

Evaluation of the Humoral Immune Response to Human Leukocyte Antigens in Brazilian Renal Transplant Candidates

Patricia Keiko Saito[1], Roger Haruki Yamakawa[1], Erica Pereira Aparecida[2], Waldir Verissimo da Silva Júnior[3], Sueli Donizete Borelli[1]*

1 Department of Basic Health Sciences, Universidade Estadual de Maringá, Maringá, Paraná, Brazil, 2 Histogene Laboratory of Histocompatibility and Genetics, Maringá, Paraná, Brazil, 3 Department of Statistics, Universidade Estadual de Maringá, Maringá, Paraná, Brazil

Abstract

Pre-transplant sensitization to human leukocyte antigens (HLA) is a risk factor for graft failure. Studies of the immunological profile related to anti-HLA antibodies in Brazilian renal transplant candidates are few. In this study, we evaluated the humoral immune response to HLA antigens in 269 renal transplant candidates, in Paraná State, Brazil. The HLA typing was performed by the polymerase chain reaction sequence-specific oligonucleotide method (PCR-SSO) combined with Luminex technology, using an SSO-LABType commercial kit (One Lambda, Inc., Canoga Park, CA, USA). The percentages of panel-reactive antibodies (PRA) and the specificity of anti-HLA antibodies were determined using the LS1PRA and LS2PRA commercial kits (One Lambda, Inc.). The PRA-positive group consisted of 182 (67.7%) patients, and the PRA-negative group of 87 (32.3%) patients. The two groups differed significantly only with respect to gender. Females were the most sensitized. Among the 182 patients with PRA- positive, 62 (34.1%) were positive for class I and negative for class II, 39 (21.4%) were negative for class I and positive for class II, and 81 (44.5%) were positive for both classes I and II. The HLA-A*02, A*24, A*01, B*44, B*35, B*15, DRB1*11, DRB1*04 and DRB1*03 allele groups were the most frequent. The specificities of anti-HLA antibodies were more frequent: A34, B57, Cw15, Cw16, DR51, DQ8 and DP14. This study documented the profile of anti-HLA antibodies in patients with chronic renal failure who were on waiting lists for an organ in Paraná, and found high sensitization to HLA antigens in the samples.

Editor: Emmanuel A. Burdmann, University of Sao Paulo Medical School, Brazil

Funding: This study was supported by National Council for Scientific and Technological Development (grant number 830008/2003-9) and Coordination for Enhancement of Higher Education Personnel – CAPES. The funders' websites are http://www.capes.gov.br/ for CAPES, and http://www.cnpq.br/ for CNPq. The funders had no role in study design, data collection and analysis, decision to publish, or preparation of the manuscript.

Competing Interests: The authors have declared that no competing interests exist.

* E-mail: sueliborelli@gmail.com

Introduction

The importance of anti-human leukocyte antigen (HLA) antibodies in organ transplantation has been known since the 1960s [1]. Many studies have shown that individuals who undergo a hyperacute rejection of an organ, or episodes of acute rejection, whether of the first or a subsequent graft, may contain anti-HLA antibodies in their serum [1–3]. These antibodies can be formed as a result of pregnancies [4–6], blood transfusions [6,7], and previous transplants [6,8].

Detection of anti-HLA antibodies is an important tool for successful transplantation [2,9], since pre-transplant sensitization to HLA antigens is a risk factor for graft failure [10,11]. Patients with high percentages of panel-reactive antibodies (PRA) have a higher probability of rejection [10–12].

Studies on the immunological profile of anti-HLA class I (A, B and Cw) and class II (DR, DQ and DP) antibodies in Brazilian renal transplant candidates are few, in particular in the state of Paraná, Brazil. This study evaluated the immune response to HLA antigens in patients with chronic renal failure, renal transplant candidates, in northern and northwestern Paraná, southern Brazil.

Materials and Methods

Patients

The study was conducted with 269 patients with chronic renal failure, renal transplant candidates, from northern and northwestern Paraná in southern Brazil. Only patients with updated records (active patients/potential recipients) were included. Data regarding demographic characteristics, and potential risk factors for the development of anti-HLA antibodies (transfusions, pregnancies and previous transplants) were obtained from the records of dialysis clinics.

According to the results for the percentage of panel-reactive antibodies (PRA), the patients were divided into two groups, PRA-negative (PRA = 0) and PRA-positive (PRA>0). Subsequently, the PRA-positive patients were divided into 2 groups according to the level of PRA class I and class II, considered separately. The first group included patients with PRA from 1% to 50%, and the second group included patients with PRA between 51% and 100%.

This study was approved by the Ethics Committee of the Universidade Estadual de Maringá, Paraná, Brazil (protocol no.

Table 1. Demographic characteristics and potential risk factors for the development of anti-HLA antibodies, according to the PRA results.

	PRA - Positive (n = 182)	PRA - Negative (n = 87)	P - value
Mean age (years)	52.0±13.2	52.4±12.0	
Gender			
Males	106 (58.2%)	66 (75.9%)	
Females	76 (41.8%)	21 (24.1%)	0.0064
Ethnic group			
White (Caucasian)	104 (57.1%)	52 (59.7%)	
Brown (Mestizo)	54 (29.7%)	16 (18.4%)	
Black	20 (11.0%)	14 (16.1%)	
Yellow (Oriental)	4 (2.2%)	5 (5.8%)	
Potential risk factors			
Mean dialysis duration (years)	7.0±3.8	6.3±3.4	
Any transfusions (no. of patients)	110 (60.4%)	50 (57.5%)	
Number of blood transfusions (units)	3.14±7.05	2.16±3.85	
Any pregnancies (no. of females)	62 (81.6%)	15 (71.4%)	
Previous transplantation history (no. of patients)	16 (8.8%)	4 (4.6%)	

333/2011). All procedures followed Resolution 196/1996 of the Brazilian Health Council, which rules on research on humans in Brazil. All procedures were explained to each subject, and written informed consent was obtained from each subject.

DNA Extraction and HLA Class I and II Typing

To perform the HLA typing, 5 mL of peripheral blood was collected by venipuncture into vacuum tubes (Vacutainer, Becton and Dickson, Oxford, England) containing ethylene diamine tetraacetic acid (EDTA) as an anticoagulant. Genomic DNA extraction was performed by the separation column method, using a Biopur commercial kit for DNA extraction (Biometrix, Curitiba, Paraná, Brazil), following the manufacturer's protocol. After the concentration of the DNA obtained was adjusted by the optical-density method, the polymerase chain reaction sequence-specific oligonucleotide method (PCR-SSO) combined with Luminex technology was carried out using SSO-LABType HLA class I (HLA-A, -B) and class II (HLA-DRB1) commercial kits (One Lambda, Inc., Canoga Park, CA, USA), which provide low-to-medium resolution typing, following the manufacturer's protocol. In this method, genomic DNA was amplified using a biotinylated sequencing primer locus-specific for HLA class I (HLA-A and -B) and class II (HLA-DRB1) in a GeneAmp PCR System 9700 thermocycler (Applied Biosystems, Foster City, CA, USA). Subsequently, hybridization was performed with complementary DNA probes conjugated to microspheres (beads) labeled with different fluorochromes to identify complementary sequences of the amplified DNA. After hybridization, the samples were read by means of the flow cytometry platform LABScan™100 (One Lambda, Inc.), followed by analysis by HLA Fusion software version 2.0 (One Lambda, Inc.).

Determination of Percentages of Panel-Reactive Antibodies (PRA) and HLA-specific Antibodies

The percentages of reactivity of panel-reactive antibodies (PRA) and HLA-specific antibodies were determined in sera from the patients, using the LS1PRA and LS2PRA commercial kits (One Lambda, Inc.) combined with the Luminex technology, following the manufacturer's protocol. In this method, percentages of PRA and HLA-specific antibodies were identified using a panel of color-coded beads coated with purified HLA antigens. The test serum was first incubated with these beads. Any HLA antibodies present in the test serum were bound to the antigens and then were labeled with R-Phycoerythrin (PE)-conjugated Goat anti-human IgG. The fluorescent emission of PE from each bead was detected using the flow cytometry platform LABScanTM100 (One Lambda, Inc.), followed by analysis in HLA Fusion version 2.0 software (One Lambda, Inc.) using the fluorescence analysis minimum recommended by the manufacturer (median fluorescence intensity equal to or greater than 500).

Statistical Analyses

All statistical analyses were performed with Statistica 7 software. Allele and phenotype frequencies were calculated by direct counting. Fisher's exact test and Student's T test were used to compare the demographic characteristics and potential risk factors for the development of anti-HLA antibodies among the study groups. The significance level of the statistical test was 5% ($P < 0.05$).

Results

The demographic characteristics and potential risk factors for the development of anti-HLA antibodies, according to the PRA results, are shown in Table 1.

The PRA-positive group consisted of 182 (67.7%) patients, and the PRA-negative group of 87 (32.3%) patients. Only gender showed a significant difference between the two groups. The females were the most sensitized.

The frequencies of the HLA-A, -B and -DRB1 allele groups of the patients are shown in Table 2. The *HLA-A*02, A*24* and *A*01* allele groups were the most common locus for A. In the B locus, the most common allele groups were *HLA-B*44, B*35*, and *B*15*;

Table 2. HLA-A, -B and -DRB1 alleles and phenotype frequencies of the total patient group.

HLA-A*	Allele frequencies	Phenotype frequencies	HLA-B*	Allele frequencies	Phenotype frequencies	HLA-DRB1*	Allele frequencies	Phenotype frequencies
01	0.1041	0.2082	07	0.0613	0.1227	01	0.0855	0.1710
02	0.2416	0.4833	08	0.0558	0.1115	03	0.1097	0.2193
03	0.0892	0.1784	13	0.0186	0.0372	04	0.1338	0.2677
11	0.0651	0.1301	14	0.0260	0.0520	07	0.1115	0.2230
23	0.0446	0.0892	15	0.0874	0.1747	08	0.0558	0.1115
24	0.1152	0.2305	18	0.0390	0.0781	09	0.0204	0.0409
25	0.0316	0.0632	27	0.0242	0.0483	10	0.0260	0.0520
26	0.0372	0.0743	35	0.1041	0.2082	11	0.1357	0.2714
29	0.0242	0.0483	37	0.0112	0.0223	12	0.0093	0.0186
30	0.0520	0.1041	38	0.0279	0.0558	13	0.1301	0.2602
31	0.0335	0.0669	39	0.0409	0.0818	14	0.0446	0.0892
32	0.0279	0.0558	40	0.0651	0.1301	15	0.1078	0.2156
33	0.0279	0.0558	41	0.0186	0.0372	16	0.0297	0.0595
34	0.0093	0.0186	42	0.0242	0.0483			
36	0.0074	0.0149	44	0.1059	0.2119			
66	0.0112	0.0223	45	0.0223	0.0446			
68	0.0576	0.1152	47	0.0019	0.0037			
69	0.0019	0.0037	48	0.0093	0.0186			
74	0.0149	0.0297	49	0.0316	0.0632			
80	0.0037	0.0074	50	0.0335	0.0669			
			51	0.0836	0.1673			
			52	0.0204	0.0409			
			53	0.0242	0.0483			
			54	0.0056	0.0112			
			55	0.0112	0.0223			
			56	0.0019	0.0037			
			57	0.0260	0.0520			
			58	0.0149	0.0297			
			81	0.0019	0.0037			
			82	0.0019	0.0037			

Table 3. Distribution of anti-HLA antibodies according to the percentage of PRA.

	Group 1 PRA = 1%–50%	Group 2 PRA = 51%–100%
Anti-Class I (N = 143)		
Anti-locus A	23	4
Anti-locus B	42	0
Anti-locus C	1	0
Anti-locus A+B	26	29
Anti-locus A+Cw	0	0
Anti-locus B+Cw	2	0
Anti-locus A+B+Cw	3	13
Anti-class II (N = 120)		
Anti-locus DR	21	4
Anti-locus DQ	10	1
Anti-locus DP	0	0
Anti-locus DR+DQ	36	38
Anti-locus DR+DP	0	0
Anti-locus DQ+DP	0	0
Anti-locus DR+DQ+DP	2	8

and in the DRB1 locus, the *HLA-DRB1*11*, *DRB1*04* and *DRB1*13* allele groups were the most common.

The distribution of anti-HLA antibodies according to the percentage of PRA is shown in Table 3.

Among the 182 patients with positive PRA, 62 (34.1%) were positive for class I and negative for class II, 39 (21.4%) were negative for class I and positive for class II, and 81 (44.5%) were positive for both classes I and II. According to the percentages of PRA class I, 97 (67.8%) patients were in group 1 and 46 (32.2%) were in group 2. For class II, 69 (57.5%) patients were in group 1 and 51 (42.5%) were in group 2.

Furthermore, according to the percentages of PRA greater or equal to 80, 28 patients were positive for class I, 27 patients for class II, and 11 patients for classes I and II.

The overall incidences of anti-HLA-A, -B, -Cw, -DR, -DQ and -DP antibodies in the group of patients with positive PRA are shown in Tables 4 and 5. The specificities of anti-HLA antibodies were most frequent: A34, B57, Cw15, Cw16, DR51, DQ8 and DP14.

Discussion

Many studies have demonstrated the importance of HLA antigens in the transplantation of organs and the effect of anti-HLA antibodies on survival and graft rejection [1–3,13]. For this reason, before transplantation, there is a need to ensure the best immunological compatibility between donor and recipient. In addition to compatibility, it is necessary to determine the existence of preformed antibodies, since the presence of these antibodies in the recipient against the donor's specific antigen, can result in a deleterious response to transplantation [1,9]. Therefore, the determination of the specificity of anti-HLA antibodies in the serum is of paramount importance for patients with renal disease and transplant candidates.

This study provides the first data on the immunological profile of anti-HLA class I (A, B and Cw) and class II (DR, DQ and DP) antibodies and the percentage of PRA in renal transplant candidates from southern Brazil. The production of anti-HLA antibodies occurs as a result of sensitizing events [4–8], and individuals may differ in the development of these antibodies. Unlike the results of studies conducted in other countries [14–16], most of the patients in this study were positive for PRA (67.7%). However, the methodologies used to determine the PRA differ among studies. The high number of patients sensitized to HLA antigens can also be explained, in part, by the practice, in Brazil, of performing blood transfusions in both hypersensitive and non-sensitized patients without regard to the high probability of generating anti-HLA antibodies.

Silva et al. [17] reported high rates of leukocyte alloimmunization (30.5%) in a study conducted with 393 patients awaiting kidney transplantation in northeastern Brazil. In the present study, the percentage of sensitized patients was higher than that found by Silva et al. [17]. One possible explanation could lie in the different methodologies used to determine the PRA. Silva et al. used a complement-dependent microlymphocytotoxicity test sensitized with human antiglobulin, and the sera were tested against panel-reactive antibodies (PRA) consisting of 50 individuals phenotyped with HLA class I antigens.

Human leukocyte antigen alloimmunization in candidates for renal transplantation is a reality [18,19] and knowledge of the incidence of sensitization to HLA antigens in the Brazilian population may be important for advances in renal transplantation and to minimize the waiting time for candidates [19].

Several studies have reported that pregnancies, blood transfusions and previous transplants are potential risk factors for development of anti-HLA antibodies [6,20]. The vast majority of patients investigated in the present study had received blood transfusions (59.5%), some patients had received previous transplants (7.4%), and most women had had pregnancies (79.4%).

Pregnancy as an immunogenic factor inducing the mother to produce antibodies against the father's antigens, which are carried by the fetus, has been reported in several studies [4,5]. Heise et al. (2001) [14], Ozdemir et al. (2004) [15], and Karahan et al. (2009) [16] found an association between pregnancy and the production

Table 4. Anti-HLA class I antibodies in patients with a positive PRA.

anti-HLA-A	frequency	anti-HLA-B	frequency	anti-HLA-Cw	frequency
anti-A1	0.1758	anti-B7	0.1484	anti-Cw1	0.0055
anti-A2	0.2143	anti-B8	0.1374	anti-Cw4	0.0220
anti-A3	0.0714	anti-B13	0.0989	anti-Cw6	0.0110
anti-A11	0.0989	anti-B18	0.1044	anti-Cw7	0.0055
anti-A23	0.1978	anti-B27	0.1703	anti-Cw9	0.0055
anti-A24	0.2308	anti-B35	0.1538	anti-Cw12	0.0110
anti-A25	0.1319	anti-B37	0.0330	anti-Cw14	0.0110
anti-A26	0.0879	anti-B38	0.0495	anti-Cw15	0.0330
anti-A29	0.0769	anti-B39	0.1044	anti-Cw16	0.0330
anti-A30	0.0769	anti-B41	0.0440	anti-Cw18	0.0055
anti-A31	0.1044	anti-B42	0.1374		
anti-A32	0.1319	anti-B44	0.0934		
anti-A33	0.1264	anti-B45	0.0934		
anti-A34	0.2473	anti-B46	0.0055		
anti-A36	0.1154	anti-B47	0.0385		
anti-A66	0.1429	anti-B48	0.1319		
anti-A68	0.2253	ant-B49	0.1154		
anti-A69	0.1868	anti-B50	0.1209		
anti-A74	0.0385	anti-B51	0.1209		
anti-A80	0.0824	anti-B52	0.1264		
		anti-B53	0.1154		
		anti-B54	0.1044		
		anti-B55	0.1044		
		anti-B56	0.1484		
		anti-B57	0.2088		
		anti-B58	0.1813		
		anti-B59	0.0604		
		anti-B60	0.1593		
		anti-B61	0.1374		
		anti-B62	0.0934		
		anti-B63	0.1319		
		anti-B64	0.0769		
		anti-B65	0.1044		
		anti-B67	0.1538		
		anti-B71	0.0659		
		anti-B72	0.0659		
		anti-B73	0.0275		
		anti-B75	0.0604		
		anti-B76	0.0659		
		anti-B78	0.0989		
		anti-B81	0.1374		
		anti-B82	0.0769		

of anti-HLA antibodies. In this study, the vast majority of female patients had been pregnant and had become sensitized in this process. However, in the present study, the PRA-positive and negative groups did not differ in this potential risk factor for the development of anti-HLA antibodies. A possible explanation could lie in the presence of maternal HLA compatibility with the father, or the degree of immunogenicity of HLA antigens that the mother may have contacted through the fetus.

Blood transfusion remains an important factor in patients on hemodialysis. Although the use of recombinant human erythropoietin in hemodialysis patients has resulted in improved hemoglobin levels and ameliorated the symptoms of anemia, significantly reducing the number of transfusions required, its use

Table 5. Anti-HLA class II antibodies in patients with a positive PRA.

anti-HLA-DR	frequency	anti-HLA-DQ	frequency	anti-HLA-DP	frequency
anti-DR1	0.2308	anti-DQ2	0.0934	anti-DP1	0.0055
anti-DR4	0.2198	anti-DQ4	0.0769	anti-DP2	0.0055
anti-DR7	0.2143	anti-DQ5	0.0714	anti-DP3	0.0110
anti-DR8	0.2198	anti-DQ6	0.0989	anti-DP4	0.0055
anti-DR9	0.2747	anti-DQ7	0.2088	anti-DP5	0.0110
anti-DR10	0.1538	anti-DQ8	0.3132	anti-DP13	0.0110
anti-DR11	0.1484	anti-DQ9	0.2967	anti-DP14	0.0165
anti-DR12	0.2802			anti-DP18	0.0055
anti-DR13	0.1923				
anti-DR14	0.1374				
anti-DR15	0.2033				
anti-DR16	0.2473				
anti-DR17	0.1868				
anti-DR18	0.1703				
anti-DR51	0.2912				
anti-DR52	0.1209				
anti-DR53	0.1868				
anti-DR103	0.1923				

does not completely eliminate the need for blood transfusions in patients [21–23].

A few patients in the study had undergone previous transplants. Great progress has been made in organ transplantation, both in immunosuppressive therapy and in pretransplant laboratory tests. This progress is reflected in the reduced number of rejections, consequently reducing the number of patients who return to the waiting queue after an unsuccessful transplantation. Phelan et al. (2012) [24] followed 2381 kidney transplants, and observed that only 190 patients suffered a rejection. The same authors reported a decrease in cases of rejection over the years, from 7% in 1990 to less than 1% in 2009.

However, in the present study, the PRA-positive and negative groups did not differ in potential risk factors for the development of anti-HLA antibodies, in contrast to findings in studies conducted in other countries [14–16]. However, this study was conducted with a sample of Brazilian patients with chronic renal failure, also differing from other studies, because of the relatively larger number of patients with a positive PRA compared with those with a negative PRA. This study also used a different methodology for determination of PRA and anti-HLA antibodies.

Among the PRA-positive patients, a high proportion were positive for both classes (I and II) of anti-HLA antibodies. Consequently, as expected, the number of HLA loci to which the antibodies were reactive was also high in the group with a PRA between 51% and 100% (group 2), in comparison with the PRA group of 1% to 50% (group 1), for the two classes of anti-HLA antibodies.

In this study also, a significant proportion of patients with a positive PRA showed values between 51% and 100%, demonstrating a high degree of sensitization to HLA in both class I and class II. The present study also found hypersensitized patients (patients with PRA greater or equal to 80). Patients with high percentages of PRA may have a higher probability of rejection [10–12].

Our study also documented the frequency anti-HLA-Cw and anti-HLA-DP antibodies, which are generally little explored in studies of antibody profiles. The clinical significance of pretransplant anti-HLA-Cw and anti-HLA-DP has not been widely investigated, although studies have now reported the effect of HLA-Cw and -DP on the survival of the renal graft. Patients with mismatched HLA-Cw showed an increase in the likelihood of acute rejection [25,26], hyperacute rejection [27], acute antibody-mediated rejection [28,29], and chronic rejection [30] in the presence of anti-HLA-Cw. Qiu et al. (2005) [31] detected a higher frequency of anti-HLA-DP in patients who rejected their grafts than in those with functioning grafts, finding anti-HLA-DP in 5.1% of 138 renal transplant recipients with functioning grafts, and 19.5% of 185 patients with rejected grafts. They called attention to the fact that 13% of patients who had rejected the graft had only anti-HLA-DP antibodies [31]. Several studies have reported acute rejection [28,32,33] and antibody-mediated chronic rejection [34] in renal transplant recipients, in the presence of anti-HLA-DP. These occurrences emphasize the importance of knowledge of the specificities of these antibodies, in order to improve graft survival.

The frequency of HLA allele groups in this study was similar to that in healthy subjects from southern Brazil [35–37]. The Brazilian population is one of the most heterogeneous in the world, consisting of various ethnic groups [38], and the frequencies of HLA alleles may vary according to the predominant ethnic group in a region [36,39,40]. The samples tested in this study were from the state of Paraná in southern Brazil. Southern Brazil was settled mainly by Europeans, but also has significant numbers of people of African descent and Native Americans in the population [39]. This influence can be observed in the results of this study, which revealed a predominant contribution of HLA allele groups of European origin, such as HLA-A*24 and -B*44 [41–43], as well as the occurrence of allele groups of African influence such as HLA-A*30 and -B*15 [44,45].

The most common HLA allele groups were HLA-A*02, -A*24, -A*01, -B*44, -B*35, -B*15, -DRB1*11, -DRB1*04 and -DRB1*13. In contrast, the specificities of anti-HLA loci for A, B and DR were frequently A34, A24, A68, B57, B58, B27, DR51, DR12 and DR9. There were similarities but also differences among the HLA allele groups, and the specificities of anti-HLA antibodies found in this study. This pattern is in agreement with the results found in another study of correlations between the frequency of HLA antigens and anti-HLA antibodies in renal transplant candidates [46]. HLA mismatch generally produces an antibody specific to that antigen. One would expect that the frequency of a specificity of anti-HLA antibody would correlate naturally with the frequency of the phenotype in the population, or if a HLA phenotype is present in low frequency in the population, antibodies specific for this phenotype would also be rare. However, Idica et al., 2006 [47] showed that immunization against low-frequency phenotypes may occur frequently, in agreement with the results found here. In the present study, relatively rare antigens such as A34, A68, B58, DR9, DR12 were among those that most induced the production of anti-HLA antibodies. This finding can also be explained by the mixture of ethnic groups, leading to a variety of combinations of HLA alleles and haplotypes in the population, and increasing the likelihood of HLA incompatibilities and sensitization to HLA antigens.

Heise et al. (2001) [14] and Karahan et al. (2009) [16] showed that certain HLA phenotypes may be associated with the development of anti-HLA antibodies in patients with chronic renal failure. Karahan et al. (2009) [16] showed that the frequencies of the HLA-A3, HLA-A66 and HLA-B18 phenotypes were significantly elevated in PRA-positive patients compared to PRA-negative patients, and the DRB1*07 allele was more frequent in patients with a history of events and no production of anti-HLA antibodies, suggesting that DRB1*07 may be associated with a low risk of formation of anti-HLA antibodies. Heise et al. (2001) [14] found a positive association for the development of anti-HLA antibodies with HLA class I phenotypes (HLA-A10, -A19, -A36, -B42 and -B53), and negative associations with HLA class I phenotypes (A1, A2, A11, B8, B12, B40) and class II phenotypes (DR1, DR4, DR7). The same study found that the DR3 phenotype was associated with high values of PRA and lower rates of graft survival, and the DR1 and DR4 phenotypes

were associated with low values of PRA and good graft survival. However, some phenotypes such as HLA-A2 and HLA-B18, which showed positive or negative associations in these studies, are common both in the chronic renal failure patients in this study and in populations of healthy individuals [36,37]. These studies emphasize the importance of knowledge of HLA diversity and the profile of antibodies to the HLA system, in the context of organ and tissue transplantation.

The limitations of this study consist particularly in the use of small sample sizes, and in the difficulties in obtaining relevant information (pregnancies, blood transfusions and previous transplants), because the majority of hemodialysis clinics and transplant centers in Brazil do not have a system for efficient data storage, updating and retrieval of this information. Despite these limitations, this study provided important data on sensitization to HLA antigens, including pre-transplant anti-HLA-Cw and anti-HLA-DP sensitization, which is little explored in studies of anti-HLA antibody profiles.

Conclusions

The data from this study document the profile of anti-HLA antibodies in chronic renal failure patients on the waiting list for an organ in northern and northwestern Paraná, showing a high proportion of sensitization to HLA antigens (positive PRA). Evaluation of the immune response to HLA antigens in the pre-transplant workup may contribute to future studies of the association of HLA alleles with the development of anti-HLA antibodies in Brazilian patients, patients with chronic kidney disease, and for the understanding of future events related to the acceptance or rejection of grafts.

Acknowledgments

We would like to thank all patients involved in this study.

Author Contributions

Conceived and designed the experiments: PKS RHY SDB. Performed the experiments: PKS RHY EPA. Analyzed the data: PKS RHY EPA WVSJ SDB. Contributed reagents/materials/analysis tools: PKS RHY WVSJ SDB. Wrote the paper: PKS RHY EPA WVSJ SDB.

References

1. Kissmeyer-Nielsen F, Olsen S, Petersen VP, Fjeldborg O (1966) Hyperacute rejection of kidney allografts, associated with pre-existing humoral antibodies against donor cells. Lancet 2: 662–665.
2. Patel R, Terasaki PI (1969) Significance of the positive crossmatch test in kidney transplantation. N Engl J Med 280: 735–739.
3. Halloran PF, Wadgymar A, Ritchie S, Falk J, Solez K, et al. (1990) The significance of the anti-class I antibody response. I. Clinical and pathologic features of anti-class I-mediated rejection. Transplantation 49: 85–91.
4. Van Rood JJ, Eernisse JG, Van Leeuwen A (1958) Leucocyte antibodies in sera from pregnant women. Nature 181: 1735–1736.
5. Payne R, Rolfs MR (1958) Fetomaternal leukocyte incompatibility. J Clin Invest 37: 1756–1763.
6. Vongwiwatana A, Tasanarong A, Hidalgo LG, Halloran PF (2003) The role of B cells and alloantibody in the host response to human organ allografts. Immunol Rev 196: 197–218.
7. Dausset J (1954) Leuco agglutinins IV. Leuco-agglutinins and blood transfusion. Vox Sang 4: 190–8.
8. Thick M, Verbi V, Kennedy L, Welsh K (1984) Sensitization following kidney graft failure and blood transfusion. Transplantation 37: 525–526.
9. Susal C, Opelz G (2002) Kidney graft failure and presensitization against HLA class I and class II antigens. Transplantation 73: 1269–1273.
10. Abe M, Kawai T, Futatsuyama K, Tanabe K, Fuchinoue S, et al. (1997) Postoperative production of anti-donor antibody and chronic rejection in renal transplantation. Transplantation 63: 1616–1619.
11. Barama A, Oza U, Panek R, Belitsky P, MacDonald AS, et al. (2000) Effect of recipient sensitization (peak PRA) on graft outcome in haploidentical living related kidney transplants. Clin Transplant 14: 212–217.
12. Matas AJ, Gillingham K, Payne WD, Humar A, Dunn DL, et al. (2000) Should I accept this kidney? Clin Transplant 14: 90–95.
13. Egfjord M, Jakobsen BK, Ladefoged J (2003) No impact of cross-reactive group human leucocyte antigen class I matching on long-term kidney graft survival. Scand J Immunol 57: 362–365.
14. Heise E, Manning C, Thacker L (2001) HLA phenotypes of ESRD patients are risk factors in the panel-reactive antibody (PRA) response. Clin Transplant 15 Suppl 6: 22–27.
15. Ozdemir FN, Sezer S, Akcay A, Arat Z, Turan M, et al. (2004) Panel reactive antibody positivity and associated HLA antibodies in Turkish renal transplant candidates. Transpl Immunol 12: 185–188.
16. Karahan GE, Seyhun Y, Oguz F, Kekik C, Onal E, et al. (2009) Anti-HLA antibody profile of Turkish patients with end-stage renal disease. Transplant Proc 41: 3651–3654.
17. da Silva SF, Ferreira GM, da Silva SL, Alves TM, Ribeiro IF, et al. (2013) Red blood cell and leukocyte alloimmunization in patients awaiting kidney transplantation. Rev Bras Hematol Hemoter 35: 185–188.
18. Krishnan NS, Zehnder D, Briggs D, Higgins R (2012) Human leukocyte antigen antibody incompatible renal transplantation. Indian J Nephrol 22: 409–414.
19. Mota MA (2013) Red cell and human leukocyte antigen alloimmunization in candidates for renal transplantation: a reality. Rev Bras Hematol Hemoter 35: 160–161.
20. Ling M, Marfo K, Masiakos P, Aljanabi A, Lindower J, et al. (2012) Pretransplant anti-HLA-Cw and anti-HLA-DP antibodies in sensitized patients. Hum Immunol 73: 879–883.

21. Kliger AS, Fishbane S, Finkelstein FO (2012) Erythropoietic stimulating agents and quality of a patient's life: individualizing anemia treatment. Clin J Am Soc Nephrol 7: 354–357.

22. Goodnough LT, Strasburg D, Riddell Jt, Verbrugge D, Wish J (1994) Has recombinant human erythropoietin therapy minimized red-cell transfusions in hemodialysis patients? Clin Nephrol 41: 303–307.

23. Tanhehco YC, Berns JS (2012) Red blood cell transfusion risks in patients with end-stage renal disease. Semin Dial 25: 539–544.

24. Phelan PJ, O'Kelly P, Tarazi M, Tarazi N, Salehmohamed MR, et al. (2012) Renal allograft loss in the first post-operative month: causes and consequences. Clin Transplant 26: 544–549.

25. Frohn C, Fricke L, Puchta JC, Kirchner H (2001) The effect of HLA-C matching on acute renal transplant rejection. Nephrol Dial Transplant 16: 355–360.

26. Tran TH, Dohler B, Heinold A, Scherer S, Ruhenstroth A, et al. (2011) Deleterious impact of mismatching for human leukocyte antigen-C in presensitized recipients of kidney transplants. Transplantation 92: 419–425.

27. Chapman JR, Taylor C, Ting A, Morris PJ (1986) Hyperacute rejection of a renal allograft in the presence of anti-HLA-Cw5 antibody. Transplantation 42: 91–93.

28. Gilbert M, Paul S, Perrat G, Giannoli C, Pouteil Noble C, et al. (2011) Impact of pretransplant human leukocyte antigen-C and -DP antibodies on kidney graft outcome. Transplant Proc 43: 3412–3414.

29. Bachelet T, Couzi L, Guidicelli G, Moreau K, Morel D, et al. (2011) Anti-Cw donor-specific alloantibodies can lead to positive flow cytometry crossmatch and irreversible acute antibody-mediated rejection. Am J Transplant 11: 1543–1544.

30. Duquesnoy RJ, Marrari M (2011) Detection of antibodies against HLA-C epitopes in patients with rejected kidney transplants. Transpl Immunol 24: 164–171.

31. Qiu J, Cai J, Terasaki PI, El-Awar N, Lee JH (2005) Detection of antibodies to HLA-DP in renal transplant recipients using single antigen beads. Transplantation 80: 1511–1513.

32. Goral S, Prak EL, Kearns J, Bloom RD, Pierce E, et al. (2008) Preformed donor-directed anti-HLA-DP antibodies may be an impediment to successful kidney transplantation. Nephrol Dial Transplant 23: 390–392.

33. Singh P, Colombe BW, Francos GC, Martinez Cantarin MP, Frank AM (2010) Acute humoral rejection in a zero mismatch deceased donor renal transplant due to an antibody to an HLA-DP alpha. Transplantation 90: 220–221.

34. Thaunat O, Hanf W, Dubois V, McGregor B, Perrat G, et al. (2009) Chronic humoral rejection mediated by anti-HLA-DP alloantibodies: insights into the role of epitope sharing in donor-specific and non-donor specific alloantibodies generation. Transpl Immunol 20: 209–211.

35. Ruiz TM, da Costa SM, Ribas F, Luz PR, Lima SS, et al. (2005) Human leukocyte antigen allelic groups and haplotypes in a brazilian sample of volunteer donors for bone marrow transplant in Curitiba, Parana, Brazil. Transplant Proc 37: 2293–2296.

36. Bortolotto AS, Petry MG, da Silveira JG, Raya AR, Fernandes SR, et al. (2012) HLA-A, -B, and -DRB1 allelic and haplotypic diversity in a sample of bone marrow volunteer donors from Rio Grande do Sul State, Brazil. Hum Immunol 73: 180–185.

37. Bardi MS, Jarduli LR, Jorge AJ, Camargo RB, Carneiro FP, et al. (2012) HLA-A, B and DRB1 allele and haplotype frequencies in volunteer bone marrow donors from the north of Parana State. Rev Bras Hematol Hemoter 34: 25–30.

38. Parra FC, Amado RC, Lambertucci JR, Rocha J, Antunes CM, et al. (2003) Color and genomic ancestry in Brazilians. Proc Natl Acad Sci USA 100: 177–182.

39. Probst CM, Bompeixe EP, Pereira NF, Dalalio MMdeO, Visentainer JE, et al. (2000) HLA polymorphism and evaluation of European, African, and Amerindian contribution to the white and mulatto populations from Parana, Brazil. Hum Biol 72: 597–617.

40. Nigam P, Dellalibera E, Mauricio-da-Silva L, Donadi EA, Silva RS (2004) Polymorphism of HLA class I genes in the Brazilian population from the Northeastern State of Pernambuco corroborates anthropological evidence of its origin. Tissue Antigens 64: 204–209.

41. Silva Carvalho A (1983) HLA-A, B and C markers in the Portuguese population. Tissue Antigens 21: 39–44.

42. Piazza A, Olivetti E, Griffo RM, Rendine S, Amoroso A, et al. (1989) The distribution of HLA antigens in Italy. Gene Geogr 3: 141–164.

43. Ribas F, Oliveira LA, Petzl-Erler ML, Bicalho MG (2008) Major histocompatibility complex class I chain-related gene A polymorphism and linkage disequilibrium with HLA-B alleles in Euro-Brazilians. Tissue Antigens 72: 532–538.

44. Assane AA, Fabricio-Silva GM, Cardoso-Oliveira J, Mabunda NE, Sousa AM, et al. (2010) Human leukocyte antigen-A, -B, and -DRB1 allele and haplotype frequencies in the Mozambican population: a blood donor-based population study. Hum Immunol 71: 1027–1032.

45. Paximadis M, Mathebula TY, Gentle NL, Vardas E, Colvin M, et al. (2012) Human leukocyte antigen class I (A, B, C) and II (DRB1) diversity in the black and Caucasian South African population. Hum Immunol 73: 80–92.

46. Fu Q, Wang C, Zeng W, Liu L (2012) The correlation of HLA allele frequencies and HLA antibodies in sensitized kidney transplantation candidates. Transplant Proc 44: 217–221.

47. Idica A, Sasaki N, Hardy S, Terasaki P (2006) Unexpected frequencies of HLA antibody specificities present in sera of multitransfused patients. Clin Transpl: 139–159.

2

Poor Long-Term Outcome in Second Kidney Transplantation: A Delayed Event

Katy Trébern-Launay[1,2], Yohann Foucher[2,1], Magali Giral[1], Christophe Legendre[3,4], Henri Kreis[3], Michèle Kessler[5], Marc Ladrière[5], Nassim Kamar[6,7], Lionel Rostaing[6,7], Valérie Garrigue[8], Georges Mourad[8], Emmanuel Morelon[9], Jean-Paul Soulillou[1]*, Jacques Dantal[1]

1 Institut de Transplantation Urologie Néphrologie (ITUN), Inserm U643, CHU Hôtel Dieu, Nantes, France, 2 Université de Nantes, EA4275 'Biostatistique, Recherche Clinique et Mesures Subjectives en Santé', Nantes, France, 3 Service de Transplantation Rénale et de Soins Intensifs, Hôpital Necker, APHP, Paris, France, 4 Universités Paris Descartes et Sorbonne Paris Cité, Paris, France, 5 Service de Transplantation Rénale, CHU Brabois, Nancy, France, 6 Service de Néphrologie, HTA, Dialyse et Transplantation d'Organes, CHU Rangueil, Toulouse, France, 7 Université Paul Sabatier, Toulouse, France, 8 Service de Néphrologie-Transplantation, Hôpital Lapeyronie, Montpellier, France, 9 Service de Néphrologie, Transplantation et Immunologie Clinique, Hôpital Edouard Herriot, Lyon, France

Abstract

Background: Old studies reported a worse outcome for second transplant recipient (STR) than for first transplant recipient (FTR) mainly due to non-comparable populations with numbers confounding factors. More recent analysis, based on improved methodology by using multivariate regressions, challenged this generally accepted idea: the poor prognosis for STR is still under debate.

Methodology: To assess the long-term patient-and-graft survival of STR compared to FTR, we performed an observational study based on the French DIVAT prospective cohort between 1996 and 2010 (N = 3103 including 641 STR). All patients were treated with a CNI, an mTOR inhibitor or belatacept in addition to steroids and mycophenolate mofetil for maintenance therapy. Patient-and-graft survival and acute rejection episode (ARE) were analyzed using Cox models adjusted for all potential confounding factors such as pre-transplant anti-HLA immunization.

Results: We showed that STR have a higher risk of graft failure than FTR (HR = 2.18, p = 0.0013) but that this excess risk was observed after few years of transplantation. There was no significant difference between STR and FTR in the occurrence of either overall ARE (HR = 1.01, p = 0.9675) or steroid-resistant ARE (HR = 1.27, p = 0.4087).

Conclusions: The risk of graft failure following second transplantation remained consistently higher than that observed in first transplantation after adjusting for confounding factors. The rarely performed time-dependent statistical modeling may explain the heterogeneous conclusions of the literature concerning second transplantation outcomes. In clinical practice, physicians should not consider STR and FTR equally.

Editor: Holger K. Eltzschig, University of Colorado Denver, United States of America

Funding: This work was partly supported by the RTRS, the 'Fondation de Co-opération Scientifique – CENTAURE' and Roche Laboratory. K. Trébern-Launay is the recipient of a grant for epidemiology and biostatistics research from the RTRS 'CENTAURE' and Novartis Pharma. The funders had no role in study design, data collection and analysis, decision to publish, or preparation of the manuscript.

Competing Interests: The authors have the following interests. This work was partly supported by Roche Laboratory, and K. Trébern-Launay is the recipient of a grant for epidemiology and biostatistics research from Novartis Pharma. There are no patents, products in development or marketed products to declare.

* E-mail: jean-paul.soulillou@univ-nantes.fr

Introduction

Nowadays, repeat transplantation provides the best chance for long-term survival and quality of life in patients facing allograft loss, as compared to maintenance dialysis therapy [1,2,3]. This concept was recently supported by Ojo et al. [2] who showed that repeat transplantation is associated with a reduced mortality compared to remaining on dialysis after a prior graft loss. This benefit is valid despite the fact that re-transplant recipients present a higher risk of death during the first month after the transplant surgery [1]. When considering short and long-term outcomes, graft survival rates following retransplantation have continuously improved in recent years [4]. There is evidence that patients undergoing a third or more transplantation have a worse prognosis [5,6,7]. However, the poor prognosis of second transplant recipients (STR) remains a matter of debate.

Some previous studies have demonstrated that STR have a lower graft survival than first transplant recipients (FTR) [2,8,9,10,11,12] leading STR to be considered as a higher risk group for graft failure, mainly related to increased levels of preformed HLA antibodies [13]. However, Coupel et al. showed that the difference in long-term graft survival was not significant between STR and FTR when an HLA-DR mismatch was avoided [14]. Recent improvements in immunosuppressive therapy may have contributed to decreasing the difference in outcomes between STR and FTR [8]. When taking into account several confounding factors such as pre-transplant immunization, evidence of an excess risk of graft failure for STR is not clear, as demonstrated by the most recent studies [1,5,15,16]. For Magee et al., after adjustment for donor and recipient factors, the risk of graft failure remained significantly higher for STR than FTR [17].

Whereas factors influencing second graft survival have been well studied [8,9,14,16,18,19,20], those related to a possible excess risk of graft failure for STR compared with FTR are not well established [15,17]. The objective of our study was not to recommend whether patients should get a second transplant or not. Addressing this important question would require a completely different study design. Indeed, the overall aim of our epidemiological observational cohort study was to provide data from a large multicenter population of kidney transplant recipients in order to clarify the relationship between the graft rank and the long term graft outcomes. For the first time, we adjusted for a large number of covariates at baseline and we modeled the time-dependent relationship between graft rank and graft survival. According to these methodological improvements, we demonstrated that STR have a poorer patient-and-graft survival (PGS) than FTR significant since four years post-transplantation.

Materials and Methods

Study population

Data were prospectively collected from the DIVAT (Données Informatisées et VAlidées en Transplantation) French multicentric database [21]. Codes were used to assure donor and recipient anonymity and blind assay. The "Comité National Informatique et Liberté" approved the study (N° CNIL 891735) and written informed consent was obtained from the participants. The data are computerized in real time as well as at each transplant anniversary and are submitted for an annual audit. The cohort consisted of 2462 FTR and 641 STR meeting the following inclusion criteria: (a) adult recipients; (b) transplantations performed between January 1996 and November 2010; and (c) maintenance therapy with calcineurin inhibitors, mammalian target of rapamycin inhibitors or belatacept, in addition to mycophenolic acid (Myfortic® Novartis, France or Cellcept® Roche, France) and steroids. Simultaneous transplantations were excluded. Among 2462 FTR meeting the inclusion criteria, 52 patients were also part of the STR group as they received two transplants during the observation period. These 52 patients, who were included in both cohorts, represented 2% and 8% of the FTR and STR groups respectively. Given the large number of covariates, it is reasonable to assume conditional independence of these patients. We did not exclude these 52 patients as this would have reduced the comparability of the two groups by under-representing the FTR patients with a rapid return-to-dialysis, which would have led to an over-estimation of FTR graft survival.

Clinical variables of interest

To guarantee the comparability between FTR and STR, adjustments were made for all of the following possible pre- or per-transplant immunological and non-immunological confounding factors: transplantation period (before or after 2005, which corresponds to the routine utilization of high sensitivity techniques for panel-reactive antibody, PRA), recipient gender and age, primary diagnosis of end stage renal disease (ESRD), comorbidities, highest historical levels of pre-transplant PRA against class I and II antigens, deceased or living donor status, donor age, cold ischemia time (CIT), HLA-A-B-DR mismatches and induction therapy. The high sensitivity techniques correspond to pre-

transplant anti-HLA identification obtained by multiplex screening test (LAT-M; One lambda, Canoga Park, CA).

French law does not authorize the storage of race information (specific authorization may be obtained in specific circumstances, such as for genetics population studies). The induction therapy was differentiated according to its effect on lymphocytes: horse or rabbit antithymocyte globulin antibodies or anti-CD3 antibody were considered as lymphocyte-depleting agents whereas anti-interleukin-2 receptor antibodies (basiliximab) were considered as a non lymphocyte-depleting agent. Since not all of the biopsies were analyzed with the recent Banff classification but as therapeutic strategies were nevertheless mostly based on a histological diagnosis regardless of the time period, and as the therapeutic strategies did not differ according to the graft rank regardless of the period, we opted to grade acute rejection episode (ARE) according to their response to steroid bolus therapy: steroid-sensitive ARE were considered as non-severe, whereas steroid-resistant ARE requiring rescue with additional therapy were considered as severe.

Statistical analysis

Comparisons of baseline characteristics between the FTR and STR were based on the chi-square test. Different times-to-event distributions were described including the time between the transplantation and: (a) the graft failure, i.e. the first event between the return to dialysis and the patient death with a functioning graft (patient-and-graft survival); (b) the return to dialysis, i.e. patient deaths were censored (graft survival); (c) the patient death with a functioning graft, i.e. the returns to dialysis were censored (patient survival); (d) the first ARE and (e) the first severe ARE, i.e. non-severe ARE were censored. Survival curves were estimated using the Kaplan-Meier estimator. Only the main outcomes, i.e. PGS and ARE/severe ARE occurrences, were analyzed in multivariate. A first selection of covariates using the Log-rank test (p<0.20) was performed before the Cox model (Wald test with p<0.05, step-by-step descending procedure). Cox models were stratified per center. Baseline parameters differentially distributed between FTR and STR were also introduced in the models. Because the Cox model was performed by using all the recipients regardless the graft rank, we did not take into account specific covariates for STR, such as the survival time of the first transplant [15,18] or the time in dialysis before retransplantation [10,15,19]. Because the definition of the duration in ESRD is different between FTR and STR, a special attention was paid to ESRD-related comorbidities.

Hazards proportionality was checked by plotting log-minus-log survival curves and by testing the scaled Schoenfeld residuals [22]. Interactions between the graft rank and all the covariates were tested. The possible colinearity between donor type and CIT was also checked. An extended Cox model with time-dependent coefficients was used for non-proportional covariates [23,24]. The change time-point of the hazard ratio was estimated by minimizing the Bayesian Information Criteria [25]. In order to evaluate graft survival for the two comparable populations of FTR and STR, we also performed a sub-analysis. According to the independent risk factors for graft failure highlighted by the previous methodology, we identified 486 pairs of FTR and STR. A Kaplan-Meier estimator and the Cox model were also used to evaluate the association between graft rank and graft survival in this sub-analysis.

Statistical analyses were performed using version 2.12.0 of the R software [26].

Results

Description of the cohort

The demographic and baseline characteristics at the time of transplantation are presented in Table 1. Among the 3103 kidney transplantations, 641 (20.7%) were STR. In both groups, the majority of patients received a transplant from a deceased donor, after a period of dialysis, and the distributions of recipient and donor gender were comparable. STR were younger (p<0.0001) and their transplants came from younger donors (p<0.0001). Recurrent nephropathies (p<0.0001), cardiac disease (p = 0.0007), hepatitis (p<0.0001) and malignancy (p<0.0001) were more frequent among STR. Compared to FTR, STR received better HLA-matched transplants (p<0.0001), but their CIT were longer (p<0.0001) and they were more sensitized, with higher positivity of anti-class I and anti-class II PRA than FTR (p<0.0001). They

were also more frequently exposed to induction therapy with a lymphocyte-depleting agent (p<0.0001).

Survival analysis

The patient-and-graft survival at 1, 5 and 10 years respectively were: 92%, 79% and 56% for STR and 94%, 83% and 66% for FTR (Figure 1-A). Without any adjustment on confounding factors, STR had a significantly higher risk of graft failure than FTR (p = 0.0127). Approximately beyond 4 years post-transplantation, the difference in survival curves appeared to increase over time. STR also had a significantly lower graft survival than FTR (Figure 1-B, p = 0.0206). However, we could not demonstrate a significant difference between the patient survival (Figure 1-C, p = 0.2890).

The univariate analysis revealed that the relationship between the graft rank and the PGS changed with post transplantation time (p = 0.0125). Assuming that the hazard ratio (HR) associated with

Table 1. Demographic and baseline characteristics of primary and second transplants performed in the DIVAT network between January 1996 and November 2010.

Characteristics	All grafts (N = 3103)		First graft (N = 2462)		Second graft (N = 641)	
	N	(%)	N	(%)	N	(%)
Transplantation period<2005	887	(28.6%)	685	(27.8%)	202	(31.5%)
Male recipient	1900	(61.2%)	1516	(61.6%)	384	(59.9%)
Recipient≥55 years of age	1295	(41.7%)	1100	(44.7%)	195	(30.4%)*
Potentially recurrent causal nephropathy	1016	(32.7%)	744	(30.2%)	272	(42.4%)*
Presence of dialysis prior transplantation	2782	(89.8%)	2197	(89.5%)	585	(91.3%)
History of diabetes	336	(10.8%)	295	(12.0%)	41	(6.4%)*
History of hypertension	2527	(81.4%)	2013	(81.8%)	514	(80.2%)
History of vascular disease	381	(12.3%)	296	(12.0%)	85	(13.3%)
History of cardiac disease	1011	(32.6%)	766	(31.1%)	245	(38.2%)*
History of dyslipemia	880	(28.4%)	731	(29.7%)	149	(23.2%)*
History of malignancy	248	(8.0%)	161	(6.5%)	87	(13.6%)*
History of B or C hepatitis	191	(6.2%)	110	(4.5%)	81	(12.6%)*
Positive recipient CMV serology	1844	(59.8%)	1413	(57.8%)	431	(67.6%)*
Positive recipient EBV serology	2886	(96.1%)	2289	(96.0%)	597	(96.8%)
Recipient BMI≥30 kg.m^{-2}	291	(9.5%)	256	(10.5%)	35	(5.5%)*
Positive anti-class I PRA	822	(26.5%)	420	(17.1%)	402	(62.7%)*
Positive anti-class II PRA	889	(28.6%)	410	(16.7%)	479	(74.7%)*
Male donor	1817	(58.9%)	1421	(58.0%)	396	(62.4%)*
Donor≥55 years of age	1265	(40.8%)	1056	(42.9%)	209	(32.6%)*
Deceased donor	2785	(89.8%)	2181	(88.6%)	604	(94.2%)*
Cerebro-vascular cause of donor death	1480	(49.7%)	1168	(49.7%)	312	(50.0%)
Donor serum creatinine≥133 µmol/l	385	(12.6%)	311	(12.9%)	74	(11.8%)
Positive donor CMV serology	1582	(51.2%)	1266	(51.6%)	316	(49.7%)
Positive donor EBV serology	2639	(94.3%)	2104	(94.6%)	535	(93.0%)
HLA-A-B-DR incompatibilities>4	432	(13.9%)	390	(15.8%)	42	(6.6%)*
HLA-A incompatibilities≥1	2437	(78.5%)	1993	(81.0%)	444	(69.3%)*
HLA-B incompatibilities≥1	2774	(89.4%)	2248	(91.3%)	526	(82.1%)*
HLA-DR incompatibilities≥1	2310	(74.4%)	1919	(77.9%)	391	(61.0%)*
Cold ischemia time≥24 h	905	(29.2%)	668	(27.1%)	237	(37.0%)*
Induction with a lymphocyte-depleting agent	1385	(44.7%)	883	(35.9%)	502	(78.3%)*

BMI, body mass index; PRA, panel reactive antibody; HLA, human leukocyte antigen; CMV, cytomegalovirus; EBV, Epstein-Barr virus.
*p<0.05.

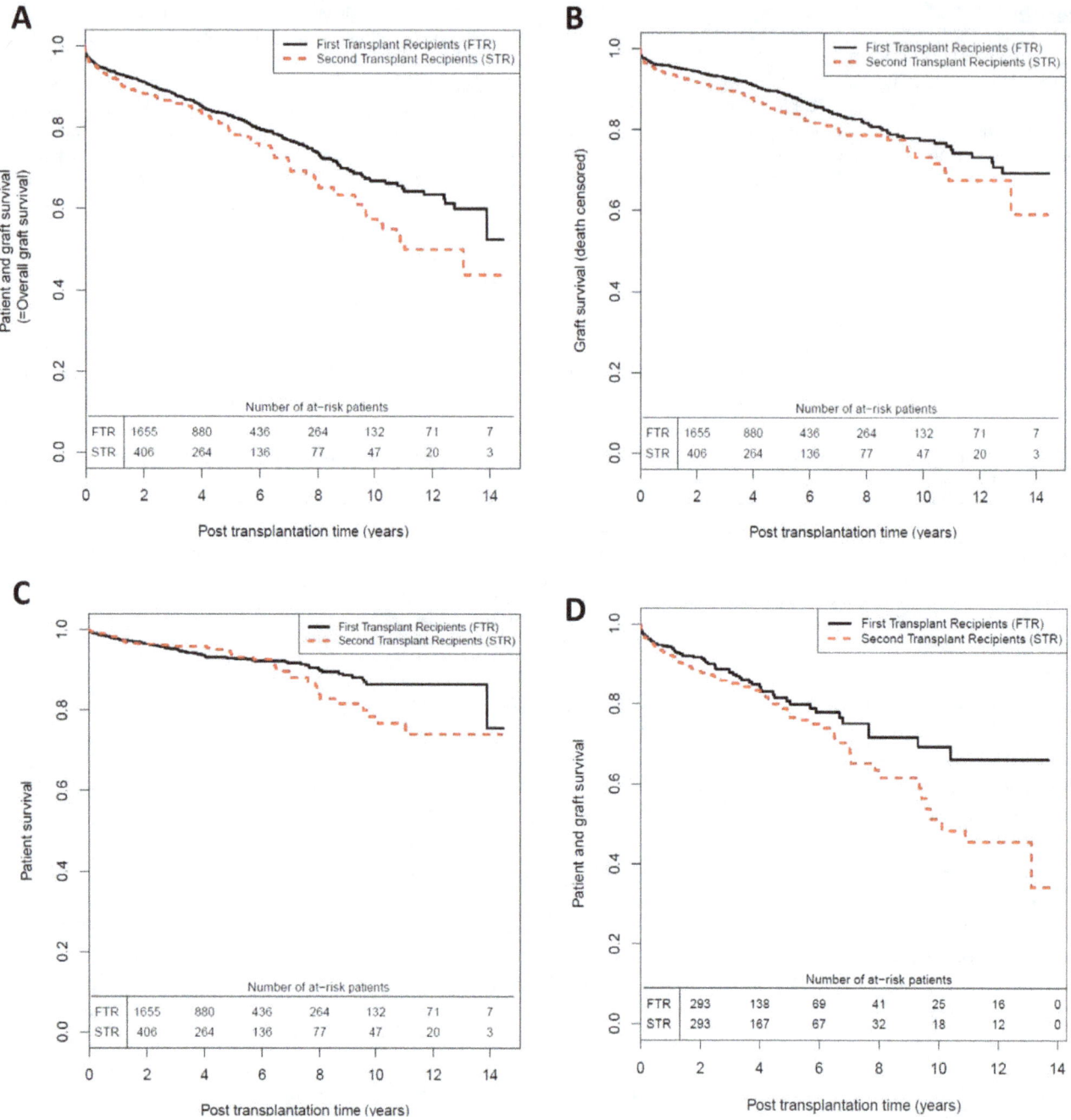

Figure 1. Unadjusted patient and/or graft survival analysis. (A) Patient-and-graft survival (= overall graft survival) : patient deaths with a functioning graft are considered as a graft failure (log-rank test: p = 0.0127) **(B)** Death-censored graft survival: patient deaths with a functioning graft are censored (log-rank test: p = 0.0206) and **(C)** Patient survival: returns to dialysis are censored (log-rank test: p = 0.2890), for first and second grafts performed in the DIVAT network between January 1996 and November 2010 (Kaplan-Meier estimates). **(D)** Patient-and-graft survival sub-analysis for a sample of matched first grafts (N = 486) and second grafts (N = 486) for the following risk factors of graft failure: transplantation period, recipient age, history of cardiac disease, anti-class I PRA, recipient/donor relationship, BMI and EBV serology.

the graft rank can be considered constant within the 2 periods; we found that the optimal cutoff point which minimized the Bayesian Information Criterion was 4 years. This model was validated by the analysis of the Schoenfeld's residuals. It was also coherent with Figure 1-A. Of note, graft failure was not significantly associated with the HLA-A-B-DR level (HR = 1.14, p = 0.274) nor with the HLA-DR level (HR = 1.03, p = 0.739).

The multivariate analysis was based on 2772 patients, as 257 FTR and 74 STR presented missing data (Table 2). The risk of graft failure was 2.18 times higher for STR after 4 years of transplantation (p = 0.0013). There was no significant difference before 4 years (HR = 1.05, p = 0.7830). The risk of graft failure was also higher for transplantation before 2005 (HR = 1.32, p = 0.0427), recipient≥55 years of age (HR = 1.49, p = 0.0012), deceased donor (HR = 2.19, p = 0.0015), cardiac disease

Table 2. Multivariate Cox model analysis of graft failure risk factors (N = 2772, as 257 first transplant recipients and 74 second transplant recipients presenting missing data for one of the covariates were deleted).

Variables	Hazard Ratio	95% CI	p
Graft rank before 4 post-transplant years (2/1)	1.05	0.75–1.47	0.7830
Graft rank after 4 post-transplant years (2/1)	2.18	1.35–3.50	0.0013
Transplantation period (<2005/≥2005)	1.32	1.01–1.72	0.0427
Recipient gender (male/female)	1.01	0.82–1.25	0.9364
Recipient age (≥55 years/<55 years)	1.49	1.17–1.89	0.0012
Causal nephropathy (recurrent/non recurrent)	1.13	0.91–1.39	0.2734
History of diabetes (positive/negative)	1.28	0.96–1.71	0.0947
History of hypertension (positive/negative)	0.86	0.67–1.12	0.2665
History of vascular disease (positive/negative)	1.05	0.80–1.38	0.7449
History of cardiac disease (positive/negative)	1.34	1.09–1.65	0.0057
History of dyslipemia (positive/negative)	1.16	0.93–1.45	0.1971
History of malignancy (positive/negative)	1.17	0.84–1.62	0.3483
History of B/C hepatitis (positive/negative)	1.06	0.72–1.57	0.7587
Number of HLA-A-B-DR mismatches (>4/≤4)	1.30	0.99–1.71	0.0639
Anti-class I PRA (positive/negative)	1.43	1.11–1.85	0.0055
Anti-class II PRA (positive/negative)	0.98	0.74–1.30	0.8970
Induction therapy (depleting/non depleting)	0.88	0.69–1.12	0.2852
Cold ischemia time (≥24 h/<24 h)	1.18	0.95–1.45	0.1370
Donor age (≥55 years/<55 years)	1.19	0.94–1.49	0.1459
Recipient/donor relationship (deceased donor/living donor)	2.19	1.35–3.57	0.0015
BMI (≥30 kg.m^{-2}/<30 kg.m^{-2})	1.54	1.14–2.09	0.0050
Donor EBV serology (positive/negative)	1.80	1.17–2.77	0.0076

CI, confidence interval; BMI, body mass index; PRA, panel reactive antibody; HLA, human leukocyte antigen; EBV, Epstein-Barr virus.

(HR = 1.34, p = 0.0057), positive anti-class I PRA (HR = 1.43, p = 0.0055), obesity (HR = 1.54, p = 0.0050) and positive donor EBV serology (HR = 1.80, p = 0.0076). Of note, no interaction with the graft rank achieved statistical significance.

The sub-analysis consisted of analyzing 486 pairs of FTR and STR with the same risk factors of graft failure (transplantation period, recipient age, history of cardiac disease, anti-class I PRA, recipient/donor relationship, BMI and EBV serology). The corresponding graft survivals are presented in Figure 1D. This confirmed the time-dependent effect of the graft rank: the risk of graft failure was 2.15 times higher for STR after 4 years of transplantation (95% CI = 1.14–4.08, p = 0.0184) but there was no significant difference before 4 years (HR = 1.11, 95% CI = 0.77–1.58, p = 0.5842).

Acute rejection episode analysis

In order to explain the previous delayed excess risk in the STR group after few years post transplantation, we first made the hypothesis of a higher frequency of ARE or severe ARE in this group, with the associated delayed consequences on the patient-and-graft survival.

The cumulative probability of ARE at 1, 3 and 12 months respectively were 10%, 13% and 19% for STR and 8%, 14% and 20% for FTR (Figure 2-A). The univariate analysis showed no trend for higher ARE occurrence in STR than FTR (p = 0.4420). The multivariate Cox model confirmed this result (Table 3, HR = 1.01, p = 0.9675). ARE occurrence was related to HLA-A-B-DR mismatches (HR = 1.46, p = 0.0004) and anti-class II PRA (HR = 1.29, p = 0.0180). Recipients≥55 years of age (HR = 0.79,

p = 0.0173) and recipients with a lymphocyte-depleting therapy (HR = 0.65, p<0.0001) had a lower risk of ARE occurrence.

The cumulative probability of severe ARE at 1 and 12 months respectively were 2% and 5% for STR, and 1% and 2% for FTR (Figure 2-B). The univariate analysis showed that STR had a higher risk of severe ARE occurrence than FTR (p = 0.0040), but this significant result was not confirmed by the multivariate Cox model (Table 4, HR = 1.27, p = 0.4087). Severe ARE occurrence was also related to anti-class II PRA (HR = 2.26, p = 0.0027). Of note, recipients transplanted before 2005 (HR = 0.52, p = 0.0329) and recipients of an old donor graft (HR = 0.59, p = 0.3470) had a significantly lower risk of severe ARE occurrence.

Discussion

Based on an overview of the literature, the prognosis of STR compared to FTR is still unclear. As the demand for kidney transplants largely exceeds the supply, it is important to evaluate the excess risk related to STR and to identify patients with the worst chances of long-term outcome.

In 2003, Coupel et al. compared 233 STR to 1174 FTR and observed no difference in the 10-year survival [14], probably as STR were younger and had a higher level of HLA-matching than FTR. In 2008, Arnol et al. reported a similar 15-year survival between 81 STR compared to 427 FTR. They also found no differences in the occurrence of ARE between the two groups [15]. From a series of 26 deceased-donor STR versus 140 FTR analyzed in 2009, Gruber et al. also reported no differences in the 8-year survival nor in the occurrence or severity of ARE [5]. In the

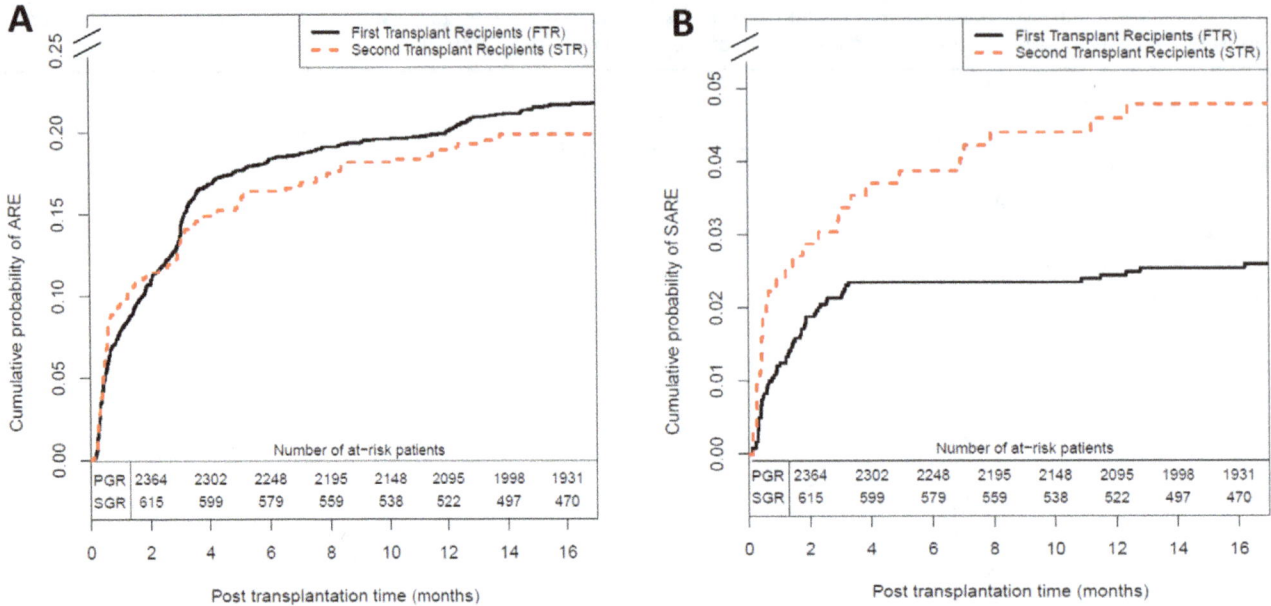

Figure 2. Cumulative probability of acute rejection episodes. (A) Cumulative probability of acute rejection episodes for FTR and STR (log-rank test: p = 0.4420) and **(B)** Cumulative probability of severe acute rejection episodes for FTR and STR (log-rank test: p = 0.0040), for first and second grafts (Kaplan-Meier estimates).

same year, Wang et al. compared the 5-year PGS of 65 deceased-donor STR versus 613 FTR and likewise, reported no difference [16]. Thus, from these former studies, it appears that STR have a long-term outcome similar to FTR. However, the interpretations of these studies are limited by several factors: the slight number of

STR (low statistical power), the monocenter design, the number of adjustment covariates or the short follow-up period. Conversely, in 2007, Magee et al. [17] compared the 5-year graft survival of a large cohort of kidney recipients (more than 2000 STR versus more than 20000 FTR), from the Organ Procurement and

Table 3. Multivariate Cox model analysis of acute rejection episode (ARE)-free time risk factors (N = 3103).

Variables	Hazard Ratio	95% CI	p
Graft rank (2/1)	1.01	0.80–1.27	0.9675
Transplantation period (<2005/≥2005)	0.80	0.64–1.01	0.0592
Recipient gender (male/female)	1.13	0.97–1.33	0.1233
Recipient age (≥55 years/<55 years)	0.79	0.65–0.96	0.0173
Causal nephropathy (recurrent/non recurrent)	1.03	0.88–1.22	0.6928
History of diabetes (positive/negative)	1.17	0.92–1.48	0.2128
History of hypertension (positive/negative)	1.18	0.96–1.45	0.1127
History of vascular disease (positive/negative)	1.16	0.91–1.48	0.2267
History of cardiac disease (positive/negative)	0.95	0.80–1.12	0.5334
History of dyslipemia (positive/negative)	0.95	0.80–1.14	0.6096
History of malignancy (positive/negative)	1.02	0.76–1.37	0.8861
History of B/C hepatitis (positive/negative)	0.75	0.53–1.08	0.1206
Number of HLA-A-B-DR mismatches (>4/≤4)	1.46	1.18–1.81	0.0004
Anti-class I PRA (positive/negative)	1.07	0.87–1.31	0.5205
Anti-class II PRA (positive/negative)	1.29	1.04–1.59	0.0180
Induction therapy (depleting/non depleting)	0.65	0.54–0.77	<0.0001
Cold ischemia time (≥24 h/<24 h)	0.88	0.73–1.07	0.1984
Donor age (≥55 years/<55 years)	1.06	0.89–1.27	0.5027
Recipient/donor relationship (deceased donor/living donor)	0.92	0.73–1.15	0.4490

CI, confidence interval; BMI, body mass index; PRA, panel reactive antibody; HLA, human leukocyte antigen.

Table 4. Multivariate Cox model analysis of severe acute rejection episode (severe ARE)-free time risk factors (N = 3103).

Variables	Hazard Ratio	95% CI	p
Graft rank (2/1)	1.27	0.72–2.21	0.4087
Transplantation period (<2005/≥2005)	0.52	0.28–0.95	0.0329
Recipient gender (male/female)	1.10	0.71–1.68	0.6762
Recipient age (≥55 years/<55 years)	1.52	0.93–2.48	0.0930
Causal nephropathy (recurrent/non recurrent)	0.97	0.63–1.51	0.9086
History of diabetes (positive/negative)	0.85	0.40–1.80	0.6769
History of hypertension (positive/negative)	1.41	0.78–2.54	0.2516
History of vascular disease (positive/negative)	0.99	0.51–1.91	0.9758
History of cardiac disease (positive/negative)	0.92	0.59–1.44	0.7299
History of dyslipemia (positive/negative)	0.81	0.49–1.33	0.4045
History of malignancy (positive/negative)	0.76	0.34–1.68	0.4952
History of B/C hepatitis (positive/negative)	0.51	0.19–1.41	0.1964
Number of HLA-A-B-DR mismatches (>4/≤4)	1.34	0.76–2.36	0.3051
Anti-class I PRA (positive/negative)	1.20	0.72–2.00	0.4911
Anti-class II PRA (positive/negative)	2.26	1.33–3.85	0.0027
Induction therapy (depleting/non depleting)	0.84	0.53–1.33	0.4545
Cold ischemia time (≥24 h/<24 h)	1.46	0.93–2.29	0.0997
Donor age (≥55 years/<55 years)	0.59	0.36–0.96	0.0347
Recipient/donor relationship (deceased donor/living donor)	0.93	0.46–1.87	0.8427

CI, confidence interval; BMI, body mass index; PRA, panel reactive antibody; HLA, human leukocyte antigen.

Transplantation Network registry, and reported that even with adjustment for donor and recipient factors, the 5-year risk of graft failure remained significantly higher for repeat kidney transplant recipients (including second transplantations and more) than for FTR. Nevertheless, adjustment factors were limited and the follow-up was short. Moreover none of these studies evaluated the possible time-dependent effect of the graft rank, which is the central assumption of the proportional hazard Cox model.

In this paper, we used a specific methodology for an accurate comparison between FTR and STR, by taking into account all the possible confounding factors and modeling the time-dependent effect of the graft rank. To our knowledge, such an analysis has never been performed. Our results, based on recipients from a large multicenter cohort under similar recent immunosuppressive maintenance therapy, show that STR have a poorer long-term prognosis than FTR. We show for the first time that this risk is delayed and appears significant beyond four years of follow-up. This cut-off definitely does not correspond to a sudden modification of the graft failure risk. We should rather retain that the excess of risk of STR appears after few years of transplantation. This time-dependent association may be a major point as it was only after its introduction that we showed the significant excess risk of graft failure for STR: it may explain that the majority of the other papers did not demonstrate significant correlation between the survival of FTR and STR.

The difference in PGS could have been due to a higher frequency of ARE or severe ARE for STR than for FTR during the follow-up. However, we did not demonstrate such a difference in ARE, nor in severe ARE occurrences. For this last endpoint, we showed that STR tended to have a higher risk of severe ARE than FTR. The lack of statistical power (only 96 severe ARE were observed in the whole cohort) may explain why this finding did not reach statistical significance.

As always in observational studies, there are several limitations to this study. (i) The use of different techniques for PRA identification may introduce a bias, limited by the fact that STR and FTR were compared over the same period/center and by adjusting on the year of transplantation. (ii) It was not possible to include the causes of graft loss in our analyses (immunologic versus non-immunologic causes) since this the collection of this information has only recently been initiated. (iii) It was unfortunately not possible to adjust for the pretransplant duration of dialysis and the duration of first transplant survival, as only covariates common to FTR and STR can be taken into account in a Cox model. To overcome this difficulty, we adjusted for the comorbidities at transplantation. (iv) Adjustment for long-term immunosuppression regimens was not done, as it is more a reflection of a therapeutic adaptation to a clinical situation and it depends on the center, on the clinician and on the therapeutic advances. (v) A possible effect of the transplantation policy might introduce some bias that is overcome by the adjustment in the multivariate model and by the matched case-control design in the sub-analysis model. (vi) Our study also failed to eliminate the effects of some confounding factors such as medication compliance; as in every large-sized cohort, this information cannot be realistically collected. (vii) Delayed graft function (DGF) was not included as a covariate in the analysis as only pre- and per-transplant covariates were taken into account. However, an additional analysis including DGF did not provide new possible explanations for the different first and second transplant outcomes (data not shown). (vii) Although all ARE were biopsy-proven, a small number were classified using the most recent Banff criteria. It will take a few years before we are able to explore the possible link between biopsy-proven antibody-mediated ARE occurrence and a worse outcome. (viii) Finally, due to the long-term follow-up period, the information about preformed DSA was available for only a very small part of our cohort, although this covariate is suspected to be related to risk of graft failure.

In conclusion, this observational study on a large multicenter cohort confirmed other findings showing that STR have a lower patient-and-graft survival compared to FTR. However, this study eliminates some confounding factors from the current literature. The excess risk of graft failure for STR was delayed after several years post transplantation. This effect did not seem to be related to a higher frequency of ARE or severe ARE for second grafts. Regardless of the limitations of such an observational cohort; the current study supports the hypothesis of a higher propensity for STR to develop donor specific antibodies post-transplantation. These findings justify further expensive systematic and prospective monitoring of antibodies in both populations. Further investigations are still needed to understand the biological/immunological mechanisms underlying graft failure, to identify patients specifically at risk of graft failure and also to provide a strategy for improving outcome in STR. But in practice, physicians should not consider second and first kidney transplant recipients equally.

Acknowledgments

We wish to thank members of the clinical research assistant team (S. Le Floch, J. Posson, C. Scellier, V. Eschbach, K. Zurbonsen, C. Dagot, F. M'Raiagh, V. Godel, X. Longy).

Author Contributions

Conceived and designed the experiments: MG JD JPS. Performed the experiments: KTL. Analyzed the data: KTL YF MG JD JPS. Contributed reagents/materials/analysis tools: CL HK MK ML NK LR VG GM EM. Wrote the paper: KTL YF MG JD JPS.

References

1. Rao PS, Schaubel DE, Wei G, Fenton SSA (2006) Evaluating the survival benefit of kidney retransplantation. Transplantation 82: 669–674.

2. Ojo A, Wolfe RA, Agodoa LY, Held PJ, Port FK, et al. (1998) Prognosis after primary renal transplant failure and the beneficial effects of repeat transplantation: multivariate analyses from the United States Renal Data System. Transplantation 66: 1651–1659.

3. Rao PS, Schaubel DE, Jia X, Li S, Port FK, et al. (2007) Survival on dialysis post-kidney transplant failure: results from the Scientific Registry of Transplant Recipients. Am J Kidney Dis 49: 294–300.

4. Sola E, Gonzalez-Molina M, Cabello M, Burgos D, Ramos J, et al. (2010) Long-term improvement of deceased donor renal allograft survival since 1996: a single transplant center study. Transplantation 89: 714–720.

5. Gruber SA, Brown KL, El-Amm JM, Singh A, Mehta K, et al. (2009) Equivalent outcomes with primary and retransplantation in African-American deceased-donor renal allograft recipients. Surgery 146: 646–652.

6. Hagan C, Hickey DP, Little DM (2003) A single-center study of the technical aspects and outcome of third and subsequent renal transplants. Transplantation 75: 1687–1691.

7. Registry UNOS (Accessed 28 January 2011) Available: www.unos.org. Accessed 2012 Sep 28.

8. Gjertson DW (2002) A multi-factor analysis of kidney regraft outcomes. Clin Transpl: 335–349.

9. Stratta RJ, Oh CS, Sollinger HW, Pirsch JD, Kalayoglu M, et al. (1988) Kidney retransplantation in the cyclosporine era. Transplantation 45: 40–45.

10. Almond PS, Matas AJ, Gillingham K, Troppmann C, Payne W, et al. (1991) Risk factors for second renal allografts immunosuppressed with cyclosporine. Transplantation 52: 253–258.

11. Kerman RH, Kimball PM, Buren CTV, Lewis RM, DeVera V, et al. (1991) AHG and DTE/AHG procedure identification of crossmatch-appropriate donor-recipient pairings that result in improved graft survival. Transplantation 51: 316–320.

12. Howard RJ, Reed AI, Werf WJVD, Hemming AW, Patton PR, et al. (2001) What happens to renal transplant recipients who lose their grafts? Am J Kidney Dis 38: 31–35.

13. Scornik JC (1995) Detection of alloantibodies by flow cytometry: relevance to clinical transplantation. Cytometry 22: 259–263.

14. Coupel S, Giral-Classe M, Karam G, Morcet JF, Dantal J, et al. (2003) Ten-year survival of second kidney transplants: impact of immunologic factors and renal function at 12 months. Kidney Int 64: 674–680.

15. Arnol M, Prather JC, Mittalhenkle A, Barry JM, Norman DJ (2008) Long-term kidney regraft survival from deceased donors: risk factors and outcomes in a single center. Transplantation 86: 1084–1089.

16. Wang D, Xu TZ, Chen JH, Wu WZ, Yang SL, et al. (2009) Factors influencing second renal allograft survival: a single center experience in China. Transpl Immunol 20: 150–154.

17. Magee JC, Barr ML, Basadonna GP, Johnson MR, Mahadevan S, et al. (2007) Repeat organ transplantation in the United States, 1996–2005. Am J Transplant 7: 1424–1433.

18. Rigden S, Mehls O, Gellert R (1999) Factors influencing second renal allograft survival. Scientific Advisory Board of the ERA-EDTA Registry. European Renal Association-European Dialysis and Transplant Association. Nephrol Dial Transplant 14: 566–569.

19. Aboujioud MS, Deierhoi MH, Hudson SL, Diethelm AG (1995) Risk factors affecting second renal transplant outcome, with special reference to primary allograft nephrectomy. Transplantation 60: 138–144.

20. Miles CD, Schaubel DE, Jia X, Ojo AO, Port FK, et al. (2007) Mortality experience in recipients undergoing repeat transplantation with expanded criteria donor and non-ECD deceased-donor kidneys. Am J Transplant 7: 1140–1147.

21. Ladrière M, Foucher Y, Legendre C, Kamar N, Garrigue V, et al. (2010) The western europe cohort of kidney transplanted recipients - the DIVAT network. Clinical transplants: 460–461.

22. Grambsch P, Therneau T (1994) Proportional hazards tests and diagnostics based on weighted residuals. Biometrika 81: 515–526.

23. Klein JP, Moeschberger ML (1997) Survival analysis: techniques for censored and truncated data. New York: Springer-verlag.

24. Therneau TM, Grambsch PM (2000) Modeling survival data: extending the cox model. New York: Springer-Verlag.

25. Volinsky CT, Raftery AE (2000) Bayesian information criterion for censored survival models. Biometrics 56: 256–262.

26. Team RDC (2010) R: A Language and Environment for Statistical Computing. Vienna, Austria: R Foundation for Statistical Computing.

3

DR^{high+}CD45RA$^-$-Tregs Potentially Affect the Suppressive Activity of the Total Treg Pool in Renal Transplant Patients

Matthias Schaier[1]*, Nicole Seissler[1], Edgar Schmitt[2], Stefan Meuer[3], Friederike Hug[1], Martin Zeier[1], Andrea Steinborn[4]

1 Department of Nephrology, University of Heidelberg, Heidelberg, Germany, 2 Institute of Immunology, University of Mainz, Mainz, Germany, 3 Institute of Immunology, University of Heidelberg, Heidelberg, Germany, 4 Department of Obstetrics and Gynecology, University of Heidelberg, Heidelberg, Germany

Abstract

Recent studies show that regulatory T cells (Tregs) play an essential role in tolerance induction after organ transplantation. In order to examine whether there are differences in the composition of the total CD4$^+$CD127$^{low+/-}$ FoxP3$^+$- Treg cell pool between stable transplant patients and patients with biopsy proven rejection (BPR), we compared the percentages and the functional activity of the different Treg cell subsets (DR^{high+}CD45RA$^-$-Tregs, DR^{low+}CD45RA$^-$-Tregs, DR$^-$CD45RA$^-$-Tregs, DR$^-$CD45RA$^+$-Tregs). All parameters were determined during the three different periods of time after transplantation (0–30 days, 31–1,000 days, >1,000 days). Among 156 transplant patients, 37 patients suffered from BPR. The most prominent differences between rejecting and non-rejecting patients were observed regarding the DR^{high+}CD45RA$^-$-Treg cell subset. Our data demonstrate that the suppressive activity of the total Treg pool strongly depends on the presence of these Treg cells. Their percentage within the total Treg pool strongly decreased after transplantation and remained relatively low during the first year after transplantation in all patients. Subsequently, the proportion of this Treg subset increased again in patients who accepted the transplant and reached a value of healthy non-transplanted subjects. By contrast, in patients with acute kidney rejection, the DR^{high+}CD45RA$^-$-Treg subset disappeared excessively, causing a reduction in the suppressive activity of the total Treg pool. Therefore, both the monitoring of its percentage within the total Treg pool and the monitoring of the HLA-DR MFI of the DR$^+$CD45RA$^-$-Treg subset may be useful tools for the prediction of graft rejection.

Editor: Aric Gregson, University of California Los Angeles, United States of America

Funding: This work was supported by the Deutsche Forschungsgemeinschaft grant STE 885/3-2 (to A. Steinborn). The funders had no role in study design, data collection and analysis, decision to publish, or preparation of the manuscript.

Competing Interests: The authors have declared that no competing interests exist.

* E-mail: matthias_schaier@med.uni-heidelberg.de

Introduction

Despite the significant improvement in the understanding of allo-immune mechanisms for graft failure and the development of innovative immune-suppressants, graft and patient survival have not increased as expected in the past decade. Prevention of graft rejection and induction of tolerance are common goals in the field of transplantation. Acute rejection has been shown to be one of the strongest negative prognostic factors for long-term graft survival after kidney transplantation [1,2]. The frequency of acute rejection episodes is highest during the first 6 months after transplantation [3]. During the second and third year post surgery, renal function becomes stable and the incidence of acute rejection and graft loss is markedly reduced [4]. After more than three years, only small changes can be observed in regard to mean GFR decline, annual incidence of graft loss and death, which all were found to represent about 1%. Currently, only limited data exist which could explain this phenomenon. Possibly, several transplant patients can develop tolerance towards the foreign allo-antigens with advancing time after transplantation.

Recent studies show that regulatory T cells (Tregs) play an essential role in tolerance induction after organ transplantation

[5,6]. The majority of such studies were done using animal models. However, in humans, the true function of Tregs in allo-immunity remains in question [7,8]. Currently, Treg cells are broadly subdivided into those that develop in the thymus (natural (n) Tregs) and those that develop from conventional T-cells in the periphery (induced (i) Tregs) [9]. A specific cell marker that differentiates human nTregs from iTregs is not yet known. Both Treg populations potentially suppress the proliferation of T effector- cells [9] and are characterized by simultaneous expression of the interleukin (IL) 2 receptor α chain (CD25) and the forkhead box P3 (FoxP3) transcription factor [10]. In addition, an inverse correlation between the expression of the IL-7 receptor α chain (CD127) and their suppressive function was observed for CD4$^+$CD25$^+$ FoxP3$^+$-Treg cells [11,12]. Currently, it is not known, to which extent each of these Treg populations contributes to the prevention of allograft rejection after transplantation. However, there is a growing body of evidence that the suppressive potency of the total Treg cell pool may depend on its composition with distinct Treg subsets. Baecher-Allan et al. have characterized a highly suppressive subset of Treg cells expressing HLA-class II (DR) antigens [13]. Such HLA-DR$^+$- Tregs were shown to express higher levels of FoxP3 and induced a more intense and a more

rapid T cell suppression than the Tregs that lack HLA-DR expression [13]. Moreover, it is known that the total Treg pool contains a population of naïve CD45RA$^+$-Treg cells. Its proportion decreases with increasing age and it was shown that naïve CD45RA$^+$-Treg cells were less proliferative than their CD45RO$^+$ counterparts [14]. Recent data demonstrate that the suppressive activity of naïve CD45RA$^+$-Treg cells is impaired in multiple sclerosis (MS) patients, suggesting that this Treg population may potentially be involved in the pathology of autoimmune diseases [15,16].

In the present study, we demonstrate that DR^{high+}CD45RA$^-$-Tregs potentially affect the suppressive activity of the total Treg pool and that the disappearance of this Treg subset gives a strong indication for acute rejection processes.

Results

The percentage of CD4$^+$CD127$^{low+/-}$FoxP3$^+$-Tregs within CD4$^+$-T cells is significantly decreased in kidney transplant patients compared to non-transplanted healthy volunteers

Both the percentage of CD4$^+$CD127$^{low+/-}$FoxP3$^+$-Treg cells of CD4$^+$-T cells and their composition with four distinct Treg cell subsets were determined in the circulation of healthy non-transplanted volunteers (Group A), stable kidney transplant patients (Group B) and kidney transplant patients with biopsy proven rejection (BPR) (Group C), (Table 1, Figure 1). PBMCs obtained from each participant were stained with anti-CD4, anti-CD127, anti-FoxP3, anti-HLA-DR and anti-CD45RA monoclonal antibodies and analyzed by five color flow cytometric analysis. Figure 2 depicts the gating strategy for these measurements. First, PBMCs were analyzed by fluorescence intensity of CD4 versus side light scatter (SSC), (Figure 2A). The CD4$^+$-T cells (P1) were gated and analyzed by fluorescence intensity of FoxP3 versus CD127, (Figure 2B). The CD4$^+$CD127$^{low+/-}$FoxP3$^+$-Tregs were gated (P2) and analyzed by their expression of HLA-DR versus CD45RA (Fig. 2C). By that, three distinct Treg cell subsets became apparent: DR$^+$CD45RA$^-$-Tregs (P3), DR$^-$CD45RA$^-$-Tregs (P4) and naïve DR$^-$CD45RA$^+$-Tregs (P5). The percentages of these distinct Treg subsets within the total CD4$^+$CD127$^{low+/-}$FoxP3$^+$-Treg cell pool were estimated for all participants. In addition, the level of HLA-DR expression (HLA-DR MFI) of the DR$^+$CD45RA$^-$-Treg subset (Fig. 2C, P3) and the percentages of DR^{low+}CD45RA$^-$-Tregs (Fig. 2D, P6) and DR^{high+}CD45RA$^-$-Tregs (Fig. 2D, P7) of the total Treg cell pool (P2) were documented.

Figure 3 shows the percentages of CD4$^+$CD127$^{low+/-}$FoxP3$^+$-Treg cells within the total CD4$^+$-T cell pool in healthy non-transplanted volunteers (Group A), in stable kidney transplant patients (Group B) and in transplant patients with biopsy proven rejection (BPR) (Group C). Compared to healthy non-transplanted volunteers, the percentage of CD4$^+$CD127$^{low+/-}$FoxP3$^+$-Tregs decreased continuously after transplantation. Significant differences concerning the percentage of CD4$^+$CD127$^{low+/-}$FoxP3$^+$-Tregs at different time points (G1–G3) after transplantation between rejecting and non-rejecting patients were not detected.

The suppressive activity of the CD4$^+$CD127$^{low+/-}$CD25$^+$-Treg cell pool is significantly reduced in patients with biopsy proven rejection (BPR)

To examine whether there were differences in the suppressive activity of the total Treg pool between rejecting and non-rejecting transplant patients we used coculture suppression assays described in the methods section. To evaluate the suppressive capacity of CD4$^+$CD127$^{low+/-}$CD25$^+$-Tregs, obtained from the different patient groups (Group A–C), we determined the maximum suppressive activity (ratio of Treg cells to responder T (Tresp) cells 1:1) and calculated the ratio of Treg cells to Tresp cells that resulted in a suppression of at least 15%. Figure 4A depicts the results of one representative experiment obtained for healthy non-transplanted volunteers (Group A), stable kidney transplant patients (Group B) and transplant patients with BPR (Group C), respectively. Figure 4B and 4C summarize the data for the individual participants in each of these three patient groups. We found that the suppressive activity of the isolated CD4$^+$CD127$^{low+/-}$CD25$^+$-Tregs, obtained from stable transplant recipients, was in the same range as that of CD4$^+$CD127$^{low+/-}$CD25$^+$-Tregs obtained from healthy non-transplanted volunteers. In contrast, the suppressive activity of Tregs obtained from patients with acute rejection was significantly reduced compared to healthy non-transplanted controls and to stable transplant patients, (Figure 4B). Furthermore, the ratio of Treg cells to responder cells (Titer Treg/Tresp) leading to a suppression of at least 15%, was significantly decreased in patients with acute rejection compared to healthy controls and stable transplant patients (Figure 4C).

After transplantation, the composition of the total Treg cell pool changes characteristically

In order to examine whether there were changes in the composition of the total Treg cell pool with distinct Treg subsets (DR^{high+}CD45RA$^-$-Tregs, DR^{low+}CD45RA$^-$-Tregs, DR$^-$CD45RA$^-$-Tregs and naïve DR$^-$CD45RA$^+$-Tregs), we determined their percentages in healthy controls and stable transplant patients. Figures 5A-4D summarize the results of these analyses. The individual ratios of the four Treg subsets showed characteristic changes over time in transplanted patients. Therefore, the transplant patients were grouped depending on the period of time after surgery (G1: 0–30 days, G2: 31–1000 days, G3: >1000 days). Non-transplanted volunteers served as healthy controls (Group A). Compared to healthy non-transplanted controls (Group A), the percentage of DR^{high+}CD45RA$^-$-Tregs decreased strongly within the first 30 days after transplantation (Fig. 5A, G1) and remained at minimum levels up to 1000 days post surgery (Fig. 5A, (G2)). The percentage of DR^{low+}CD45RA$^-$-Tregs increased initially (Fig. 5B, G1), but decreased subsequently and reached the lowest levels between 31 and 1000 days post transplantation (Fig. 5B, (G2)). After a period of 1000 days (G3) both the percentages of DR^{high+}CD45RA$^-$-Tregs and DR^{low+}C-D45RA$^-$-Tregs returned to levels in the range of healthy non-transplanted controls (Group A), (Figures 5A and 5B). As the differentiation between DR^{high+}CD45RA$^-$-Tregs and DR^{low+}C-D45RA$^-$-Tregs was difficult, we additionally estimated the HLA-DR mean fluorescence intensity (MFI) of the DR$^+$CD45RA$^-$-Treg cell subset for all participants (Fig. 5E). We found a dramatic decrease within the first days after surgery (Fig. 5E, G1), it is likely due to a strong decrease of the DR^{high+}CD45RA$^-$-Treg subset and an increase of the DR^{low+}CD45RA$^-$-Treg subset. However, subsequently a continuous increase of the HLA-DR MFI could be documented (Fig. 5E, G2–G3), because in the period between 30–1000 days post surgery (Fig. 4E, G2), the percentage of the DR^{low+}CD45RA$^-$-Treg subset decreased while the percentage of DR^{high+}CD45RA$^-$-Treg subset did not change. After 1000 days post surgery (Fig. 5E, G3), both the percentages of the DR^{high+}CD45RA$^-$- and the DR^{low+}CD45RA$^-$-Treg subsets increased strongly.

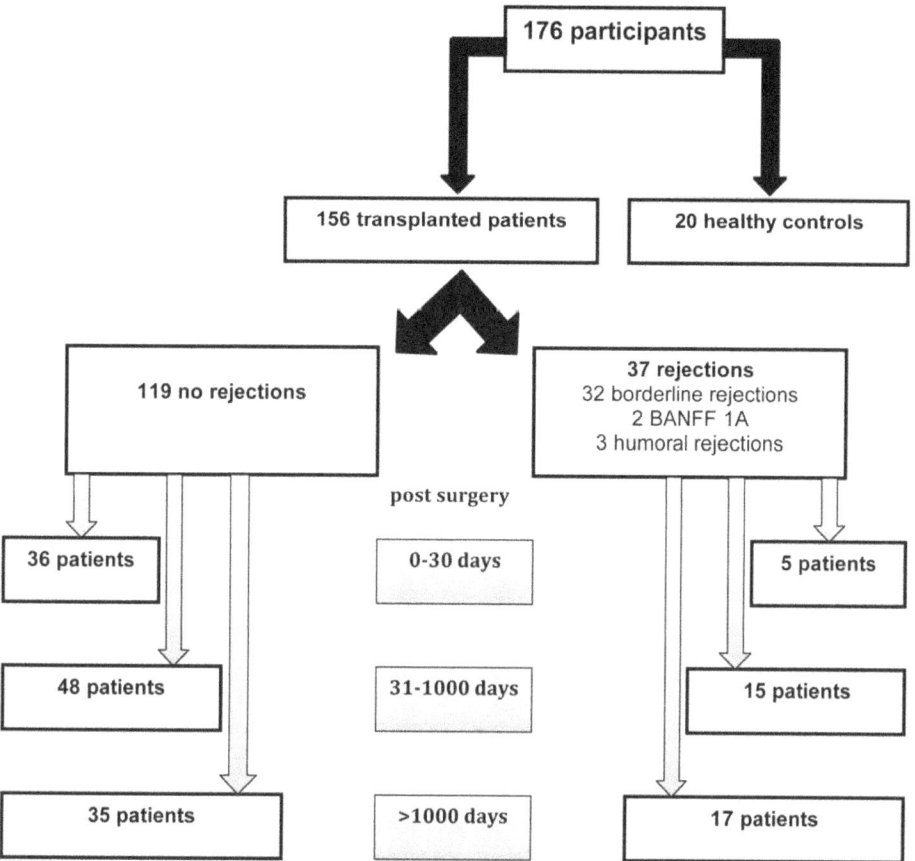

Figure 1. Flow diagram of the different patient groups.

The percentage of the naïve $DR^-CD45RA^+$ -Treg subset decreased significantly during the first 30 days after transplantation (Fig. 5C, G1), but afterwards, it increased strongly and reached maximum levels between 31 and 1000 days post surgery (Fig. 5C, G2). After 1000 days post surgery, a significant decrease of this Treg subset was observed (Fig. 5C, G3).

The percentage of the $DR^-CD45RA^-$ -Treg subset increased immediately after transplantation (Fig. 5D, G1) and revealed the highest levels between 31 and 1000 days after surgery (Fig. 5D, G2). After more than 1000 days post transplantation (Fig. 5D, G3), a slight but significant decrease was observed.

The percentage of the $DR^{high+}CD45RA^-$ -Treg subset within the total Treg pool and the HLA-DR MFI of the $DR^+CD45RA^-$ -Treg subset are strongly reduced in patients with BPR after 31 days post surgery

In order to examine whether there are differences in the composition of the total Treg cell pool between stable transplant patients (Group B) and patients with BPR (Group C), we compared the percentages of the different Treg cell subsets ($DR^{high+}CD45RA^-$ -Tregs, $DR^{low+}CD45RA^-$ -Tregs, $DR^-CD45RA^-$ -Tregs, $DR^-CD45RA^+$ -Tregs) and the HLA-DR MFI of the $DR^+CD45RA^-$ -Treg cell subset. All parameters were determined during the three different periods of time after transplantation (G1: 0–30 days, G2: 31–1000 days, G3: >1000 days). Figure 5A–5E and Table 2 show the results of these measurements.

Among 156 transplant patients, 37 patients suffered from BPR. The most prominent differences between non-rejecting (Group B)

and rejecting BPR patients (Group C) were seen regarding the $DR^{high+}CD45RA^-$ -Treg cell subset. BPR patients showed a 32% reduction of this Treg subset within the total Treg cell pool after 31–1000 days (G2) and a 44% reduction after more than 1000 days post surgery (G3) versus patients without rejection. Differences concerning the $DR^{low+}CD45RA^-$ -Treg subset could not be detected. In parallel, the HLA-DR MFI of the $DR^+CD45RA^-$ -Treg cell subset was strongly reduced in patients with BPR versus no BPR (31% after 31–1000 days (G2); 38% after 1000 days (G3)). Figure 4E shows the relationship of the HLA-DR MFI of the $DR^+CD45RA^-$ -Treg cell subset and the time after transplantation for stable transplant patients (Group B) and for patients with BPR (Group C). A positive linear correlation was found for stable transplant patients (r = 0.569, p<0.00001) and for patients with BPR (r = 0.664, p<0.00001). Comparison of these two regression lines revealed significant differences (p<0.001) between rejecting and non-rejecting transplant patients.

Moreover, contrary to stable transplant patients, BPR patients revealed a significantly higher proportion of $DR^-CD45RA^-$ -Tregs after 30 days post surgery. Their percentage within the total Treg cell pool was 21% higher after 31 days (G2) and 39% higher after 1000 days post transplantation (G3). The percentage of the naïve $DR^-CD45RA^+$ -Treg subset was lower in patients with BPR after 30 days post surgery, compared to patients with stable transplant function (G2 and G3). With regard to all examined parameters, there were no differences between rejecting and non-rejecting transplant patients during the first 30 days after surgery (G1).

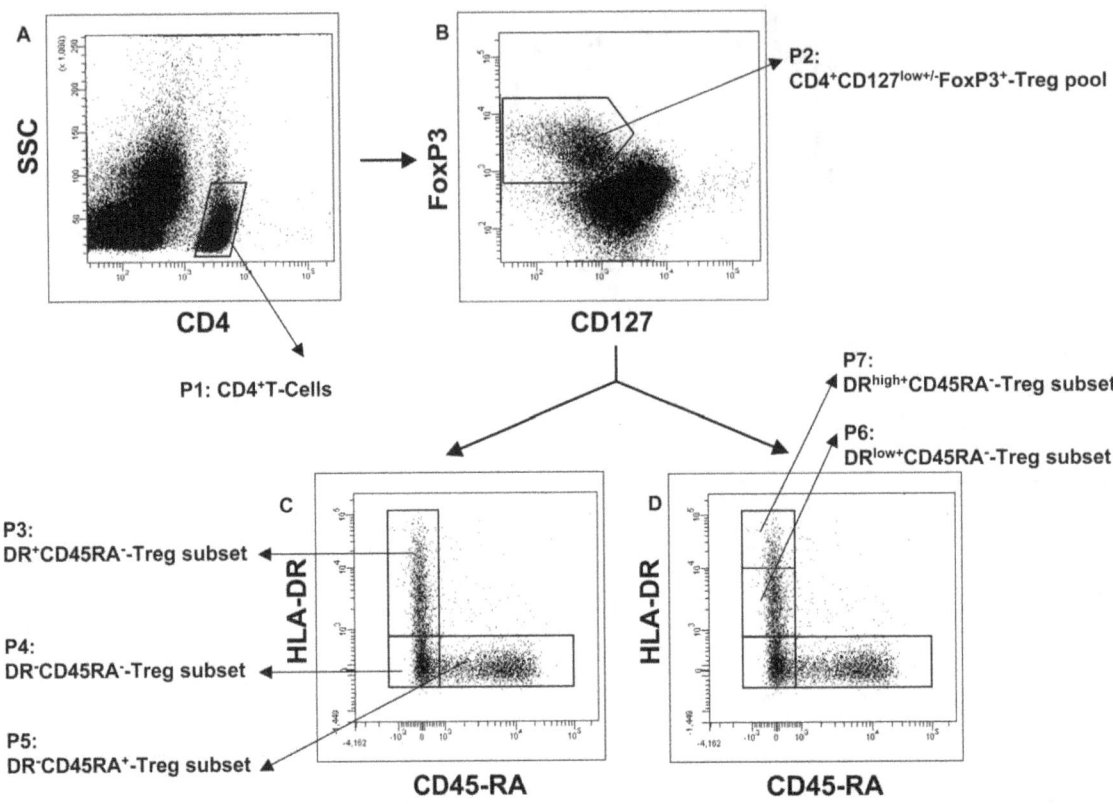

Figure 2. Gating strategy for five color flow cytometric detection of the total CD4$^+$CD127$^{low+/-}$FoxP3$^+$-Treg cell pool and its composition with four different Treg-subsets. A: CD4$^+$-T cells (P1) were gated by fluorescence intensity of CD4 versus side light scatter (SSC). B: CD4$^+$CD127$^{low+/-}$FoxP3$^+$-Treg cells were gated by fluorescence intensity of FoxP3 versus CD127 (P2). C–D: The percentage of the DR^{high+}CD45RA$^-$- (P6), the DR^{low+}CD45RA$^-$- (P7), the DR$^-$CD45RA$^-$- (P4) and the naïve DR$^-$CD45RA$^+$- (P5) Treg subset was estimated by analyzing CD4$^+$CD127$^{low+/-}$CD25$^+$Foxp3$^+$-Treg cells (P2) for their expression of HLA-DR and CD45RA. In addition, the MFI of HLA-DR expression of the DR$^+$CD45RA$^-$FoxP3$^+$-Treg subset (P3) was estimated for all participants. MFI = mean fluorescence intensity.

The low suppressive capacity of CD4$^+$CD127$^{low+/-}$CD25$^+$-Tregs observed in BPR patients correlates with a decline of the HLA-DR MFI of the DR$^+$CD45RA$^-$-Treg subset

We examined whether there was a correlation between the HLA-DR MFI of the DR$^+$CD45RA$^-$-Treg subset and the suppressive activity of the total Treg cell pool. Figure 6 shows the positive correlation (r = 0.546, p<0.001) between the HLA-DR MFI of the DR$^+$CD45RA$^-$-Treg subset and the titer (Treg/Tresp) of Tregs, with which a minimum suppressive activity of 15% was achieved. Thereby, CD4$^+$CD127$^{low+/-}$CD25$^+$-Tregs were obtained from healthy controls, BPR patients and patients without BPR. In summary, our data clearly demonstrate that the low suppressive activity of CD4$^+$CD127$^{low+/-}$CD25$^+$-Tregs observed in BPR patients correlates with a low HLA-DR MFI of the DR$^+$CD45RA$^-$-Treg cells subset. Otherwise, the high suppressive activity assessed in healthy controls and stable transplant patients correlate with a high HLA-DR MFI of the DR$^+$CD45RA$^-$-Treg subset.

The DR^{high+}CD45RA$^-$-Treg subset has the highest suppressive capacity within the total CD4$^+$CD127^{low+}CD25$^+$-Treg cell pool

Our data demonstrate that the level of HLA-DR expression of the DR$^+$CD45RA$^-$-Treg cell subset correlated positively with the suppressive activity of the total Treg cell pool from healthy controls, stable transplant patients and patients with BPR,

respectively. These findings suggested that the DR^{high+}CD45RA$^-$-Treg subset has the highest suppressive activity within the total Treg cell pool. Thus, magnetically isolated CD4$^+$CD127$^{low+/-}$CD25$^+$-Treg cells were separated via FACSort into four different Treg cell subsets consisting of DR^{high+}CD45RA$^-$-, DR^{low+}CD45RA$^-$-, DR$^-$CD45RA$^-$- and naïve DR$^-$CD45RA$^+$-Treg cells (Figure 7A). Subsequently, the suppressive activity of these different Treg subsets was analyzed. Both the maximum suppressive activity (Figure 7B) and the titer (Treg/Tresp) with which a minimum suppressive activity of 15% could be achieved (Figure 7C) were highest for the DR^{high+}CD45RA$^-$-Treg subset. For the DR^{low+}CD45RA$^-$-Treg subset, the suppressive activity was slightly reduced compared to the DR^{high+}CD45RA$^-$-Treg subset. An even less suppressive activity was found for the DR$^-$CD45RA$^-$-Tregs and the lowest suppressive activity was assessed for the naïve DR$^-$CD45RA$^-$-Treg subset. Thus, the DR^{high+}CD45RA$^-$-Treg subset was shown to exhibit the highest suppressive activity of the total CD4$^+$CD127$^{low+/-}$CD25$^+$-Treg cell pool.

Discussion

Therefore, Tregs play an important role in transplantation [5,17] and pregnancy [18,19], but also influence infectious diseases [20], autoimmunity [21], and anti-tumor immunity [22]. Meanwhile, promising data in regard to solid organ transplantation are increasingly available. Considering the potential role of Tregs in

Table 1. Clinical characteristics of kidney transplant patients.

Group	n	Median time after Transplantation [days]	Median Creatinine [mg/dl]	Results of Biopsy	Immunosuppression
A	20	-	-	-	-
B	119	181 [5–9155]	1.84 [0.74–11.6]	no rejection	
					27 Tac+MPA+steroids
					80 CsA+MPA+steroids
					5 mTor+MPA+steroids
					4 mTor+CsA+MPA+steroids
					3 others+MPA+steroids
C	37	793 [6–6938]	2.41 [1.34–6.93]	acute rejection	
				32 borderline rejections	
					8 Tac+MPA+steroids
					22 CsA+MPA+steroids
					1 mTor+CsA+MPA+steroids
					1 Azathioprin+MPA+steroids
				2 BANFF 1A rejections	
					1 CsA+MPA+steroids
					1 mTor+CsA+MPA+steroids
				3 acute humoral rejections	
					1 CsA+MPA+steroids
					1 mTor+MPA+steroids
					1 mTor+CsA+MPA+steroids

the control of allo-responses in renal transplant patients, one of the aims of this study was to examine whether quantitative and functional monitoring of Tregs could be used as markers of immunological tolerance. We demonstrated that in post-transplant patients the proportion of CD4+CD127$^{low+/-}$FoxP3+-Tregs decreased continuously in comparison to healthy volunteers over an

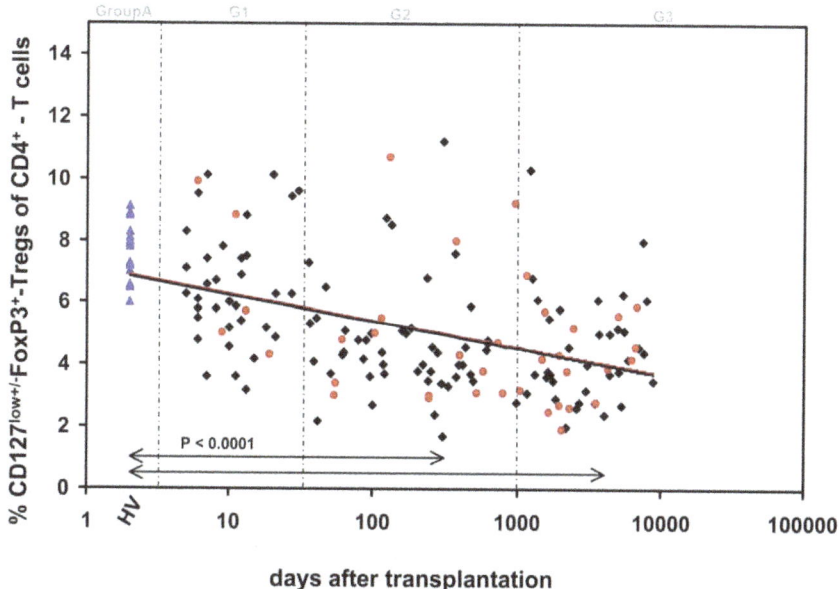

Figure 3. Detection of the percentage of CD4+CD127$^{low+/-}$FoxP3+-Treg cells of total CD4+-T cells in rejecting and non-rejecting patients after kidney transplantation. The percentage of CD4+CD127$^{low+/-}$FoxP3+-Tregs of total CD4+-T cells was estimated in healthy non-transplanted volunteers (▲), in kidney transplant patients with stable transplant function (◆) and in kidney transplant patients with biopsy proven rejection (BPR), (●). The percentage of CD4+CD127$^{low+/-}$FoxP3+-Tregs decreased continuously after transplantation. Significant differences between rejecting and non-rejecting patients were not detected.

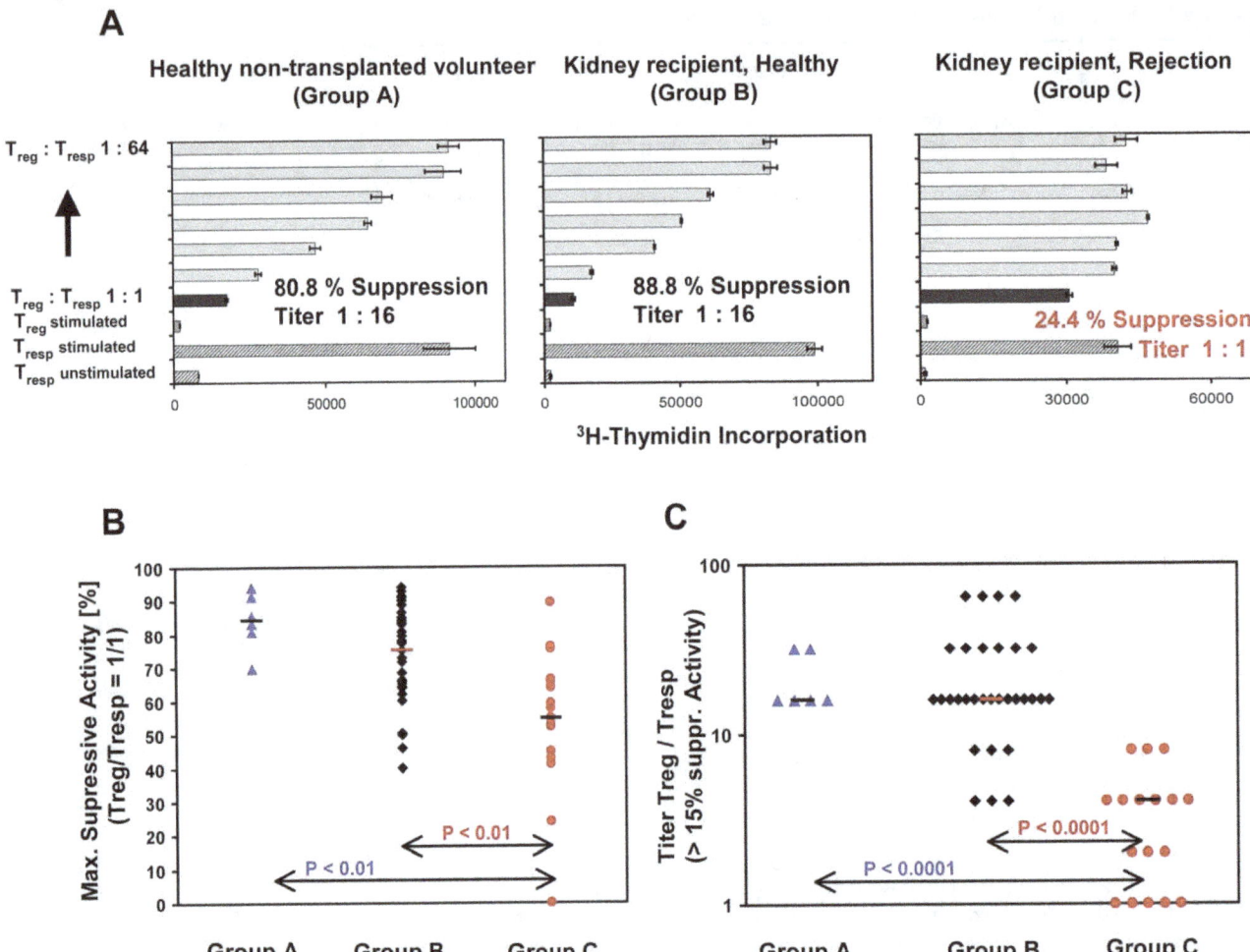

Figure 4. Evaluation of the suppressive activity of CD4$^+$CD127$^{low+/-}$CD25$^+$-Treg cells obtained from healthy non-transplanted volunteers and kidney transplant patients with stable transplant function or acute rejection. A: CD4$^+$CD127$^{low+/-}$CD25$^+$-Treg cells were isolated by the MACS technique and their suppressive activity was examined using suppression assays (see methods). One representative experiment is shown for healthy volunteers, kidney recipients with stable transplant function and kidney recipients with acute rejection. The maximum suppressive activity (Treg/Tresp = 1/1) (B) and the ratio of Treg/Tresp (titer) up to which the purified Treg cells could be diluted to achieve a minimum suppressive activity of at least 15% (C), were estimated for all participants. The figures show the individual and median data obtained for all patients groups.

observation period of almost 25 years after transplantation. In contrast to the results obtained with smaller studies [23,24,25], we demonstrated in our cohort that the percentage of CD4$^+$CD127$^{low+/-}$FoxP3$^+$-Tregs within the CD4$^+$-T cells was not different between rejecting and non-rejecting patients. Such differences may be based on inconsistent characterization of the total Treg pool, different gating strategies and small numbers of participants in many studies.

In addition, we demonstrated that the suppressive activity of the total CD4$^+$CD127$^{low+/-}$CD25$^+$-Treg cell pool from patients with biopsy proven rejection (BPR) was significantly reduced compared to patients with stable graft function and compared to healthy non-transplanted volunteers. Currently, limited data exist concerning the suppressive activity of Tregs from transplant patients with BPR. Dijke et al. demonstrated that CD4$^+$CD25$^+$FoxP3$^+$ Tregs of heart transplant patients who experienced acute rejection had a reduced regulatory function compared to those obtained from non-rejecting patients [26]. These and our results are contrary to the findings of a smaller study performed by Kreijveld et al. who

did not find any differences concerning the suppressive activity between renal transplant recipients with rejection and those without rejection [27].

Moreover, recent data revealed that the total Treg pool seems to be inconsistent. Different Treg subsets such as naïve CD45RA$^+$- or HLA-DR$^+$- expressing Treg cells were shown to be important for the functional activity of the total Treg cell pool [13,15]. We demonstrated that differential expression of HLA-DR and CD45RA distinguished four different Treg subsets, which showed characteristic changes concerning their percentages within the total Treg pool during the time after transplantation. Initially after transplantation, the proportion of the naïve DR$^-$CD45RA$^+$- and the DR^{high+}CD45RA$^-$-Tregs decreased strongly while the proportion of the DR^{low+}CD45RA$^-$- and the DR$^-$CD45RA$^-$-Tregs showed a considerable increase. In consequence, the HLA-DR MFI of the DR$^+$CD45RA$^-$-Treg subset was also dramatically reduced. Such findings may propose that there is a strong conversion of naïve Tregs into DR$^-$CD45RA$^-$- and DR^{low+}C-D45RA$^-$-Tregs shortly after transplantation. In addition, we

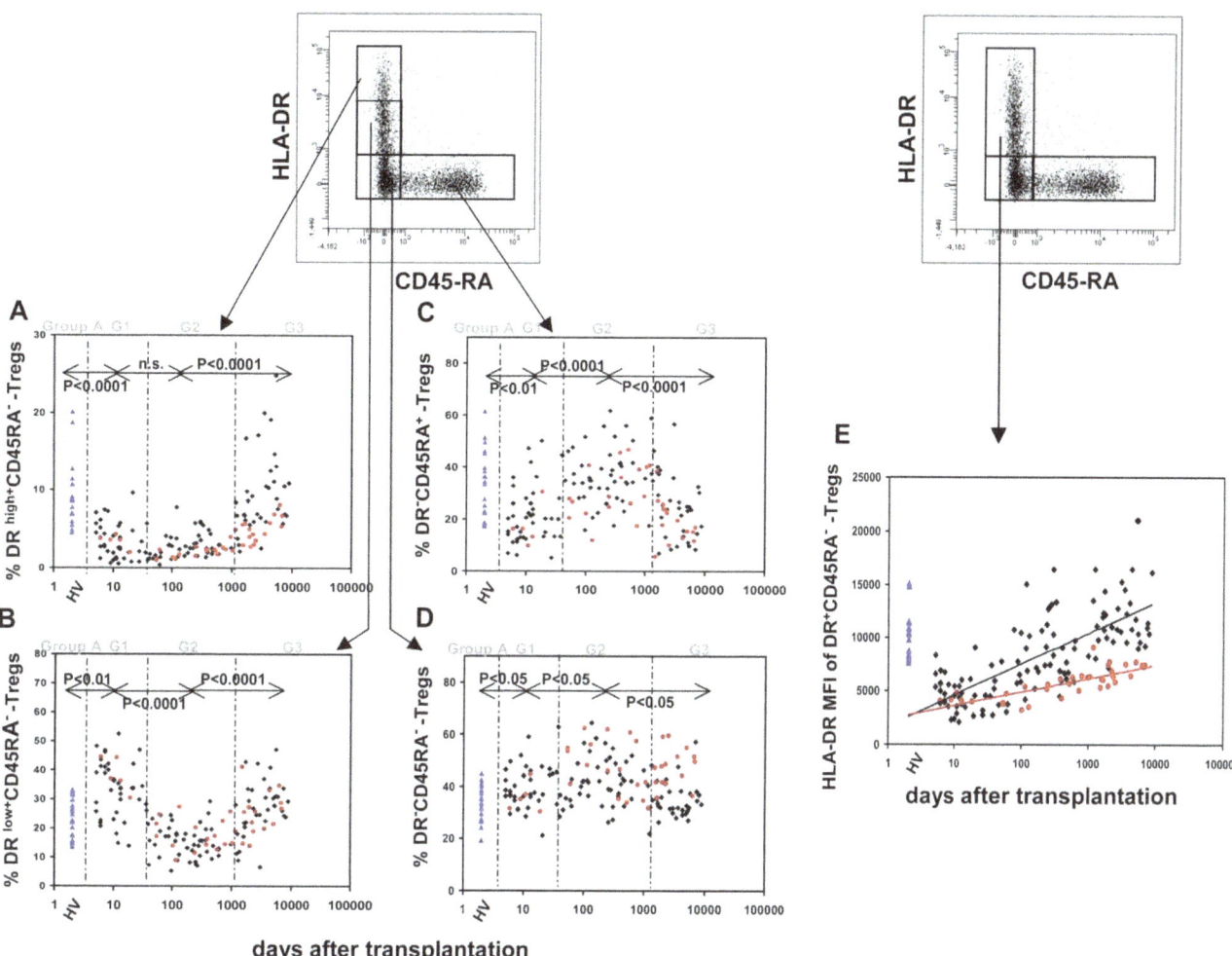

Figure 5. Detection of the changes in the composition of the total CD4$^+$CD127$^{low+/-}$FoxP3$^+$-Treg cell pool with four different Treg subsets during the time after transplantation. The percentage of the DR^{high+}CD45RA$^-$ (A), the DR^{low+}CD45RA$^-$ (B), the DR$^-$CD45RA$^+$ (C), and the DR$^-$CD45RA$^-$ (D) Treg subset within the total Treg cell pool was estimated in healthy non-transplanted volunteers (▲) and in non-rejecting (♦) and rejecting kidney transplant patients (●) at different time points after transplantation. In addition the HLA-DR MFI of the DR$^+$CD45RA$^-$-Treg subset was determined for all participants in all patient groups (E). Monitoring the HLA-DR MFI allowed a significant discrimination between rejecting and non-rejecting patients, due to a significantly reduced percentage of the DR^{high+}CD45RA$^-$-Treg subset within the total Treg pool. MFI = mean fluorescence intensity.

Table 2. Percentage of different Treg subsets of the total Treg pool obtained from healthy non-transplanted volunteers and kidney transplant patients in the presence or absence of BPR.

	Time after Tx [days]	n	DR$^-$CD45RA$^+$ [% Tregs]	DR$^-$CD45RA$^-$ [% Tregs]	DR^{low+} CD45RA$^-$ [% Tregs]	DR^{high+} CD45RA$^-$ [% Tregs]	HLA-DR MFI
Controls		20	34 (17–61)	33 (19–45)	25 (14–33)	7.5 (4.5–20.1)	10470 (7607–15090)
No BPR	0–30	36	20 (5–50)	37 (21–59)	34 (14–53)	2.8 (0.5–9.6)	4604 (2112–9076)
	31–1000	48	35 (13–62)	42 (27–65)	16 (5–29)	2.5 (0.4–7.8)	7431 (2782–16440)
	>1000	35	24 (7–59)	33 (22–57)	28 (7–47)	8.4 (2.1–24.8)	11102 (7219–21025)
BPR	0–30	5	16 (10–30)	35 (30–45)	37 (30–47)	3.6 (2.0–4.3)	4058 (4002–4817)
	31–1000	15	28 (12–47)*	51 (34–62)*	16 (9–27)	1.7 (1.0–2.8)*	5151 (3230–6401)*
	>1000	17	21 (6–41)	46 (32–60)***	26 (14–41)	4.7 (2.2–8.1)***	6843 (5312–9105)***

*: p<0.05; no BPR versus BPR.
***: p<0.001; no BPR versus BPR.

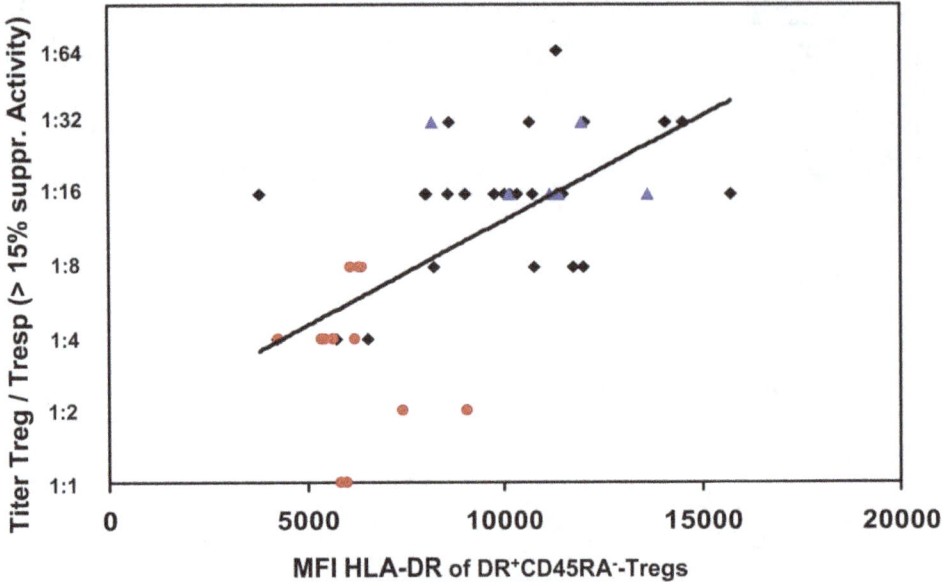

Figure 6. Correlation between the HLA-DR MFI of the DR⁺CD45RA⁻-Treg subset and the ratio of Treg/Tresp (titer) up to which a significant suppression could be achieved. CD4⁺CD127$^{low+/-}$CD25⁺-Tregs were purified from healthy non-transplanted volunteers (▲), kidney transplant patients with stable transplant function (◆) and kidney transplant patients with BPR (●). Their suppressive activity concerning the ratio of Treg/Tresp (titer) up to which the purified Treg cells could be diluted to achieve a minimum suppressive activity of at least 15% was related to the HLA-DR MFI of the DR⁺CD45RA⁻-Treg subset. The figure shows the positive correlation (r = 0.546, p<0.001) between the HLA-DR MFI of the DR⁺CD45RA⁻-Treg subset and the ratio of Treg/Tresp (titer). MFI = mean fluorescence intensity.

observed the striking effect that the naïve DR⁻CD45RA⁺-Treg subset increased strongly during the first year but decreased considerably during the time afterwards. Complementary to the naïve DR⁻CD45RA⁺-Treg subset the DR^{low+}CD45RA⁻-Treg subset decreased significantly during the first year but increased during the time afterwards. Such findings may propose that naïve DR⁻CD45RA⁺-Treg cells may be increasingly released by the thymus during the first year after transplantation. Presumably, after that time, the thymic output of Treg cells is exhausted. As HLA-DR⁺-Treg cells are known to represent highly activated mature Treg cells [13], it seems likely that during the first year after transplantation such cells were preferentially eliminated, presumably due to permanent allogenic stimulation of the immune system. After that time, the maturation of the HLA-DR⁺-Treg cells outnumbers their elimination and the percentage of the HLA-DR⁺-Treg cells again increases to the level of healthy non-transplanted volunteers. In either case it seems that the changes in the percentages of the DR^{high+}- and DR^{low+}CD45RA⁻-Treg cells occur in the way that the HLA-DR MFI increases continuously after transplantation. Such findings may explain why transplant outcome studies have shown markedly reduced rejection rates after three years post surgery [3,4].

To determine whether there were differences in the composition of the total Treg cell pool between transplant patients with and without BPR, we determined the proportion of the different Treg cell subsets for both patient collectives. Comparable to previous works [27], we found a reduction of the naïve DR⁻CD45RA⁺-Treg subset in regard to the total Treg pool in patients with BPR compared to patients with stable transplant function. Rejecting patients showed significantly higher proportions of DR⁻CD45RA⁻-Treg cells, but the most prominent difference between rejecting and non-rejecting patients was seen regarding the HLA-DR MFI of the DR⁺CD45RA⁻-Treg cell subset. This effect may be explained by the fact that patients with allograft

rejection showed a highly significant decrease of the DR^{high+}CD45RA⁻-Treg subset within the total Treg cell pool.

The evaluation of the suppressive activity of each of the four different Treg subsets (DR^{high+}CD45RA⁻-, DR^{low+}CD45RA⁻-, DR⁻CD45RA⁻- and DR⁻CD45RA⁺-Tregs) revealed that the DR^{high+}CD45RA⁻-Treg subset had the highest suppressive activity compared to the other Treg subsets.

Similar to findings documented by Baecher-Allan [13], the populations of DR^{high+}CD45RA⁻-Tregs and DR^{low+}CD45RA⁻-Tregs had a higher suppressive capacity than the populations of DR⁻CD45RA⁻- and DR⁻CD45RA⁺-Tregs. Therefore, specifically the loss of DR^{high}CD45RA⁻-Tregs obviously impaired the suppressive activity of the total Treg cell pool. Our data clearly demonstrate that the determination of the HLA-DR MFI allows a precise evaluation of the ratio between DR^{high+}CD45RA⁻-Tregs and DR^{low+}CD45RA⁻-Tregs within the DR⁺CD45RA⁻-Treg cell subset. We found a significant correlation between the level of HLA-DR expression of the DR⁺CD45RA⁻-Treg subset and the suppressive activity of the total Treg pool, determined both in healthy non-transplanted volunteers, healthy transplanted patients and transplanted patients with BPR. The lowest suppressive activity of the CD4⁺CD127$^{low+/-}$CD25⁺-Treg pool which correlated with a low HLA-DR MFI of the DR⁺CD45RA⁻-Treg cell subset was observed in patients with BPR.

During pregnancy the "fetal semi-allograft" is perfectly tolerated by the maternal immune system. In a recent published study we demonstrated that women with preterm labor necessitating preterm delivery showed significantly reduced HLA-DR expression of CD4⁺CD127$^{low+/-}$CD25⁺FoxP3⁺-Tregs, indicating that the immunologic mechanisms leading to preterm labor may be similar to those leading to allograft rejection after transplantation [28]. The underrepresentation of HLA-DR⁺-Treg cells in the neonatal compared with the adult circulation indicates that the presumed nTreg population gains HLA-DR expression upon

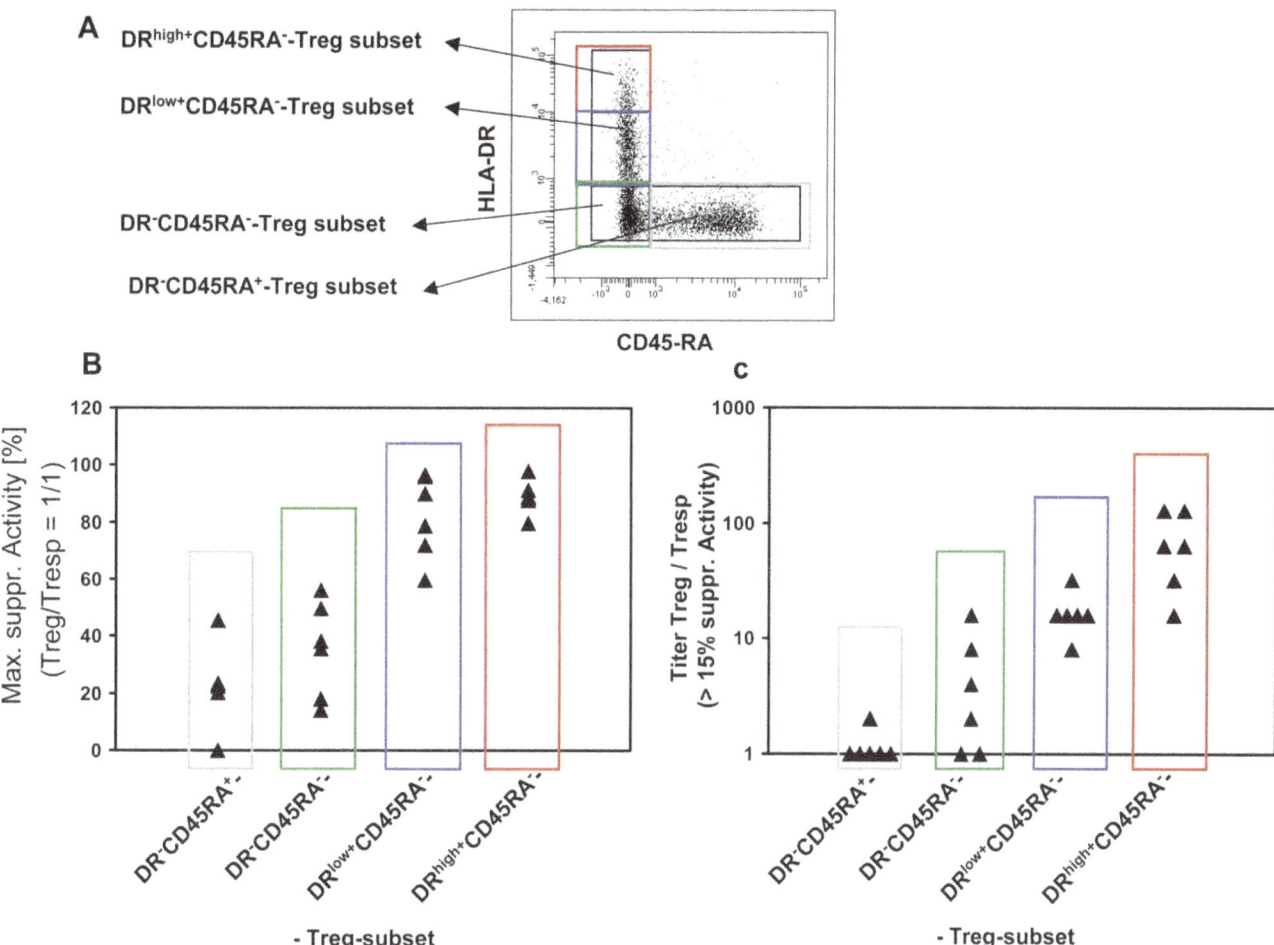

Figure 7. Positive selection and functional testing of four different Treg subsets within the total CD4$^+$CD127$^{low+/-}$CD25$^+$-Treg pool. A: Magnetically isolated CD4$^+$CD127$^{low+/-}$CD25$^+$-Treg cells were stained with anti-HLA-DR and anti-CD45RA specific monoclonal antibodies and sorted into a population of DR^{high+}CD45RA$^-$-, DR^{low+}CD45RA$^-$-, DR$^-$CD45RA$^-$-, and naïve DR$^-$CD45RA$^+$-Treg cells. Subsequently the different Treg populations obtained from six different healthy non-transplanted volunteers were analyzed concerning their maximum suppressive activity (Treg/Tresp = 1/1) (B) and the minimum ratio of Treg/Tresp (titer) up to which the purified Tregs could be diluted to achieve a minimum suppressive activity of at least 15% (C).

differentiation [29]. Ashley et al. suggest that the CD127^{low}DR$^+$-Tregs are terminally differentiated effector Tregs, as they do not proliferate and are highly sensitive to apoptosis [30]. It was shown that Granzyme B, which was produced by strongly stimulated non-regulatory responder CD4$^+$-T cells, reduced especially the suppressive capacity of the non-proliferating HLA-DR$^+$-Tregs cells [30]. On the other hand, the proliferation-competent HLA-DR$^-$-Treg cells remained viable [30] and were shown to be more sensitive to Fas-L induced apoptosis [31]. Therefore, it may be hypothesized that the decrease in the MFI of the DR$^+$CD45RA$^-$-Treg cell subset obtained from rejecting kidney recipients may be caused by the increased Granzyme B induced apoptosis of DR$^+$CD45RA$^-$-Treg cells which express the HLA-DR molecules very strongly. As it was ascertained that the Granzyme B induced apoptosis of the highly suppressive HLA-DR$^+$-Treg cells happened preferentially in the case of strong responder T-cell stimulation [30], it may be assumed that acute rejection episodes after transplantation that are characterized by strong stimulation of CD4$^+$-T cells lead to a loss of the strongly suppressive DR^{high+}-Treg-subset.

In summary, we clearly demonstrated that patients with biopsy proven rejection (BPR) show deficiencies concerning the functional activity of their Treg pool. Thereby, its composition was changed in the way that the DR^{high+}CD45RA$^-$-Treg subset, which was shown to possess the highest suppressive activity, was decreased. In contrast, the DR$^-$CD45RA$^-$-Treg subset with lower suppressive capacity was increased in transplanted patients with acute rejection. Especially the determination of the HLA-DR MFI of the DR$^+$CD45RA$^-$-Treg subset allowed a significant discrimination between patients with acute graft rejection and those without rejection. The clinical usefulness of the monitoring of these peripheral blood parameters after solid organ transplantation and its relation to clinical outcomes needs to be investigated in large prospective cohort studies of transplant patients.

Materials and Methods

Study population

The study was approved by the Ethics Committee of the Medical Faculty Heidelberg. All patients and healthy controls were fully informed of the aim of the study and written informed consent was obtained from all participants.

The study included 20 non-transplanted healthy volunteers (Group A) and 156 kidney transplant patients (Groups B and C) (Table 1). Forty-seven patients received a graft obtained from a living donor and 109 patients received a graft from a cadaveric donor. The mean age of our transplant cohort was 45 years (20–73 years). The causes of end-stage renal failure in our transplant cohort were diabetes mellitus (38%, n = 59), vascular nephopathy (26%, n = 41), glomerulonephritis (15%, n = 23), autosomal dominant polycystic kidney disease (8%, n = 12), autoimmune diseases (5%, n = 8) like systemic lupus erythematosus and systemic vasculitis and 8% (n = 13) were unknown. Blood samples were obtained on the same day when kidney transplant recipients admitted to the Department of Nephrology for kidney biopsy. Kidney biopsies were classified according to the BANFF-classification [32,33]. Biopsy proven rejection was defined as rising creatinine over 30% above the last three measurements and further pathological findings according to the BANFF-classification (Table 1). Patients with acute graft failure because of infection, postrenal obstruction or drug induced renal failure were excluded. All transplant patients were further subdivided into three different groups. The first group (G1) contains transplant recipients before the 30th day after transplantation. The second group (G2) contains recipients between the 31st and the 1000th day after transplantation and the third group (G3) contains recipients more than 1000 days post transplantation. The 156 transplant patients received an immunosuppressive regime with Mycophenolic acid (MPA), Methylprednisolone and Calcineurininhibitors (Ciclosporin: 104 patients; Tacrolimus: 35 patients) or mTOR-Inhibitors (Everolimus: 13 patients, whereas 7 recipients received a combination of Cyclosporine and Everolimus) and 4 recipients received other immunosuppressive drugs (Table 1).

Fluorescence-activated cell sorter (FACS) staining

Venous blood samples (9 ml) from all patients were collected into EDTA-containing tubes. Whole peripheral blood mononuclear cells (PBMCs) were isolated by Ficoll-Hypaque (Amersham Bioscience) gradient centrifugation and analyzed by five color flow cytometric analysis. Briefly, PBMCs (4×10^6 cells) were surface-stained with 10 µl PerCP-conjugated-anti-CD4 (BD Bioscience), 10 µl PE-conjugated anti-CD127 (eBioscience), 5 µl PE-Cy7-conjugated anti-HLA-DR (BD Bioscience) and 20 µl APC-conjugated anti-CD45RA (BD Bioscience) mouse monoclonal antibodies. Intracellular staining for the detection of FoxP3 was achieved using a FITC labeled anti-human FoxP3 staining set (clone PCH101, eBioscience) according to the manufacturer's instructions. Both the percentage of $CD4^+CD127^{low+/-}FoxP3^+$-Treg cells of total $CD4^+$-T cells and the percentage of $DR^{high+}CD45RA^-$-Tregs, $DR^{low+}CD45RA^-$-Tregs, $DR^-CD45RA^-$-Tregs and naïve $DR^-CD45RA^+$-Tregs within the total Treg pool were estimated for all participants. In addition the mean fluorescence intensity (MFI) of HLA-DR expression of the $DR^+CD45RA^-$-Treg cell subset was estimated for all participants. Negative control samples were incubated with isotype-matched antibodies. Dead cells were excluded by forward and side scatter characteristics. Cells were analyzed by a FACS Canto cytometer (BD Bioscience). Cells were analyzed by a FACS Canto cytometer (BD Bioscience) which is equipped with a 488-nm blue laser and a 633-nm red laser. The following standard filter set-ups were used: PerCP: 655 Longpass/670 LP Bandpass; PE: 556 Longpass/585/42 Bandpass; FITC: 502 Longpass/530/30 Bandpass; PE-Cy7: 735 Longpass/780/60 Bandpass; APC: 660/20 Bandpass). Statistical analysis was based on at least 100,000 gated $CD4^+$-T cells.

Positive selection and staining of $CD4^+CD127^{low+/-}CD25^+$-Treg cells

Whole peripheral blood mononuclear cells (PBMCs) were isolated from 45 ml EDTA-blood samples by Ficoll-Hypaque (Amersham Bioscience) gradient centrifugation. The $CD4^+CD127^{low+/-}CD25^+$-Treg cells were purified using the $CD4^+CD127^{low+/-}CD25^+$-Regulatory T cell Isolation Kit II (Miltenyi Biotec) according to the manufacturer's instructions. First $CD4^+CD127^{low+/-}$-T-cells were isolated by magnetic depletion of non-$CD4^+CD127^{high+}$-T-cells. In a second step, the $CD4^+CD127^{low+/-}CD25^+$-Treg cells were isolated by positive selection over two consecutive columns. The $CD4^+CD127^{low+/-}CD25^-$-T cells were obtained in the flow-through fraction and used as responder T cells. The $CD4^+CD127^{low+/-}CD25^+$-Treg cells were subsequently retrieved from the columns. The purified $CD4^+CD127^{low+/-}CD25^+$-Treg cell fraction was analyzed using four color flow cytometry. Briefly, 1×10^5 cells were stained with 10 µl PerCP-conjugated-anti-CD4, PE-conjugated anti-CD25, FITC-conjugated FoxP3 and biotin-conjugated anti-CD127 monoclonal antibodies. Positive staining for CD127 was detected using APC-conjugated streptavidin molecules. On average, 85% of the isolated $CD4^+CD127^{low+/-}CD25^+$-Treg cells were shown to be within the $CD4^+CD127^{low+/-}CD25^+Foxp3^+$-Treg cell population.

Co-culture suppression assay

Whole peripheral mononuclear cells (PBMCs) were isolated from 45 ml peripheral blood drawn in EDTA tubes by Ficoll-Hypaque (Amersham Bioscience) gradient centrifugation. $CD4^+CD127^{low+/-}CD25^+$-Treg cells were purified using the $CD4^+CD127^{low+/-}CD25^+$-Regulatory T cell Isolation Kit II (Miltenyi Biotec) described above. In all assays, 2×10^4 responder-T-cells were co-cultured with the purified $CD4^+CD127^{low+/-}CD25^+$-Treg cells at ratios 1:1 to 1:256 in 96-well v-bottom plates. Suppression assays were performed in a final volume of 100 µl/well of X-VIVO15 medium (Bio Whittaker). For T-cell stimulation, the medium was supplemented with 1 µg/ml anti-CD3 and 2 µg/ml anti-CD28 antibodies (eBioscience). As controls, $CD4^+CD127^{low+/-}CD25^+$-Treg cells and responder T cells alone were cultured both with and without any stimulus. Cells were incubated at 37°C and 5% of CO_2. After four days, 1 µCi ^3H-thymidine was added to the cultures and cells were further incubated for 16 hours. Then, cells were harvested and ^3H incorporation was measured by scintillation counting. All assays exhibited <10% SEM and were performed a minimum of six times using blood from 6 different healthy non-transplanted volunteers, 32 healthy non-rejecting transplant patients and 17 transplant patients with acute rejection. In order to compare the suppressive capacity of the isolated $CD4^+CD127^{low+/-}CD25^+$-Tregs between the different patient groups, we calculated the maximum suppressive activity (ratio of Treg cells to responder T cells 1:1) and the minimum ratio of Treg cells to responder cells, with which a suppression of at least 15% could be achieved.

Sorting and functional testing of the four different Treg cell subsets

Venous blood samples (100 ml) from six different healthy, non-transplanted volunteers were collected into EDTA-containing tubes. The whole peripheral blood mononuclear cells (PBMCs) were isolated by Ficoll-Hypaque (Amersham Bioscience) gradient centrifugation. For fluorescence activated cell sorting of the four different Treg cell subsets, $CD4^+CD127^{low+/-}CD25^+$-Treg cells were purified using the $CD4^+CD127^{low+/-}CD25^+$-Regulatory T cell Isolation Kit II (Miltenyi Biotec) as described above. Respectively, 5×10^5 cells of the isolated $CD4^+CD127^{low+/-}$ $CD25^+$-Treg cells were stained with 15 µl PE-Cy7-conjugated anti-HLA-DR (BD Bioscience) and 50 µl FITC-conjugated anti-CD45RA mouse monoclonal antibodies. Dead cells were excluded, while the remaining $CD4^+CD127^{low+/-}CD25^+$-Treg cells were sorted using a FACS-VantageSE-Sorter (BD Bioscience). Thereby, the $CD4^+CD127^{low+/-}CD25^+$-Treg cell population was divided into four Treg subsets: $DR^{high+}CD45RA^-$-, $DR^{low+}CD45RA^-$-, $DR^-CD45RA^-$-, and naïve $DR^-CD45RA^+$-Treg cells. Subsequently, the suppressive activity of each Treg population was analyzed using the above described suppression assay.

Statistical analysis

Statistical comparison of the percentages of $CD4^+CD127^{low+/-}$ $FoxP3^+$-Treg cells of $CD4^+$-T cells, of the percentages of the different Treg subsets ($DR^{high+}CD45RA^-$-Tregs, $DR^{low+}C$-$D45RA^-$-Tregs, $DR^-CD45RA^-$-Tregs and naïve DR^-CD45-RA^+-Tregs) within the total $CD4^+CD127^{low+/-}FoxP3^+$-Treg cell pool and of the HLA-DR MFIs between the different patient populations was done using the non-parametric H test of Kruskal and Wallis, which is used for simultaneous comparison of more than two sample populations. Each H test was followed by a Dunn test. Comparison of the suppressive activity of the purified $CD4^+CD127^{low+/-}FoxP3^+$-Tregs cells was also done using the Kruskal-Wallis-Test. $P<0.05$ was considered significant. Statistical analyses and graphs were performed using GraphPad Prism version 5 (San Diego, CA, USA) and BiAS 9.14 for windows (Frankfurt, Germany).

Acknowledgments

We would like to thank Dieter Stefan (Institute of Immunology, Heidelberg, Germany) for professional help with FACS sorting of Treg cell subsets.

Author Contributions

Conceived and designed the experiments: MS AS MZ. Performed the experiments: NS FH. Analyzed the data: MS AS NS SM ES MZ. Contributed reagents/materials/analysis tools: NS AS FH ES SM. Wrote the paper: MS AS.

References

1. Tesi RJ, Elkhammas EA, Henry ML, Davies EA, Salazar A, et al. (1993) Acute rejection episodes: best predictor of long-term primary cadaveric renal transplant survival. Transplant Proc 25: 901–902.
2. Pirsch JD, Ploeg RJ, Gange S, D'Alessandro AM, Knechtle SJ, et al. (1996) Determinants of graft survival after renal transplantation. Transplantation 61: 1581–1586.
3. Meier-Kriesche HU, Schold JD, Srinivas TR, Kaplan B (2004) Lack of improvement in renal allograft survival despite a marked decrease in acute rejection rates over the most recent era. American journal of transplantation 4: 378–383.
4. Ekberg H, Bernasconi C, Tedesco-Silva H, Vitko S, Hugo C, et al. (2009) Calcineurin inhibitor minimization in the Symphony study: observational results 3 years after transplantation. American journal of transplantation 9: 1876–1885.
5. Joffre O, Santolaria T, Calise D, Al Saati T, Hudrisier D, et al. (2008) Prevention of acute and chronic allograft rejection with CD4+CD25+Foxp3+ regulatory T lymphocytes. Nat Med 14: 88–92.
6. Noris M, Casiraghi F, Todeschini M, Cravedi P, Cugini D, et al. (2007) Regulatory T cells and T cell depletion: role of immunosuppressive drugs. Journal of the American Society of Nephrology: JASN 18: 1007–1018.
7. Li XC, Turka LA (2010) An update on regulatory T cells in transplant tolerance and rejection. Nature reviews Nephrology 6: 577–583.
8. Boros P, Bromberg JS (2009) Human FOXP3+ regulatory T cells in transplantation. American journal of transplantation 9: 1719–1724.
9. Curotto de Lafaille MA, Lafaille JJ (2009) Natural and adaptive foxp3+ regulatory T cells: more of the same or a division of labor? Immunity 30: 626–635.
10. Banham AH, Powrie FM, Suri-Payer E (2006) FOXP3+ regulatory T cells: Current controversies and future perspectives. Eur J Immunol 36: 2832–2836.
11. Liu W, Putnam AL, Xu-Yu Z, Szot GL, Lee MR, et al. (2006) CD127 expression inversely correlates with FoxP3 and suppressive function of human CD4+ T reg cells. The Journal of experimental medicine 203: 1701–1711.
12. Seddiki N, Santner-Nanan B, Tangye SG, Alexander SI, Solomon M, et al. (2006) Persistence of naive CD45RA+ regulatory T cells in adult life. Blood 107: 2830–2838.
13. Baecher-Allan C, Wolf E, Hafler DA (2006) MHC class II expression identifies functionally distinct human regulatory T cells. Journal of immunology 176: 4622–4631.
14. Booth NJ, McQuaid AJ, Sobande T, Kissane S, Agius E, et al. (2010) Different proliferative potential and migratory characteristics of human CD4+ regulatory T cells that express either CD45RA or CD45RO. Journal of immunology 184: 4317–4326.
15. Haas J, Fritzsching B, Trubswetter P, Korporal M, Milkova L, et al. (2007) Prevalence of newly generated naive regulatory T cells (Treg) is critical for Treg suppressive function and determines Treg dysfunction in multiple sclerosis. Journal of immunology 179: 1322–1330.
16. Venken K, Hellings N, Broekmans T, Hensen K, Rummens JL, et al. (2008) Natural naive CD4+CD25+CD127low regulatory T cell (Treg) development and function are disturbed in multiple sclerosis patients: recovery of memory Treg homeostasis during disease progression. Journal of immunology 180: 6411–6420.
17. Lopez-Hoyos M, Segundo DS, Fernandez-Fresnedo G, Marin MJ, Gonzalez-Martin V, et al. (2009) Regulatory T cells in renal transplantation and modulation by immunosuppression. Transplantation 88: S31–39.
18. Steinborn A, Haensch GM, Mahnke K, Schmitt E, Toermer A, et al. (2008) Distinct subsets of regulatory T cells during pregnancy: is the imbalance of these subsets involved in the pathogenesis of preeclampsia? Clin Immunol 129: 401–412.
19. Aluvihare VR, Kallikourdis M, Betz AG (2004) Regulatory T cells mediate maternal tolerance to the fetus. Nat Immunol 5: 266–271.
20. Rouse BT, Sarangi PP, Suvas S (2006) Regulatory T cells in virus infections. Immunological reviews 212: 272–286.
21. Sakaguchi S, Ono M, Setoguchi R, Yagi H, Hori S, et al. (2006) Foxp3+ CD25+ CD4+ natural regulatory T cells in dominant self-tolerance and autoimmune disease. Immunol Rev 212: 8–27.
22. Beyer M, Schultze JL (2006) Regulatory T cells in cancer. Blood 108: 804–811.
23. Stenard F, Nguyen C, Cox K, Kambham N, Umetsu DT, et al. (2009) Decreases in circulating CD4+CD25hiFOXP3+ cells and increases in intragraft FOXP3+ cells accompany allograft rejection in pediatric liver allograft recipients. Pediatr Transplant 13: 70–80.
24. Louis S, Braudeau C, Giral M, Dupont A, Moizant F, et al. (2006) Contrasting CD25hiCD4+T cells/FOXP3 patterns in chronic rejection and operational drug-free tolerance. Transplantation 81: 398–407.
25. Braudeau C, Racape M, Giral M, Louis S, Moreau A, et al. (2007) Variation in numbers of CD4+CD25highFOXP3+ T cells with normal immuno-regulatory properties in long-term graft outcome. Transpl Int 20: 845–855.
26. Dijke IE, Korevaar SS, Caliskan K, Balk AH, Maat AP, et al. (2009) Inadequate immune regulatory function of CD4+CD25bright+FoxP3+ T cells in heart transplant patients who experience acute cellular rejection. Transplantation 87: 1191–1200.
27. Kreijveld E, Koenen HJ, van Cranenbroek B, van Rijssen E, Joosten I, et al. (2008) Immunological monitoring of renal transplant recipients to predict acute allograft rejection following the discontinuation of tacrolimus. PloS one 3: e2711.
28. Kisielewicz A, Schaier M, Schmitt E, Hug F, Haensch GM, et al. (2010) A distinct subset of HLA-DR+regulatory T cells is involved in the induction of preterm labor during pregnancy and in the induction of organ rejection after transplantation. Clin Immunol 137: 209–220.
29. Baecher-Allan CM, Costantino CM, Cvetanovich GL, Ashley CW, Beriou G, et al. (2011) CD2 costimulation reveals defective activity by human CD4+CD25 hi regulatory cells in patients with multiple sclerosis. Journal of immunology 186: 3317–3326.
30. Ashley CW, Baecher-Allan C (2009) Cutting Edge: Responder T cells regulate human DR+ effector regulatory T cell activity via granzyme B. J Immunol 183: 4843–4847.
31. Yolcu ES, Ash S, Kaminitz A, Sagiv Y, Askenasy N, et al. (2008) Apoptosis as a mechanism of T-regulatory cell homeostasis and suppression. Immunology and cell biology 86: 650–658.
32. Racusen LC, Solez K, Colvin RB, Bonsib SM, Castro MC, et al. (1999) The Banff 97 working classification of renal allograft pathology. Kidney international 55: 713–723.
33. Sis B, Mengel M, Haas M, Colvin RB, Halloran PF, et al. (2010) Banff '09 meeting report: antibody mediated graft deterioration and implementation of Banff working groups. American journal of transplantation 10: 464–471.

4

CD154 Blockade Alters Innate Immune Cell Recruitment and Programs Alloreactive CD8+ T Cells into KLRG-1high Short-Lived Effector T Cells

Ivana R. Ferrer, Maylene E. Wagener, Mingqing Song, Mandy L. Ford*

Emory Transplant Center and Department of Surgery, Emory University, Atlanta, Georgia, United States of America

Abstract

CD154/CD40 blockade combined with donor specific transfusion remains one of the most effective therapies in prolonging allograft survival. Despite this, the mechanisms by which these pathways synergize to prevent rejection are not completely understood. Utilizing a BALB/c (H2-Kd) to B6 (H2-Kb) fully allogeneic skin transplant model system, we performed a detailed longitudinal analysis of the kinetics and magnitude of CD8+ T cell expansion and differentiation in the presence of CD154/CD40 pathway blockade. Results demonstrated that treatment with anti-CD154 vs. DST had distinct and opposing effects on activated CD44high CD62Llow CD8+ T cells in skin graft recipients. Specifically, CD154 blockade delayed alloreactive CD8+ T cell responses, while DST accelerated them. DST inhibited the differentiation of alloreactive CD8+ T cells into multi-cytokine producing effectors, while CD40/CD154 blockade led to the diminution of the KLRG-1low long-lived memory precursor population compared with either untreated or DST treated animals. Moreover, only CD154 blockade effectively inhibited CXCL1 expression and neutrophil recruitment into the graft. When combined, anti-CD154 and DST acted synergistically to profoundly diminish the absolute number of IFN-γ producing alloreactive CD8+ T cells, and intra-graft expression of inflammatory chemokines. These findings demonstrate that the previously described ability of anti-CD154 and DST to result in alloreactive T cell deletion involves both delayed kinetics of T cell expansion and differentiation and inhibited development of KLRG-1low memory precursor cells.

Editor: Mehrdad Matloubian, University of California, San Francisco, United States of America

Funding: This work was supported by National Institutes of Health grants AI073707 and AI079409 to Mandy L. Ford. The funders had no role in study design, data collection and analysis, decision to publish, or preparation of the manuscript.

Competing Interests: The authors have declared that no competing interests exist.

* E-mail: mandy.ford@emory.edu

Introduction

Current immunosuppressive regimens in organ transplantation require life-long administration and result in off-target toxicities such as nephrotoxicity and cardiovascular and metabolic complications [1]. Considering these significant co-morbidities, much work over the years has focused on the development of novel modes of immunosuppression. The development of costimulation blocking molecules has been the basis for research by several groups to specifically target and inhibit the full activation of alloantigen-specific T cells at the time of transplantation. One of the most effective pathways for therapeutic intervention is the CD154/CD40 pathway, blockade of which results in profound inhibition of graft rejection and in some models the induction of transplantation tolerance [2–4]. However, translation of therapeutic blockade of this pathway has been stymied by the observation of thromboembolic complications in pilot clinical trials as a result of the expression of CD154 on platelets [5]. Nevertheless, understanding the altered differentiation programs initiated in alloreactive T cell populations under conditions of CD154 blockade remains an important goal in the ongoing pursuit to harness the therapeutic potential of this pathway.

In order to study the effects of CD40/CD154 pathway blockade on donor-reactive T cell responses to a transplant, we employed an allogeneic skin graft (SG) model in which anti-CD154 monoclonal antibodies (mAb) were administered in combination with donor specific transfusion (DST) as previously described [4,6,7]. DST provides a large bolus of antigen presented by relatively inert APCs [8], stimulating antigen-specific T cell activation by providing "signal one." Other groups have also demonstrated the potent effects of combined DST and costimulation blockade in the prolongation of islet, cardiac, skin and kidney allograft survival in murine and nonhuman primate models [4,6–11]. Although it has been generally accepted that CD154 costimulation blockade leads to anergy [12] or deletion [13,14] of recently activated T cells, the mechanism by which DST and anti-CD154 mAb synergize to induce these effects on the alloreactive T cell population remains incompletely understood.

In order to assess the differential impact of DST and anti-CD154 mAb on the programming of donor-reactive CD8+ T cell expansion, contraction, and differentiation over time, we performed longitudinal analyses on the donor-reactive CD8+ T cell responses. We hypothesized that the previously observed deletion of graft-reactive CD8+ T cells following anti-CD154/DST treatment was the result of differential programming of these cells following encounter with alloantigen [8,12]. Recently, studies of viral-specific CD8+ T cell responses have revealed programmed differentiation of antigen-specific T cells into either long-lived memory precursors or short-lived effectors as early as four days post-infection [15]. These differentially programmed cells can be segregated on the basis of their expression of KLRG-1 (killer cell lectin-like receptor G-1), in that KLRG-1[high] cells represent short-lived effectors, while KLRG-1[low] antigen-specific CD8[+] T cells distinguish the long-lived memory precursors [15,16]. As compared to KLRG-1[low] cells, KLRG-1[high] cells go on to express lower levels of Bcl-2, CD27, and CD62L, and higher levels of GzmB. Functionally, KLRG-1[high] cells are compromised in their ability to produce IL-2, an important T cell autocrine growth factor [15,16]. Finally, adoptive transfer recipients of KLRG-1[high] cells have been shown to have poorer recall potential upon secondary rechallenge as compared to those receiving KLRG-1[low] cells, consistent with diminished ability to survive and differentiate into long-lived memory cells [15]. Here, we assessed the impact of anti-CD154 and DST to induce distinct differentiation programs in graft-reactive CD8[+] T cell responses. Specifically, anti-CD154 treatment functioned to reduce the magnitude of the alloreactive T cell response by delaying CD8[+] T cell expansion and increasing the proportion of KLRG-1[high] short-lived effector cells. In contrast, DST treatment prevented alloreactive CD8[+] T cells differentiation into multi-cytokine producing effectors.

In addition to its potent effects on adaptive immune responses, CD154 can play a major role in the activation of innate immunity. For example, in the setting of tissue injury and inflammation, CD154-expressing platelets are activated and have been shown to induce upregulation of adhesion molecules on and chemokine secretion by endothelial cells in a CD40-dependent manner [17]. Because chemokines that recruit innate immune cells are expressed early in the wound healing process of skin grafts [18], we aimed to determine whether blockade of CD154 also influences the chemotactic signals delivered to graft-infiltrating leukocytes. In this study, we observed that animals treated with CD154 blockade had significantly impaired expression of CXCL1/KC, CCL3/MIP-1α (macrophage inflammatory protein-1α), and CCL5/RANTES (regulated upon activation normal T cell expressed and secreted) in the allografts compared to untreated controls. Thus, blockade of CD154 impacts both innate and adaptive immunity to prolong allograft survival.

Materials and Methods

Ethics Statement

This research was approved by the Emory University Institutional Animal Care and Use Committee. All animals were treated ethically according to Emory University IACUC protocol 2001175.

Mice

B6-Ly5.2/Cr (H2-K[b], CD45.1) and BALB/c (H2-K[d], CD45.2) mice were obtained from the National Cancer Institute (Charles River, Frederick, MD).

Skin Transplantation, Donor Specific Transfusion and Antibody Treatment

Full thickness BALB/c tail and ear skins were transplanted onto dorsal thorax of recipient mice and secured with adhesive bandages for 6 days. DST was the adoptive transfer of whole splenocytes, given as a single dose of 10^7 splenocytes i.v. on the day of transplantation. Anti-CD154 treatment (MR1, BioExpress, West Lebanon, NJ) was administered i.p. at 500µg/ dose on the day of transplantation as well as on days 2, 4, 6 post-transplantation, where indicated. Skin grafts were monitored over time and declared rejected when <10% viable graft remained.

Activated T Cell Surface Staining and TruCount Analysis

At indicated time points, splenocytes were removed and disrupted with glass slides. Cells were stained with antibodies against CD4 and CD8 (Invitrogen), CD62L (BD Pharmingen), CD44 (eBiosciences), and KLRG-1 PE (Southern Biotech). Absolute counts were obtained by using TruCount tubes (BD Pharmingen). Samples were run on a LSR II Flow Cytometer (BD Pharmingen). Data were analyzed using FlowJo software (Treestar, San Carlos, CA).

Histology and IHC Quantification

Skin grafts were removed and placed in cryomolds with OCT Embedding Compound (Tissue-Tek, Hatfield, PA) and frozen on dry ice on day 7 post transplantation. Longitudinal sections of skin grafts were cut 5 µm thick with a cryostat (Leica CM 1850, Leica Microsystems, Wetzlar, Germany) and mounted on Superfrost Plus microscope slides. Slides were fixed with 100% acetone and used for H&E as well as immunohistochemical staining. CD8a (BD Biosciences) and Neutrophil Marker, Ly6b, (Santa Cruz Biotechnology, Santa Cruz, CA) antibodies were used for CD8[+] T cell and neutrophil immunohistochemical detection, respectively, by 3,3 diaminobenzidine (DAB) peroxidation and counterstained with haematoxylin. An Olympus BX43 microscope was used for visualization.

The whole slide digital images were captured using the Aperio ScanScope XT Slide Scanner (Aperio Technologies, Vista, CA) system with a 20× objective. Images were viewed and analyzed with ScanScope software using positive pixel count algorithm (Aperio). Several fields (8–10) of epidermis and dermis areas were measured in each section. The ratio of total strong positive vs. area measured was used as the quantifying parameter.

RNA Isolation and Chemokine RT-PCR

Mice were sacrificed and skin grafts were extracted and placed in RNA*later* (Qiagen) at 4°C until ready for use. RNA was isolated from skins using RNeasy Fibrous Tissue kit (Qiagen), according to manufacturer's instructions. Reverse transcription of RNA into cDNA was performed using TaqMan reverse transcription kit (Roche). CXCL1, CCL3, CCL5 real-time PCR assays (Applied Biosystems) were run on a 7900HT Real-Time PCR System (ABI).

T Cell Intracellular Cytokine Staining

To measure IFN-γ (eBiosciences) and TNF (BD Pharmingen) production by donor reactive cells, single cell suspensions of responder splenocytes from transplanted mice were stimulated with BALB/c splenocytes in the presence of 10µg/mL Brefeldin A for 4 hours *ex vivo*. An intracellular staining kit (BD Biosciences) was used according to manufacturer's instructions. Samples were run on a LSR II Flow Cytometer (BD Pharmingen). Data were analyzed using FlowJo software (Treestar, San Carlos, CA).

Statistical Analysis

GraphPad, Inc. Prism software was used to perform log-rank Kaplan-Meier statistical analyses on skin graft survival curves. For longitudinal analysis of T cell expansion and differentiation, two-way ANOVA tests were performed, followed by Tukey post-test on significant results. For analysis of cytokine producing cells and KLRG-1 expression, one-way ANOVA tests were performed, followed by Tukey post-test on significant results.

Results

Anti-CD154 and DST interact to protect allogeneic grafts from rejection

Combined DST/MR-1 administration function in concert to prolong graft survival, but the independent contributions of these treatments to the innate and adaptive immune responses are still incompletely understood. Here, we examined the individual contributions of DST and anti-CD154 on innate and adaptive cell recruitment, the accumulation of inflammatory chemokines within the allograft, and the programming of alloreactive CD8+ T cell responses. This well-established regimen consists of BALB/c DST administered in conjunction with anti-CD154 monoclonal antibody treatment at the time of BALB/c skin transplantation onto naïve B6 recipients [6]. Using this protocol, untreated animals rapidly reject their skin grafts (MST 13d), while anti-CD154 mAb monotherapy results in a modest, but significant, delay in graft rejection as compared to untreated mice (MST 17d, p = 0.039), and DST monotherapy results in rapid allograft rejection, similar to untreated animals (MST 13d). In contrast, combined treatment with anti-CD154 mAb and DST results in significant prolongation of skin graft survival, as treated animals exhibited a MST of 50 days (p = 0.0002, compared to untreated mice) (Figure 1B).

Anti-CD154 treatment alters recruitment of graft-infiltrating cells following transplantation

In order to assess the impact of DST and/or CD154 blockade on cellular infiltration into the graft, we measured the level of

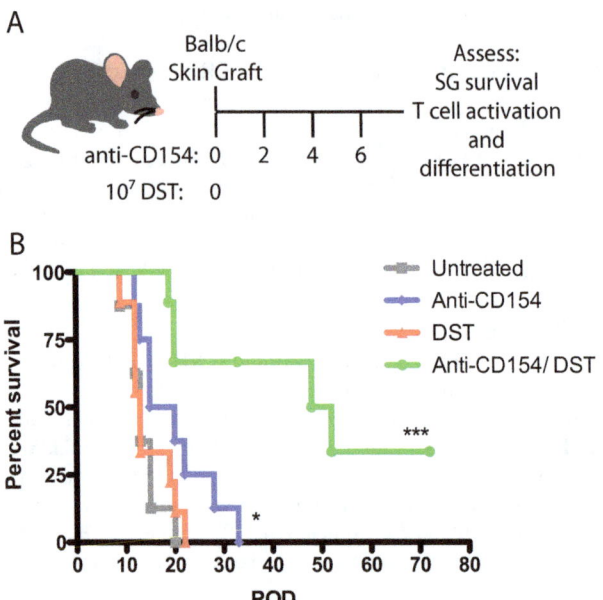

Figure 1. Anti-CD154 and DST interact to protect allogeneic grafts from rejection. A. B6-Ly5.2/Cr mice were transplanted with BALB/c skin grafts and were treated with 10^7 BALB/c splenocytes (DST) and/ or anti-CD154 monoclonal antibody (500 µg on D0, 2, 4, 6), where indicated. B. Allo-skin grafts in untreated mice had an MST of 13 days. Monotherapy with either CD40/CD154 pathway blockade or DST led to rapid rejection of the allograft with MSTs of 17.5d (p = 0.039) and 13d (p = n.s.), respectively. Anti-CD154 and DST combined treated significantly prolonged allograft survival to 50 days (p = 0.0002). Data are summary of two experiments of 4–5 mice per group. *p<0.05, ***p<0.001.

infiltrating CD8+ T cells and neutrophils in explanted allografts on day 7 post-transplantation via immunohistochemical staining for CD8+ T cells (Figure 2A) and neutrophils (Figure 2C). Quantification of the number of strongly positive pixels per µm² revealed that either DST or CD154 blockade individually or in combination diminished CD8+ T cell infiltration into allografts (Figure 2B). In contrast, only anti-CD154 treatment resulted in profound diminution of neutrophil-specific anti-Ly6b staining in the transplanted allografts (Figure 2D).

CD154 blockade decreases CXCL1, CCL3, and CCL5 expression in allografts

Given the differential migration of neutrophils into the transplanted allografts in the presence of CD154 blockade vs. DST, we aimed to determine whether CD40/CD154 pathway blockade and DST differentially influenced the expression of chemokines in graft tissue. We interrogated the expression of CXCL1 (KC), CCL3 (MIP-1α), and CCL5 (RANTES) in allografts on day 7 post-transplantation by real-time PCR (Figure 3). The relative expression of KC/CXCL1, a primary neutrophil chemoattractant [19], was significantly attenuated in skin grafts of all animals treated with anti-CD154 mAb either as a monotherapy (0.21±0.09, p<0.0001) or in combination with DST (0.26±0.11, p<0.0001) when compared to untreated animals. In contrast, DST alone did not significantly reduce CXCL1 expression compared to untreated controls (Figure 3A).

Similarly, our results demonstrated that both MIP-1α and RANTES, molecules associated with the recruitment of both innate and adaptive immune cells including monocytes and T cells [19], were significantly attenuated in animals treated with CD154-blockade (Figure 3B, 3C). Again, DST did not statistically significantly diminish the expression of either MIP-1α or RANTES in the explanted grafts. Taken together, these results suggest that DST alone impairs adaptive CD8+ T cell responses but that only CD154 blockade attenuates expression of chemokines within the graft, thereby inhibiting neutrophil infiltration.

Anti-CD154 and DST independently alter the expansion kinetics of activated CD44^high CD62L^low CD8+ T cells

Next, we investigated the independent effects of DST and CD154 blockade on the magnitude and kinetics of the donor-reactive CD8+ T cell response following transplantation by tracking the absolute number of antigen-experienced CD44^high CD62L^low CD8+ T cells over time. In naïve B6 animals, approximately 0.45±0.07×10^6 cells of the peripheral CD8+ T cell compartment were CD62L^low and CD44^high cells. Untreated recipients of allogeneic skin grafts developed large numbers of antigen-experienced cells with a peak of expansion at day 10 post-transplantation (2.36±0.55×10^6) (representative flow cytometry data shown in Figure 4A). Following resolution of this effector cell population into memory, untreated recipients maintained 1.0±0.32×10^6 effector/ memory phenotype T cells at day 50. Anti-CD154 mAb monotherapy resulted in a delayed expansion of activated CD8+ T cells, with a peak at day 14 (0.95±0.16×10^6). Furthermore, the magnitude of this peak was significantly reduced compared with the peak response of untreated mice (day 10) (p = 0.0133). In contrast, DST monotherapy modestly accelerated the expansion of activated CD8+ T cells starting at day 7 (0.83±0.13×10^6, p = 0.059), but also significantly reduced the peak expansion of activated CD8+ T cells compared to untreated controls (day 10: 0.98±0.07×10^6, p<0.001). The combination of CD154 blockade and DST led to a significantly greater diminution of both the magnitude and kinetics of expansion of

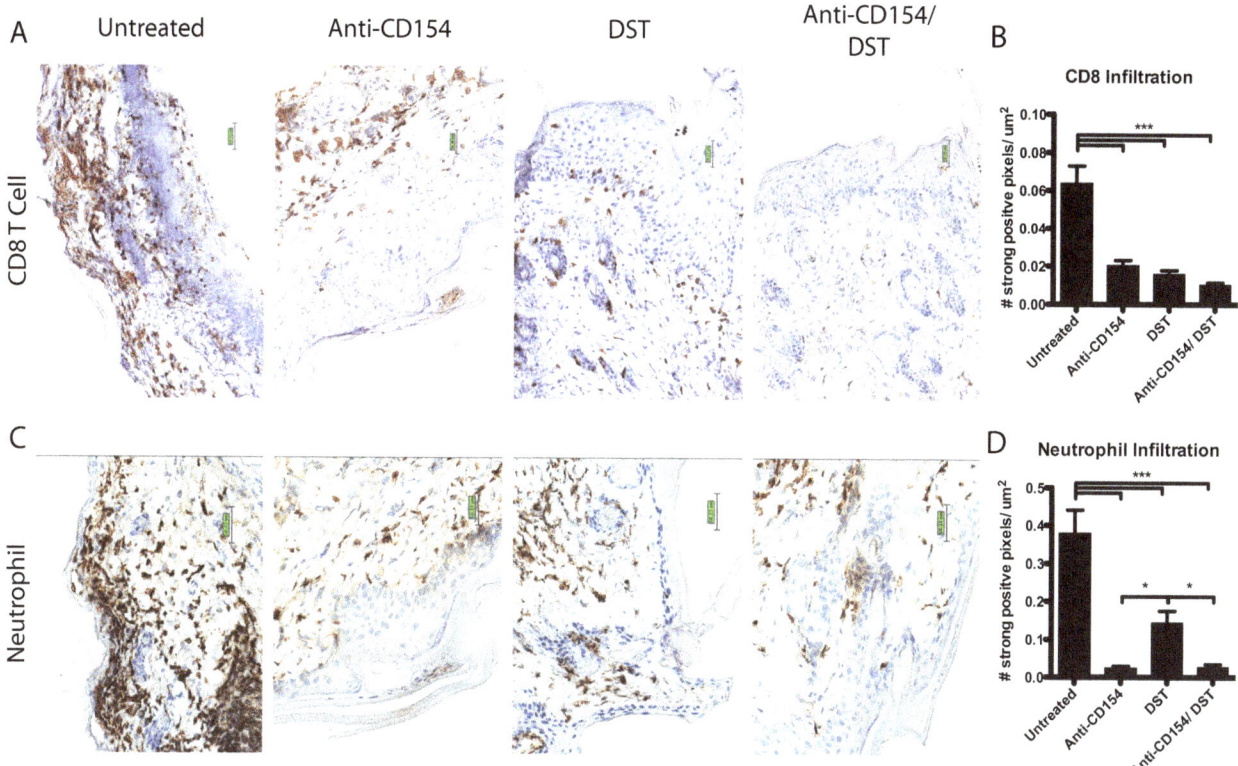

Figure 2. Anti-CD154 treatment alters recruitment of graft-infiltrating cells following transplantation. B6.SJL mice were transplanted with BALB/c skin grafts and were treated with 10^7 BALB/c DST and/ or anti-CD154 mAb, where indicated. Day 7 explanted allo-skin grafts were stained for (A) CD8 and (C) Ly6b to determine the level of CD8$^+$ T cell and neutrophil infiltration, respectively. Histological analyses of (B) CD8$^+$ T cell and (D) neutrophil infiltration were digitally measured in 8–17 fields of epidermis and dermis. The ratio of total strongly positive pixels to total area was determined. Data are a summary of two experiments with three mice per group. Values are mean $\pm$ SEM. **p$<$0.01, ***p$<$0.001.

graft-reactive CD8$^+$ T cells. In particular, the peak of expansion of these cells was delayed (day 14) compared with untreated controls. Furthermore, the magnitude of the peak of the alloreactive CD8$^+$ T cell response following combined anti-CD154 and DST (day 14) was significantly diminished compared with the peak expansion of untreated mice (day 10) ($0.62\pm0.08\times10^6$ vs. $2.36\pm0.55\times10^6$, respectively; p = 0.0026) (Figure 4B, C). In addition, compared with untreated animals, anti-CD154 and DST also significantly diminished the persistence of antigen-experienced CD44^{high} CD62L^{low} CD8$^+$ T cells at memory time points (day 50) ($1.01\pm0.32\times10^6$ vs. $0.32\pm0.03\times10^6$, respectively; p$<$0.05) (Figure 4B, C).

Anti-CD154 and DST distinctly alter alloreactive CD8$^+$ T cell programming into cytokine-producing effector cells

To assess the effects of anti-CD154 and DST on the programmed differentiation of alloreactive CD8$^+$ T cells into cytokine-producing effectors, splenocytes from skin grafted animals treated with anti-CD154, DST, or the combination were stimulated *ex vivo* with BALB/c splenocytes and subjected to intracellular cytokine staining (Figure 5). Data showed that as early as day 7 post-transplantation, splenic CD8$^+$ T cells from untreated animals began to differentiate into multi-functional TNF and IFN-γ producing T cells. At day 10, untreated mice developed a peak of IFN-γ producing donor-reactive CD8$^+$ T cells ($1.96\pm0.70\times10^5$) (Figure 5A, B). DST mediated an early expansion of IFN-γ producing graft-specific CD8$^+$ T cells with a peak response at day 7 ($0.90\pm0.05\times10^5$) (Figure 5B). In contrast, anti-CD154 mAb

monotherapy delayed CD8$^+$ T cell differentiation into IFN-γ producing cells, such that a modest peak was observed 14 days post-transplantation ($0.22\pm0.21\times10^5$) (Figure 5B). Finally, combined treatment with anti-CD154 and DST significantly impaired the differentiation of antigen-specific CD8$^+$ T cells into cytokine-producing donor-reactive T cells compared to untreated controls, such that IFN-γ^+ alloreactive CD8$^+$ T cells were virtually undetectable (Figure 5A, B).

We observed similar numbers of alloreactive IFN-γ-producing effectors in the untreated and DST treated groups on day 7 post-transplantation (Figure 5B). However, by day 10, this population expanded in the untreated animals, while it contracted in the DST treated animals. In order to understand the nature of the T cell programming that led to these disparate outcomes, we sought to determine the fraction of CD44^{high} CD62L^{low} activated T cells in these animals that produced cytokines following *ex vivo* restimulation with alloantigen. On day 7, $17.10\pm3.49\%$ of antigen-experienced CD44^{high} CD62L^{low} CD8$^+$ T cells isolated from untreated animals produced IFN-γ (Figure 5C, left). In contrast, although DST resulted in early accumulation of CD44^{high} CD62L^{low} CD8$^+$ T cells, a significantly lower fraction of these cells had differentiated into IFN-γ producers on day 7 compared with untreated animals ($8.08\pm0.64\%$, p$<$0.05) (Figure 5C, right).

These results indicated that DST decreased the frequency of differentiated IFN-γ producers as a percentage of the total activated T cell population. Therefore, we next interrogated whether this treatment also affected T cell differentiation into multi-cytokine producing effectors. To test this, IFN-γ producing

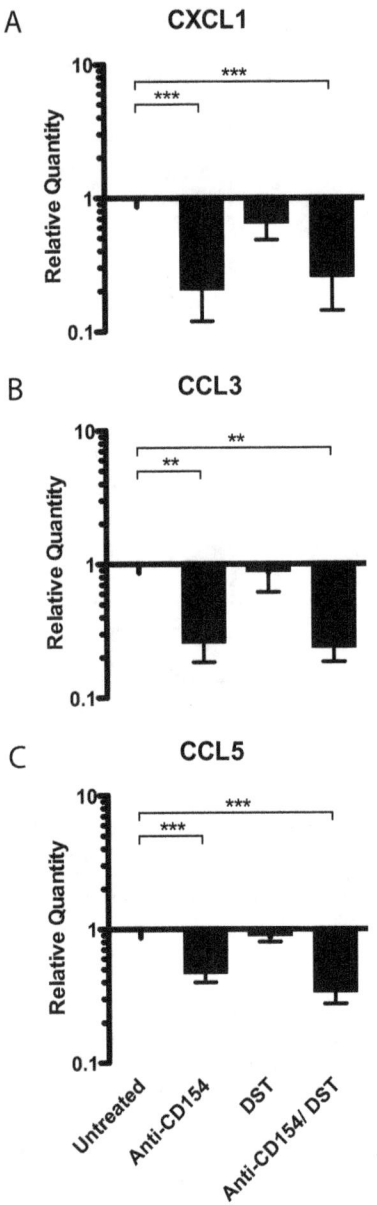

Figure 3. CD154 blockade decreases CXCL1, CCL3, and CCL5 expression in allografts. B6.SJL mice were transplanted with BALB/c skin grafts and were treated with 10^7 BALB/c DST and/ or anti-CD154 mAb, where indicated. On day 7, skin grafts were explanted and processed for RNA extraction. Real time PCRs for chemokines CXCL1/ KC, CCL3/ MIP-1α, and CCL5/ RANTES were performed from cDNA. Data are summary of two experiments with three mice per group. Values are mean ± SEM. **p<0.01, ***p<0.0001.

CD8$^+$ T cells were analyzed for their co-production of TNF. In untreated animals, the large majority of IFN-γ producing CD8$^+$ T cells co-produced TNF (77.89±3.04%) upon restimulation. However, DST treatment significantly impaired the ability of graft-reactive CD8$^+$ T cells to differentiate into IFN-γ$^+$ TNF$^+$ multi-cytokine producers compared with untreated controls (53.27±2.17%, p = 0.0028) (Figure 5D).

Similar to the effect on total burst size and differentiation of T cells, CD40/CD154 pathway blockade also impaired the development of alloreactive CD8$^+$ memory T cells. Specifically, treatment with anti-CD154 resulted in a reduced accumulation of

IFN-γ producing alloreactive CD8$^+$ T cells at day 50 post-transplantation compared with untreated controls (0.45±0.17×10^4 vs. 7.35±0.84×10^4, respectively; p<0.0001). Similarly, DST monotherapy also diminished the persistence of IFN-γ producing alloreactive memory CD8$^+$ T cells (1.07±0.03×10^4, p<0.0001) at day 50 compared with untreated animals. Finally, the combination of CD154 blockade and DST reduced the alloreactive CD8$^+$ memory T cell population more profoundly compared with untreated controls (0.02±0.02×10^4 vs. 7.35±0.84×10^4, respectively; p<0.0001) (Figure 5B).

Anti-CD154 treatment increases the frequency of KLRG-1^{high} short-lived CD8$^+$ effectors

These results indicate that CD154 blockade delays and diminishes the accumulation of alloreactive CD8$^+$ T cells during the immune response to a transplant. In order to interrogate the molecular mechanisms underlying this effect, we examined the expression of a cell surface protein known to be associated with the differentiation of short-lived effector T cells that exhibit rapid contraction *in vivo*. The increased expression of KLRG-1 early during T cell responses has recently been shown to be upregulated on short-lived effector cells following antigen stimulation while the lower expression of KLRG-1 is associated with a long-lived memory T cell program [15]. We analyzed the expression of KLRG-1 on alloreactive CD8$^+$ T cells on day 7 post-transplantation. In untreated animals, 44.12±2.30% of antigen-experienced CD44^{high} CD62L^{low} CD8$^+$ T cells expressed increased levels of KLRG-1 by day 7. In contrast, CD154 blockade led to a marked reduction in the long-lived memory precursor KLRG-1^{low} CD8$^+$ T cell population, and a commensurate increase in the frequency of KLRG-1^{high} short-lived effectors compared with untreated controls (KLRG-1^{high}: 58.68±4.62% vs. 44.12±2.30%, respectively; p<0.05) (Figure 6A, B). DST monotherapy did not significantly alter the frequency of KLRG-1^{high} alloreactive CD8$^+$ T cells (35.15±1.20%) (Figure 6A, B). Finally, the addition of anti-CD154 treatment to DST significantly increased the frequency of KLRG-1^{high} short-lived alloreactive CD8$^+$ T cells compared with DST monotherapy (57.87±3.97% vs. 35.15±1.20%, respectively; p<0.001) (Figure 6A, B).

Lack of CD4$^+$ T cell help has been associated with reduced memory CD8$^+$ T cell development and survival following pathogen infection [20,21]. Because we observed both an increase in KLRG-1^{high} CD8$^+$ T cells early on and a diminution of alloreactive CD8$^+$ T cells during memory timepoints, we hypothesized that anti-CD154-mediated inhibition of CD4$^+$ T cell help may underlie these observations. We assessed the accumulation of alloreactive CD4$^+$ T cells on day 7 post-transplantation by analysis of IFN-γ production following *ex vivo* restimulation. Results demonstrated that CD40/CD154 pathway blockade significantly reduced the accumulation of alloreactive IFN-γ$^+$ CD4$^+$ T cells compared with untreated controls (0.46±0.16×10^4 vs. 1.75±0.18 10^4, respectively; p<0.01) (Figure 6C). Furthermore, when anti-CD154 treatment was combined with DST, IFN-γ-producing CD4$^+$ T cells were significantly reduced compared to DST monotherapy (0.49±0.09×10^4 vs. 4.78±0.23×10^4, respectively; p<0.001) (Figure 6C).

Discussion

In this manuscript, we assessed the impact of CD154 blockade and DST on the programmed differentiation of alloreactive CD8$^+$ T cell responses longitudinally following transplantation. We interrogated the effects of CD40/154 pathway blockade and DST

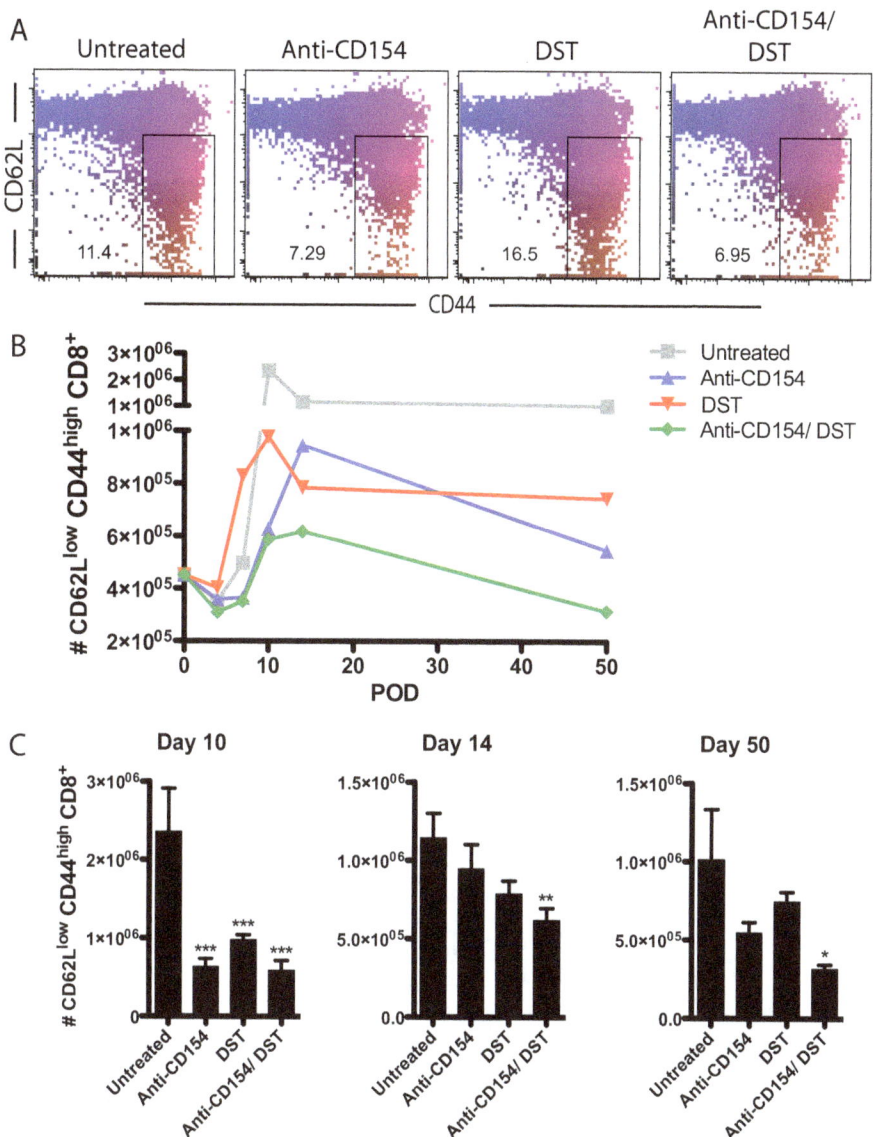

Figure 4. Anti-CD154 and DST independently alter the expansion kinetics of activated CD44high CD62Llow CD8+ T cells. B6-Ly5.2/Cr mice were transplanted with BALB/c skin grafts and were treated with 10^7 BALB/c DST and/ or anti-CD154 mAb, where indicated. A. Representative flow plots of CD44high and CD62Llow CD8+ T cells isolated from spleens of mice on day 7 post-transplantation. B. Expansion kinetics of activated CD8+ T cells after allo-transplantation. C. Accumulation of CD44high CD62Llow CD8+ T cells on day 10, 14, and 50 post-transplantation. Data are summary of two experiments with three mice per group. Values are mean ± SEM. *p<0.05, **p<0.01, ***p<0.001.

treatment on adaptive and innate immune cell involvement in graft rejection. We demonstrated that treatment with anti-CD154 and DST induces distinct differentiation programs in alloreactive T cell populations; specifically that treatment with anti-CD154 not only delayed the expansion and accumulation of activated CD62Llow CD44high CD8+ T cells, but also delayed and reduced CD8+ T cell differentiation into IFN-γ producing cells. Although the eventual emergence of alloreactive CD8+ T cells in anti-CD154 treated animals could be attributed to the waning effects of the antibody following cessation of treatment, this is not likely since *in vivo* administration of MR-1 has been shown to persist in animals with a half-life of 10.4 days [22]. Therefore, the delayed CD8+ T cell response in animals treated with CD40/CD154 blockade monotherapy is likely due to a CD154-independent breakthrough response, and not due to incomplete blockade of the pathway in this system.

Importantly, this study revealed a novel effect of CD40/CD154 pathway blockade on T cell differentiation, specifically the ability of CD154 blockade to increase the frequency of KLRG-1high short-lived effector cells among CD8+ CD44high CD62low alloreactive effectors, and correspondingly decrease the frequency of KLRG-1low long-lived memory precursors. KLRG-1 expressed early during an immune response is associated with a short-lived effector cell that is destined to die during the contraction phase of the response [15]. CD8+ T cell populations in CD154/DST treated animals contained fewer numbers of CD44high CD62Llow activated effectors; therefore, these data suggest that one mechanism by which CD154 blockade might mediate deletion of this subset is through the induction of KLRG-1 expression. Previous studies have shown that increased expression of KLRG-1 can be attributed to increased antigen duration and increased inflammation [16,23]. Further investigation into the mechanisms

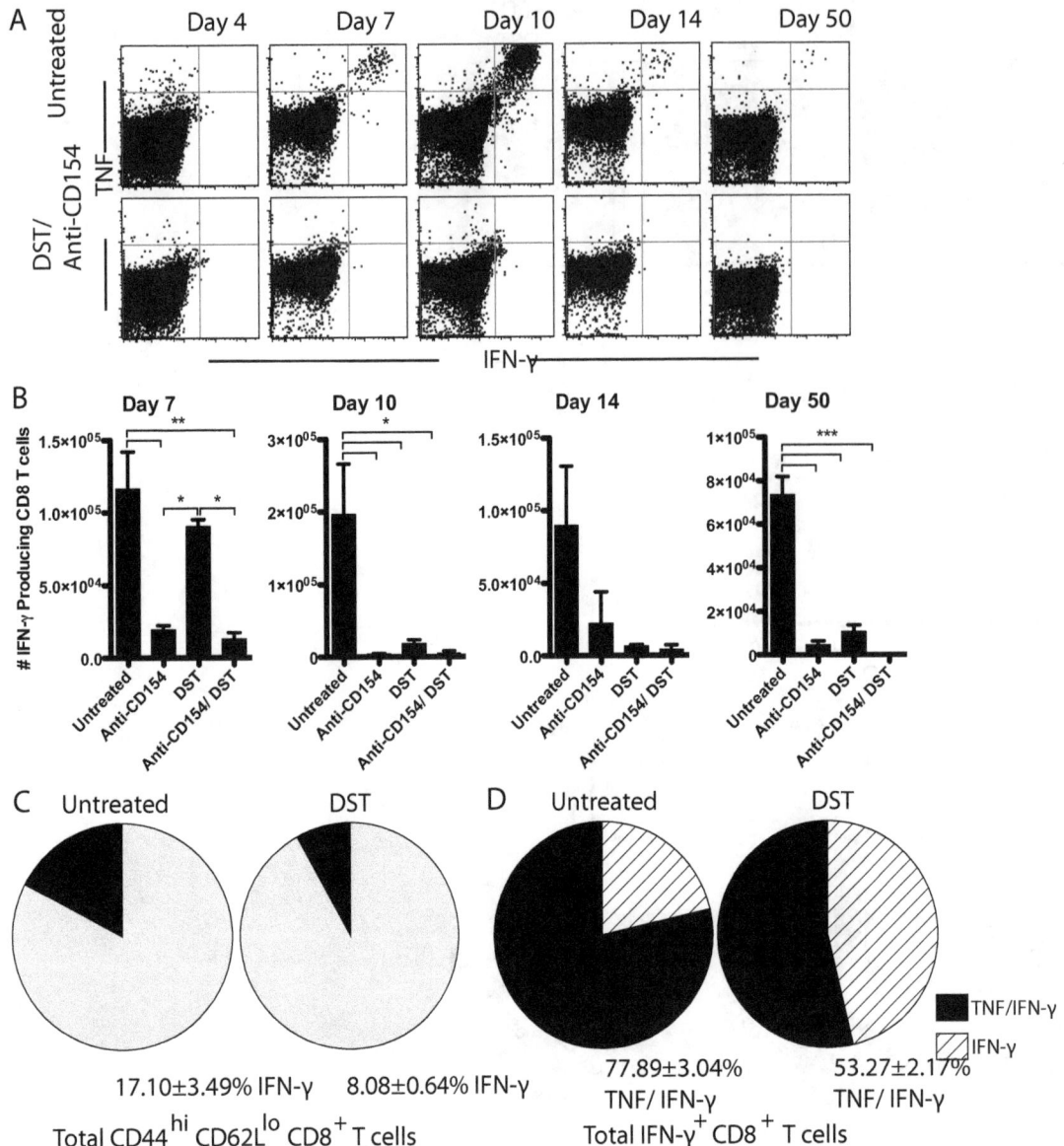

Figure 5. Anti-CD154 and DST distinctly alter alloreactive CD8+ T cell programming into cytokine-producing effector cells. B6-Ly5.2/Cr mice were transplanted with BALB/c skin grafts and were treated with 10^7 BALB/c DST and/ or anti-CD154 mAb, where indicated. A. Representative flow plots of TNF and IFN-γ producing CD8+ T cells after *ex vivo* restimulation with BALB/c splenocytes, isolated from spleens of mice at day 7 post-transplantation. B. Absolute count of total IFN-γ producing CD8+ T cells in the spleen over time following *ex vivo* restimulation. C. Pie charts represent total activated CD44high CD62Llow CD8+ T cells. The black wedges represent the frequency of activated CD44high CD62Llow CD8+ T cells that produce IFN-γ on day 7 post-transplantation (p<0.05). D. Pie charts represent all IFN-γ producing CD8+ T cells. The striped wedges represent the IFN-γ-only producing population and black segments represent the TNF/IFN-γ double producing population in untreated vs. DST treated mice on day 7 (p = 0.0028). Data are summary of two experiments with three mice per group. Values are mean ± SEM. *p<0.05, **p<0.01, ***p<0.001.

by which CD154 blockade also increases KLRG-1 expression in the context of transplantation is warranted.

In contrast, DST treatment significantly inhibited CD8+ T cell differentiation into competent IFN-γ secreting effectors, and of these IFN-γ-producing cells, a lower percentage of IFN-γ+ TNF+ double producers was observed compared with untreated controls. This pattern of cytokine expression is reminiscent of CD8+ T cell exhaustion, wherein T cells first lose the ability to make TNF, followed by the loss of IFN-γ, before being deleted altogether [24]. Because CD8+ T cell exhaustion is facilitated by exposure to high dose antigen, we posit that DST could be initiating a process

similar to T cell exhaustion by exposing the cells to high dose antigen presented on relatively inert APCs [8].

Overall, our results suggest that the distinct effects of anti-CD154 and DST on T cell programming, namely to skew the antigen-specific population towards KLRG-1hi short lived effectors and to induce a cytokine secretion pattern reminiscent of T cell exhaustion, respectively, functioned in concert to profoundly attenuate antigen-specific T cell responses. This was true both in terms of numbers of activated alloreactive CD8+ T cells and IFN-γ producers, at all time points over the course of the immune response to the allograft. Thus, our data suggest that the blunted T cell differentiation observed in DST treated recipients, when

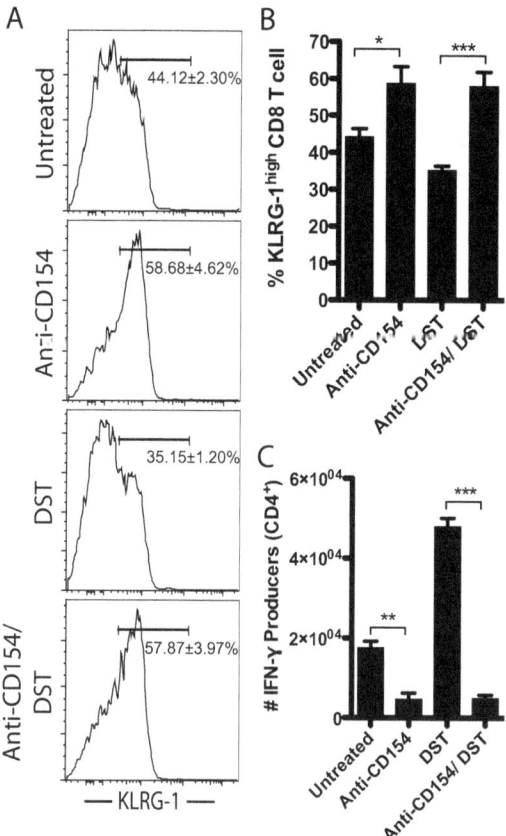

Figure 6. Anti-CD154 treatment increases the frequency of KLRG-1^{high} short-lived CD8$^+$ effectors. B6-Ly5.2/Cr mice were transplanted with BALB/c skin grafts and were treated with 10^7 BALB/c DST and/ or anti-CD154 mAb, where indicated. A. Flow plots of KLRG-1 expression on antigen experienced CD44^{high} CD62L^{low} CD8$^+$ T cells at day 7 post-transplantation. B. Frequency of KLRG-1^{high} antigen experienced CD44^{high} CD62L^{low} CD8$^+$ T cells on day 7. C. Absolute count of alloreactive CD4$^+$ T cells producing IFN-γ on day 7. Data are summary of two experiments with three mice per group. Values are mean ± SEM. *p<0.05, **p<0.01, ***p<0.001.

combined with the inhibitory signals associated with CD40/CD154 pathway blockade, produces a catastrophic exhaustive event for the cell, resulting in failure to mount and maintain an effective CD8$^+$ T cell response followed by prolonged protection of the graft.

In addition, we investigated the effects of CD40/CD154 pathway blockade on neutrophil recruitment in the graft, as other studies have previously demonstrated that depletion of PMNs alleviates cellular infiltration and prevents cardiac allograft rejection [25], and observed that CD154 costimulation blockade resulted in reduced intra-graft infiltration of neutrophils. The ability of CD154 blockade to impair innate immunity has also been observed in other systems. For example, in a murine model of arterial vessel injury, treatment with anti-CD154 monoclonal antibodies significantly impaired innate immune cell infiltration into the carotid arteries [26]. In an antigen non-specific model of ischemia and reperfusion injury in liver transplants, Shen *et al.* demonstrated that animals treated with anti-CD154 had reduced injury to livers compared to untreated or anti-IFN-γ treated animals [27]. Taken together, our data demonstrate that not only are CD8$^+$ T cell responses inhibited by CD154 blockade, but also innate immune cell trafficking into allografts may be dependent on CD40-CD154 interactions.

From these data, we conclude that anti-CD154 and DST work through distinct mechanisms to inhibit the expansion and differentiation of donor-reactive CD8$^+$ T cells and recruitment of innate immune cells, resulting in prolonged graft survival following transplantation. While the use of intact FcR-binding anti-CD154 is not a clinically applicable approach due to the concerns for thromboembolism, blockade of this pathway remains a uniquely effective method of inhibiting graft rejection in experimental models. Current work to translate this approach to a clinically viable strategy has included the development of anti-CD40 monoclonal antibodies and RNAi-based approaches to inhibit CD40 expression [28,29]. This RNAi approach could also be adapted for CD154 inhibition. Alternatively, non-cross-linking mAbs could be developed to antagonize CD154, similar to the development of nonactivating single chain F$_V$-based reagents as a substitute for cross-linking anti-CD28 mAbs [30].

Thus, as renewed interest in therapeutic blockade of the CD154/CD40 pathway gains momentum due to promising results using anti-CD40 monoclonal antibodies in translational models [31], understanding the cellular and molecular mechanisms by which blockade of the CD154/CD40 pathway functions to inhibit alloreactive T cell responses is critical to guide rational development of immunosuppressive regimens incorporating these therapeutics for use in transplantation.

Author Contributions

Conceived and designed the experiments: IRF MLF. Performed the experiments: IRF MEW MS. Analyzed the data: IRF MS MLF. Wrote the paper: IRF MLF.

References

1. Halloran PF (2004) Immunosuppressive drugs for kidney transplantation. N Engl J Med 351: 2715–2729.
2. Kirk AD, Harlan DM, Armstrong NN, Davis TA, Dong Y, et al. (1997) CTLA4-Ig and anti-CD40 ligand prevent renal allograft rejection in primates. Proc Natl Acad Sci U S A 94: 8789–8794.
3. Larsen CP, Elwood ET, Alexander DZ, Ritchie SC, Hendrix R, et al. (1996) Long-term acceptance of skin and cardiac allografts after blocking CD40 and CD28 pathways. Nature 381: 434–438.
4. Parker DC, Greiner DL, Phillips NE, Appel MC, Steele AW, et al. (1995) Survival of mouse pancreatic islet allografts in recipients treated with allogeneic small lymphocytes and antibody to CD40 ligand. Proc Natl Acad Sci U S A 92: 9560–9564.
5. Kawai T, Andrews D, Colvin RB, Sachs DH, Cosimi AB (2000) Thromboembolic complications after treatment with monoclonal antibody against CD40 ligand. Nat Med 6: 114.
6. Markees TG, Phillips NE, Gordon EJ, Noelle RJ, Shultz LD, et al. (1998) Long-term survival of skin allografts induced by donor splenocytes and anti-CD154 antibody in thymectomized mice requires CD4(+) T cells, interferon-gamma, and CTLA4. J Clin Invest 101: 2446–2455.

7. Zheng XX, Markees TG, Hancock WW, Li Y, Greiner DL, et al. (1999) CTLA4 signals are required to optimally induce allograft tolerance with combined donor-specific transfusion and anti-CD154 monoclonal antibody treatment. J Immunol 162: 4983–4990.
8. Phillips NE, Markees TG, Mordes JP, Greiner DL, Rossini AA (2003) Blockade of CD40-mediated signaling is sufficient for inducing islet but not skin transplantation tolerance. J Immunol 170: 3015–3023.
9. Hancock WW, Sayegh MH, Zheng XG, Peach R, Linsley PS, et al. (1996) Costimulatory function and expression of CD40 ligand, CD80, and CD86 in vascularized murine cardiac allograft rejection. Proc Natl Acad Sci U S A 93: 13967–13972.
10. Pearl JP, Xu H, Leopardi F, Preston E, Kirk AD (2007) CD154 blockade, sirolimus, and donor-specific transfusion prevents renal allograft rejection in cynomolgus monkeys despite homeostatic T-cell activation. Transplantation 83: 1219–1225.
11. Preston EH, Xu H, Dhanireddy KK, Pearl JP, Leopardi FV, et al. (2005) IDEC-131 (anti-CD154), sirolimus and donor-specific transfusion facilitate operational tolerance in non-human primates. Am J Transplant 5: 1032–1041.

12. Quezada SA, Fuller B, Jarvinen LZ, Gonzalez M, Blazar BR, et al. (2003) Mechanisms of donor-specific transfusion tolerance: preemptive induction of clonal T-cell exhaustion via indirect presentation. Blood 102: 1920–1926.

13. Margenthaler JA, Kataoka M, Flye MW (2003) Donor-specific antigen transfusion-mediated skin-graft tolerance results from the peripheral deletion of donor-reactive CD8+ T cells. Transplantation 75: 2119–2127.

14. van Maurik A, Fazekas de St Groth B, Wood KJ, Jones ND (2004) Dependency of direct pathway CD4+ T cells on CD40-CD154 costimulation is determined by nature and microenvironment of primary contact with alloantigen. J Immunol 172: 2163–2170.

15. Sarkar S, Kalia V, Haining WN, Konieczny BT, Subramaniam S, et al. (2008) Functional and genomic profiling of effector CD8 T cell subsets with distinct memory fates. J Exp Med 205: 625–640.

16. Joshi NS, Cui W, Chandele A, Lee HK, Urso DR, et al. (2007) Inflammation directs memory precursor and short-lived effector CD8(+) T cell fates via the graded expression of T-bet transcription factor. Immunity 27: 281–295.

17. Henn V, Slupsky JR, Grafe M, Anagnostopoulos I, Forster R, et al. (1998) CD40 ligand on activated platelets triggers an inflammatory reaction of endothelial cells. Nature 391: 591–594.

18. Kondo T, Novick AC, Toma H, Fairchild RL (1996) Induction of chemokine gene expression during allogeneic skin graft rejection. Transplantation 61: 1750–1757.

19. Rollins BJ (1997) Chemokines. Blood 90: 909–928.

20. Sun JC, Williams MA, Bevan MJ (2004) CD4+ T cells are required for the maintenance, not programming, of memory CD8+ T cells after acute infection. Nat Immunol 5: 927–933.

21. Sun JC, Bevan MJ (2003) Defective CD8 T cell memory following acute infection without CD4 T cell help. Science 300: 339–342.

22. Pearson T, Markees TG, Wicker LS, Serreze DV, Peterson LB, et al. (2003) NOD congenic mice genetically protected from autoimmune diabetes remain resistant to transplantation tolerance induction. Diabetes 52: 321–326.

23. Floyd TL, Koehn BH, Kitchens WH, Robertson JM, Cheeseman JA, et al. (2011) Limiting the amount and duration of antigen exposure during priming increases memory T cell requirement for costimulation during recall. J Immunol 186: 2033–2041.

24. Wherry EJ, Blattman JN, Murali-Krishna K, van der Most R, Ahmed R (2003) Viral persistence alters CD8 T-cell immunodominance and tissue distribution and results in distinct stages of functional impairment. J Virol 77: 4911–4927.

25. El-Sawy T, Belperio JA, Strieter RM, Remick DG, Fairchild RL (2005) Inhibition of polymorphonuclear leukocyte-mediated graft damage synergizes with short-term costimulatory blockade to prevent cardiac allograft rejection. Circulation 112: 320–331.

26. Li G, Sanders JM, Bevard MH, Sun Z, Chumley JW, et al. (2008) CD40 ligand promotes Mac-1 expression, leukocyte recruitment, and neointima formation after vascular injury. Am J Pathol 172: 1141–1152.

27. Shen X, Reng F, Gao F, Uchida Y, Busuttil RW, et al. (2010) Alloimmune activation enhances innate tissue inflammation/injury in a mouse model of liver ischemia/reperfusion injury. Am J Transplant 10: 1729–1737.

28. Pluvinet R, Petriz J, Torras J, Herrero-Fresneda I, Cruzado JM, et al. (2004) RNAi-mediated silencing of CD40 prevents leukocyte adhesion on CD154-activated endothelial cells. Blood 104: 3642–3646.

29. Ripoll E, Pluvinet R, Torras J, Olivar R, Vidal A, et al. (2011) In vivo therapeutic efficacy of intra-renal CD40 silencing in a model of humoral acute rejection. Gene Ther 18: 945–952.

30. Zhang T, Fresnay S, Welty E, Sangrampurkar N, Rybak E, et al. (2011) Selective CD28 blockade attenuates acute and chronic rejection of murine cardiac allografts in a CTLA-4-dependent manner. Am J Transplant 11: 1599–1609.

31. Badell IR, Thompson PW, Turner AP, Russell MC, Avila JG, et al. (2012) Nondepleting Anti-CD40-Based Therapy Prolongs Allograft Survival in Nonhuman Primates. Am J Transplant 12: 126–135.

5

Oligodendrocyte Precursor Cell Transplantation into Organotypic Cerebellar Shiverer Slices: A Model to Study Myelination and Myelin Maintenance

Jenea M. Bin, Soo Yuen Leong, Sarah-Jane Bull, Jack P. Antel, Timothy E. Kennedy*

Department of Neurology and Neurosurgery, Montreal Neurological Institute, McGill University, Montreal, Quebec, Canada

Abstract

Current *in vitro* models to investigate the consequence of oligodendrocyte-specific loss-of-function mutations on myelination are primarily limited to co-culture experiments, which do not accurately recapitulate the complex *in vivo* environment. Here, we describe the development of an *in vitro* model of myelination and myelin maintenance in which oligodendrocyte precursor cells are transplanted into organotypic cerebellar slice cultures derived from dysmyelinated shiverer mice. Compared to neuron-oligodendrocyte co-cultures, organotypic slices more closely mimic the environment *in vivo*, while utilizing a genetic background that allows for straight-forward identification of myelin generated by transplanted cells. We show at the ultrastructural level that the myelin generated by wild-type transplanted oligodendrocytes is compact and terminates in cytoplasmic loops that form paranodal junctions with the axon. This myelination results in the appropriate sequestering of axonal proteins into specialized domains surrounding the nodes of Ranvier. We also demonstrate the applicability of this approach for xenograft transplantation of oligodendrocyte precursor cells derived from rat or human sources. This method provides a time-efficient and cost-effective adjunct to conditional knockout mouse lines or *in vivo* transplantation models to study oligodendrocyte-specific loss-of-function mutations. Furthermore, the approach can be readily used to assess the effect of pharmacological manipulations on myelin, providing a tool to better understand myelination and develop effective therapeutic strategies to treat myelin-related diseases.

Editor: Martin Stangel, Hannover Medical School, Germany

Funding: This project was supported by operating grants from Multiple Sclerosis Society of Canada (http://mssociety.ca/en/research/default.htm). JMB is supported by a Vanier Canada Graduate Scholarship and SJB is supported by a Multiple Sclerosis Society of Canada Studentship. TEK is a Killam Foundation Scholar and holds a Chercheur National award from the Fonds de la Recherche en Santé du Québec. The funders had no role in study design, data collection and analysis, decision to publish, or preparation of the manuscript.

Competing Interests: The authors have declared that no competing interests exist.

* E-mail: timothy.kennedy@mcgill.ca

Introduction

Myelination of axons by oligodendrocytes is critical for achieving appropriate saltatory signal conduction in the central nervous system (CNS). Failure to properly myelinate during development, or remyelinate after injury, is characteristic of several myelin-related diseases including leukodystrophies and multiple sclerosis. Efforts to gain a better understanding of the complex process of myelination and to develop effective therapeutic treatments require the use of both *in vitro* and *in vivo* models. While techniques to study the development of oligodendrocyte precursor cells (OPCs) into mature oligodendrocytes have been well established *in vitro*, current models to study myelination *in vitro* pose several technical challenges and limitations that have restricted their utility.

Currently, two of the most commonly used *in vitro* methods to study CNS myelination are the organotypic slice culture and the neuron-glia co-culture systems (reviewed in [1]). Organotypic slice cultures, which can be grown either in a roller tube or on a semi-porous membrane, involve preparing slices of tissue from the postnatal brain [2]. Over a period of 2–4 weeks, endogenous OPCs within the slice mature and myelinate axons [3,4]. In the co-culture method, isolated OPCs are seeded onto purified

neuronal cultures, which the OPCs that successfully mature then proceed to myelinate. Several variations of myelinating co-cultures have been developed, which differ primarily in the type of neurons utilized [1]. Both of these systems have their advantages and limitations. For example, organotypic slice cultures maintain a microenvironment that more closely resembles the *in vivo* environment and achieve more robust myelination than the co-culture system. On the other hand, the co-culture system provides the flexibility to use oligodendrocytes and neurons from different genetic backgrounds, which can be useful to study cell-specific defects arising from loss- or gain-of-function mutations. Here, we describe the development of a new protocol that combines these advantages from both systems to study oligodendrocyte-specific defects in myelination and myelin maintenance *in vitro*.

Transplantation of OPCs into the shiverer mouse brain is a well established technique employed to study cell replacement and myelination *in vivo* (reviewed in [5]). The shiverer mouse genome contains a large deletion in the myelin basic protein (MBP) gene that results in the failure to produce all six classic protein isoforms of MBP, and consequently causes extensive CNS dysmyelination [6]. Thus, any myelin produced by wild-type OPCs transplanted into a shiverer CNS can be unambiguously identified by positive immunohistochemical staining for MBP. Using a similar principle *in vitro*, we show that allogenic OPCs transplanted into homozygous shiverer organotypic cerebellar slice cultures achieve robust myelination, and further show that this myelin results in the proper sequestering of axonal proteins into specialized domains that surround nodes of Ranvier. We have maintained such slices in culture for more than 64 days post-transplant, making this model useful for studying both myelination and myelin maintenance.

Materials and Methods

Ethics Statement

All procedures with animals were approved by the Montreal Neurological Institute Animal Care Committee (approval ID #4330) and performed in accordance with the Canadian Council on Animal Care guidelines for the use of animals in research. Studies using human fetal CNS tissue or human adult CNS tissue were approved by the Albert Einstein College of Medicine Institutional Review Board (approval ID #1993-042) and the Montreal Neurological Institute and Hospital Research Ethics Board (approval ID # ANTJ 1988/3). Informed written consent was received from all tissue donors.

Animals

Shiverer mice [6] were obtained from Dr. Alan Peterson (McGill University) and bred into a C57/Bl6 background. For the isolation of wild-type OPCs, newborn CD1 mouse pups and Sprague-Dawley rat pups were obtained from Charles River Canada (Montreal, Canada).

Preparation and culture of organotypic slices from shiverer mice

Organotypic cerebellar slice cultures were prepared from P0 shiverer pups as previously described [3,4]. Briefly 200 μm sagittal slices of cerebellum were sectioned using a McIlwain tissue chopper and transferred onto Millicell cell culture inserts (Millipore, MA, USA) in a 6-well plate containing 1 mL of serum-containing medium (SCM; 50% MEM with Earle's Salts, 25% heat inactivated horse serum, and 25% Earle's balanced salt solution supplemented with glutamax, penicillin-streptomycin, 6.5 mg/mL glucose, and fungizone). The media was changed every two days during the culture period. For all experiments, except where specified, beginning with the second media change the cultures were gradually switched to serum-free medium (SFM; 50% DMEM and 50% F12 supplemented with 1% B27, 0.5% N2, glutamax, penicillin-streptomycin, and fungizone) [7]. This was done by mixing 1/3 SFM with 2/3 SCM on day 4 *in vitro* and 2/3 SFM with 1/3 SCM of day 6 *in vitro*. From 8 days *in vitro* (DIV) onward, SFM was used.

Preparation of mouse glial cultures

Mixed glial cultures were prepared from P0 CD1 wild-type mouse pups as described [8]. In brief, cortices were dissected in ice cold MEM/HEPES and digested with papain (1.2 U/mL), L-cysteine (0.24 mg/mL) and DNAseI type IV (40 μg/mL). Dissociated cells were plated in PDL-coated T25 flasks (cortices from one pup/flask) with DMEM media supplemented with 10% FBS, penicillin-streptomycin, and glutamax. Media was changed on the fourth day, and every three days thereafter. Beginning with the second media change, 5 μg/mL of insulin was also added to the media to enhance the number of OPCs.

Preparation of rat glial cultures

Mixed glial cultures were prepared from P0 Sprague Dawley rat pups as described [9]. In brief, cortices were dissected in ice

cold HBSS and digested with tryspin-EDTA and DNAseI. Dissociated cells were plated in 10 PDL-coated T75 flasks with DMEM media supplemented with 10% FBS, penicillin-streptomycin, and glutamax. Media was changed every 2–3 days.

Isolation of mouse and rat oligodendrocyte precursor cells

OPCs were collected by shake-off and differential adhesion after 8–14 DIV as described [10]. Cultures were agitated on an orbital shaker for 1 hr at 150 rpm, 37°C to remove loosely adherent microglia. All of the media was replaced and flasks were then allowed to equilibrate in the tissue culture incubator for 1 hr. Flasks were then shaken for 14–16 hrs at 180 rpm to detach the OPCs. Detached cells were plated in uncoated petri dishes for 30 min, during which time the majority of contaminating microglia attached to the surface of the plate, while the OPCs remained floating in the medium. In some experiments, 10 μM of CMFDA cell-tracker dye (Invitrogen, ON, Canada) was added to the media during this incubation period to label the cells. Floating cells were then collected, pelleted and resuspended to a density of 20,000 cells/μL in oligodendrocyte defined medium (OLDEM; DMEM, 5 μg/mL insulin, 100 μg/mL transferrin, 30 nM sodium selenite, 30 nM triiodothyronine, 100 μg/mL penicillin-streptomycin, 2 mM glutamax) in preparation for transplantation. Fluorescent activated cell sorting identified >95% of isolated mouse OPCs to be PDGFαR+.

Isolation of human fetal and adult oligodendrocyte precursor cells

Human fetal CNS tissue was obtained from 15- to 16-week-old embryos provided by the Human Fetal Tissue Repository (Albert Einstein College of Medicine, NY, USA). Human adult CNS tissue was collected via surgical resection performed as treatment for non-tumour-related intractable epilepsy in accordance with guidelines from Biomedical Ethics Unit of McGill University. Tissues were dissociated with 0.25% trypsin and 25 μg/mL DNase I at 37°C for 30 min and then passed through a nylon mesh. Adult CNS cell suspension was subjected to an additional cell separation step using a linear 30% Percoll gradient (Pharmacia Biotech, NJ, USA) to remove myelin debris and red blood cells. Fetal cells were collected from pre-myelinating brain and hence did not required Percoll gradient separation. Total neural cells were cultured overnight (fetal cells) or for 48 hrs (adult cells) in DMEM/F12 media supplemented with N1 and BSA. Floating cells were harvested and labelled with PE-conjugated mouse anti-O4 (FAB1326P, R&D systems, MN, USA) and collected by fluorescence activated cell sorting.

Transplantation of OPCs into shiverer slices

Transplantations were performed into shiverer$^{-/-}$ slices that had been cultured 10–21 DIV. 20,000 cells were injected into each slice in two 0.5 μl injections using a broken glass-pulled pipette tip. Slices were cultured for 3–9 weeks before fixing for further analysis.

Immunohistochemistry

Slices were fixed in 4% paraformaldehyde (PFA) in PBS at pH 7.4 for 1 hr on ice (or for 15 min at room temperature for Na$^+$ channel or Kv1.2 immunostaining). Slices were blocked in 3% heat-inactivated horse serum, 2% bovine serum albumin (BSA), 0.25% triton X-100 for a minimum of 2 hrs. Primary antibody was prepared in 2% BSA, 0.25% triton X-100 PBS and incubated on the slices for 36–48 hrs, after which they were washed

1×10 min, 2×1 hr in PBS. Secondary antibody was prepared in 2% BSA PBS and incubated on the slices for 16–24 hrs. Slices were washed 1×10 min, 2×1 hr, 1 × overnight in PBS before mounting with Fluoromount G. Primary antibodies used included: rat anti-MBP (1:100; Millipore, MA, USA), chicken anti-MBP (1:1000; Aves Labs, OR, USA), mouse anti-caspr (1:50; Neuro-Mab, CA, USA), rabbit anti-caspr (1:1000; gift from Dr. David Coleman, Quebec, Canada), mouse anti-Na$^+$ channel (1:300; Sigma, MO, USA), rabbit anti-Kv1.2 (1:300; Alomone Labs, Jerusalem, Israel), chicken anti-NFM (1:1000; Aves Labs, OR, USA), and mouse anti-axonal neurofilaments (SMI-312; 1:500; Covance, NJ, USA). Secondary antibodies used included: Alexa 488 or 555 donkey anti-rabbit, alexa 488 donkey anti-rat, alexa 546 goat anti-chicken, alexa 488, 555, or 647 donkey anti-mouse (1:1000, Molecular Probes, OR, USA).

Electron Microscopy

Slices were fixed in 2.5% gluteraldehyde in 0.1 M sodium cacodylate buffer for a minimum of 24 hrs to a maximum of 2 weeks. Samples were then osmicated with potassium ferrocyanide-reduced 1% osmium tetraoxide solution for 1 hr, dehydrated with successive rinses of increasing concentrations of ethanol, then infiltrated and embedded in Epon. 70–100 nm sections were mounted onto 200 mesh copper grids and stained with 4% uranyl acetate for 5 min followed by Reynold's lead citrate for 3 min. The sections were examined using a FEI Technai 12 transmission electron microscope at 120 kV and images collected using a Gatan Ultrascan 4k×4k digital (CCD) camera system.

Results

Optimization of the transplant protocol

In order to generate an *in vitro* model of myelination with the capacity to use neurons and oligodendrocytes from different genetic backgrounds, while maintaining an environment that closely resembles that *in vivo*, we transplanted isolated mouse OPCs into organotypic cerebellar slices generated from shiverer mutant mice. Homozygous shiverer mutant mice do not express MBP. As

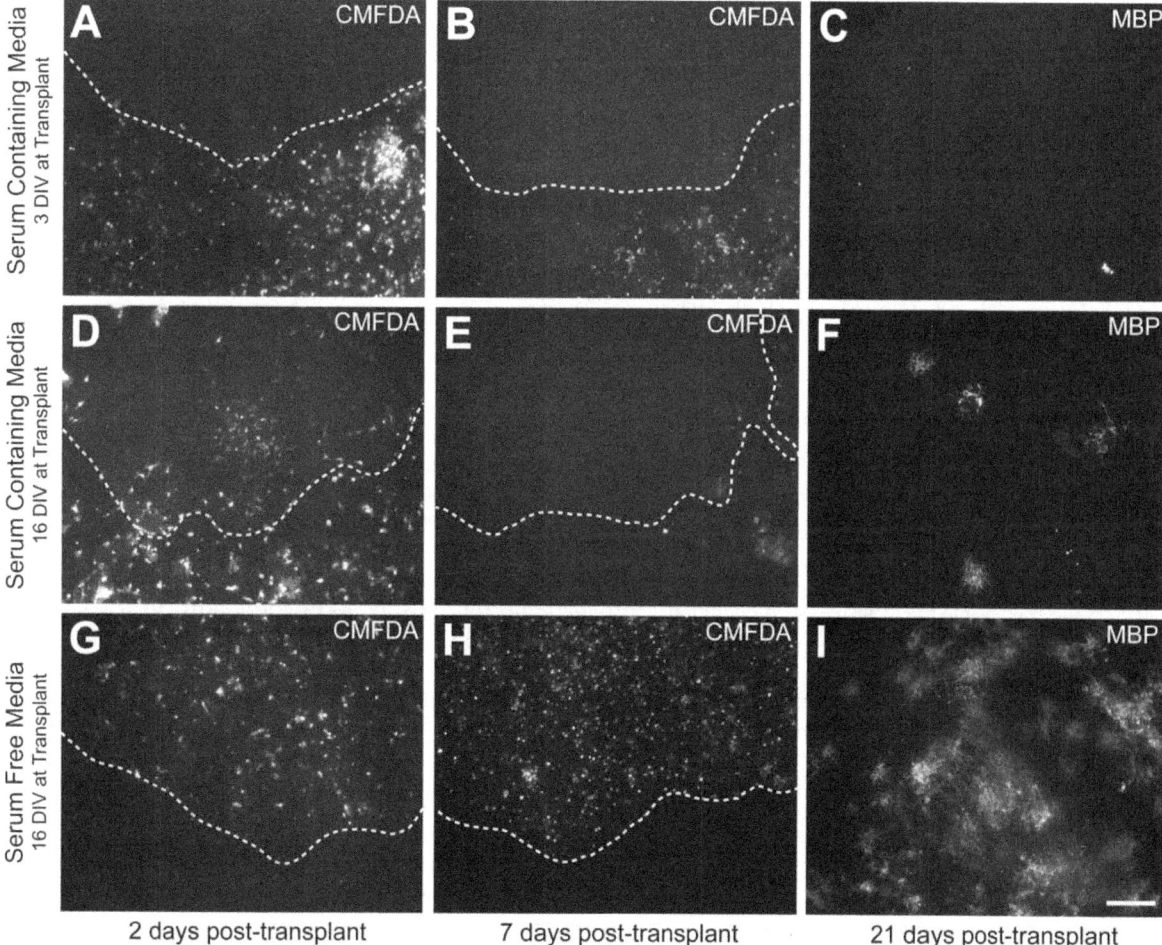

Figure 1. Increased myelination efficiency by transplanted OPCs in older slices and serum-free media. Representative images comparing transplantation of CMFDA-labelled OPCs into 3 DIV organotypic slices cultured in serum-containing media (A–C), 16 DIV organotypic cerebellar slices cultured in serum-containing media (D–F), and 16 DIV organotypic cerebellar slices cultured in serum-free media (G–I). In both of the serum-containing media conditions, substantial migration of the labelled OPCs out of the slices onto the surrounding membrane could be observed by two days post-transplant (A,D). More cells remained in the slices transplanted at 16 DIV (D), compared to the slices transplanted at 3 DIV (A); however, by 7 days post-transplant few of these labelled cells remained (B,E). In contrast, when transplanting into slices cultured in serum-free media, the majority of cells remained within the slices at both 2 and 7 days post-transplant (G,H). After 3 weeks, substantially more MBP-positive myelin was present in the serum-free media condition (I), compared to both serum-containing media conditions (C,F). The dashed line shows the boundary between the slice (above) and the culture membrane (below). Scale bar = 200 μm.

a result, oligodendrocytes mature and sometimes ensheath axons, but are unable to form compact myelin [6]. This provides an ideal background to quickly and unambiguously identify myelin generated by transplanted cells using immunohistochemical staining for MBP. In addition, any compact myelin with major dense lines detected by electron microscopy can be concluded to have been generated by transplanted oligodendrocytes.

In initial studies, we transplanted wild-type OPCs into organotypic cerebellar slices prepared from P0 shiverer mice that were cultured for 2–5 DIV in standard organotypic slice culture media, which typically contains 25% serum. However, at 21 days post-transplant, we found few, if any, MBP-positive myelinating oligodendrocytes in the cultures, suggesting that the OPCs had either failed to be incorporated into the slice, failed to survive, or failed to mature into oligodendrocytes. Using a fluorescent cell-tracker dye to follow the fate of the transplanted cells, two factors were found to play a critical role in the efficiency of myelination: (1) the age of the slice at transplantation and (2) the composition of the media.

Unsuccessful incorporation of OPCs into the slice was identified to be the principle cause for the failure of these cells to myelinate. While at twelve hours post-transplant, labelled OPCs were dispersed throughout the slice, when examined two days post-transplant, virtually all labelled cells had migrated out of the slice onto the surrounding membrane (Figure 1A–C). Transplanting into slices that had been cultured for a longer period of time *in vitro* increased the number of cells that remained within the slice, as well as the amount of myelination; however, the majority of cells still migrated out of the slices (Figure 1D–F).

Replacing the standard serum-containing media (SCM) with a serum-free defined media (SFM) (see Material and Methods for detailed description of media) was crucial to prevent OPC migration out of the slice, and resulted in a robust increase in the amount of myelination by the transplanted cells. At two days post-transplant, while the majority of OPCs had migrated out of the slice in the SCM condition (Figure 1D), in the SFM condition, transplanted OPCs remained distributed throughout the slice (Figure 1G). By seven days post-transplant, a large number of transplanted cells were still readily observed in the SFM condition, whereas in the SCM condition few labelled cells remained (Figure 1E,H). Immunostaining fixed slices for MBP-positive myelin three weeks post-transplant revealed a greater amount of myelin generated by the transplanted cells in the SFM condition compared to the SCM condition (Figure 1F,G). We concluded that SFM was more conducive to OPC incorporation into the slice, and consequently, all subsequent experiments were conducted using slices cultured in SFM, as outlined in Figure 2.

Robust production of compact myelin by transplanted OPCs

Initial ensheathment of axons by MBP-positive myelin membrane could be observed in transplanted slices at two days post-transplant. By two to three weeks post-transplant, the majority of MBP-positive cells within slices exhibited the morphology of mature myelinating oligodendrocytes, based on the presence of multiple tubular shaped MBP-positive segments that surrounded axons and on the absence of superfluous non-myelinating MBP-positive processes (Figure 3A,B). The presence of compact myelin in the transplanted slices was confirmed by electron microscopy at both five and nine weeks post-transplant (Figure 3C,D). In agreement with previous studies, no compact myelin was found in the untransplanted shiverer organotypic slices [6,11]. Paranodes also formed properly, with compact myelin terminating in cytoplasmic loops in close contact with both the

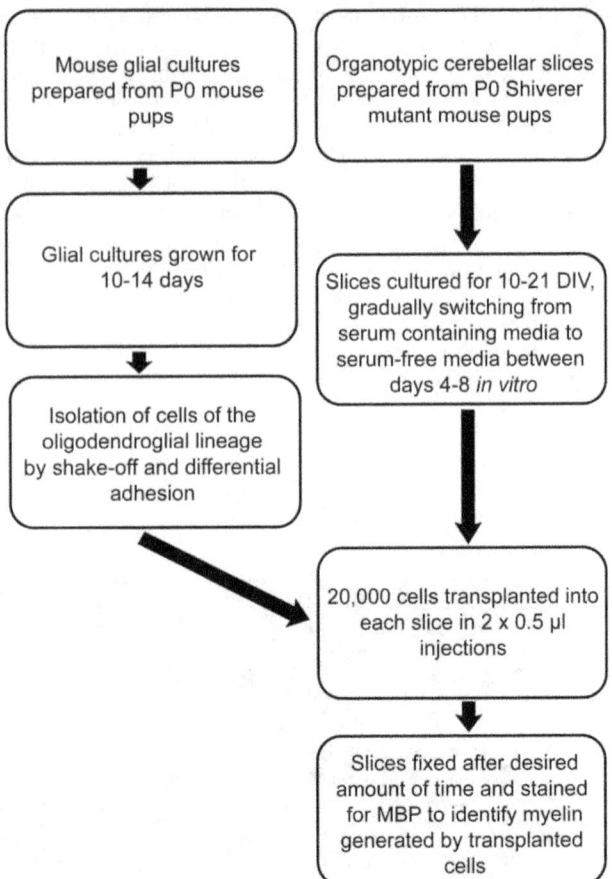

Figure 2. Overview of the OPC – organotypic cerebellar slice culture transplant protocol.

axon and with neighbouring glial loops (Figure 3E). Transverse bands, which are specialized contacts that link paranodal loops to the axon, were also readily detected (Figure 3F).

Formation of specialized domains along axons myelinated by transplanted oligodendrocytes

Myelination results in the formation of specialized domains along the axon: nodes of Ranvier, paranodes, juxtaparanodes, and internodes [12]. Using immunohistochemical staining and confocal microscopy, we determined that myelin formed by the transplanted oligodendrocytes resulted in the appropriate sequestering of sodium channels at the node of Ranvier, caspr at the paranode, and Kv1.2 channels at the juxtaparanode (Figure 4A,B). Sodium channel sequestering was readily observed by four days post-transplant, while caspr channel sequestering appeared complete by approximately ten days post-transplant. Maintenance of these molecular domains was observed for at least 64 days post-transplant. This axonal domain specialization, taken together with the correct paranodal ultrastructure, makes this a useful model for examining the specific contribution of oligodendrocytes to the formation and maintenance of paranodes and the neighbouring domains found along axons.

Xenotransplantation of OPCs derived from rat and human brain

In some experimental paradigms it may be of interest to transplant OPCs generated from species other than mouse. For

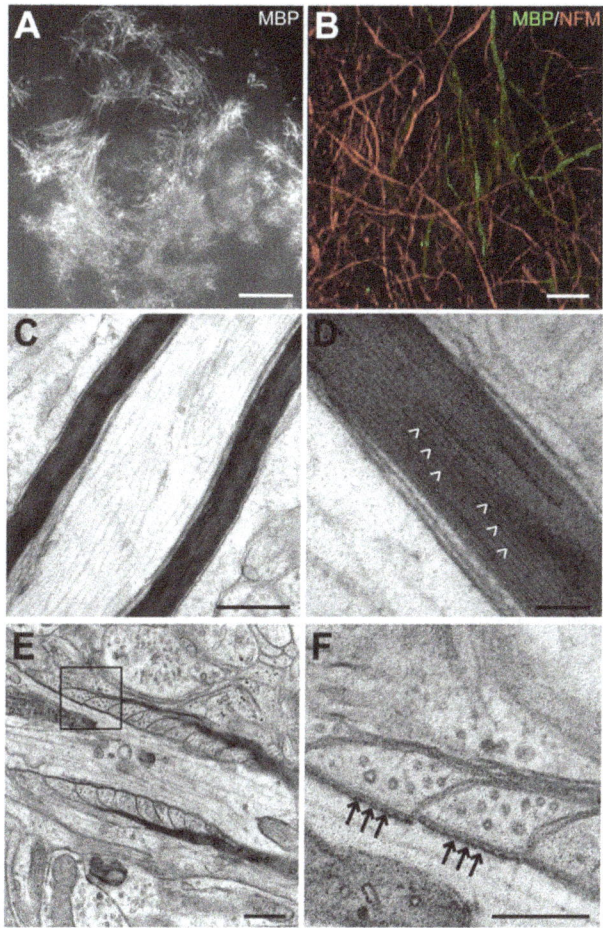

Figure 3. Myelin formed by the transplanted cells is compact and has appropriate paranode ultrastructure. (A) Low magnification epifluorescent and (B) high magnification confocal images showing that at three weeks post-transplant, the majority of MBP-positive oligodendrocytes exhibited the morphology of mature myelinating oligodendrocytes based on the presence of tubular shaped MBP-positive segments that surrounded NFM-labeled axons. (C,D) Electron microscopy of shiverer mutant organotypic slices transplanted with wild-type mouse OPCs showing that myelin formed by the transplanted OPCs is compact. This myelin contains major dense lines (D; white arrowheads), which differentiates it from membrane ensheathments made by shiverer oligodendrocytes. (E) Paranodes of myelin formed by transplanted cells appear ultrastructurally normal by electron microscopy. (F) Magnification of boxed area in E, displaying that transverse bands (black arrows) are present and regularly spaced. Scale bars: A = 100 μm; B = 20 μm; C = 500 nm; D = 100 nm; E = 500 nm; F = 250 nm.

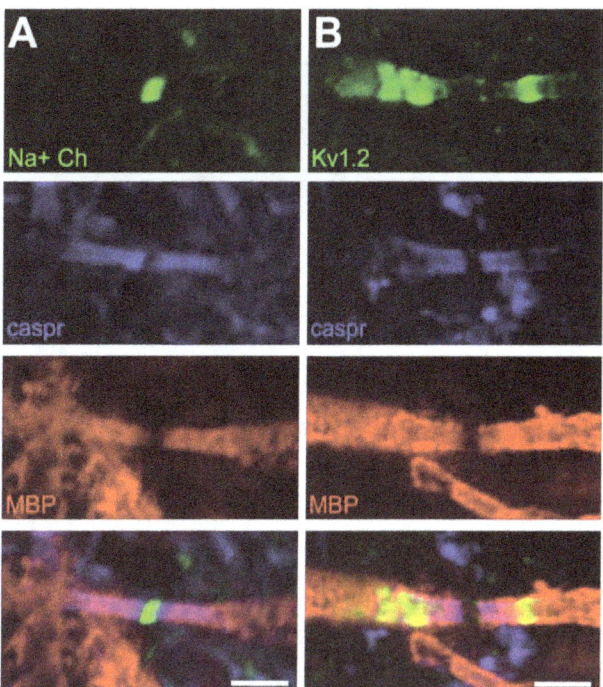

Figure 4. Axons myelinated by transplanted OPCs display appropriate specialized domain structure around nodes of Ranvier. (A) Sodium channels sequestered at the node. (B) Kv1.2 channels sequestered at the juxtaparanode. (A,B) Caspr sequestered at the paranode. Flanking MBP staining indicates myelin is generated by transplanted OPCs. Scale bar = 3 μm.

example, when the use of transgenic mice is not necessary, it may be advantageous to use wild-type rat OPCs, which, when compared with mouse OPCs, can be obtained in higher numbers per litter (approximately 5x more in our experience) and cultured more readily *in vitro*. Transplantation of OPCs obtained from newborn rat pups into shiverer organotypic cerebellar slices resulted in robust myelination and appropriate sequestering of proteins surrounding the nodes of Ranvier (Figure 5A,C,D). In all experimental trials, rat OPCs generated more MBP-positive myelin (71% compared to control) than mouse OPCs (22% compared to control), with some transplanted slices displaying amounts of myelination that resembled what was typical for untransplanted wild-type control slices (Figure 5B). Thus, our

findings indicate that rat OPCs can be substituted for mouse OPCs in this protocol.

We also assessed whether human oligodendrocyte lineage cells could be utilized in this *in vitro* model of myelination. Transplantation of either human fetal or adult-derived O4-positive oligodendrocyte lineage cells resulted in the successful generation of myelin internodes in the shiverer organotypic cerebellar slices (Figure 6), but this myelination was limited in comparison to that obtained with mouse OPCs. Further optimization of the protocol with these cell types may increase the efficiency of myelination. However, the limited amount of myelin generated may be useful for testing the capacity of compounds to promote myelination by transplanted human oligodendrocyte progenitors.

Discussion

Our findings demonstrate that OPCs transplanted into organotypic cerebellar slices derived from homozygous shiverer mutant mice generate MBP-positive compact myelin that can be readily distinguished from the MBP-negative membrane ensheathments produced by the shiverer oligodendrocytes. The compact myelin and flanking paranodal domains appear ultrastructurally normal by electron microscopy, although some axons were surrounded by fewer wraps of compact myelin than expected for their given diameter, reminiscent of myelin formed during remyelination [13]. The myelin formed by the transplanted oligodendrocytes resulted in the sequestering of Kv1.2 channels, caspr, and sodium channels into distinct domains at the juxtaparanode, paranode, and node, which were maintained for more than 64 days post-transplant. Taken together, we conclude that this transplant model is applicable to study both myelination

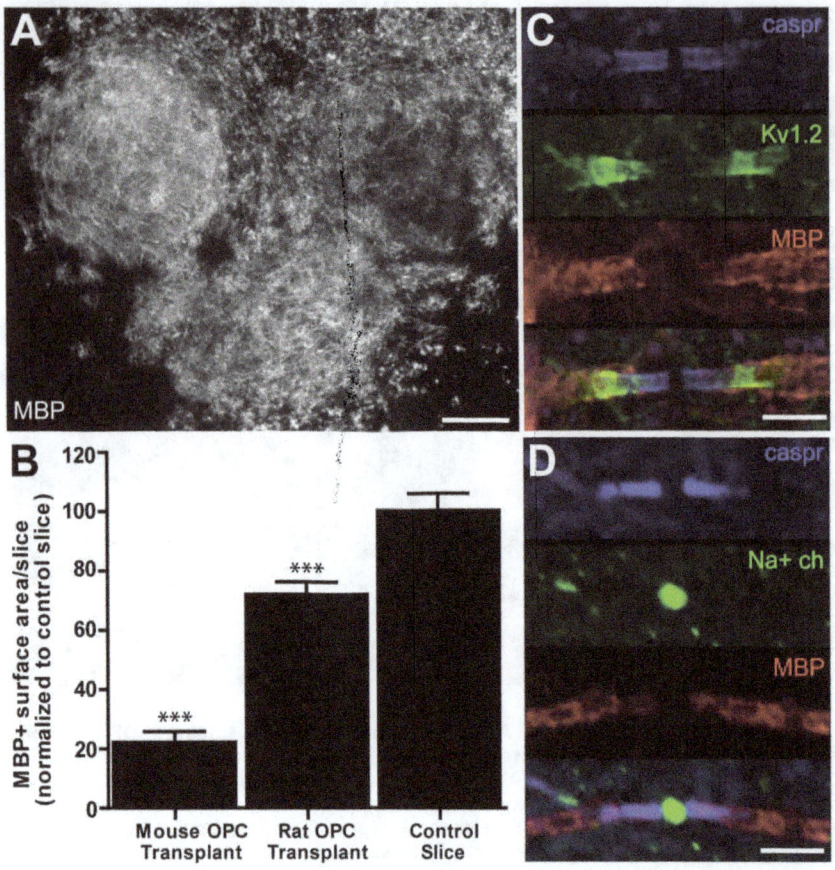

Figure 5. Rat OPCs myelinate shiverer organotypic cerebellar slices with high efficiency. (A) Extensive myelination throughout a shiverer organotypic slice by transplanted rat OPCs. (B) Quantification of MBP-positive surface area in shiverer organotypic slices transplanted with wild-type mouse OPCs and with wild-type rat OPCs, compared to myelinated control organotypic slices. (C) Sequestering of Kv1.2 at juxtaparanode and caspr at paranode of axons myelinated by rat OPCs. (D) Sequestering of sodium channels at the node and caspr at the paranode of axons myelinated by rat OPCs. Scale bars: A = 400 μm; C & D = 3 μm. *** p<0.0001 one-way ANOVA with Tukey's post-hoc test.

and myelin maintenance *in vitro*, providing a time- and cost-effective adjunct to *in vivo* approaches.

A key factor in achieving robust myelination by the transplanted cells was the composition of the organotypic slice culture media. We observed that the commonly used slice culture media containing 25% serum is not optimal for incorporation of transplanted OPCs into the slice. Instead, we utilized a serum-free defined medium, which resulted in a robust increase in the amount of myelination observed. In addition, while the age of the slice at transplant was a flexible variable in this protocol (we transplanted into slices that had been in culture up to 30 days with success), we noted that transplanting into slices that had matured for less than 8 DIV resulted in considerably reduced levels of myelination by the exogenous OPCs. This time point corresponds with when the majority of cell death associated with preparing the slices is complete, suggesting that a stabilized slice environment is beneficial for OPC incorporation into the slice. We also found that mouse OPCs isolated from mixed glial cultures after 8–10 DIV more robustly myelinated the shiverer organotypic slices than mouse OPCs isolated after 12–14 DIV, consistent with younger, less differentiated OPCs, having a greater capacity to myelinate.

Previous studies have reported similar experimental paradigms to myelinate shiverer organotypic slices *in vitro*. Billings-Gagliardi and colleagues [14] showed that organotypic shiverer cerebellar slices injected with explants of wild-type optic nerve exhibited axons surrounded by apparently normal myelin. Additionally,

transplantation of rodent and human embryonic stem-cell derived O4-positive oligodendrocyte progenitors into the hippocampus of whole brain organotypic shiverer slices has been used to determine how different pre-treatments of the transplanted cells enhanced myelination [7,15]. However, in these two studies, the baseline amount of myelination present without treatment was very low in comparison to what we report here, which could be explained by differences both in the source of transplanted OPCs and in the tissue area into which the OPCs were transplanted. Furthermore, while one study did confirm the presence of compact myelin by electron microscopy [15], neither addressed the formation of paranodal junctions or the specialized axonal domains that surround the node of Ranvier.

As a proof of principle we have transplanted wild-type OPCs. However, this model is well-suited to study how mutations or genetic modifications carried specifically by the transplanted oligodendrocytes influence the formation and maintenance of myelin. This will be of utility in scenarios where conventional, but not conditional, knock-out mice are available for study, particularly for mutations that are lethal before myelination is normally well established *in vivo*. While using immunohistochemistry for MBP is an extremely useful tool to identify and study myelin generated by transplanted oligodendrocytes, it is also a potential limitation. MBP is not a practical marker for counting the number of myelinating oligodendrocytes. Traditional markers to label and count oligodendrocyte cells bodies, such as CC1 or olig2, will not

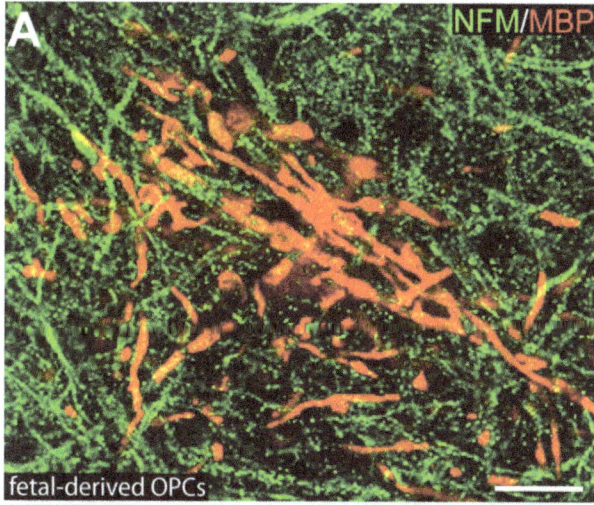

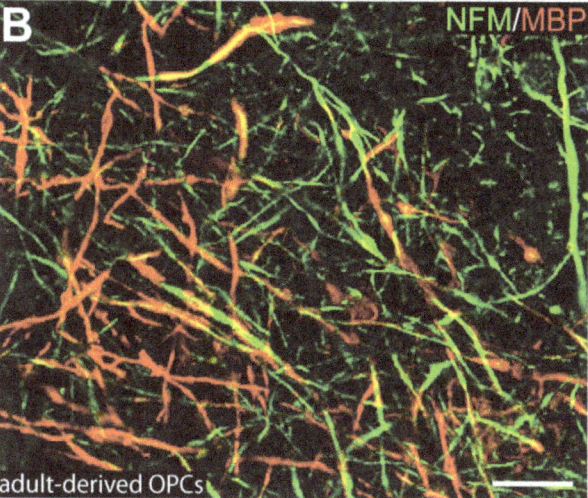

Figure 6. Human-derived OPCs can myelinate shiverer organotypic cerebellar slices. (A) Myelin generated by human fetal-derived O4+ oligodendrocyte lineage cells. (B) Myelin generated by human adult-derived O4+ oligodendrocyte lineage cells. Scale bars: 20 μm.

distinguish between endogenous shiverer oligodendrocytes and the exogenous transplanted oligodendrocytes. In addition, since MBP

expression begins during terminal differentiation of oligodendrocytes [16], this limits observations to after this time point. To examine effects on pre-myelinating oligodendrocytes prior to terminal differentiation, OPCs would need an alternative method to be identified, such as genetic modification to express green fluorescent protein.

In addition to studying genetic mutations, this model could also be used to investigate the effect of pharmacological manipulations on myelination. *In vitro* models of myelination are of particular interest for drug studies targeting autoimmune CNS demyelinating diseases, such as multiple sclerosis, as the absence of the peripheral immune system allows for an assessment of the direct effect of therapies on CNS myelination, which may be confounded using *in vivo* models. Furthermore, the method provides the opportunity to compare and translate findings from rodents to humans using xenotransplantation of oligodendrocyte lineage cells. Transplantation into shiverer slices could be advantageous over testing drugs on regular organotypic slices since transplantation adds the ability to temporally control the onset of the myelination being quantified. In wild-type organotypic slices, endogenous oligodendrocytes express MBP by 3 DIV with myelination following shortly after [3]. During this initial time in culture, the slices undergo a period of cell death and reorganization [4], which could be affected by the addition of a drug and make the effect on myelination more difficult to interpret. This can be avoided by transplanting and treating the slices after they have stabilized in culture. Quantitative measures to screen for agents that promote or inhibit myelination can be readily carried out, for example, by assessing the co-localization of MBP and neurofilament heavy chain using immunohistochemistry [1,17], complemented by using electron microscopy to verify compact myelin ultrastructure. We anticipate that this model will be beneficial to advance our understanding of the mechanisms that underlie myelin formation and maintenance, with the ultimate goal of promoting remyelination in demyelinating diseases.

Acknowledgments

We thank Katherine Horn and Karen Lai Wing Sun for assistance in performing the transplant procedures.

Author Contributions

Conceived and designed the experiments: JMB SYL JPA TEK. Performed the experiments: JMB SYL SJB. Analyzed the data: JMB SYL. Contributed reagents/materials/analysis tools: JPA TEK. Wrote the paper: JMB TEK.

References

1. Jarjour AA, Zhang H, Bauer N, Ffrench-Constant C, Williams A (2012) In vitro modeling of central nervous system myelination and remyelination. Glia 60: 1–12.
2. Gahwiler BH, Capogna M, Debanne D, McKinney RA, Thompson SM (1997) Organotypic slice cultures: a technique has come of age. Trends in neurosciences 20: 471–477.
3. Jarjour AA, Bull SJ, Almasieh M, Rajasekharan S, Baker KA, et al. (2008) Maintenance of axo-oligodendroglial paranodal junctions requires DCC and netrin-1. The Journal of neuroscience : the official journal of the Society for Neuroscience 28: 11003–11014.
4. Notterpek LM, Bullock PN, Malek-Hedayat S, Fisher R, Rome LH (1993) Myelination in cerebellar slice cultures: development of a system amenable to biochemical analysis. Journal of neuroscience research 36: 621–634.
5. Duncan ID, Kondo Y, Zhang SC (2011) The myelin mutants as models to study myelin repair in the leukodystrophies. Neurotherapeutics : the journal of the American Society for Experimental NeuroTherapeutics 8: 607–624.
6. Readhead C, Hood L (1990) The dysmyelinating mouse mutations shiverer (shi) and myelin deficient (shimld). Behavior genetics 20: 213–234.
7. Zhang PL, Izrael M, Ainbinder E, Ben-Simchon L, Chebath J, et al. (2006) Increased myelinating capacity of embryonic stem cell derived oligodendrocyte precursors after treatment by interleukin-6/soluble interleukin-6 receptor fusion protein. Molecular and cellular neurosciences 31: 387–398.
8. O'Meara RW, Ryan SD, Colognato H, Kothary R (2011) Derivation of enriched oligodendrocyte cultures and oligodendrocyte/neuron myelinating co-cultures from post-natal murine tissues. Journal of visualized experiments : JoVE.
9. Chen Y, Balasubramaniyan V, Peng J, Hurlock EC, Tallquist M, et al. (2007) Isolation and culture of rat and mouse oligodendrocyte precursor cells. Nature protocols 2: 1044–1051.
10. Armstrong RC (1998) Isolation and characterization of immature oligodendrocyte lineage cells. Methods 16: 282–292.
11. Windrem MS, Nunes MC, Rashbaum WK, Schwartz TH, Goodman RA, et al. (2004) Fetal and adult human oligodendrocyte progenitor cell isolates myelinate the congenitally dysmyelinated brain. Nature medicine 10: 93–97.
12. Poliak S, Peles E (2003) The local differentiation of myelinated axons at nodes of Ranvier. Nature reviews Neuroscience 4: 968–980.
13. Blakemore WF (1974) Pattern of remyelination in the CNS. Nature 249: 577–578.

6

Natural Killer Cell Mediated Missing-Self Recognition can Protect Mice from Primary Chronic Myeloid Leukemia *In Vivo*

Mika Kijima¤, Noémie Gardiol, Werner Held*

Ludwig Center for Cancer Research of the University of Lausanne, Epalinges, Switzerland

Abstract

Background: Natural Killer (NK) cells are thought to protect from residual leukemic cells in patients receiving stem cell transplantation. However, multiple retrospective analyses of patient data have yielded conflicting conclusions regarding a putative role of NK cells and the essential NK cell recognition events mediating a protective effect against leukemia. Further, a NK cell mediated protective effect against primary leukemia *in vivo* has not been shown directly.

Methodology/Principal Findings: Here we addressed whether NK cells have the potential to control chronic myeloid leukemia (CML) arising based on the transplantation of BCR-ABL1 oncogene expressing primary bone marrow precursor cells into lethally irradiated recipient mice. These analyses identified missing-self recognition as the only NK cell-mediated recognition strategy, which is able to significantly protect from the development of CML disease *in vivo*.

Conclusion: Our data provide a proof of principle that NK cells can control primary leukemic cells *in vivo*. Since the presence of NK cells reduced the abundance of leukemia propagating cancer stem cells, the data raise the possibility that NK cell recognition has the potential to cure CML, which may be difficult using small molecule BCR-ABL1 inhibitors. Finally, our findings validate approaches to treat leukemia using antibody-based blockade of self-specific inhibitory MHC class I receptors.

Editor: Clive M. Gray, University of Cape Town, South Africa

Funding: This work was supported in part by a grant from the Swiss Cancer League to W.H. The funders had no role in study design, data collection and analysis, decision to publish, or preparation of the manuscript. No additional external funding received for this study.

Competing Interests: The authors have declared that no competing interests exist.

* E-mail: Werner.Held@unil.ch

¤ Current address: Max Planck Institute of Immunobiology and Epigenetics, Freiburg, Germany

Introduction

Chronic myeloid leukemia (CML) is a myeloproliferative disorder characterized by a reciprocal translocation between chromosome 9 and 22, the so-called Philadelphia (Ph) chromosome. This translocation juxtaposes the genes encoding the ABL1 tyrosine kinase and BCR (Breakpoint cluster region), resulting in a BCR-ABL1 fusion protein with constitutive tyrosine kinase activity. This activity is critically involved in the initial chronic phase of CML disease and the subsequent disease progression. Indeed, the BCR-ABL1 inhibitor imatinib has become the standard therapy in newly diagnosed CML patients. Based on multiple clinical studies, a majority of patients (52–69%) achieve a complete cytogenic response (i.e. no Ph+ metaphases in 20/20 cells) but only a minority of patients (12–40%) achieve a major molecular response (i.e. a 3-log reduction in BCR-ABL1 mRNA) by 12 months of treatment [1]. Nilotinib and desatinib are second-generation inhibitors that exhibit considerably higher activity against BCR-ABL1 and that show further increased response rates [1]. Despite the impressive ability to control disease, there are CML patients that do not respond to BCR-ABL1 inhibitors or in which the disease progresses, some times based on mutations in

BCR-ABL1. Finally, recurrence has been observed in a significant fraction of patients when BCR-ABL1 inhibitor treatment is discontinued [2], suggesting that leukemia initiating cells may persist and be refractory to inhibitor treatment. Thus additional treatment options, which are able to target leukemia-propagating cells, are needed to treat certain CML patients.

Haematopoietic stem cell transplantation has the potential to cure CML [3]. This is in part due to immune cells present in the graft and/or developing from grafted stem cells, which mediate a graft versus leukemia (GvL) effect to eliminate residual leukemic cells. Unrelated HLA-matched and partially HLA-mismatched transplants may contain T cells, which recognize minor histocompatibility antigens or HLA molecules on residual leukemic cells, respectively. However, such T cell recognition bears the significant risk of graft versus host disease (GvHD), a life threatening complication of (partially) HLA mismatched stem cell transplantation, in which donor-derived T cells attack non-haematopoietic, healthy tissues of the recipient. A partial HLA mismatch can also be recognized by NK cells and it has been suggested that alloreactive NK cells can prevent leukemia relapse following stem cell transplantation [4]. In contrast to T cells, NK cells do not seem to cause GvHD [5,6].

NK cells can react to allogeneic cells based on various recognition events. First some NK cells can be activated using receptors, which are specific for allogeneic MHC-I [7,8]. In addition, many NK cells express inhibitory receptors specific for MHC-I [9,10]. MHC-I receptors counteract NK cell activation by receptors specific for ligands that are constitutively expressed on healthy host cells. This dual receptor system allows the killing of diseased host cells, which display aberrantly low levels of MHC-I molecules (missing-self recognition) [11]. Since inhibitory MHC-I receptors (KIR (Killer Immunoglobulin-like Receptors) in human and Ly49 family receptors in mice) do not recognize all MHC-I alleles, the dual receptor system can confer reactivity to allogeneic cells that express the wrong MHC-I (KIR ligand mismatch). NK cell alloreactivity is further dependent on NK cell education [12] i.e. activation receptors on NK cells, which express a KIR/Ly49 specific for self-MHC-I respond more efficiently to stimulation [13,14,15,16]. Consequently, NK cell alloreactivity depends on the expression of a KIR/Ly49 and its MHC-I ligand in the donor (for education) and the absence of MHC-I ligand in the recipient (for the relieve from inhibition). Conversely, the activation receptors on NK cells that do not express a KIR/Ly49 specific for self-MHC-I respond poorly stimulation [13,14,15,16]. However, the function of these activation receptors can improve when these uneducated NK cells are exposed to inflammatory cytokines [14,17]. Consequently, it is possible that uneducated NK cells acquire reactivity due to the peculiar inflammatory environment during stem cell transplantation [18]. In addition to NK cell alloreactivity, there is evidence that the upregulation of stress induced self ligands, such as those engaging the NKG2D activation receptor [19], represents an important NK cell recognition strategy for transformed cells [20]. The importance of this pathway in the context of GvL is not known.

A role of NK cells to protect from leukemia has been inferred from the retrospective analysis of data from patients receiving unrelated HLA matched or partially HLA mismatched hematopoietic stem cell transplantation. A reduced relapse and improved disease free survival of leukemia patients receiving partially mismatched transplants has been attributed to NK cell alloreactivity mediated by the absence of KIR ligand in the recipient (KIR-ligand mismatch i.e. missing-self recognition) [4]. However, certain studies have either found no beneficial effect of KIR ligand mismatch or reported even worse outcomes following partially HLA mismatched stem cell transplantation [21,22]. Moreover, other studies have proposed protective roles for NK cell recognition of allogenic HLA using activating KIR [23,24] or they suggested a role for uneducated NK cells [25,26,27] (for review see [28,29]). Some of these discrepancies may be due to distinct conditioning regimens, differences in the preparation, the source and the dose of the transplanted stem cells and/or the fact that the cohorts included patients with distinct hematological malignancies that are based on different primary genetic lesions.

Despite some of the above correlations, it has not been shown directly that NK cells control primary leukemic cells arising in vivo and, if so, it is not clear which NK cell recognition strategy would be most effective against leukemic cells. Finally it is not known whether NK cells can target leukemia initiating stem cells and thus whether NK cells have the potential to contribute to curing leukemia.

Here we have addressed whether NK cells do have the potential to control primary CML in vivo. To this end, we used a well-established mouse model, in which bone marrow (BM) precursor cells are transduced with the BCR-ABL1 oncogene. Infected BM cells are transplanted into lethally irradiated recipient mice, which develop a fatal CML disease [30,31]. This disease model was combined with the classical model of BM graft rejection mediated by host NK cells [32], which allowed us to determine whether there was a difference in the efficacy of NK cells against normal and leukemic cells. Our analyses reveal that NK cell-mediated missing-self recognition, but none of the other NK cell recognition strategies, significantly impacts the outgrowth of CML cells in vivo. The NK cell mediated effect is based at least in part on the targeting of leukemia initiating stem cells, which suggests that NK cell recognition may contribute to cure CML disease.

Results

Lack of NK cell recognition of MHC-I matched BCR-ABL1+ myeloid cells in vivo

To determine whether NK cells can protect against primary BCR-ABL1+ cells in vivo, BM progenitor cells were infected with a retrovirus encoding the BCR-ABL1 (p210) oncogene plus green fluorescent protein (GFP) or with a control retrovirus expressing only GFP. Transduced BM precursor cells (usually around 10% GFP+) were transplanted into lethally irradiated recipient mice. Polymorphisms in the CD45 molecule were utilized to discriminate hematopoietic cells of donor (CD45.1) and recipient (CD45.2) origin.

To address whether NK cells protect against MHC-I matched BCR-ABL1+ cells, we estimated the abundance of GFP+ myeloid cells (CD11b+) in recipient spleens 8 days (d8) after transplantation (**Fig. 1**). B6 (H-2^b)-derived BM precursors transduced with the control virus yielded low numbers of GFP+ myeloid cells in spleens of MHC-I matched B6 recipients (H-2^b) (10^5 cells/spleen) (**Fig. 1A, B**). Transduction with the BCR-ABL1 virus resulted in significantly elevated numbers of GFP+ CD11b+ cells (5×10^6 cells) (**Fig. 1A, B**), confirming that BCR-ABL1 expression induces an expansion of myeloid cells. The depletion of NK1.1+ cells prior to BM transplantation did not impact the abundance of BCR-ABL1 expressing CD11b+ cells (**Fig. 1B**), indicating that NK cells do not react to MHC-I-matched BCR-ABL1 transformed cells.

NK cell mediated missing-self recognition reduces the expansion of BCR-ABL1+ myeloid cells

We next addressed whether a partial MHC-I mismatch, which results in NK cell mediated missing-self recognition, impacts the expansion of BCR-ABL1 expressing cells. Control infected B6 BM precursors yield myeloid cells in B6 hosts (10^5 cells) (**Fig. 1B**) but not in B6 hosts expressing a H-$2D^d$ transgene (H-2^bD^d)($<10^4$ cells) (**Fig. 1D**), illustrating NK cell mediated rejection of normal BM grafts based on missing-self recognition [33,34]. The transplantation of BCR-ABL1 B6 BM progenitors into B6D^d hosts yielded a large number of BCR-ABL1+ myeloid cells ($>10^6$ cells) when NK1.1+ cells had been depleted (**Fig. 1C, D**). When NK cells were present, the number of BCR-ABL1+-CD11b+ cells was approximately 30 fold lower (**Fig. 1C, D**). Thus a partial MHC-I mismatch significantly diminished the expansion of BCR-ABL1+ cells in vivo due to the presence of NK cells. This is likely mediated by NK cells expressing inhibitory Ly49A+ and Ly49G2+ receptors, which are inhibited by H-$2D^d$ but not H-2^b molecules [35].

We next tested whether complete MHC-I deficiency further accentuated the protective effect. Indeed, the abundance of BCR-ABL1+ myeloid cells that developed from β2m-deficient (β2m-ko, MHC-I^{low}) BM precursors was reduced 500 fold in the presence of NK cells in B6 recipient mice (H-2^b) (**Fig. 1E, F**). We conclude that NK cell mediated missing-self recognition can efficiently

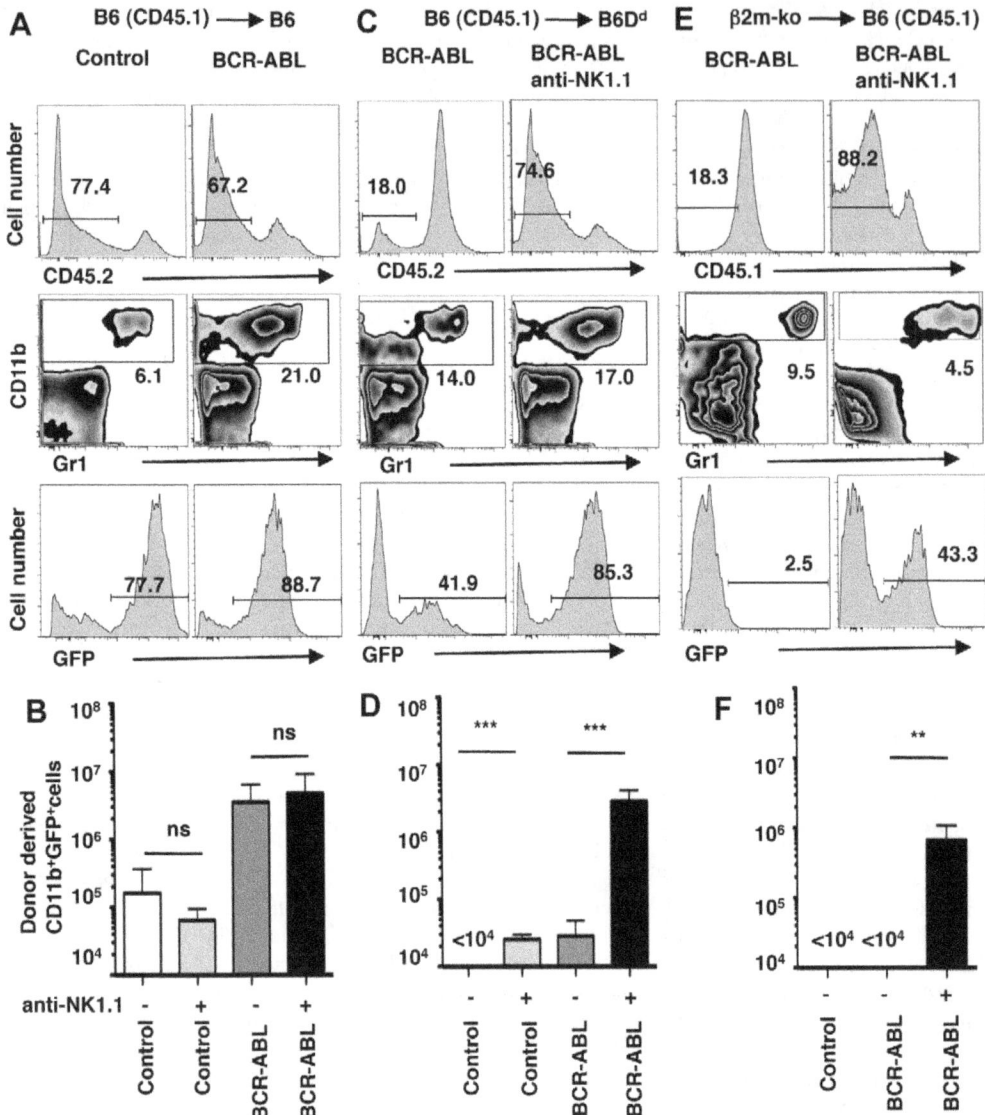

Figure 1. NK cell mediated missing-self recognition reduces the expansion of BCR-ABL1+ myeloid cells *in vivo*. BM cells from 5-FU treated B6 mice (H-2^b, CD45.1) were transduced with retroviral vectors encoding GFP (Control) or BCR-ABL1 plus GFP (BCR-ABL1) followed by transplantation into lethally irradiated, MHC-I matched B6 (H-2^b, CD45.2) mice (**A, B**) or MHC-I-different B6 D^d mice (H-2^{b}D^d, CD45.2) (**C, D**). In addition, BM cells from 5-FU treated β2m-deficient (β2m-ko) mice (MHC-I^{low}, CD45.2) were transduced with retroviral vectors encoding BCR-ABL1 plus GFP followed by transplantation into B6 (H-2^b, CD45.1) mice (**E, F**). Some recipient mice had been depleted of NK1.1+ cells by the injection of mAb PK136 (anti-NK1.1). Histograms show the identification of donor-derived cells at day 8 after transplantation (upper panel). Donor-derived cells were further analyzed for the presence of myeloid cells (CD11b+)(middle panel) and GFP expression in donor-derived myeloid cells (lower panel). Numbers indicate the percentage of cells in the respective gate. Bar graphs show the mean absolute number ($\pm$SD) of donor-derived myeloid cells expressing GFP (either control or BCR-ABL1) in recipient spleens at day 8 after transplantation. Donor-recipient mouse strain combinations were (**B**) B6 (H-2^b, CD45.1)->B6 (H-2^b, CD45.2) (MHC-I identical) and (**D**) B6 ((H-2^b, CD45.1) into B6D^d (H-2^{b}D^d, CD45.2) (MHC-I different, partial missing-self) and (**F**) β2m-ko (MHC-1^{low}, CD45.2)−>B6 (H-2^b, CD45.1) (MHC-I deficient, complete missing-self). The significance of the difference between indicated data sets is depicted as *** p<0.001, ** p<0.01 and ns not significantly different p>0.05.

control myeloid expansion driven by the BCR-ABL1 oncogene *in vivo*. The improved protective effect is likely due to a higher number of mismatches between inhibitory receptors and MHC-I ligands as observed for the NK cell mediated rejection of MHC-I-different normal cells [36].

NK cell mediated "non-self" or "induced-self" recognition fails to control BCR-ABL1+ cells

To address whether NK cell activation by non-self MHC-I conferred a protective effect, we transplanted BCR-ABL1

expressing B6D^d BM precursors into B6 recipients. In this donor/recipient combination, host NK cells partially reject normal B6D^d BM allografts based on the H-2D^d-specific Ly49D activation receptor [37]. However, NK cells in B6 recipients failed to impact the expansion of BCR-ABL1+ B6D^d myeloid cells (**Fig. 2A**), indicating that NK cell mediated non-self recognition is not effective against primary BCR-ABL1+ cells *in vivo*.

There is considerable evidence that the engagement of the NKG2D activation receptor by stress-induced ligands plays an

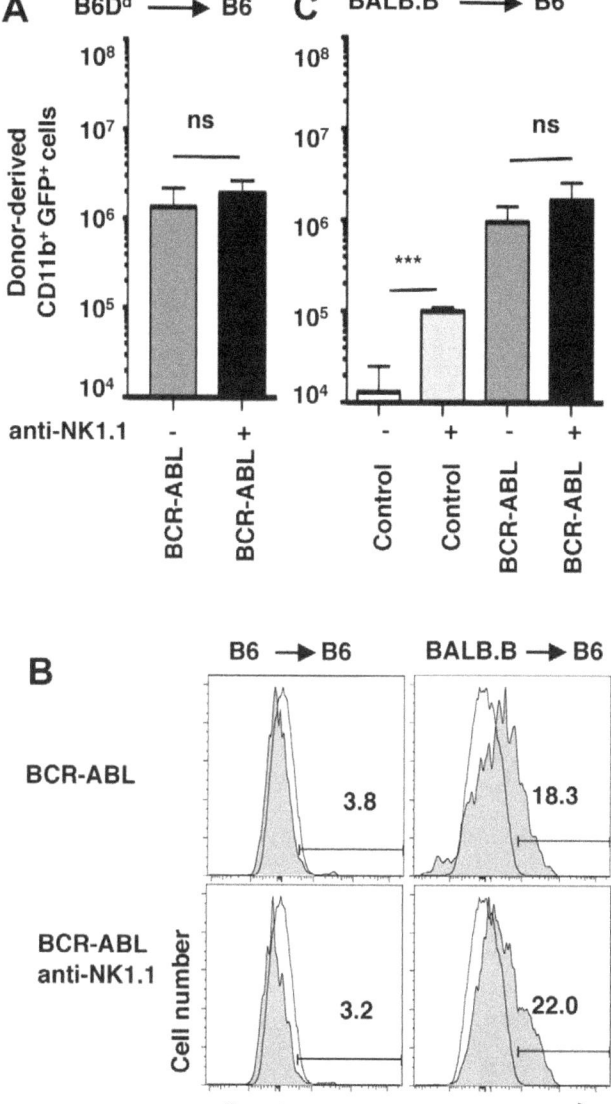

Figure 2. NK cell mediated non-self or induced-self recognition does not impact the expansion of BCR-ABL1+ cells. (**A**) The bar graph shows the mean absolute number (±SD) of B6 D^d (H-2^{b}D^d, CD45.1)-derived myeloid cells expressing BCR-ABL1 (GFP) in B6 (H-2^b, CD45.2) recipients at day 8 after transplantation (MHC-I different, non-self recognition). (**B**) The expression of Rae-1 NKG2D ligands was determined on B6 (left) or BALB.B (right)-derived myeloid cells (CD11b+) expressing BCR-ABL1 on day 8 after transplantation into B6 mice (gray fill). Open histograms depict background staining on BM-derived CD11b+ cells of normal B6 mice. (**C**) The bar graph shows the mean absolute number (±SD) of BABL.B (H-2^b, CD45.2)-derived myeloid cells expressing GFP (either control or BCR-ABL1) in B6 (H-2^b, CD45.1) recipients at day 8 after transplantation (MHC-I matched, unrelated, induced-self recognition).

important role for the recognition of transformed cells by NK cells [20]. While B6-background BCR-ABL1+ myeloid cells do not express the NKG2D ligands Rae-1 (**Fig. 2B**) or Mult1 (**not shown**), myeloid cells from certain mouse strains upregulate Rae-1 following BM transplantation and this results in graft rejection in specific recipient mouse strains [38]. Accordingly, we used the MHC-I matched, unrelated strain combination of BALB.B (H-2^b)−>B6 (H-2^b) to address whether induced-self

recognition can control BCR-ABL1+ cells. However, despite significant expression of Rae-1 (but not MULT1 or H60) (**Fig. 2B** and **data not shown**) we failed to observe a significant NK cell-mediated effect on BALB.B BCR-ABL1+ myeloid cells (**Fig. 2C**). Of note, though, we observed a significant NK cell-dependent rejection of normal BALB.B myeloid cells (**Fig. 2C**), in agreement with [38]. Thus, despite the expression of NKG2D ligand, induced-self recognition of BCR-ABL1+ cells *in vivo* is impaired.

NK cell mediated missing-self recognition can protect from CML disease *in vivo*

Since NK cell mediated missing-self recognition impacted myeloid expansion at d8 post transplantation, we next determined whether recipient mice were protected from CML disease *in vivo*. Since NK cell rejection of normal BM allografts is lethal between d12 and d14 post transplantation we ensured the long-term survival of host mice by co-transplanting MHC-I matched rescue BM (**Fig. 3A**). Similar to the transplantation with a single type of BM, such mixed BM grafts rapidly induced CML disease, which is characterized by weight loss, increased numbers of peripheral-blood cells (with a predominance of mature granulocytes), splenomegaly and pulmonary hemorrhage, owing to granulocyte infiltration into the lung (**Fig. 3B**) [31].

When BCR-ABL1+ BM was transplanted into MHC-I matched recipients, the presence of NK cells did not improve the survival of recipient mice, delay the onset of disease (**Fig. 4A**) or alter any of the symptoms associated with CML disease (**data not shown**). Corresponding observations were made when BCR-ABL1+ B6 BM was transplanted into NK cell-sufficient RAG-1-knock out mice (H-2^b) and into NK cell-deficient RAG-1 common γ chain double-knock-out mice (**data not shown**). Thus, as expected, NK cells do not impact MHC-I matched CML disease.

The transplantation of B6 BCR-ABL1+ BM into B6D^d hosts, from which NK1.1+ cells had been depleted, resulted in CML disease in 100% of recipient mice (mean onset day 11.0±1.3, n = 14) (**Fig. 4B**). The presence of host NK cells significantly delayed disease onset (mean onset day 13.7±3.1, n = 12)(p<0.01). In addition, in the presence of NK cells, only 12 of 14 mice (86%) succumbed to CML disease. The remaining recipients (2/12, 14%) remained disease free (>50d) (**Fig. 4B**). Thus a partial Ly49 ligand mismatch reduced CML disease *in vivo*.

In contrast to the early time point after transplantation (d8) (**Fig. 1C, D**), animals with CML disease had comparable numbers of BCR-ABL1+ myeloid cells, irrespective of whether NK cells were deleted or not (**Fig. 5A**). The eventual failure to prevent disease progression was not due to a loss of NK cells. On the contrary, NK cells were actually slightly more abundant at later time points (**Fig. 5B**). Thus the initial control of leukemic cells is incomplete and BCR-ABL1+ myeloid cells eventually escaped NK cell-mediated missing-self recognition.

Finally we tested whether complete MHC-I mismatch provided an improved protection against CML disease. In the absence of NK cells, the majority of B6 recipients receiving β2m-ko BCR-ABL1+ BM developed disease symptoms (70%, 7/10) (**Fig. 4C**). In contrast, when NK cells were present most recipients of β2m-ko BCR-ABL1+ BM remained disease free (89%, 8/9) for >45d (**Fig. 4C**). Interestingly, the only recipient that developed disease, had symptoms characteristic of B-ALL (B cell acute lymphocytic leukemia) rather than CML. B-ALL is characterized by a moderate splenomegaly and enlarged lymph nodes due to an expansion of B220+ B cells and such mice do not have the extensive infiltration of the lung and liver characteristic of CML

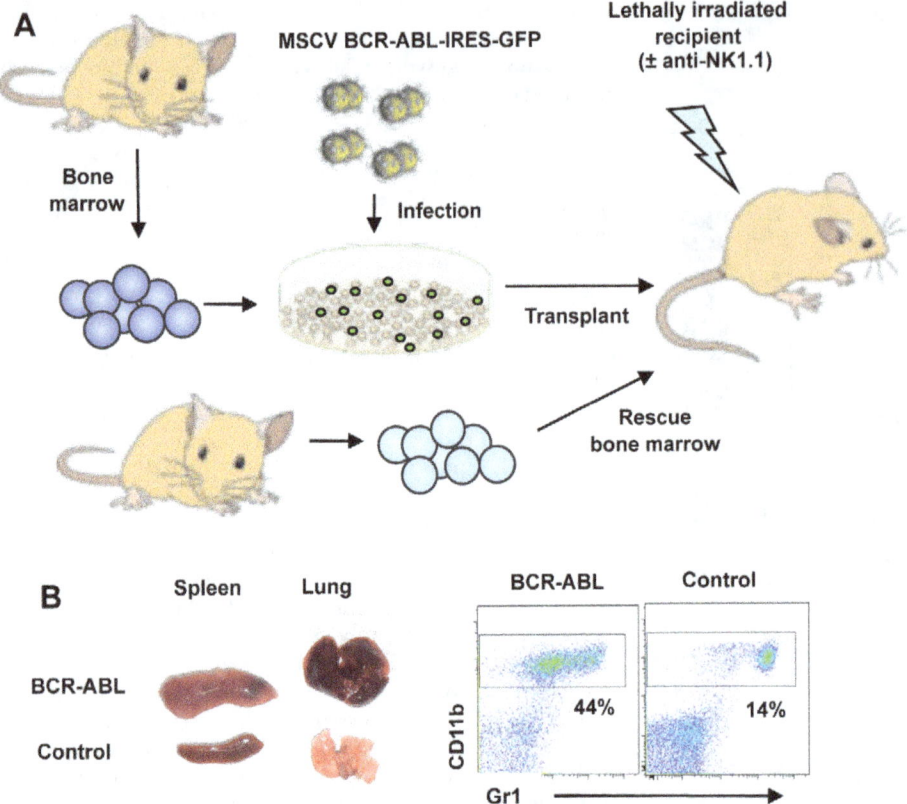

Figure 3. Schematic representation of CML protection assays. (A) NK cell rejection of normal BM allografts is lethal between d12 and d14 post transplantation. To ensure the survival of host mice beyond this time point, lethally irradiated recipient mice were transplanted with mixtures of MHC-I matched rescue BM plus MHC-I-different BCR-ABL1 transduced BM. **(B)** Mixed BM grafts rapidly induces CML disease, which is characterized by pulmonary hemorrhage, splenomegaly and increased numbers of mature granulocytes in peripheral blood.

(data not shown). In the absence of NK cells, some B6 recipients of BCR-ABL1+ β2m-ko BM also developed B-ALL (2/7 mice that were diseased). However most recipients developed CML (5/7). These experiments formally show that following BM transplantation, NK cell mediated missing-self recognition can protect from CML disease.

NK cell recognition of BCR-ABL1+ leukemia initiating cells

Finally we addressed whether NK cells exerted their protective effect by targeting mature BCR-ABL1+ myeloid cells, immature myeloid precursors or the small population of leukemia initiating cells, which propagate CML disease [39]. As mentioned above, NK cell mediated missing-self recognition strongly reduced the abundance of mature BCR-ABL1+ myeloid cells (**Fig. 1**). Moreover, myeloid/erythroid progenitor cells (Lin- Kit+ Sca-1- (LKS-)) GFP+ were also strongly reduced (**Fig. 6A, B, D**), suggesting that NK cells efficiently target immature myeloid progenitors. Finally, the abundance of leukemia initiating cells, which are present in the haematopoietic stem cell compartment (Lin- Sca-1+ c-kit+) (LSK) expressing BCR-ABL1 [40], was significantly reduced based on a partial MHC-I deficiency of the graft relative to the host (**Fig. 6A, C**). Leukemia initiating cells were essentially absent when the graft lacked MHC-I molecules (**Fig. 6E**). These data show that NK cell-mediated missing-self recognition can target leukemia initiating cancer stem cells and that this correlates with protection from CML disease.

Discussion

A potential role of NK cells to prevent leukemia relapse has been suggested based on the retrospective analysis of data from patients receiving unrelated HLA matched or partially HLA mismatched bone marrow transplantation. However, direct evidence that NK cells can prevent leukemia relapse is lacking and it has remained unclear what NK cell recognition events might be effective. Here we provide direct evidence that NK cells can be effective against primary CML *in vivo*. Unexpectedly, a protective effect was only observed for NK cell mediated missing-self recognition whereby an increased MHC-I receptor-ligand mismatch improved the protective effect *in vivo*. In contrast, the positive recognition of allogeneic MHC-I exerted no measurable effect on the abundance of BCR-ABL1-expressing myeloid cells *in vivo*. Further, it was possible that lethal irradiation/BM transplantation produced a cytokine milieu that reversed the reduced responsiveness of activation receptors on non-educated NK cells (i.e. Ly49A+ and Ly49G2+ NK cells in H-2^b mice), which are not inhibited by the MHC-I of the tumor. However, the absence of an effect of NK cells upon MHC-I matched transplantation provides circumstantial evidence that uneducated NK cells do not become reactive against BCR-ABL1+ cells. Finally, the recognition of stress-induced ligands by NKG2D also failed to mediate a significant protective effect against leukemia, even in a situation where the respective ligand(s) are expressed. Since normal BM cells that express NKG2D ligand are rejected, the data raise the possibility that BCR-ABL1 expression impairs

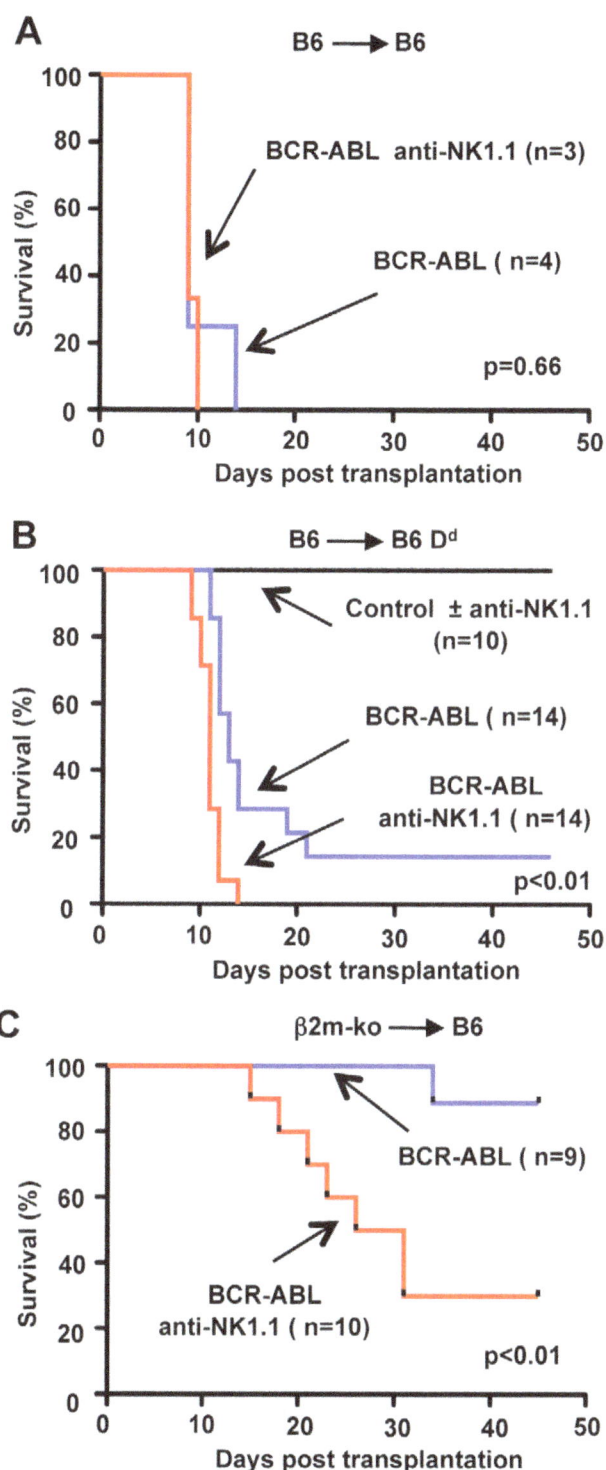

Figure 4. NK cell-mediated missing-self recognition can protect from BCR-ABL1 induced CML disease. A Survival graph of B6 recipients (H-2^b) transplanted with a mixture of BCR-ABL1 transduced B6 BM cells (H-2^b) and non-transduced B6 rescue BM (H-2^b). Some recipient mice had been depleted of NK1.1+ cells by the injection of mAb PK136 (anti-NK1.1). These data are derived from a single experiment. **B** Survival graph of B6D^d recipients (H-2^{b}D^d) transplanted with mixtures of control transduced B6 BM (H-2^b) and non-transduced B6D^d rescue BM (H-2^{b}D^d). All recipient mice survived independent of the presence or absence of NK1.1+ cells (±anti-NK1.1). Survival of B6D^d recipients (H-2^{b}D^d) transplanted with mixtures of BCR-ABL1 transduced B6 BM (H-2^b) and non-transduced B6D^d rescue BM (H-2^{b}D^d). In the

presence of NK cells, the survival of recipients is significantly improved ($p<0.01$). The data have been compiled from three independent experiments. **C** Survival graph of B6 recipients (H-2^b) transplanted with mixtures of BCR-ABL1 transduced β2m-ko (MHC-I^{low}) BM and non-transduced B6 rescue BM (H-2^b). In the presence of NK cells, the survival of recipients is significantly improved ($p<0.01$). The data have been compiled from two independent experiments.

the recognition of cells expressing NKG2D ligand. This defect was not based on a down-regulation or loss of the NKG2D receptor on NK cells (data not shown). Collectively, we have been unable to identify NK cell recognition events that allow the selective detection of BCR-ABL1+ as compared to normal host cells. Rather this study has identified NK cell recognition events that are impaired due to the expression of BCR-ABL1. Missing-self recognition was the only NK cell recognition strategy, which was not impaired and which significantly impacted the course of CML disease.

The NK cell activation receptors (and their ligands) mediating missing-self recognition remain incompletely defined. It is clear, however, that NK cells are activated by multiple receptors specific for constitutively expressed ligands on healthy host cells. The predominant reactivity of NK cells for cells of haematopoietic origin is explained in part by the expression of SLAM family receptors/ligands by haematopoietic cells [41]. Such restricted expression of ligands may also explain the observation that NK cells do not mediate GvHD [42]. The identification of all the activating receptors and their ligands will be required to explain why missing-self recognition is particularly effective against CML and whether the recognition of CML is dependent on the same or partially distinct activation receptors. Moreover, this knowledge will be essential to understand how CML eventually escapes NK cell mediated missing-self recognition. In addition to specific receptor-ligand interactions, it is also possible that the particular cytokine milieu generated in the course of conditioning and BM transplantation favors missing-self reactivity.

Here we have aimed at determining the potential of NK cells to protect from CML following BM transplantation. The advantage of our set-up is that the efficacy of NK cells against BCR-ABL1+ cells can be compared to that against normal cells, which is well established based on classical BM graft rejection experiments. Indeed, as detailed above, we did identify significant differences between the control of normal and BCR-ABL1+ BM progenitors. It is clear, however, that GvL is mediated by donor-derived and not by host-derived NK cells. Thus future studies will verify whether missing-self recognition by donor-derived NK cells is equally effective. While missing-self recognition has the potential to protect from CML disease, the efficacy of host NK cells against partially mismatched CML was limited. Despite a delay in disease onset, the majority of recipient mice (12/14; 86%) eventually succumbed to CML disease. While NK cells largely controlled BCR-ABL1+ myeloid cells at an early time-point after transplantation (day 8), in diseased animals the abundance of CML cells and their precursors was comparable, independent of the presence of NK cells. The eventual lack of control was not due to a complete loss host NK cells. On the contrary, host NK cells were slightly more abundant in the spleen of diseased mice. In agreement with these data, normal allogeneic BM induces the expansion of adoptively transferred NK cells [43]. Irrespective of this, BCR-ABL1+ cells eventually escape NK cell mediated control. The limited efficacy of NK cells may be

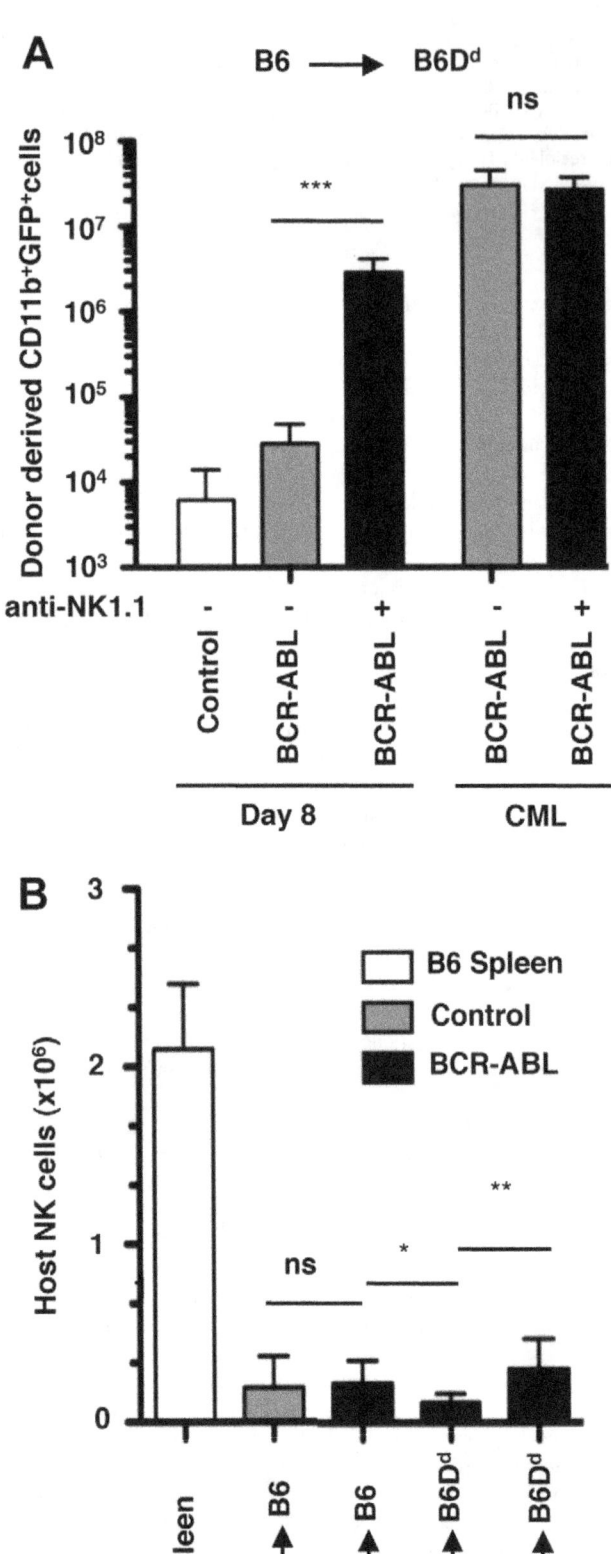

recipient mice at d8 after transplantation (left) and when CML disease had developed (right). Some recipient mice had been depleted of NK1.1+ cells by the injection of mAb PK136 (anti-NK1.1). (B) Mean number (±SD) of host-derived NK cells in the spleen of recipient mice at d8 after transplantation and when CML disease had developed (right). Significant differences between groups is indicated as * p<0.05, ** p<0.01 and *** p<0.001; (ns) not significantly different p>0.05.

explained by irradiation damage to host NK cells. Indeed, we have noted that lethal and even sub-lethal irradiation significantly reduces the abundance of splenic NK cells (5 fold). Moreover, within the first few days after transplantation residual host NK cells do not proliferate [44] (and our unpublished data). As donor-derived or adoptively transferred NK cells should not be damaged, it will be of interest to see whether these NK cell populations are more effective against CML. On the other hand, recent data suggest that the systemic exposure of mature NK cells to a large number of MHC-I-deficient normal cells profoundly reduces NK cell function [45]. Induction of NK cell hyporesponsiveness seems to be the outcome when mature NK cells are persistently stimulated under non-inflammatory conditions. Indeed, when NK cells are stimulated in the context of an inflammatory environment their function can stably improve [46,47]. If so, approaches to keep stimulated NK cells functional in a non-inflammatory environment may be needed to obtain protective effect against leukemia. The mouse models used here should be useful to address these issues.

Significantly we provide evidence that NK cells can impact the course of CML disease by targeting leukemia initiating stem cells that are refractory to the control by BCR-ABL1 tyrosine kinase inhibitors. These data suggest that NK cell recognition has the potential to cure CML. Finally, our findings validate approaches to treat leukemia using mAb-based blockade of self-specific inhibitory MHC-I receptors [48,49] and they may influence the selection of optimal donor/recipient combinations for stem cell transplantation to treat leukemia.

Materials and Methods

Mice

C57BL6 (B6) mice (H-2^b; CD45.2) were purchased from Harlan Olac (The Netherlands), CD45.1 congenic B6 mice (H-2^b; CD45.1). BALB.B (H-2^b; CD45.2) and β2m-deficient B6 mice (MHC-I^{low}; CD45.2) were originally purchased from The Jackson lab (Bar Harbor, ME) and maintained at the LICR. H-2D^d transgenic mice, backcrossed >10 generation to B6 (B6 D^d) (H-2^{b}D^d; CD45.2) have been described before [34]. Animal experimentation followed protocols reviewed and approved by the Service Vétérinaire du Canton de Vaud (authorization number 1124).

Retroviral infection and bone marrow transplantation

Retroviral infection and BM transplantation was performed essentially as described in [31]. Briefly, plasmids containing MSCV IRES GFP and MSCV BCR-ABL1 (p210) IRES GFP were transiently transfected into 293T cells for high titer virus production using standard procedures. BM donor mice were injected with 5-Fluorouracil (5-FU) (0.15 mg/ml) and BM cells were harvested 4 days later. BM cells were cultured in DMEM (plus 10% FCS, 50 mM 2-ME, 50 U/ml penicillin/50 μg/ml streptomycin, 10 mM HEPES) supplemented with IL-3 (10 ng/ml), IL-6 (10 ng/ml) and SCF (50 ng/ml) for 48 h and infected

Figure 5. BCR-ABL1+ myeloid cells escape NK cell mediated control. (A) The bar graph shows the mean number (±SD) of donor-derived GFP+ (control or BCR-ABL1) myeloid cells in the spleen of

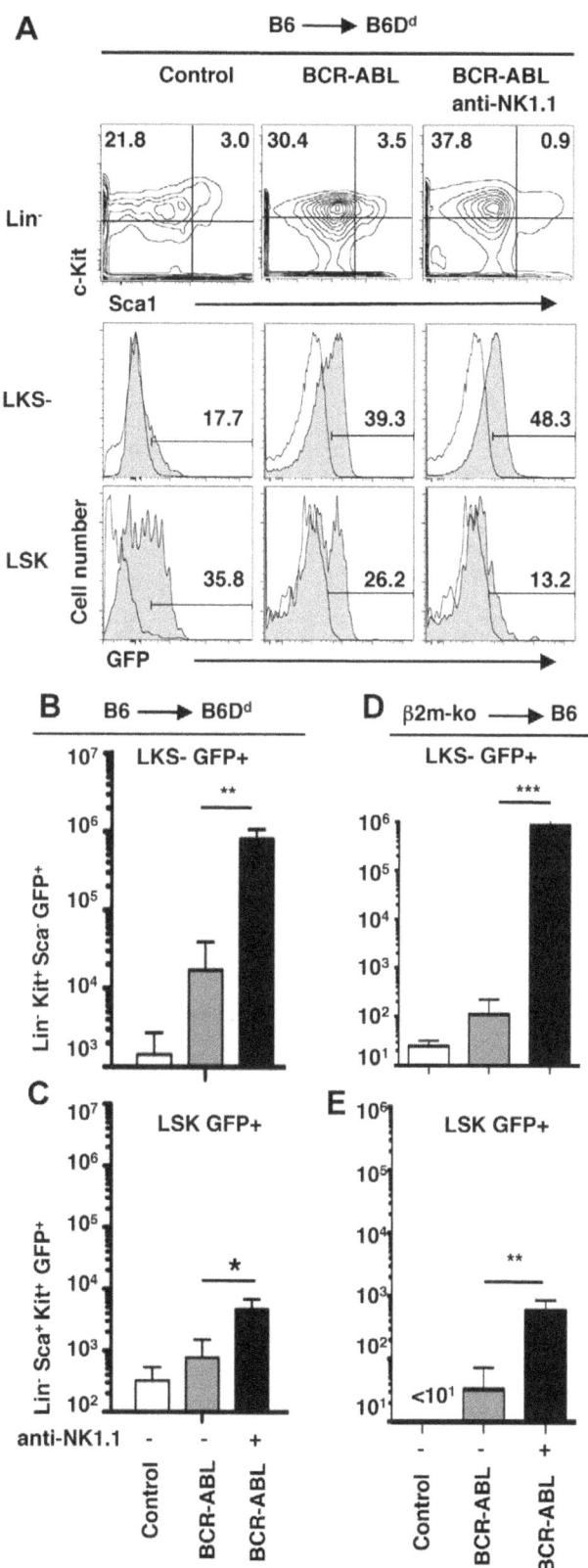

cells lacking markers of mature lineage cells (Lin-) were analyzed for the expression of c-kit and Sca-1 (top row). Histograms (gray filled) depict GFP expression (Control or BCR-ABL1) in gated Lin- c-kit+ sca-1- (LKS-) cells (myeloid/erythroid progenitors) (middle row) and in Lin- c-kit+ sca-1+ (LSK) cells (haematopoietic stem cell compartment) (bottom row). Open histograms depict background staining using BM precursor cells from normal B6 mice. Numbers indicate the percentage of cells in the respective gate. Some recipient mice had been depleted of NK1.1+ cells (anti-NK1.1). The bar graphs show the mean absolute number ($\pm$SD) of donor-derived GFP+ (Control or BCR-ABL1) LKS- cells (myeloid/erythroid progenitors) (**B**) and LSK cells (haematopoietic stem cell compartment) (**C**) at d8 after transplantation. (**D, E**) The bar graphs show the mean absolute number ($\pm$SD) of $\beta2$m-ko-derived GFP+ (Control or BCR-ABL1) LKS- cells (**D**) and LSK cells (**E**) at d8 after transplantation into B6 (H-2^b) recipients. Significant differences between groups are indicated as * $p<0.05$, ** $p<0.01$ and *** $p<0.001$; (ns) not significantly different $p>0.05$.

with retrovirus in the presence of polybrene (8 μg/ml). After 24 h, 10^5 cells (usually around 10% GFP+) were injected i.v. into lethally irradiated recipient mice (2 doses of 480rad 4 h apart from a ^{137}Cs source). One day prior to irradiation, some recipient mice were injected i.p. with 200 μg of mAb PK136 (anti-NK1.1) to deplete NK1.1+ cells. Recipient mice were sacrificed at day 8 after transplantation and analyzed by flow cytometry (see below). Alternatively, for leukemia induction experiments, irradiated recipient mice were transplanted with a mixture of infected BM and non-infected (MHC-I-matched) rescue BM (10^5 each), both derived from 5-FU treated donors. Recipient mice were monitored daily for weight loss and failure to thrive. Pre-morbid animals were sacrificed and relevant tissues were harvested and analyzed visually and by flow cytometry (see below). For continuous depletion of NK1.1+ cells, recipient mice were injected i.p. with 200 μg of mAb PK136 (anti-NK1.1) one day prior to irradiation and mAb injection was repeated every 2 weeks.

Flow cytometry

Spleen and BM cells were incubated with 2.4G2 (anti-CD16/32) hybridoma supernatant (to block Fc receptors) before staining for multi-color flow cytometry. The following mAbs were used: CD3ε (17A2), CD4 (GK1.5), CD8 (53.6.7), CD11b (Mac1)(M1/70), CD41 (MWReg30), CD45R (B220) (RA3-6B2), CD45.1 (A20.1), CD45.2 (104), CD117 (ACK2), CD127 (A7R34), CD135 (FLT3R)(A2F10.1), CD161 (NK1.1) (PK136), GR1 (RB6-8C5), TCRβ (H57), TCRγδ (GL3) and Ter119, Rae-1 (186107: R&D), Mult-1 (5D10: eBiosciences). Abs were conjugated with appropriate fluorochromes at the LICR or purchased from BD PharMingen (San Diego, CA) or eBioscience (San Diego, CA).

A cocktail of FITC-conjugated mAbs to TCRβ, TCRγδ, CD3ε, CD4, CD8, Mac-1, B220, NK1.1, Ter119 and GR1 was used to gate out cells expressing markers of mature lineage-cells (Lin) cells. Samples were run on a FACSCanto flow cytometer and analyzed with Cell Quest or FACS Diva software (Becton Dickinson, San Jose, CA).

Statistical analysis

A two-tailed student's t-test was used to determine significant differences between data sets and a Gehan-Wilcoxon test was used to compare survival curves. Data sets were considered significantly different when $p<0.05$.

Figure 6. NK cell mediated missing-self recognition reduces the abundance of BCR-ABL1+ leukemia initiating cells. (A) B6 BM cells (H-2^b) were transduced with a retrovirus expressing GFP (Control) or BCR-ABL1 plus GFP (BCR-ABL1) and transplanted into lethally irradiated B6D^d recipient mice (H-2^{b}D^d). Recipient spleens were analyzed by flow cytometry at d8 post transplantation. Donor-derived

Acknowledgments

We thank Stéphanie Bessoles and Giorgi Angelov for critical reading of the manuscript.

Author Contributions

Conceived and designed the experiments: MK WH. Performed the experiments: MK NG WH. Analyzed the data: MK WH. Contributed reagents/materials/analysis tools: NG. Wrote the paper: WH.

References

1. Shami P, Deiniger M (2011) Evolving treatment strategies for patients newly diagnosed with chronic myeloid leikemia: the role of second-generation BCR-ABL inhibitors as first-line therapy. Leukemia. doi: 10.1038/leu.2011.217. [Epub ahead of print].

2. Mahon FX, Réa D, Guilhot J, Guilhot F, Huguet F, et al. (2010) Discontinuation of imatinib in patients with chronic myeloid leukaemia who have maintained complete molecular remission for at least 2 years: the prospective, multicentre Stop Imatinib (STIM) trial. Lancet Oncol 11: 1029–1035.

3. Gratwohl A, Heim D (2009) Current role of stem cell transplantation in chronic myeloid leukaemia. Best Pract Res Clin Haematol 22: 431–443.

4. Ruggeri L, Capanni M, Casucci M, Volpi I, Tosti A, et al. (1999) Role of natural killer cell alloreactivity in HLA-mismatched hematopoietic stem cell transplantation. Blood 94: 333–339.

5. Miller JS, Soignier Y, Panoskaltsis-Mortari A, McNearney SA, Yun GH, et al. (2005) Successful adoptive transfer and in vivo expansion of human haploidentical NK cells in patients with cancer. Blood 105: 3051–3057.

6. Ruggeri L, Mancusi A, Burchielli E, Aversa F, Martelli MF, et al. (2007) Natural killer cell alloreactivity in allogeneic hematopoietic transplantation. Curr Opin Oncol 19: 142–147.

7. Moretta A, Sivori S, Vitale M, Pende D, Morelli L, et al. (1995) Existence of both inhibitory (p58) and activatory (p50) receptors for HLA-C molecules in human natural killer cells. J Exp Med 182: 875–884.

8. Nakamura MC, Linnemeyer PA, Niemi EC, Mason LH, Ortaldo JR, et al. (1999) Mouse Ly49D recognizes H-2D^d and activates natural killer cell cytotoxicity. J Exp Med 189: 493–500.

9. Karlhofer FM, Ribaudo RK, Yokoyama WM (1992) MHC class I alloantigen specificity of Ly-49+ IL-2 activated natural killer cells. Nature 358: 66–70.

10. Colonna M, Samaridis J (1995) Cloning of immunoglobulin-superfamily members associated with HLA-C and HLA-B recognition by human natural killer cells. Science 268: 405–408.

11. Ljunggren HG, Kärre K (1990) In search of the 'missing self': MHC molecules and NK cell recognition. Immunol Today 11: 237–244.

12. Ohlen C, Kling G, Höglund P, Hansson M, Scangos G, et al. (1989) Prevention of allogeneic bone marrow graft rejection by H-2 transgene in donor mice. Science 246: 666–668.

13. Fernandez NC, Treiner E, Vance RE, Jamieson AM, Lemieux S, et al. (2005) A subset of natural killer cells achieve self-tolerance without expressing inhibitory receptors specific for self MHC molecules. Blood 105: 4416–4423.

14. Kim S, Poursine-Laurent J, Truscott SM, Lybarger L, Song YJ, et al. (2005) Licensing of natural killer cells by host major histocompatibility complex class I molecules. Nature 436: 709–713.

15. Anfossi N, Andre P, Guia S, Falk CS, Roetynck S, et al. (2006) Human NK cell education by inhibitory receptors for MHC class I. Immunity 25: 331–342.

16. Chalifour A, Scarpellino L, Back J, Brodin P, Devèvre E, et al. (2009) A role for cis interaction between the inhibitory Ly49A receptor and MHC class I for NK cell education. Immunity 30: 337–347.

17. Orr MT, Murphy WJ, Lanier LL (2010) 'Unlicensed' natural killer cells dominate the response to cytomegalovirus infection. Nat Immunol 11: 321–327.

18. Hill GR, Crawford JM, Cooke KR, Brinson YS, Pan L, et al. (1997) Total body irradiation and acute graft-versus-host disease: the role of gastrointestinal damage and inflammatory cytokines. Blood 90: 3204–3213.

19. Bauer S, Groh V, Steinle A, Phillips JH, Lanier LL, et al. (1999) Activation of NK cells and T cells by NKG2D, a receptor for stress-inducible MICA. Science 285: 727–729.

20. Guerra N, Tan YX, Joncker NT, Choy A, Gallardo F, et al. (2008) NKG2D-deficient mice are defective in tumor surveillance in models of spontaneous malignancy. Immunity 28: 571–580.

21. Davies SM, Ruggieri L, DeFor T, Wagner JE, Weisdorf DJ, et al. (2002) Evaluation of KIR ligand incompatibility in mismatched unrelated donor hematopoietic transplants. Killer immunoglobulin-like receptor. Blood 100: 3825–3827.

22. Brunstein CG, Wagner JE, Weisdorf DJ, Cooley S, Noreen H, et al. (2009) Negative effect of KIR alloreactivity in recipients of umbilical cord blood transplant depends on transplantation conditioning intensity. Blood 113: 5628–5634.

23. Cooley S, Trachtenberg E, Bergemann TL, Saeteurn K, Klein J, et al. (2009) Donors with group B KIR haplotypes improve relapse-free survival after unrelated hematopoietic cell transplantation for acute myelogenous leukemia. Blood 113: 726–732.

24. Pende D, Marcenaro S, Falco M, Martini S, Bernardo ME, et al. (2009) Anti-leukemia activity of alloreactive NK cells in KIR ligand-mismatched haploidentical HSCT for pediatric patients: evaluation of the functional role of activating KIR and redefinition of inhibitory KIR specificity. Blood 113: 3119–3129.

25. Leung W, Iyengar R, Turner V, Lang P, Bader P, et al. (2004) Determinants of antileukemia effects of allogeneic NK cells. J Immunol 172: 644–650.

26. Hsu KC, Gooley T, Malkki M, Pinto-Agnello C, Dupont B, et al. (2006) KIR ligands and prediction of relapse after unrelated donor hematopoietic cell transplantation for hematologic malignancy. Biol Blood Marrow Transplant 12: 828–836.

27. Miller JS, Cooley S, Parham P, Farag SS, Verneris MR, et al. (2007) Missing KIR ligands are associated with less relapse and increased graft-versus-host disease (GVHD) following unrelated donor allogeneic HCT. Blood 109: 5058–5061.

28. Benjamin JE, Gill S, Negrin RS (2010) Biology and clinical effects of natural killer cells in allogeneic transplantation. Curr Opin Oncol 22: 130–137.

29. Pegram HJ, Ritchie DS, Smyth MJ, Wiernik A, Prince HM, et al. (2011) Alloreactive natural killer cells in hematopoietic stem cell transplantation. Leuk Res 35: 14–21.

30. Daley GQ, Van Etten RA, Baltimore D (1990) Induction of chronic myelogenous leukemia in mice by the P210bcr/abl gene of the Philadelphia chromosome. Science 247: 824–830.

31. Pear WS, Miller JP, Xu L, Pui JC, Soffer B, et al. (1998) Efficient and rapid induction of a chronic myelogenous leukemia-like myeloproliferative disease in mice receiving P210 bcr/abl-transduced bone marrow. Blood 92: 3780–3792.

32. Murphy WJ, Kumar V, Bennett M (1987) Acute rejection of murine bone marrow allografts by natural killer cells and T cells. J Exp Med 166: 1499–1509.

33. Öhlén C, Kling G, Höglund P, Hansson M, Scangos G, et al. (1989) Prevention of allogeneic bone marrow graft rejection of H-2 transgene in donor mice. Science 246: 666–668.

34. Ioannidis V, Zimmer J, Beermann F, Held W (2001) Cre recombinase-mediated inactivation of H-2Dd transgene expression: evidence for partial missing-self recognition by Ly49A NK cells. J Immunol 167: 6256–6262.

35. Hanke T, Takizawa H, McMahon CW, Busch DH, Pamer EG, et al. (1999) Direct assessment of MHC class I binding by seven Ly49 inhibitory NK cell receptors. Immunity 11: 67–77.

36. Brodin P, Lakshmikanth T, Johansson S, Karre K, Hoglund P (2009) The strength of inhibitory input during education quantitatively tunes the functional responsiveness of individual natural killer cells. Blood 113: 2434–2441.

37. Raziuddin A, Longo AL, Mason L, Ortaldo JR, Bennett M, et al. (1998) Differential effects of the rejection of bone marrow allografts by the depletion of activating versus inhibiting Ly-49 natural killer cell subsets. J Immunol 160: 87–94.

38. Ogasawara K, Benjamin J, Takaki R, Phillips JH, Lanier LL (2005) Function of NKG2D in natural killer cell-mediated rejection of mouse bone marrow grafts. Nat Immunol.

39. Hu Y, Liu Y, Pelletier S, Buchdunger E, Warmuth M, et al. (2004) Requirement of Src kinases Lyn, Hck and Fgr for BCR-ABL1-induced B-lymphoblastic leukemia but not chronic myeloid leukemia. Nat Genet 36: 453–461.

40. Hu Y, Swerdlow S, Duffy TM, Weinmann R, Lee FY, et al. (2006) Targeting multiple kinase pathways in leukemic progenitors and stem cells is essential for improved treatment of Ph+ leukemia in mice. Proc Natl Acad Sci U S A 103: 16870–16875.

41. Dong Z, Cruz-Munoz ME, Zhong MC, Chen R, Latour S, et al. (2009) Essential function for SAP family adaptors in the surveillance of hematopoietic cells by natural killer cells. Nat Immunol 10: 973–980.

42. Ruggeri L, Capanni M, Urbani E, Perruccio K, Shlomchik WD, et al. (2002) Effectiveness of donor natural killer cell alloreactivity in mismatched hematopoietic transplants. Science 295: 2097–2100.

43. Olson JA, Zeiser R, Beilhack A, Goldman JJ, Negrin RS (2009) Tissue-specific homing and expansion of donor NK cells in allogeneic bone marrow transplantation. J Immunol 183: 3219–3228.

44. Prlic M, Kamimura D, Bevan MJ (2007) Rapid generation of a functional NK-cell compartment. Blood 110: 2024–2026.

45. Joncker NT, Shifrin N, Delebecque F, Raulet DH (2010) Mature natural killer cells reset their responsiveness when exposed to an altered MHC environment. J Exp Med 207: 2065–2082.

46. Sun JC, Beilke JN, Lanier LL (2009) Adaptive immune features of natural killer cells. Nature 457: 557–561.

47. Cooper MA, Elliott JM, Keyel PA, Yang L, Carrero JA, et al. (2009) Cytokine-induced memory-like natural killer cells. Proc Natl Acad Sci U S A 106: 1915–1919.

48. Sola C, Andre P, Lemmers C, Fuseri N, Bonnafous C, et al. (2009) Genetic and antibody-mediated reprogramming of natural killer cell missing-self recognition in vivo. Proc Natl Acad Sci U S A 106: 12879–12884.

49. Vahlne G, Lindholm K, Meier A, Wickstrom S, Lakshmikanth T, et al. (2010) In vivo tumor cell rejection induced by NK cell inhibitory receptor blockade: maintained tolerance to normal cells even in the presence of IL-2. Eur J Immunol 40: 813–823.

7

Significance and Suppression of Redundant IL17 Responses in Acute Allograft Rejection by Bioinformatics based Drug Repositioning of Fenofibrate

Silke Roedder[1,9], **Naoyuki Kimura**[2,9], **Homare Okamura**[2], **Szu-Chuan Hsieh**[1], **Yongquan Gong**[2], **Minnie M. Sarwal**[1]*

1 Transplant Research Program Sutter Health Care, California Pacific Medical Center, San Francisco, California, United States of America, 2 Department of Cardiothoracic Surgery, Stanford University School of Medicine, Stanford, California, United States of America

Abstract

Despite advanced immunosuppression, redundancy in the molecular diversity of acute rejection (AR) often results in incomplete resolution of the injury response. We present a bioinformatics based approach for identification of these redundant molecular pathways in AR and a drug repositioning approach to suppress these using FDA approved drugs currently available for non-transplant indications. Two independent microarray data-sets from human renal allograft biopsies (n = 101) from patients on majorly Th1/IFN-y immune response targeted immunosuppression, with and without AR, were profiled. Using gene-set analysis across 3305 biological pathways, significant enrichment was found for the IL17 pathway in AR in both data-sets. Recent evidence suggests IL17 pathway as an important escape mechanism when Th1/IFN-y mediated responses are suppressed. As current immunosuppressions do not specifically target the IL17 axis, 7200 molecular compounds were interrogated for FDA approved drugs with specific inhibition of this axis. A combined IL17/IFN-y suppressive role was predicted for the antilipidemic drug Fenofibrate. To assess the immunregulatory action of Fenofibrate, we conducted *in-vitro* treatment of anti-CD3/CD28 stimulated human peripheral blood cells (PBMC), and, as predicted, Fenofibrate reduced IL17 and IFN-γ gene expression in stimulated PMBC. *In-vivo* Fenofibrate treatment of an experimental rodent model of cardiac AR reduced infiltration of total leukocytes, reduced expression of IL17/IFN-y and their pathway related genes in allografts and recipients' spleens, and extended graft survival by 21 days (p<0.007). In conclusion, this study provides important proof of concept that meta-analyses of genomic data and drug databases can provide new insights into the redundancy of the rejection response and presents an economic methodology to reposition FDA approved drugs in organ transplantation.

Editor: Lucienne Chatenoud, Université Paris Descartes, France

Funding: This work was supported by Beta-Sigma Phi Northern California Chapter. The funders had no role in study design, data collection and analysis, decision to publish, or preparation of the manuscript.

Competing Interests: The authors have declared that no competing interests exist.

* E-mail: Msarwal@psg.ucsf.edu

9 These authors contributed equally to this work.

Introduction

There is an unmet clinical need for novel immunmodulatory drugs in transplantation, as redundant alloimmune mechanisms, not adequately targeted by current immunosuppressive drugs, require additional modulation to mitigate the development of graft injury, chronic allograft damage and premature graft loss. Better understanding of some of these redundant immune responses may allow for the identification of novel drug targets and drugs for improved post-transplant patient care.

We hypothesized, that the application of a bioinformatics based genomic drug target discovery that uses publicly available functional data in conjunction with the concept of repositioning already FDA approved drugs, represents a promising approach for transplantation medicine which has a finite market size, to identify novel treatment options. This approach has been previously successfully applied by us in inflammatory bowel disease [1], and is now focused on human renal acute allograft rejection (AR).

Initial discovery of escape mechanisms in transplant rejection was done by whole genome microarray analyses of renal transplant recipient biopsies with AR. Analyses focused on bio-databases of functional gene-sets and pathways and discovered biologically relevant transcriptional changes in kidney allograft AR. We identified the Interleukin- (IL) 17 pathway as a pivotal redundant pathway in transplant rejection under the umbrella of Calcineurin inhibitor based immunosuppression (Tacrolimus, Cyclosporine). Recent evidence has hypothesized IL17 as a potential escape mechanism in AR if IFN-y mediated/Th1 responses are suppressed as is with Calcineurin inhibitors [2].

IL17 acts as pro-inflammatory cytokine promoting neutrophil and monocyte recruitment to sites of inflammation usually under the influence of IL-1β, IL-6, and tumor necrosis factor (TNF), and interferon (IFN)-γ [3]. Transcription and production of IL17 during AR occurs in multiple cell-types and is not limited to the Th-subpopulation: IL17 can be expressed by innate and adaptive immune cells, particularly by neutrophils, macrophages, dendritic

A. IN-SILICO NOVEL DRUG DISCOVERY

B. IN-VITRO & IN-VIVO DRUG ASSESSMENT

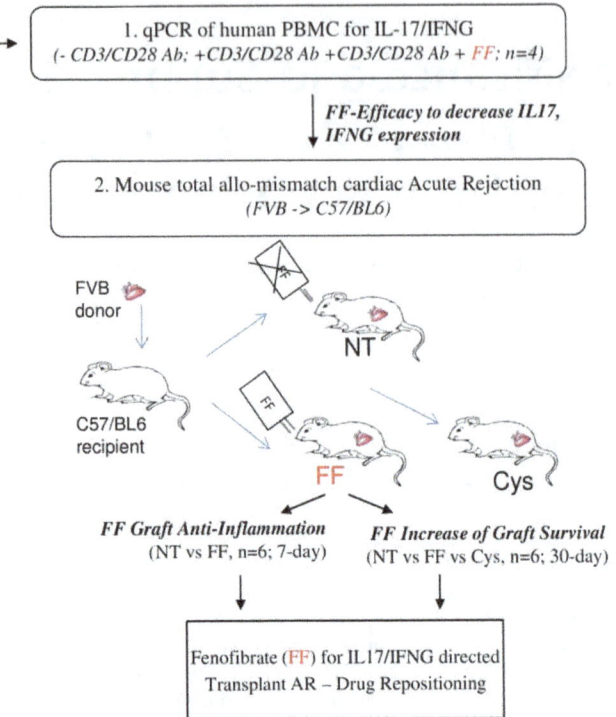

Figure 1. Study Design. Whole genome microarrays from 66 pre- and post-transplant kidney graft biopsies and from 35 post-transplant kidney graft biopsies were analyzed for rejection specific injury pathways using 3 computational databases comprising 3305 independent gene-sets. AR specific IL17 pathway (FDR = 0.3, p = 0.011) and activated IL17+ T-helper cells cell (FDR = 0.5; p = 0.008) gene-sets were aligned to a database of 7200 compounds with proven interactions with the input genes (MetaCore[TM], GeneGo, Thomson Reuters) resulting in the identification of Fenofibrate for drug repositioning in AR. Efficacy of Fenofibrate was tested in vitro using human PBMC and in vivo in mouse total allo-mismatch cardiac rejection for anti-inflammatory and for its potency to prolong graft survival.

cells, CD4+ and CD8+ T-cells, in addition to endothelial and epithelial cells [4–7]. IL17+ cells in biopsies from kidney transplant recipients correlated with the degree of inflammation during AR and independently predicted graft dysfunction at the last follow up [6]. Our results together with other previously published data suggested that IL17 could be an attractive drug target for transplant medicine [8,9]. Currently, there is no FDA approved small molecule drug to regulate IL17 responses and antagonizing IL17 in transplantation is not an approved indication.

Bioinformatic analyses of the genomic and drug databases identified Fenofibrate as a drug with established human safety that regulates IL17 and IFN-γ responses and thus could be repositioned for treatment of the IL17 mediated axis of allograft AR. Fenofibrate previously attenuated IFN-γ and IL17 mediated experimental colitis [10] and has also reduced systemic inflammatory effects in patients with metabolic syndrome [11] within clinical studies. In addition, we selected Fenofibrate for our drug repositioning studies as it is a small molecule drug for oral application, with proven administration, distribution, metabolism and excretion (ADME) profile, and has extensive human safety data with tolerable side effects.

Study Design

The study was based on human tissue-specific acute rejection (AR) injury pathway discovery, their application towards inferred drug targets, and the validation of selected drugs for abrogation of experimental graft rejection by in vitro and in vivo methods (Figure 1). The first phase of this study consisted of a whole

genome microarray discovery phase in humans for rejection specific transcriptional analyses of implantation (33 D0) and their paired post-transplant rejecting (17 AR) and non-rejecting (16 STA) biopsies. All 66 biopsies were blindly scored by the same pathologist (Neeraja Kambham, Stanford University, CA) and rejection was graded by the Banff criteria [12]. Three computational databases (MSigDb = molecular Signatures database; SMD = Stanford Microarray database; AcIc = activated immune cells) were analyzed for significant enrichment of pathways and networks (GSA = Gene set analysis) that were redundant in AR. For validation, an additional microarray data-set from 35 renal allograft biopsies (21 STA, 14 AR) from adult recipients post transplantation was interrogated which was downloaded from Gene Expression Omnibus (GEO, GSE9493). The IL17 rejection-specific pathway, chosen as one of the most significant pathway in AR in both data-sets was aligned to a drug database with PubMed proven interactions to the input target genes, resulting in the selection of an FDA approved small molecule drug, Fenofibrate, for possible drug repositioning. Fenofibrate was identified to additionally target the IFN-γ pathway. Initial validation of the effect of Fenofibrate was done to examine its regulation of IL17 and IFN-γ in vitro in human peripheral blood mononuclear cells (PBMC) stimulated with anti CD3/anti CD28. Next, Fenofibrate was tested for its efficacy to improve acute tissue rejection and prolong allograft survival in vivo in an experimental model of heterotopic cardiac AR. End-points examined were reduction of inflammation in the graft, and extension of graft survival compared to non-treatment (NT) and standard immunosuppression (Cyclosporine, Cys) applying Flow cytometry (FACS), histology and assessment of graft function by palpation. Local and systemic efficacy of Fenofibrate to regulate IL17 pathway and IFN-y pathway response genes was characterized by quantitative PCR (QPCR) in mice grafts and spleens at post-operative day (POD) 7 and compared to NT and Cys (Figure 1).

Materials

Patients and Transplant Biopsies

In our data-set of 66 renal transplant biopsies from 33 unique pediatric and young adult patients (age range 4–22) were examined. To minimize baseline confounders inclusion criteria were young donor age (7–30 years), no delayed graft function, unsensitized recipients (peak panel reactive antibody <20%), and similar immunosuppression (Daclizumab induction, mycophenolate mofetil (MMF), tacrolimus (Tac)) (Table 1). Excluded were expanded criteria donor kidneys, as they are not used for pediatric and adolescent recipients. Each patient had a biopsy profiled at time of engraftment (D0) prior to reperfusion of the donor kidney, and within the first year post-transplantation, either for cause or as part of protocol surveillance. Biopsies were blindly read for histological evaluation by a single pathologist resulting in 17 patients with Banff graded [12] acute rejection (AR), and 16 patients with essentially normal biopsy reads (no substantive pathology, negative C4d, CD20 staining) (STA). In the rejection cohort, 4 biopsies showed relevant cellular infiltrates that were suspicious for but did not reach the threshold for diagnosis of acute T-cell mediated rejection and were thus diagnosed as borderline rejection (BL), 7 biopsies were graded as ARIA and 6 biopsies as ARIB. All patients gave written informed consent, and the study was approved by the institutional review board of Stanford University and adhered to the Declarations of Istanbul and Helsinki. Written informed consent was obtained and documented on the consent form from the next of kin, caretakers, or guardians on the behalf of the minors/children participants involved in the study and was approved by the ethics committee [13,14]. Demographics and clinical information are summarized in Table 1. The publicly available data-set (GSE9493) downloaded from Gene Expression Omnibus (GEO) included data from 35 renal allograft biopsies from adult recipients post transplantation. This data-set included 21 STA, and 14 rejection cases. Within the rejection group, 4 cases showed abnormalities which were graded as BL rejection according to Banff [15]. Demographics of these patients can be found here [16].

Mice for Experimental Transplant Rejection

For in vivo experimental heart transplantation, recipient C57BL/6J (H2b) and donor FVB (H2q) mice were used (SM and [8]). All animal experiments were approved by Stanford University Institutional Animal Care and performed in accordance with the Guide for the Care and Use of Laboratory Animals (Ref; National Research Council 1996; Guide for the Care and Use of Laboratory Animals, Washington D.C., National Academy Press). All surgery was performed under sodium pentobarbital anesthesia, and all efforts were made to minimize suffering. In brief, FVB donor hearts were implanted into the abdomen of C57BL/6 WT mice representing a complete MHC-class 1 and -2 mismatch [17,18]. Animals were divided into treatment (Fenofibrate, FF) and no-Treatment (NT) groups, each consisting of 6 animals in the in the 7-day treatment model and consisting of 6 animals in the NT group, 9 animals in the FF group in the 30-day graft survival study. In the graft survival study, we additionally added a group of 6 animals that were treated with standard

immunosuppression, Cyclosporine (Cys). Animal activity, body weight and graft function were assessed daily. The latter was measured by direct abdominal palpation and expressed as graft beating score (BS) using the Stanford cardiac surgery laboratory graft scoring system (0: no contraction; 1: contraction barely palpable; 2: obvious decrease in contraction strength, but still contracting in a coordinated manner, rhythm disturbance; 3: strong, coordinated beat but noticeable decrease in strength or rate, distention/stiffness; or 4: strong contraction of both ventricles, regular rate, no enlargement or stiffness).

Concise Methods

Human Tissue Microarray Experiments

Total RNA extraction, quality control, complementary (c)-DNA amplification and microarray hybridization for human renal allograft biopsies was essentially performed as published [19] and described in SM. In brief, total RNA was extracted from biopsies stored in RNAlater (Ambion, Texas, TX) using TRIzol Reagent (Invitrogen, Carlsbad, CA). After quality control, RNA was amplified to cDNA, biotin labeled and hybridized onto Affymetrix GeneChip Human Genome U133 plus 2.0 Arrays.

Human PBMC Stimulation

Human PBMC for in-vitro drug efficacy assays were isolated from whole blood of 5 healthy individuals (2 female, 3 males, mean age 31+/−14 years) using Ficoll gradient centrifugation (Ficoll-Paque™ PLUS, Amersham Biosciences, Uppsala, Sweden). Isolated PBMCs were pretreated with 100 μMol Fenofibrate (Sigma Aldrich, St. Luis, MO) for 2 hours and then stimulated with anti-human CD3/CD28 antibodies for 65 hours. Thereafter cells were harvested and snap frozen at −80°C until downstream analysis of gene expression. In vitro experiments are described in detail in SM.

Mouse Treatment

Fenofibrate (F6020; Sigma Aldrich, St. Louis, MO) was dosed at 100 mg/kg body weight/day and administered daily either by i.p. injection in the 7-day inflammatory model, or by oral gavage in the 30-day graft survival study. Treatment started the day prior to transplantation and lasted until the day before sacrifice (SM). Cyclosporine (Cys) was dosed at 20 mg/kg/day and was administered daily by i.p. injection. The dosage of Cyclosporine was based on published literature in experimental cardiac allograft rejection [20], the dosage of Fenofibrate was based on literature of an experimental mouse model of atherosclerosis that showed efficacy but no toxicity during the treatment [21]. A 1:1 translation of either Cyclosporine or of Fenofibrate dosages used to treat humans were not possible, as the ADME profiles between mice and humans are not comparable.

Treatment Efficacy Endpoints

Murine cardiac allograft survival. To investigate cardiac graft survival in transplanted mice, graft beating scores were determined daily for a maximum of 30 days in Fenofibrate (FF, n = 9) treated mice, and was compared to non-treated animals (NT, n = 6), as well as to standard immunosuppression, Cyclosporine (CSA, n = 6) treated animals. Significance between graft survival between the FF, CSA, and NT groups were assessed by Wilcoxon log rank test in GraphPad Prism 5.04 (GraphPad Software Inc., La Jolla, CA). A p-value <0.05 was considered significant.

Murine cardiac allograft inflammation. To study anti-inflammatory effects of Fenofibrate in cardiac AR, animals

Table 1. Patient Demographics.

Score	D0	STA	BL	ARIA	ARIB
Number	33	16	4	7	6
Histological diagnosis (Banff)	Pre-transplant donor biopsy	No significant graft abnormalities	Borderline acute rejection	Mild-moderate cellular acute rejection	Severe cellular acute rejection
% non-protocol	/	25%	50%	57%	33.3%
Time post Transplantation [months]	/	25.4 (+71/−25)	10.2 (+8/−5)	12.6 (+19/−7)	5.8 (+8/−3)
# C4D	/	0	0	2	1
# CD20	/	0	0	0	3
Serum Creatinine [mg/mL]	/	0.5275	1.075	0.924	0.72
Recipient age	8.3 (+10/−6.7)	16.6 (+2/−4)	12.3 (+6/−4)	11.8 (+6/−8)	13.4(+5/−10)
Recipient gender [%male]	75%	75%	50%	28.6%	66.7%
Donor age	29.5(+23/−15)	31.1 (+16/−17)	26.5 (+12/−26)	26.7 (+17.3/−19)	26.7 (+17/−11)
Donor gender [%male]	40.9%	50%	50%	57.1%	83.3%
Immunosuppression	/	MMF+Tac (9)/Sir (1)/ Aza (1) +/−SB (5)[b]	MMF+Tac+SB	MMF+Tac (4)/Sir (1)+/−SB (2)	MMF+Tac(2)/Aza (1)+/−SB (3)
HLA MM [a]	/	1.5	0	0	0

[a]HLA MM = human leukocyte antigen mismatch;
[b]Sir = Sirolimus; SB = steroid based; Aza = Azathioprine;

underwent Fenofibrate treatment for 7 days and the following assays were performed:

Graft histology at POD7 was evaluated by light microscopy of hematoxylin and eosin (H&E) stained formalin fixed and paraffin embedded tissue sections using a Nikon E600 light microscope (Nikon Instruments Inc., Melville, NY) at 10× magnification and Spot V4.6 imaging software (Spot Imaging, Sterling Heights, MI). See SM for details.

Fluorescence Activated Cell Sorting (FACS) of graft infiltrating cells was performed to determine the number of infiltrating cells in recipient cardiac allografts (CD4+, CD8+, B220+, CD11b+, F4/80, Gr1.1) at POD7 and has been described by us [8] and can be found in detail in SM.

Human in vitro and murine in vivo QPCR. For quantification of gene expression in in-vitro and in-vivo experiments by quantitative PCR (QPCR), total RNA from human PBMC was isolated using the Pico Pure RNA isolation Kit (Arcturus, Life Technologies, Foster City, CA). Total RNA from mice allograft and spleen tissues was extracted using TRIzol® Reagent (Invitrogen, Life Technologies, Carlsbad, CA) [8]. Each time, 250 ng of total RNA were reverse transcribed using Superscript II (Invitrogen, Life Technologies, Carlsbad, CA). In human PBMC, expression of 7 genes plus 18S as endogenous control was analyzed in duplicates by TaqMan QPCR (ABI HT7900 Instrument, Applied Biosystems, Life Technologies, CA, USA) according to standard protocols. Data was analyzed using SDS 2.3 software (Applied Biosystems, Life Technologies, Foster City, CA). Mouse allograft and recipient spleen gene expression was assessed using the high throughput Fluidigm BioMark instrument (BioMark; Fluidigm, San Francisco, CA) as described in detail in SM. In brief, cDNA was amplified for 14 target genes using Applied Biosystems primers and probes. Preamplified cDNA was loaded into a Dynamic 96.96 chip (Fluidigm) for a 40 cycle QPCR. Expression of 18S served as endogenous control, and data was analyzed in the Biomark RT-PCR analysis software V.2.0. Assay IDs are listed in SM.

Data Analysis

Microarray data analysis. Affymetrix HG U133 plus2.0 gene chip CEL files from 66 pre-transplant donor samples (D0, n = 33) and post-transplant Banff graded renal allograft biopsy samples (STA, n = 16; BL, n = 4; ARIA, n = 7; ARIB, n = 6) were uploaded into dChip 2006 software [22] for processing and normalization. Perfect match only for background correction was performed and arrays were checked for single, array and probe outliers before quantile normalization and computing of model based expression values [23]. Only genes with expression values present on each array were used for analyses. Raw data are stored in gene expression omnibus (GEO) under GSE34437, sample IDs used for microarray analyses are listed in Table S1.

To expand the number of patients and to validate the findings in our data-set an additional microarray data-set (Affymetrix HG U133 plus2.0) was downloaded from GEO (GSE9493) consisting of whole genome expression profiles from 21 STA, 4 BL and 10 AR renal allograft biopsies. Data had been preprocessed and normalized (RMA, Quantile normalization, log2 transformation) as described [16,24].

Computational analyses of databases for rejection pathway analysis. Significance analysis of microarrays (SAM, [25]) for two-class and for quantitative gene-set analysis (GSA) [26] was performed to detect rejection specific gene-sets in patient biopsies with AR. Enrichment in AR compared to STA was identified by two-class GSA. To identify pathways with increasing enrichment from D0>STA>BL>ARIA>ARIAB quantitative GSA was applied. GSA uses maxmean statistics and applies a restandardization of genes and sample permutations to estimate false discovery rate (FDR) which means that a gene-set must be unusual both as compared to gene-sets of the same size sampled at random from the set of genes represented by the gene-set, and as compared to itself, when the outcome labels are permuted [27,28]. Here, the FDR was calculated in 1000 permutations, and significance level was set at an FDR of 0.5. Correlation between gene expression values and phenotype was based on T-test for 2-class GSA and on regression for quantitative GSA. A total of 3307

Table 2. GSA identifies increasing enrichment of IL-17 gene-sets in human renal allograft acute rejection across independent Patient Data-Sets.

	Analysis	Gene-Sets	p-value	FDR
Discovery Data-Set (n = 66)				
	AR vs. STA	IL17-Pathway	0.007	0.3
		Th17 gene set	0	0.2
	D0> STA> BL>ARIA> ARIB	IL17-Pathway	0.011	0.3076
Verification Data-Set (n = 35)				
	AR vs. STA	IL17-Pathway	0.011	0.33
		Th17 gene set	0.026	0.39
	STA> BL>AR	IL17-Pathway	0.008	0.5

There were total 140 gene-sets significantly enriched in AR in both Data-Sets (FDR = 0.5), the IL-17 pathway and Th17 gene-sets are listed above. Other significant gene-sets that reached the threshold of FDR = 0.5 included gene-sets associated with innate immune cells (Dendritic Cell, Natural Killer Cell, Granulocyte, Monocyte), and innate immune responses (CTLA4 pathway, Toll-like receptor pathway, NFKB targets, PD1 signaling), with Cytokine Signaling (IL-10, IL-2, IL-5, IL-22BP, IL-12) as well as with gene-sets related to Th-differentiation and activation (CD40 signaling, Costimulation, Th1/Th2, Th-Differentiation). Th1 (FDR = 0.3, p = 0.007) and IL-12 (FDR = 0.3, p = 0.011) had higher FDR and p-values compared to the Th17 and IL-17 gene-sets in our data-set and similar values compared to GSE 9493. Other gene-sets were Graft versus Host Disease, Autoimmune Thyroiditis, and Antigen processing.

publicly available and manually curated gene-sets, containing a total of 839,839 genes (= 20,930 unique genes) were tested.

From the Molecular Signature Database (MSigDb v2.0, Broad Institute) we downloaded 3272 gene-sets curated using seven online pathway databases (KEGG; BioCarta, BioScience Corp., Reactome, Sigma-Aldrich, Signal transduction knowledge environment and signaling gateway), PubMed publications, and knowledge of domain experts. From the Stanford microarray database (SMD, http://smd.stanford.edu) 24 gene-sets for cellular processes were downloaded, and an additional dataset of Activated Immune Cells (AcicDb) consisting of 9 gene-sets were manually created by us using publicly available microarray gene expression data of in-vitro activated T-helper lymphocytes (Th) (Th1, Th2, IL17+ T-helper cells), antigen presenting cells (dendritic cells (DC), natural killer (NK) cells) and cells of the innate immune system (monocytes, neutrophils). Detailed gene-set descriptions are listed in Table S2.

Multivariate analysis of gene expression for IL17 pathway and IL17+ T-helper cells genes. To confirm GSA results, unsupervised Principal Component Analysis (PCA) and hierarchical clustering were performed for the IL17 pathway and Th17 gene-set genes in AR and STA (Partek Genomics Suite V.6.6, Partek Inc. USA). In case of multiple array probe-sets for the same gene, the probe-set with the lowest deviation (standard error of mean) across the AR and STA samples was used for the analyses. In cases where different probe-sets for AR and STA revealed lower deviation, both probe-sets were used. In addition we evaluated if there were any specific transcriptional changes in biopsies that were C4d$^+$ AR (n = 3) versus C4d$^-$ AR (n = 10).

Drug discovery targeting IL17 pathway and IL17+ T-helper cells genes. Affymetrix unique probe-IDs for selected IL17 pathway and Th17 gene-set genes were uploaded into MetaCore^{TM}, an interactive platform of biologically relevant data to integrate rejection specific genes with annotated functional data of gene-protein, protein-protein, and protein-compound interactions, together with compound and drug content, and gene disease relationships (MetaCore^{TM}; GeneGo, Thomson Reuters, St. Joseph, MI). The Drug Lookup feature in MetaCore^{TM} correlated input genes with deposited data from therapeutic, non-therapeutic, and secondary drug interactions that had an underlying data entry in PubMed. Resulting compounds were then filtered for direct

inhibition of target genes, number of genes targeted and their FDA status. In addition, the underlying PubMed entry was carefully checked.

QPCR data analysis. Relative gene expression in in-vitro and in-vivo experiments was assessed by the delta delta Ct method and fold changes were calculated to either a human or a mouse universal RNA (Stratagene). Significance was calculated in Excel (Microsoft Office 2007, Microsoft Inc. USA) and GraphPad Prism 5.04 (GraphPad Software Inc., La Jolla, CA) using a 2-sided Student T-test and a p-value of 0.05 as threshold for significance.

Results

Discovery of Acute Rejection Specific Redundant IL17 Pathway Enrichment in Human Kidney Transplant Biopsies Across Independent Patient-Sets

Significance Analysis of Microarray Data (SAM) based two-class and quantitative Gene Set Analysis (GSA) [25,29] across 3307 curated biologically relevant gene-sets and across 66 whole genome microarrays identified significantly increasing enrichment of IL17 pathway genes and genes which had shown significant 2-fold upregulation (p-value <0.05) in T-cells experimentally differentiated into Th17 cells and which were summarized in the "Th17 gene-set" in AR based on false discovery rate (FDR) and p-value (Table 2).

Across 13 AR graded ARIA or higher and 16 STA two-class GSA revealed enrichment of the Th17 gene-set with an FDR = 0.2, p = 0, as well as of the IL17 pathway gene-set with FDR = 0.3, p = 0.007. Quantitative GSA (qGSA) across D0, matched STA, and rejection biopsies separated by grade of rejection into borderline (BL), ARIA and ARIB showed that the IL17 pathway gene-set additionally was increasingly enriched with D0<STA<BL<ARIA<ARIB (IL17 pathway gene-set FDR = 0.3 p = 0.011) supporting the relevance of the IL17 pathway in AR. To validate these findings, we investigated an independent microarray data-set from 21 STA, and 14 rejection renal allograft biopsy cases which was publicly available in Gene Expression Omnibus (GEO, GSE9493). Two-class GSA across the STA and biopsy confirmed AR (n = 10) showed significant enrichment of both gene-sets IL17-pathway and Th17 sets in these AR (IL17-pathway, FDR = 0.33, p-value = 0.011; Th17 gene-set,

FDR = 0.39, p-value = 0.026). Overall, there were 140 gene-sets common in both data-sets which were significantly enriched in AR (FDR = 0.5). As the publicly downloaded data-set also included 4 cases among their 14 rejection cases that were defined as borderline acute rejection, we added a quantitative GSA analysis which revealed that the IL17 pathway was significantly enriched following STA<BL<AR (FDR = 0.5, p-value 0.008). Due to the small numbers of BL cases in comparison to the numbers of STA and AR cases in this data-set, these analyses might be skewed.

Additional QGSA across 10 gene-sets representing the transcriptome of innate and adaptive immune cells (Monocytes, Natural Killer Cells, Dendritic Cells, Th1-cells, Th2-cells, Th17-cells, T-regulatory cells, gamma delta T-cells) in response to experimental activation, and T-cell differentiation (Th-Differenti-ation, Anergy/Regulation) identified enrichment of the IL17+ T-helper cell gene-set (Th17, 157 unique genes) [30] in increasing AR (FDR 0.1, p = 0.047; Table 2). The Th17 gene-set response was more redundant in the AR biopsies than the Th1 gene-set response [31] (FDR = 0.1, p = 0.05). Genes regulated in the IL17 pathway and the Th17 gene-sets allowed for almost complete separation of rejecting renal allograft biopsies from non-rejecting biopsies by hierarchical clustering (Euclidean Distance and Cosine Dissimilarity) (Figure 2A, 2B). A total of 8 genes (Il-17 pathway, n = 1; Th17 gene-set, n = 8) were significantly different expressed between C4d$^+$ AR vs. C4d$^-$ AR cases (Student T-test, p<0.05). Interleukin 8 was common in both gene-sets and showed significant different expression between C4d$^+$ and C4d$^-$ AR cases. Unsupervised Principal Component Analysis (PCA) for IL17 pathway and Th17 gene-set genes explained 45.1% and 44.7% respectively of the differences between AR and STA in the first of three principal components (Figure 2C, 2D). PCA did not segregate the C4d$^+$ AR from C4d$^-$ AR.

Identification of Drugs for Repositioning for IL17 Pathway Directed Inhibition of AR

AR specific IL17 pathway and IL17+ T-helper cell genes were interrogated against the MetaCore^{TM} (GeneGo, St. Joseph, MI) Compound Database evaluating the interaction of rejection specific genes against data of 7200 different therapeutic and non-therapeutic compounds in the drug lookup interface. The resulting 297 therapeutic and non-therapeutic compounds identified to interact with one or more of the input genes from the IL17 and IL17+ T-helper cell gene sets were filtered for direct inhibition and targeting at least 5 genes in the rejection input data-set, including IL17. Fenofibrate, an FDA approved small molecule drug for the treatment of hypertriglyceridemia and hypercholes-terolemia, was inferred to directly inhibit IL17A the major IL17 pathway cytokine and was also suggested to act via the Th1 response directly inhibiting expression of IFN-γ the major Th1 inducing cytokine [10]. In addition to Fenofibrate, our approach also identified three corticosteroids (Prednisolone, Budesonid and Flunisolide). Steroids are currently used as standard immunosuppression and are the mainstay treatment for an AR episode. This result provided confidence for the validity of our approach. However, the steroids were not predicted to directly act via IL17A. As Fenofibrate was hypothesized to directly act on IL17A as well as on the Th1 cytokine IFN-γ, was an FDA approved small molecule drug with known human safety and side-effect profiles and established drug delivery and administration frequency, and with known pleiotropic anti-inflammatory effects [11], Fenofibrate was selected as drug candidate for AR repositioning. The subsequent in vitro and in vivo experiments in our study support likely efficacy for AR in human renal transplant rejection.

Attenuation of IL17 and IFN-γ Gene Expression by Fenofibrate in CD3/CD28 Stimulated Human PBMC

Anti-CD3/CD28 stimulation of human PBMC from independent healthy volunteers upregulated expression of IL17 and IFN-γ in all five individual PBMC; the average fold change for IL17 was 12.15 (p = 0.01), of IFN-γ 96.58 (p<0.0001) compared to non-stimulated PBMC (n = 5). Fenofibrate treatment of stimulated PBMC significantly reversed the upregulation in all cases but one with respect to IL17 and in all cases with respect to IFN-γ: the average fold change for down regulation was 1.38 and 2.17 for IL17 (p = 0.02) and IFN-γ (p = 0.001) respectively (Figure 3). Shown are relative fold changes (RQ) in gene expression levels normalized to 18S and universal RNA for non-stimulated (NS), stimulated (S) and stimulated and Fenofibrate treated (S+FF) PBMC.

Experimental in-vivo Evaluation of Fenofibrate for Efficacy in AR and Characterization of its Immune Regulatory Effects

Prolonged graft survival in a rodent heart transplant model of AR by Fenofibrate treatment. A 30-day graft survival study in BL6/C57 mice heterotropically transplanted with an allogenic FVB donor heart resulted in significantly prolonged survival of total allo-mismatch donor hearts transplanted into Fenofibrate-treated (100 mg/kg/d) recipients (median survival: 25 days; n = 6) compared to non-treated recipients (NT, median survival: 9.5 days; n = 6) (Wilcoxon log-rank test, p = 0.0007) (Figure 4) and led to allograft beating beyond day 30 (study end-point) in two animals. Mice tolerated the Fenofibrate dose well; no change in total body weight during the treatment was observed. Allografts in the NT control group were rejected within an average of 12 days after transplantation. Comparison to standard immunosuppression (Cyclosporine, Cys, 20 mg/kg/d i.p.) re-vealed equivalent efficacy of Fenofibrate for extending graft survival (median survival Cys 30 days) (Figure 4).

Significantly improved graft function with Fenofibrate. Seven days daily treatment with Fenofibrate-using the same acute rejection model used for graft survival, resulted in significantly higher average BS' (mean BS = 3.5) compared to NT (mean BS = 2, p<0.001) (Figure 5A). The chosen dosage of 100 mg/kg/d Fenofibrate was well tolerated by the mice as there was no change in body weight, liver function and serum Creatinine (Materials and Methods S1).

Reduction in cellular infiltrates and myocyte damage with Fenofibrate. Graft tissue from POD7 was assessed by a single blinded pathologist by microscopic evaluation of H&E staining applying ISHLT criteria [32,33]. Grafts from Fenofibrate treated animals revealed decreased cellular infiltrates either uni- or multifocal but never diffuse, and with- or without myocyte damage compared to grafts from untreated animals which always showed diffuse multifocal cellular infiltrates and were always associated with myocyte damage (Figure 5B).

Significantly reduced numbers of graft infiltrating innate and adaptive immune cells with Fenofibrate. FACS analysis of graft infiltrating cells not only confirmed histological evaluation but further quantified the anti-inflammatory effect of Fenofibrate. Assessed were total numbers of graft infiltrating total leukocytes (CD45+), and of differential innate Dendritic- (DC,CD11c), Natural Killer (ND, NK1.1), Macrophages (F4/80), Neutrophils (Gr1+)) and adaptive immune Cytotoxic-(CD8), Helper T-(CD4), and B-(CD220)) cells in Fenofibrate and no-treated grafts at POD7 (Figure 5C). Numbers of cells were corrected for total graft weight. Fenofibrate significantly decreased the number of CD45+ graft

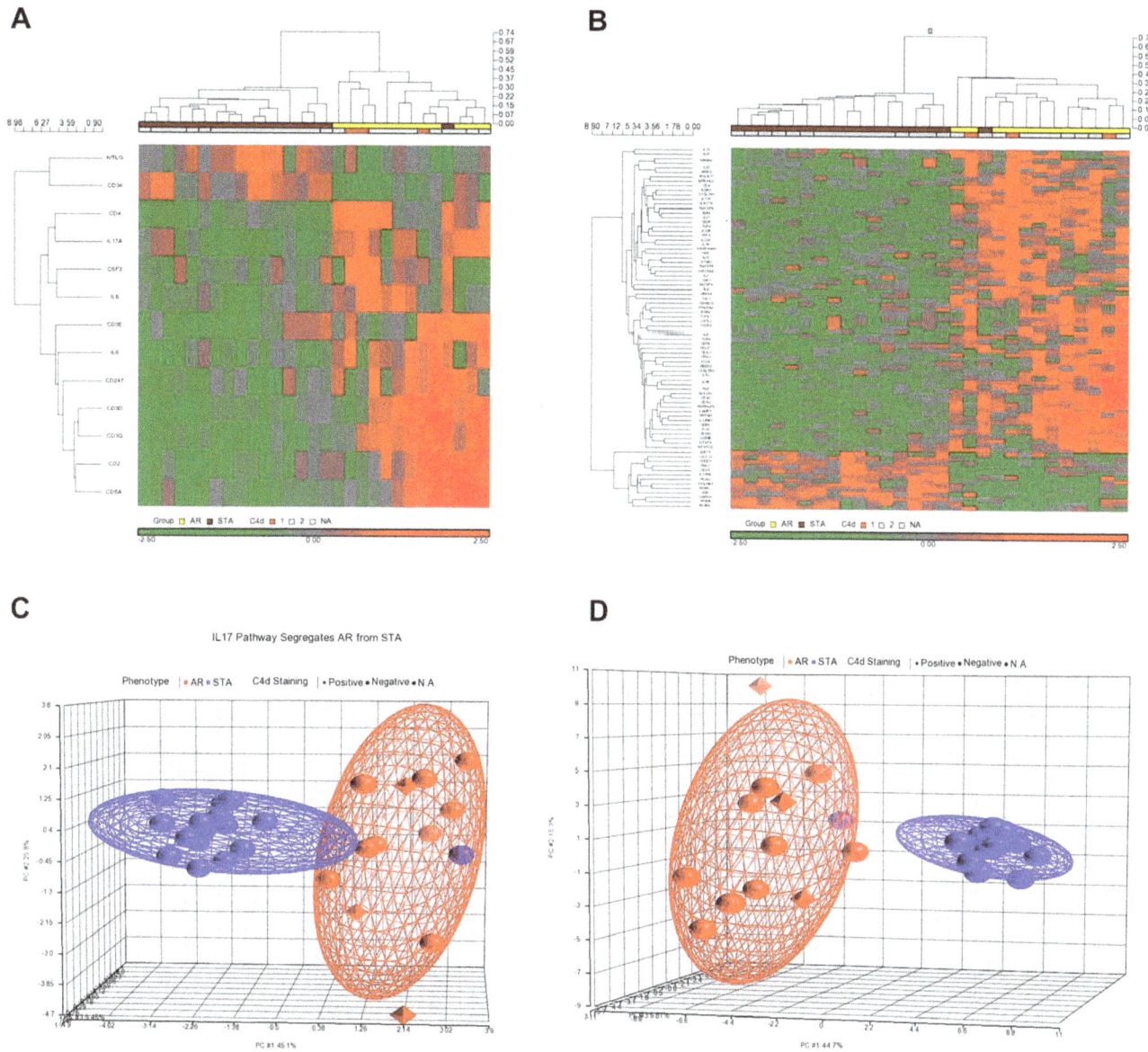

Figure 2. IL17 pathway- and IL17⁺ Th- gene sets in human AR: Segregation of AR and STA. Genes from the IL17 pathway gene-set (2a) and from the Th17 gene-set (2b) were used for hierarchical clustering of post-transplant biopsies and resulted in clear separation of AR and STA after mean centering arrays and genes (Euclidean Distance, Cosine Dissimilarity). Unsupervised principal component analysis (PCA) of the same samples using the same genes confirmed the separation of AR and STA (2c, d). A separation of the AR group into C4d+ and C4d- cases was not seen.

infiltrating total leukocytes (p<0.001); more specifically, there was a significant reduction in antigen presenting DC (p<0.01), in CD4+ T-helper and CD8+ cytotoxic T-cells, as well as in infiltrating neutrophils (p<0.01) and NK cells. As IL17 is known to promote neutrophil infiltration, the observed reduction of neutrophils in the graft of Fenofibrate treated mice potentially reflects the IL17 pathway inhibition by Fenofibrate. Infiltrating macrophages and B-cells were also reduced but numbers did not reach significance.

Significant inhibition of graft and spleen IL17 and Th1 genes in vivo with Fenofibrate. Corroborating the findings of Fenofibrate on anti-CD3/CD28 stimulated human PBMCs, Fenofibrate treatment in vivo in cardiac transplanted mice resulted in reduced gene expression levels of IFN- γ and IL17A (Figure 6A, 6B). IL17A expression in the Fenofibrate treated mice

was only detectable in the transplanted hearts and did not reach the threshold of detection by QPCR in the recipients' spleens at POD7. In grafts IL17 was significantly lower compared to no treatment (6a, p = 0.0462). In spleens, Fenofibrate significantly reduced IFN-γ expression (6b, p = 0.0094) whereas reduction of graft IFN-y expression did not quite reach the significance threshold of p = 0.05 when compared to no-treatment by two sided Student T-test (6a). Next, we further elucidated the efficacy of Fenofibrate and expanded graft (Figure 6A) and spleen (Figure 6B) gene expression analyses to genes up- and downstream of the Th1 response and IL17 pathway: Fenofibrate reduced the IL17 stimulating cytokines IL-1β, and TGF-β, as well as of IL-17 downstream TNF in both mice allografts and spleens. IL-6 which also is upstream of IL17 and together with IL1-β and TGF-β important for activating the IL17 response was significantly

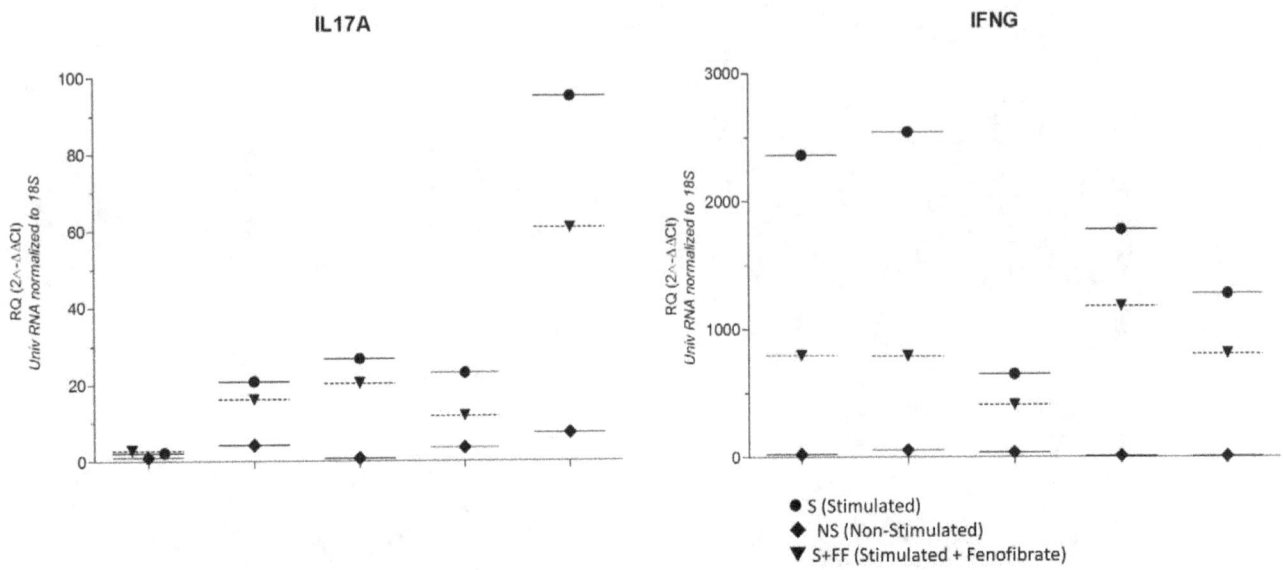

Figure 3. Fenofibrate gene expression in human PBMC: Fenofibrate regulates IL17 and IFN-γ gene expression in CD3/CD28 stimulated human PBMC. PBMC from healthy individuals (n = 5) were stimulated with CD3/CD28 antibodies (S) leading to significant upregulation of IL17 and IFN-γ which was inhibited by Fenofibrate (S+FF). Values represent mean fold changes versus non-stimulated (NS) cells plus Standard error of mean calculated using ΔΔCt method and 18S as endogenous control gene; experiments were performed in triplicates. Student T-test for paired data: * p-value <0.05. Individual p-values are displayed in Table 3.

reduced by Fenofibrate in mice allografts only. The Th1 response was further investigated quantifying the stimulating IL-12 cytokine expression as well as the Th1 transcription factor STAT4. Fenofibrate significantly decreased expression of both genes in mouse spleens, STAT4 was additionally significantly decreased in the in the graft as compared to mice that were not-treated with Fenofibrate for AR. QPCR in grafts and spleens from Cys treated mice at POD7 validated the preferential inhibition of Th1 responses by Cys seen in reduced graft IFN-y (p = 0.0101) and STAT4 (p = 0.0091) expression, whereas IL17A was not affected by Cys (p = 0.2180) but even showed a trend towards higher expression. To address the question, whether the effect of Fenofibrate to inhibit the IL17 pathway is more dependent on the related orphan receptors RORγ/RORα or on STAT3 (which induce Th17 cell differentiation), we performed additional QPCR for RORγ, RORα and STAT3 expression in grafts and spleens from untreated and Fenofibrate treated mice at POD7. There was no significant difference with treatment in expression of either RORγ (p = 0.26 in the graft; p = 0.59 in the spleen) or RORα

(p = 0.96 in the graft; p = 0.076 in the spleen), but there was a significant reduction for STAT3 expression in the spleen of Fenofibrate treated mice at POD7 (p = 0.026), but not in the graft (p = 0.72). Our results indicate that there is bias towards STAT3 targeted IL17 pathway inhibition by Fenofibrate. Additionally, there may be differential immune responses in spleen and graft.

Single network formation of rejection specific Fenofibrate regulated genes. Rejection specific genes which were upregulated in AR and down regulated again by Fenofibrate could be assembled into a single-network of direct interactions in MetaCore™ network analyses. In this analysis, c-Jun and downstream of c-Jun, IL-7 receptor (IL7R) were detected as additional genes interacting with the genes that were regulated by Fenofibrate (Figure 6C). Our subsequent analyses of c-Jun and IL7R by QPCR of mice graft and spleen RNA showed that both genes were upregulated in mice which did not receive Fenofibrate and that both were down regulated again in mice treated with Fenofibrate. Specifically, Fenofibrate significantly regulated c-Jun (p = 0.0293) in mice spleens, and IL7R (p = 0.0162) in mice allografts. Interestingly, Fenofibrate did not show efficacy on ROR-α, a transcription factor relevant for IL17 expression in IL17+ T-helper cells (Figure 6C).

Discussion

The present study elucidates a process of microarray-based and bioinformatics-driven discovery of transplant rejection specific functional gene-sets and pathways that are highly relevant to redundant acute renal allograft rejection, in combination with a process by which FDA approved drugs can be tested for repositioning for immunomodulation in human organ transplantation. While most microarray data analysis methods focus on the identification of individual differentially expressed genes in two or more conditions, we focused here on sets of biologically relevant genes in our initial discovery applying gene set analysis (GSA) as a more robust method with reduced false positive results and more likely to reveal redundant biologically relevant pathways

Table 3. Effects of Fenofibrate on IFNG and IL17A expression in human PBMC: Fold changes (Fc) comparing stimulated (S) to no-stimulated (NS) PBMC (upper part) and comparing stimulated (S) to stimulated and Fenofibrate treated (S+FF) PBMC (lower part); direction of the gene expression change and p-values calculated by two-sided Student T-test.

		Fc	Direction	P-value
S vs. NS	IFNG	96.58	Up	*** <0.0001
	IL17A	12.15	Up	* 0.0142
S vs. S+FF	IFNG	2.17	Down	** 0.0014
	IL17A	1.38	Down	* 0.0224

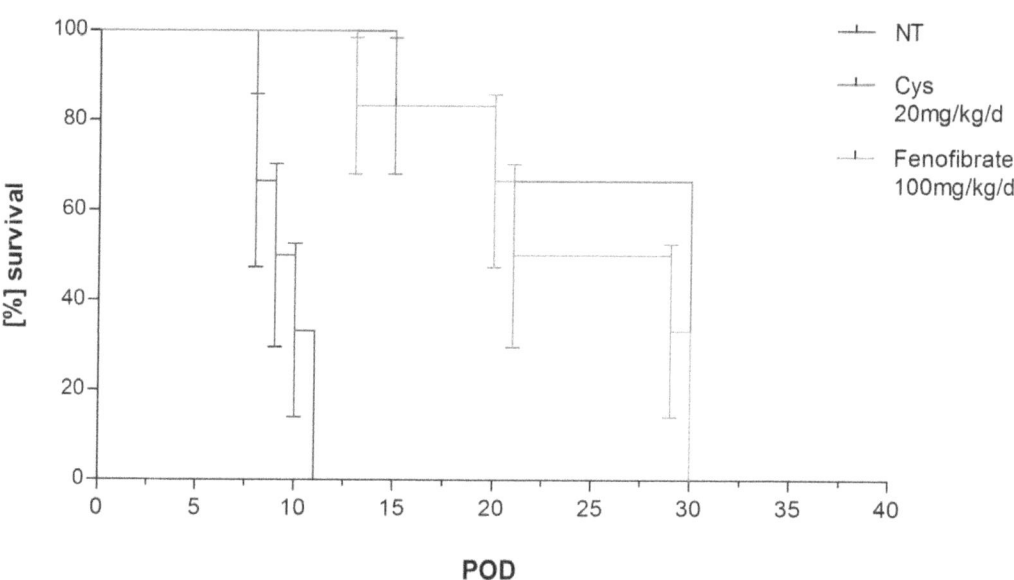

Figure 4. Graft Survival with Fenofibrate: Fenofibrate treatment alone prolonged cardiac graft survival in transplanted mice. Kaplan Meyer curve for graft survival data after total allo-mismatch murine heart transplantation was assessed by determining the number of post operational days (POD) on which transplanted mice showed a palpatable graft beating score (BS). The median number of days grafts of Fenofibrate treated animals (FF, n = 6) showed beating was 25 compared to 9.5 days in non-treated animals (NT, n = 6). Significance of graft survival was assessed by Wilcoxon log-rank test (p = 0.0007).

underlying graft rejection and describing potential novel drug targets [26,30,33]. Next, we investigated drugs that already passed the costly clinical phases of drug development and drug safety in humans for indications unrelated to organ transplantation, but could inhibit identified critical gene-sets and pathways in the allo-immune response. We hypothesized that these target drugs could be repositioned for suppressing the acute allo-immune response, providing a more cost effective means of introducing novel drugs for treatment of acute rejection in organ transplant recipients.

The role of IL17 in innate and adaptive auto- and allo-immune responses has been investigated by several groups, but is still not fully understood. Clearly, IL17 was increased in human acute lung, liver and kidney rejection [4,34,35] and promoted early graft inflammation [36]. Results in experimental mouse models of cardiac AR reported that in Th1 transcription factor T-bet deficient mice, an IL17 response was mounted leading to acute graft rejection [2,5]. In another study IL17 was also involved in the acceleration of AR in a T-bet positive background with a full Th1 response [8]. The role of T-bet for IL17 mediated acute rejection remains controversial, yet most recent evidence suggests, that IL17 plays an accelerated role in a Th1 response suppressed environ-ment [2]. Our results for IL17 expression in grafts from transplanted mice treated with Cys which majorly affects the Th1 response showed higher IL17 expression compared to not-treatment, whereas IFN-y was significantly lower. As current immunosuppressive drugs used in transplantation majorly act via the Th1 response, a potential increased emergence of IL17 in redundant acute rejection seems to be likely, and our microarray analyses provides further evidence for the role of IL17 pathway as an important mechanism of escape in more aggressive acute allograft rejection in patients on standard immunosuppression where IL17 appears to drive the intensity of allograft inflamma-tion. Thus synergistic inhibition of Th1 and IL17 pathways could

be very promising and has been suggested by others [5]. On the contrary, Huh et al. found that cardiac glycosides inhibited differentiation of Th17 cells in vitro with high specificity by binding to the transcription factor RORyt [37]. This did not only result in a decreased IL17 transcription and production, but the isolate inhibition of RORyt by cardiac glycosides additionally resulted in reciprocal increased T-cell IFN-y and FOXP3 expression. The results by Huh et al further support our findings that a synergistic inhibition of both IFN-y and IL17 pathways as seen with Fenofibrate may be especially relevant in diseases where both immune axes play a significant role such as in acute allograft rejection.

Despite this evidence, IL17 inhibitors are not currently used in transplantation and in the absence of any available synthetic IL17 inhibitors, we thus pursued the approach of drug repositioning Fenofibrate, a commercially available FDA approved drug, used for treatment of hyperlipidemia, and inferred from our study, to simultaneously inhibit the IL17 pathway and the Th1 mediated IFN-γ pathway in acute graft rejection. Although Fenofibrate has never been used in transplantation, several studies including the FIELD study [11], indicated general anti-inflammatory pleiotropic effects in patients who were treated with Fenofibrate. In addition to Fenofibrate, steroids currently used in the post-transplant management of AR, were noted to also regulate many of the input AR genes in our dataset, supporting the reliability of our approach, though it is important to note that steroids did not regulate IL17. As Fenofibrate had been shown to inhibit expression of both the IL17 and the Th1 response gene IFN-γ [10], Fenofibrate represented a very promising candidate for repositioning in transplantation. Thus, we characterized the anti-inflammatory effects of Fenofibrate in organ transplant rejection related to the inhibition of the IL17 and IFN-γ/Th1 responses, both locally in the allograft and systemically in the spleen of

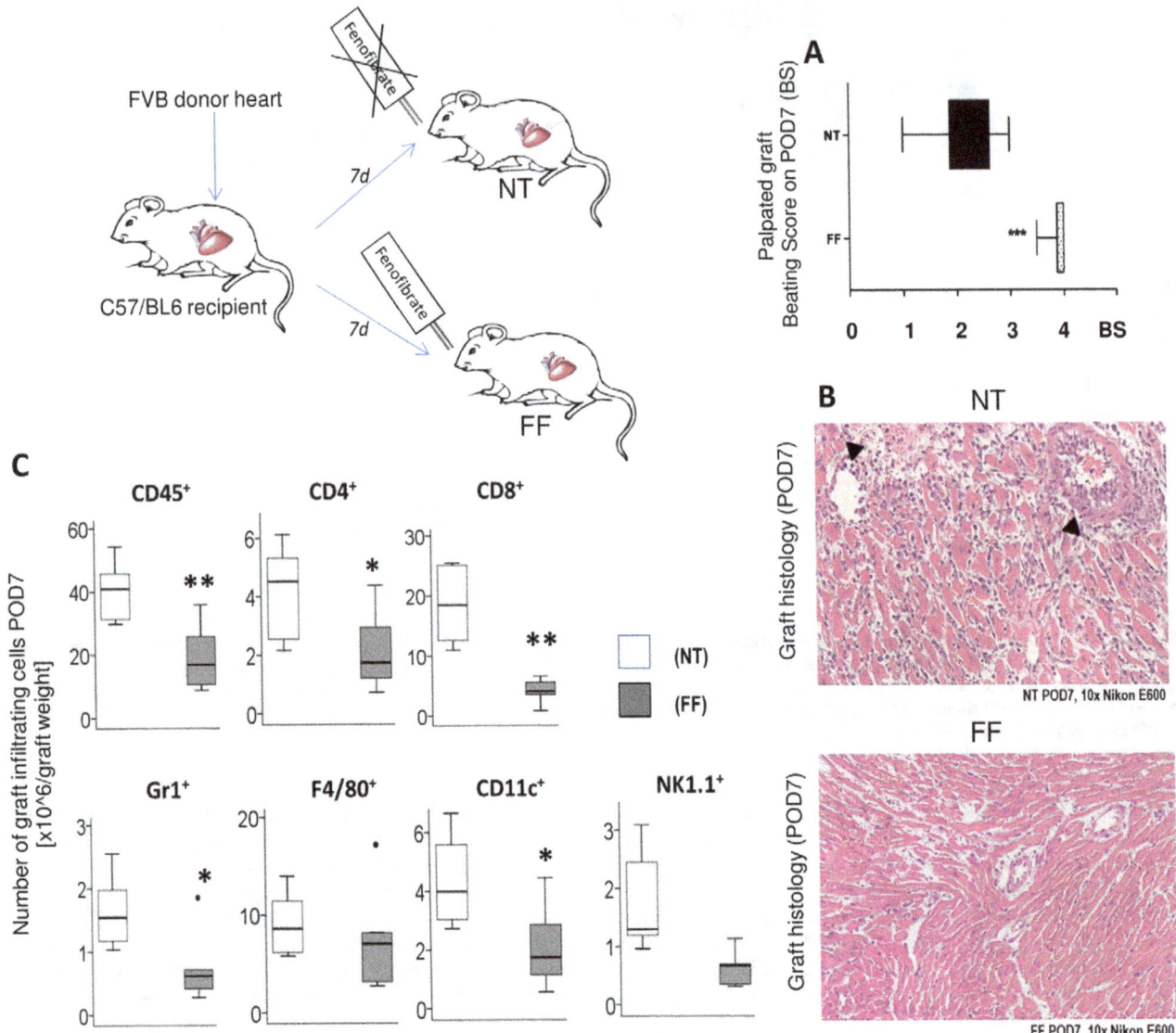

Figure 5. Significant improvement of graft function, graft histology and significant reduction in graft cell infiltration with Fenofibrate treatment. Palpated graft beating in transplanted mice was assessed daily and assigned a beating score (BS). Transplanted mice BS were significantly improved when treated with Fenofibrate (FF) compared to non- treated ones (NT) (n = 6, p<0.001; shown are mean BS plus SEM), (a). H&E stainings of mice grafts at POD7 revealed decreased cellular infiltrates and histological damage upon Fenofibrate treatment (b). FACS of infiltrating cells from the same grafts showed significantly reduced numbers of infiltrating innate and adaptive immune cells in the Fenofibrate treated mice (*p<0.05, **p<0.01, 2-sided Student T-test, n = 6). Box Plots show median and first and third quartiles of infiltrating cells corrected for total number of infiltrating cells and total graft weight.

rejecting animals. We could show profound attenuation of graft rejection and most importantly Fenofibrate extended graft survival by 11 days over no-treatment and was almost as efficient as standard immunosuppression.

The exact mechanism by which Fenofibrate inhibited the IL17 and the Th1 response in our model is not clear, but our gene expression analyses both in PBMC and in mouse grafts and spleens suggested an effect upstream of IL17, as the IL17 pathway activating genes IL1-β, TGF-β and IL6 were significantly decreased by Fenofibrate. IL6 is known to induce the IL17 pathway promoting the differentiation of IL17 producing T-cells [38], and was also increased in human AR [35,39]. Importantly inhibition of the Th1 response in IL-6 deficient mice had a synergistic effect on attenuating AR [39], similarly to inhibition

of IL-6 in T-bet deficient mice [2], both also leading to decreased IL17. Here, we showed that Fenofibrate treatment of experimental AR resulted in simultaneous inhibition of Th1 response genes and of IL6. Our results further suggest that Fenofibrate also regulates the IL17 pathway independent from the IL17+ T-helper cell specific transcription factors ROR-α and −γ, as these were not significantly reduced in mice treated with Fenofibrate. On the other hand, there was significant down regulation of STAT3 in spleens from mice treated with Fenofibrate. Only very recently, an experimental study of murine in-vitro Th-cell differentiation showed that Fenofibrate inhibited a differentiation of IL17 producing CD4+ T-cells, providing another line of evidence for Fenofibrate on the IL17-pathway [40]. In this study, the authors were able to show a dose response curve on IL17 producing T-

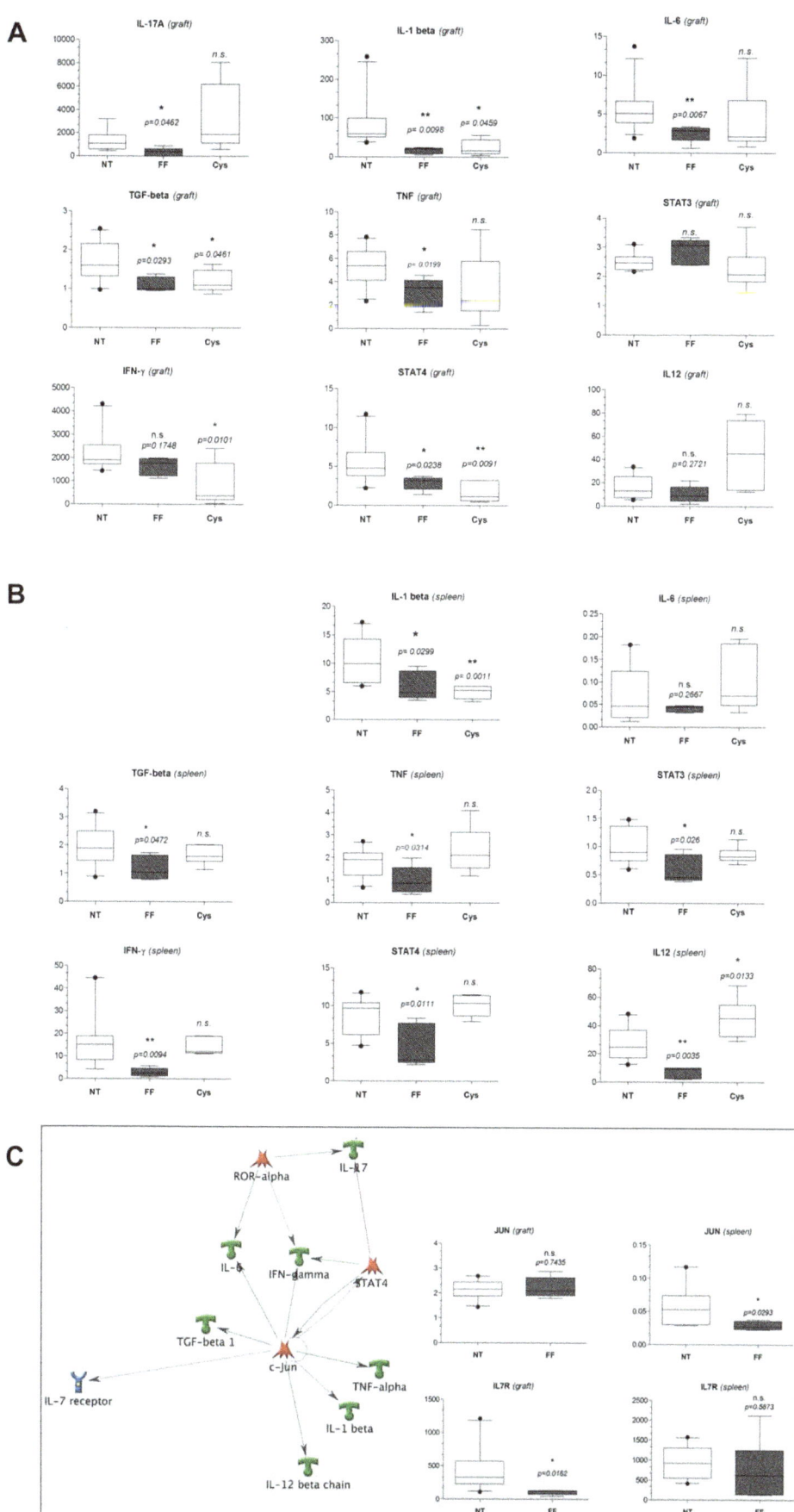

Figure 6. Gene Expression Profiles of Fenofibrate Effects in mouse grafts and spleens: significant repression of IL17 and Th1 genes in vivo in spleens and grafts and formation of a single network of direct interactions. PCR of RNA from mice cardiac allografts (5a) and recipient spleens (b) corroborated in vitro findings and further characterized the mechanism of Fenofibrate to regulate the IL17 pathway and Th1 response (c). Gene expression results in mice recipient grafts (a,c) and spleens (b,c) at POD7 are displayed as box and whisker plots of mean relative fold changes with 10th and 90th percentile to universal RNA after 18S normalization using the $\Delta\Delta Ct$ method. Significance between Fenofibrate (FF) treatment over no treatment (NT) and between Cyclosporine (Cys) treatment over no treatment were calculated by a 2-sided Student t-test and a p-value of $p<0.05$ considered as significant. Results of our additional network analyses in MetaCore revealed a central role for the transcription factor c-jun (c). Subsequent PCR for c-jun and its associated cytokine receptor IL7R showed decreased expression by Fenofibrate and suggested different sites of actions in spleen and grafts (c).

cells with Fenofibrate [40]. They used TGF-β, IL6, IL4 and IFN-γ to induce the IL17 producing CD4+ T-cells, all of which were upregulated in our study of experimental AR, and again down regulated with Fenofibrate.

We also provided additional data on the mechanism of Fenofibrate by our network analyses, where c-Jun was found to actually act on all genes regulated by Fenofibrate, either directly or indirectly. The protein c-Jun in combination with c-Fos forms the activator protein 1 (AP-1) early response transcription factor. Inhibition of AP-1 using decoy oligonucleotides at day of transplantation was efficient in attenuating cardiac vasculopathy in rats [41]. Here, c-jun was significantly upregulated in mice allografts with AR, and Fenofibrate treatment led to significant down regulation of c-Jun in cardiac grafts compared to no treatment, suggesting a potential central anti-inflammatory mechanism of Fenofibrate on T-cells.

A retrospective analysis of human transplant recipients receiving Fenofibrate is currently under way to evaluate any synergistic protective role of Fenofibrate on acute and chronic graft rejection (Roedder et al, manuscript under preparation). Additional analysis of the genome wide association study of inflammatory biomarker changes in response to Fenofibrate treatment [42] can shed additional light on selecting patients prior to transplantation that can benefit from a combination of Fenofibrate treatment with standard immunosuppression. This data supports that, in addition to standard immunosuppression, the inhibition of the IL17 pathway, may be effective in reducing the incidence and severity of acute rejection and thus positively impact on long term outcomes after organ transplantation and can potentially be achieved using Fenofibrate.

Acknowledgments

We thank Sarwal Lab (CPMCRI) and Fischbein Lab (Stanford University) for constructive discussion.

Author Contributions

Conceived and designed the experiments: SR NK MS. Performed the experiments: SR NK HO YG SH. Analyzed the data: SR NK. Contributed reagents/materials/analysis tools: MS. Wrote the paper: SR MS NK.

References

1. Dudley JT, Sirota M, Shenoy M, Pai RK, Roedder S, et al. (2011) Computational repositioning of the anticonvulsant topiramate for inflammatory bowel disease. Sci Transl Med 3: 96ra76.

2. Burrell BE, Csencsits K, Lu G, Grabauskiene S, Bishop DK (2008) CD8+ Th17 mediate costimulation blockade-resistant allograft rejection in T-bet-deficient mice. J Immunol 181: 3906–3914.

3. Kish DD, Li X, Fairchild RL (2009) CD8 T cells producing IL-17 and IFN-gamma initiate the innate immune response required for responses to antigen skin challenge. J Immunol 182: 5949–5959.

4. Loverre A, Tataranni T, Castellano G, Divella C, Battaglia M, et al. (2011) IL-17 expression by tubular epithelial cells in renal transplant recipients with acute antibody-mediated rejection. Am J Transplant 11: 1248–1259.

5. Yuan X, Paez-Cortez J, Schmitt-Knosalla I, D'Addio F, Mfarrej B, et al. (2008) A novel role of CD4 Th17 cells in mediating cardiac allograft rejection and vasculopathy. J Exp Med 205: 3133–3144.

6. Yapici U, Kers J, Bemelman FJ, Roelofs JJ, Groothoff JW, et al. (2011) Interleukin-17 positive cells accumulate in renal allografts during acute rejection and are independent predictors of worse graft outcome. Transpl Int 24: 1008–1017.

7. Li L, Huang L, Vergis AL, Ye H, Bajwa A, et al. (2010) IL-17 produced by neutrophils regulates IFN-gamma-mediated neutrophil migration in mouse kidney ischemia-reperfusion injury. J Clin Invest 120: 331–342.

8. Itoh S, Kimura N, Axtell RC, Velotta JB, Gong Y, et al. (2011) Interleukin-17 accelerates allograft rejection by suppressing regulatory T cell expansion. Circulation 124: S187–196.

9. Vokaer B, Van Rompaey N, Lemaitre PH, Lhomme F, Kubjak C, et al. (2010) Critical role of regulatory T cells in Th17-mediated minor antigen-disparate rejection. J Immunol 185: 3417–3425.

10. Lee JW, Bajwa PJ, Carson MJ, Jeske DR, Cong Y, et al. (2007) Fenofibrate represses interleukin-17 and interferon-gamma expression and improves colitis in interleukin-10-deficient mice. Gastroenterology 133: 108–123.

11. Belfort R, Berria R, Cornell J, Cusi K (2010) Fenofibrate reduces systemic inflammation markers independent of its effects on lipid and glucose metabolism in patients with the metabolic syndrome. The Journal of clinical endocrinology and metabolism 95: 829–836.

12. Solez K, Colvin RB, Racusen LC, Haas M, Sis B, et al. (2008) Banff 07 classification of renal allograft pathology: updates and future directions. American journal of transplantation : official journal of the American Society of Transplantation and the American Society of Transplant Surgeons 8: 753–760.

13. World Medical Association I (2009) Declaration of Helsinki. Ethical principles for medical research involving human subjects. J Indian Med Assoc 107: 403–405.

14. Kuri AD (2008) The law and the ethic in human transplantation. The Declaration of Istanbul. Rev Med Inst Mex Seguro Soc 46: 581–582.

15. Racusen LC, Halloran PF, Solez K (2004) Banff 2003 meeting report: new diagnostic insights and standards. Am J Transplant 4: 1562–1566.

16. Rodder S, Scherer A, Korner M, Eisenberger U, Hertig A, et al. (2010) Meta-analyses qualify metzincins and related genes as acute rejection markers in renal transplant patients. Am J Transplant 10: 286–297.

17. Corry R, Russell P (1973) New possibilities for organ allografting in the mouse. Immunological aspects of transplantation surger. New York: Wiley. 279.

18. Fischbein MP, Ardehali A, Yun J, Schoenberger S, Laks H, et al. (2000) CD40 signaling replaces CD4+ lymphocytes and its blocking prevents chronic rejection of heart transplants. J Immunol 165: 7316–7322.

19. Sarwal M, Chua MS, Kambham N, Hsieh SC, Satterwhite T, et al. (2003) Molecular heterogeneity in acute renal allograft rejection identified by DNA microarray profiling. The New England journal of medicine 349: 125–138.

20. Tanaka M, Mokhtari GK, Balsam LB, Cooke DT, Kofidis T, et al. (2005) Cyclosporine mitigates graft coronary artery disease in murine cardiac allografts: description and validation of a novel fully allogeneic model. J Heart Lung Transplant 24: 446–453.

21. Duez H, Chao YS, Hernandez M, Torpier G, Poulain P, et al. (2002) Reduction of atherosclerosis by the peroxisome proliferator-activated receptor alpha agonist fenofibrate in mice. J Biol Chem 277: 48051–48057.

22. Li C, Wong WH (2001) Model-based analysis of oligonucleotide arrays: expression index computation and outlier detection. Proceedings of the National Academy of Sciences of the United States of America 98: 31–36.

23. Oikawa M, Yoshiura KI, Kondo H, Miura S, Nagayasu T, et al. (2011) Significance of Genomic Instability in Breast Cancer in Atomic Bomb Survivors: Analysis of Microarray-Comparative Genomic Hybridization. Radiat Oncol 6: 168.

24. Rodder S, Scherer A, Raulf F, Berthier CC, Hertig A, et al. (2009) Renal allografts with IF/TA display distinct expression profiles of metzincins and related genes. Am J Transplant 9: 517–526.

25. Tusher VG, Tibshirani R, Chu G (2001) Significance analysis of microarrays applied to the ionizing radiation response. Proceedings of the National Academy of Sciences of the United States of America 98: 5116–5121.

26. Shahbaba B, Tibshirani R, Shachaf CM, Plevritis SK (2011) Bayesian gene set analysis for identifying significant biological pathways. J R Stat Soc Ser C Appl Stat 60: 541–557.

27. Ma S, Kosorok MR, Huang J, Xie H, Manzella L, et al. (2006) Robust semiparametric microarray normalization and significance analysis. Biometrics 62: 555–561.

28. Olson NE (2006) The microarray data analysis process: from raw data to biological significance. NeuroRx 3: 373–383.

29. Subramanian A, Tamayo P, Mootha VK, Mukherjee S, Ebert BL, et al. (2005) Gene set enrichment analysis: a knowledge-based approach for interpreting genome-wide expression profiles. Proceedings of the National Academy of Sciences of the United States of America 102: 15545–15550.

30. Cosmi L, De Palma R, Santarlasci V, Maggi L, Capone M, et al. (2008) Human interleukin 17-producing cells originate from a CD161+CD4+ T cell precursor. J Exp Med 205: 1903–1916.

31. Nagai S, Hashimoto S, Yamashita T, Toyoda N, Satoh T, et al. (2001) Comprehensive gene expression profile of human activated T(h)1- and T(h)2-polarized cells. Int Immunol 13: 367–376.

32. Rodriguez ER, International Society for H, Lung T (2003) The pathology of heart transplant biopsy specimens: revisiting the 1990 ISHLT working formulation. J Heart Lung Transplant 22: 3–15.

33. Billingham M, Kobashigawa JA (2005) The revised ISHLT heart biopsy grading scale. J Heart Lung Transplant 24: 1709.

34. Fabrega E, Lopez-Hoyos M, San Segundo D, Casafont F, Pons-Romero F (2009) Changes in the serum levels of interleukin-17/interleukin-23 during acute rejection in liver transplantation. Liver Transpl 15: 629–633.

35. Vanaudenaerde BM, De Vleeschauwer SI, Vos R, Meyts I, Bullens DM, et al. (2008) The role of the IL23/IL17 axis in bronchiolitis obliterans syndrome after lung transplantation. Am J Transplant 8: 1911–1920.

36. Gorbacheva V, Fan R, Li X, Valujskikh A (2010) Interleukin-17 promotes early allograft inflammation. The American Journal of pathology 177: 1265–1273.

37. Huh JR, Leung MW, Huang P, Ryan DA, Krout MR, et al. (2011) Digoxin and its derivatives suppress TH17 cell differentiation by antagonizing RORgammat activity. Nature 472: 486–490.

38. Korn T, Bettelli E, Oukka M, Kuchroo VK (2009) IL-17 and Th17 Cells. Annu Rev Immunol 27: 485–517.

39. Zhao X, Boenisch O, Yeung M, Mfarrej B, Yang S, et al. (2012) Critical role of proinflammatory cytokine IL-6 in allograft rejection and tolerance. Am J Transplant 12: 90–101.

40. Zhou Z, Sun W, Liang Y, Gao Y, Kong W, et al. (2012) Fenofibrate Inhibited the Differentiation of T Helper 17 Cells In Vitro. PPAR Res 2012: 145654.

41. Stadlbauer TH, Wagner AH, Holschermann H, Fiedel S, Fingerhuth H, et al. (2008) AP-1 and STAT-1 decoy oligodeoxynucleotides attenuate transplant vasculopathy in rat cardiac allografts. Cardiovasc Res 79: 698–705.

42. Aslibekyan S, Kabagambe EK, Irvin MR, Straka RJ, Borecki IB, et al. (2012) A genome-wide association study of inflammatory biomarker changes in response to fenofibrate treatment in the Genetics of Lipid Lowering Drug and Diet Network. Pharmacogenet Genomics 22: 191–197.

8

Distinct Innate Immune Gene Expression Profiles in Non-Melanoma Skin Cancer of Immunocompetent and Immunosuppressed Patients

Beda Muehleisen[1,2], Shang Brian Jiang[1], Julie A. Gladsjo[1], Monika Gerber[1], Tissa Hata[1], Richard L. Gallo[1,3,4]*

1 Division of Dermatology, University of California San Diego, La Jolla, California, United States of America, 2 Department of Dermatology, Zurich University Hospital, Zurich, Switzerland, 3 Department of Medicine, University of California San Diego, La Jolla, California, United States of America, 4 Veterans Administration San Diego Healthcare System, San Diego, California, United States of America

Abstract

Squamous cell carcinoma (SCC) and basal cell carcinoma (BCC) are the most frequent skin cancers in humans. An intact immune system is critical for protection against SCC since organ transplant recipients (OTR) have a 60- to 100-fold higher risk for developing these tumors. The role of the innate immune system in tumor immunosurveillance is unclear. Our aim was to determine the expression of selected innate immune genes in BCC and SCC arising in immunocompetent and OTR patients. Lesional and peri-lesional skin from 28 SCC and 19 BCC were evaluated for mRNA expression of toll-like receptors (TLR) 1–9, downstream TLR signaling molecules, and antimicrobial peptides. 11 SCC occurring in OTR patients were included in the analysis. We found that SCC but not BCC showed significantly elevated expression of TLRs 1–3, 5–8, TRIF and TRAF1. TNF was increased in SCC compared to normal skin. BCC showed increased IFNγ. hBD1, hBD2 and psoriasin mRNA and protein expression were significantly higher in SCC than in normal skin and higher than in BCC. SCC from OTR showed only an increase in hBD2 but no increase in hBD1 or psoriasin. We conclude that innate immune gene expression in SCC is distinct from normal skin and BCC. BCC shows lesser induction of innate immune genes. SCC from OTR patients have depressed expression of hBD1 and psoriasin compared to SCC from immunocompetent patients.

Editor: Amanda Ewart Toland, Ohio State University Medical Center, United States of America

Funding: This work was supported by United States National Institutes of Health grants R01 AR052728, R01 AI052453, R01 AI0833358, and the Swiss National Science Foundation (PBZHP3-125571, PASMP3_140073) to B.M. The funding institutions had no role in study design, data collection and analysis, decision to publish, or preparation of the manuscript.

Competing Interests: The authors have declared that no competing interests exist.

* E-mail: rgallo@ucsd.edu

Introduction

Basal cell carcinoma (BCC) and squamous cell carcinoma (SCC) are the most frequent non-melanoma skin cancers (NMSC) in humans [1]. In the U.S.A. more than 3 million cases of BCC and SCC are estimated to occur annually [2–3]. However, although significant progress has been made in understanding the pathogenesis of NMSC, the host immune defense mechanisms that predict patient outcome are still largely unknown. The highly increased incidence of skin cancers in immunosuppressed patients such as organ transplant recipients (OTRs) [4] has clearly shown the importance of the immune system in controlling the development of NMSC. Furthermore, because ultraviolet (UV) radiation has important immunomodulatory properties [5–6], its contribution as a major risk factor for NMSC is amplified.

Currently, most research on tumor immunosurveillance in NMSC, including those within the framework of cancer immunoediting [7–8], have focused mainly on T-cell mediated, adaptive immune mechanisms. However, there is evidence that innate immune mechanisms are also important in NMSC. Early studies by William Coley demonstrated spontaneous tumor regression after developing postsurgical infections [9], and experimental administration of *Streptococcus pyogenes* has also

resulted in tumor regression [10]. Today it is well known that infectious agents can be recognized by keratinocytes and other immune cells through various genes of the innate immune system such as toll-like receptors (TLRs). Recognition of microbes results in expression of antimicrobial peptides (AMPs), cytokines and chemokines [11–15].

The activation of an innate immune response has diverse consequences. AMPs can kill microbes and prevent infection [13,16–17]. Furthermore, AMPs can act in a manner similar to chemokines and have pro- and anti-inflammatory effects, stimulate angiogenesis and induce cell death [12,14,18] - effects that might be relevant also in carcinogenesis. Prior work in tumors such as oral squamous cell carcinoma showed enhanced expression of the AMPs human β-defensin 2 and psoriasin and this correlated with the clinicopathological features [19–20]. Furthermore, the expression of cathelicidin by NK cells has been directly shown to limit the growth rate of melanoma in mouse models [21]. More evidence for a role of the innate immune system in NMSC stems from treatment with TLR7 agonist imiquimod which is effective against superficial primary skin tumors and cutaneous metastases, including BCC, actinic keratosis and Bowen's disease [22].

Since very little data has been published on innate immune responses in NMSC we wished to provide an overview of innate immune gene expression in a population of patients with SCCs and BCCs, focusing on TLRs, TLR-signaling intermediates, cytokines and antimicrobial peptides. Since OTRs have a significantly higher risk for SCC [4], this study also included 11 SCCs from OTRs to characterize innate immune gene expression in that high risk population. We report that NMSCs have distinct expression patterns of several genes critical to innate immunity.

Results

Enhanced mRNA Expression of Epidermal Differentiation Genes in SCC

A total population of 37 patients was included in this study, comprising 28 patients with SCC and 19 with BCC. SCCs came from 17 immunocompetent patients and 11 that were OTR. Patient demographics in each group were similar with the exception of OTR who were generally younger (**Figure 1a,b**). Samples for analysis were taken from distant normal skin, peritumoral skin, at the tumor margin, and from central tumor tissue (See methods and **Figure 1c**).

Cutaneous SCC typically retains characteristics of squamous differentiation. To further characterize the specimens in our study, we measured mRNA expression of several epidermal differentiation genes. Samples within the central tumor tissue of SCC showed significantly elevated mRNA expression of filaggrin (13.60 ± 4.52-fold (mean $\pm$ SEM), $p<0.05$) and keratin 10 (10.83 ± 0.51-fold, $p<0.001$) compared to normal skin. Filaggrin and keratin 10 expression in the tumor center was also higher compared to the tumor margin (0.44 ± 0.22, $p<0.001$; 1.56 ± 0.51, $p<0.05$) and to peritumoral tissue (0.62 ± 0.18, $p<0.001$; 1.19 ± 0.34, $p<0.01$). Filaggrin and keratin 10 expression in the tumor center of SCC was also significantly higher than in the tumor center of BCC (5.50 ± 2.98, $p<0.05$; 0.39 ± 0.09, $p<0.001$). For loricrin, reduced mRNA expression in the tumor margin of SCC was observed compared to normal skin (0.073 ± 0.021, $p<0.001$), the tumor center (8.29 ± 5.29, $p<0.001$) and peritumoral tissue (0.33 ± 0.08, $p<0.05$) (**Figure 2**).

Enhanced TLR Expression in SCC

TLR1 mRNA expression in the SCC tumor center was 5.49 ± 1.21-fold higher ($p<0.01$) than in normal skin and also significantly higher than in the tumor center of BCCs (1.82 ± 1.21, $p<0.001$). TLR2 mRNA expression in the SCC tumor center was 7.90 ± 1.76-fold higher ($p<0.01$) than in normal skin and also higher than in the tumor center of BCCs (1.41 ± 0.35, $p<0.001$). TLR3 mRNA expression in the SCC tumor center was 8.51 ± 2.11-fold higher ($p<0.01$) than in normal skin and also higher than in peritumoral tissue (1.61 ± 0.70, $p<0.05$). TLR5 mRNA expression in the SCC tumor center showed the largest magnitude difference and was 30.8 ± 22.9-fold higher ($p<0.05$) than in normal skin and also significantly higher than in the tumor center of BCCs (0.92 ± 0.46, $p<0.01$). TLR6 mRNA expression was significantly higher in the SCC tumor center (4.48 ± 1.44) than in the tumor margin (0.96 ± 0.48, $p<0.05$). TLR7 mRNA expression in the SCC tumor center was 15.6 ± 3.70-fold higher than in normal skin ($p<0.001$) and also significantly higher than in peritumoral tissue (3.37 ± 1.35, $p<0.01$) and than in the tumor center of BCCs (1.98 ± 0.53, $p<0.001$).

Of note, TLR8 mRNA expression was significantly higher in the peritumoral tissue of SCC (13.93 ± 0.57) as well as in the tumor center (7.46 ± 4.99) compared to normal skin ($p<0.05$ for both)

and significantly higher compared to BCC peritumoral (0.36 ± 0.21) and BCC tumor center tissue (0.35 ± 0.14) ($p<0.01$ for both) (**Figure 3**).

Enhanced TRIF, TRAF1 and TNF Expression in SCC. Enhanced TNF and IFNγ Expression in BCC

Consistent with the increased expression of TLRs in SCC, gene products that are either downstream of the TLR signaling cascade, or inducible by TLR activation, were also elevated in SCC. TRIF mRNA expression in the SCC tumor center was 17.11 ± 5.14-fold higher than in normal skin ($p<0.01$), in peritumoral tissue (3.89 ± 2.51, $p<0.05$) and also significantly higher than in the tumor center of BCCs (3.13 ± 1.36, $p<0.001$). TRAF1 mRNA expression in the SCC tumor center was 9.62 ± 2.18-fold higher than in normal skin ($p<0.01$) and also significantly higher than in the tumor center of BCCs (3.40 ± 2.36, $p<0.05$). TNF mRNA expression in the SCC tumor center was 515 ± 144-fold higher than in normal skin ($p<0.001$) and also significantly higher than in the tumor center of BCCs (55.5 ± 29.3, $p<0.001$). In SCC, TNF mRNA expression was also significantly elevated in the tumor margin compared to normal skin (176.2 ± 89.4, $p<0.05$). BCC showed also significantly higher TNF expression (55.5 ± 29.3 vs. 1.02 ± 0.55, $p<0.05$) and higher IFNγ expression (17.1 ± 4.1 vs. 1.01 ± 0.04, $p<0.05$) than in normal skin (**Figure 4**).

Enhanced Expression of hBD1 and 2 and Psoriasin in SCC. BCC Shows Less Expression of CAMP, hBD1-3, RNase7 and Psoriasin than SCC

hBD1 mRNA expression in the SCC tumor center was 50.36 ± 28.90-fold higher than in normal skin ($p<0.05$), in the tumor margin (0.93 ± 0.44, $p<0.05$) and also significantly higher than in the tumor center of BCCs (1.08 ± 0.45, $p<0.001$). In BCC hBD1 mRNA expression was significantly lower in the tumor margin than in the tumor center (0.15 ± 0.04 vs. 1.08 ± 0.45, $p<0.05$). hBD2 mRNA expression in the SCC tumor center was 4748 ± 3934-fold higher than in normal skin ($p<0.005$), in the tumor margin (5.02 ± 2.11, $p<0.01$) and also significantly higher than in the tumor center of BCCs (58.36 ± 40.56, $p<0.05$). In BCC hBD2.

mRNA expression was significantly higher in the tumor center (58.36 ± 40.56) than in the tumor margin (0.61 ± 0.26, $p<0.05$) or in the peritumoral tissue (0.30 ± 0.11, $p<0.01$). Psoriasin(S100A7) is an abundant protein in the epidermis with much different antimicrobial activity than hBDs or cathelicidins. At protein concentrations exceeding 100 ug/ml psoriasin can partially inhibit the growth of Gram negative bacteria while hBDs and cathelicidins act at low micromolar concentrations against a broad range of bacteria, viruses and fungi [12,23–26]. mRNA expression for psoriasin in the SCC tumor center was 1334 ± 690-fold higher than in normal skin ($p<0.05$) and also significantly higher than in the tumor center of BCCs (27.41 ± 14.50, $p<0.001$). Cathelicidin and hBD3 mRNA expression were significantly lower in the tumor center of BCC compared to SCC (0.72 ± 0.14 vs. 1.71 ± 0.39, $p<0.05$; 9.59 ± 5.15 vs. 2497 ± 1447, $p<0.001$) (**Figure 5**). In line with elevated mRNA expression, immunofluorescence staining also revealed enhanced protein expression for hBD1, hBD2 and psoriasin in SCC compared to normal skin or BCC (**Figure 6**).

Lack of an Increase of hBD1 and psoriasin Expression in OTR

A direct comparison was made between the expression of all target genes in OTR and immunocompetent patients (ICP).

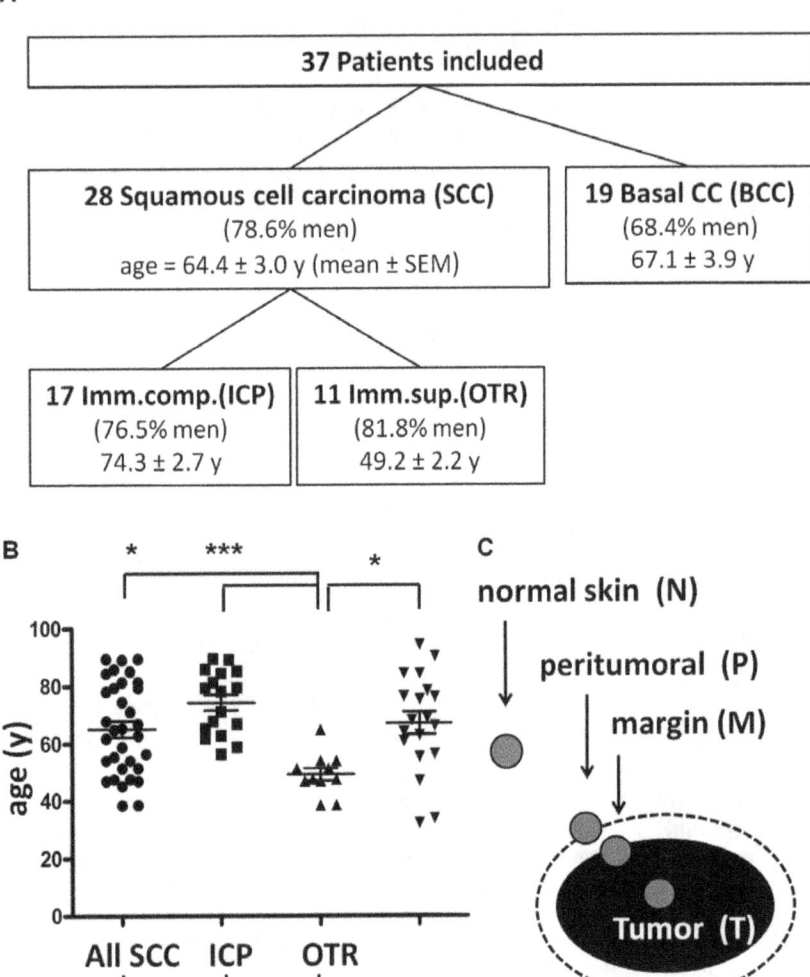

Figure 1. Patients enrolled and sample collection. 1A) Patients enrolled in the study, tumor diagnoses and immune status. SCC = squamous cell carcinoma. BCC = basal cell carcinoma. Imm'comp. (ICP) = immunocompetent patients. Imm.sup.(OTR) = organ transplant recipients (immunosuppressed patients). Gender (percentage male) and age (mean ± SEM) distribution in each group of patients is shown. 1 B) Age distribution in patient groups. Scatter plots including mean ± SEM are shown. *p < 0.05, ***p < 0.005 (one-way ANOVA with Bonferroni's post-test). 1 C) From each case, a specimen was collected from the center of the tumor (T), from the tumor margin (M) including tumor cells as well as non-tumor cells, from peritumoral tissue (P) that does not contain any tumor cells, and from normal control skin (N) in far distance from the tumor.

Differences in gene expression between OTR and ICP were only found for antimicrobial peptide genes and are displayed in **figure 7**. For all other genes in this study with similar expression between ICP and OTR, both patient categories were merged (n = 28 SCC) for statistical comparison to BCCs and for presentation in figures 2–4.

As in ICPs, SCC in OTRs showed enhanced hBD2 mRNA expression in the tumor center (233.5±149.2) compared to the tumor margin (3.11±2.16, p<0.05), peritumoral tissue (1.22±0.95, p<0.01) and normal skin (2.14±1.61, p<0.05). However, in contrast to ICPs, SCC in OTRs did not overexpress hBD1 or psoriasin. Psoriasin mRNA expression in the tumor center of SCC in OTRs was significantly lower than in ICPs (71.9±49.1 vs. 1334±690, p<0.01) (**Figure 7**). Further supporting these findings were our results from immunohistofluorescence staining showing also lower hBD1 and psoriasin protein expression in SCC from OTRs compared to ICPs (Figure 6).

Discussion

This study sought to provide an in depth analysis of innate immune gene expression in NMSC. The goal of this work was to further understand how our skin responds to the development of tumors and thus gain essential information that can help guide therapy. The candidate genes evaluated represented those such as TLRs that are involved in the innate immune recognition of danger, cytoplasmic molecules such as TRIF and TRAF that transmit information detected by these receptors, and molecules triggered by this process. These last groups of effector molecules are the AMPs and cytokines responsible for mediating the host response once danger is detected. Results show a dramatic difference in expression of many of these critical molecules in SCC, suggesting that this tumor type has enhanced many elements of innate immune response compared to normal skin. Since many of the effector molecules may play a role in the growth of the tumor or resistance to infection, and some are further altered in

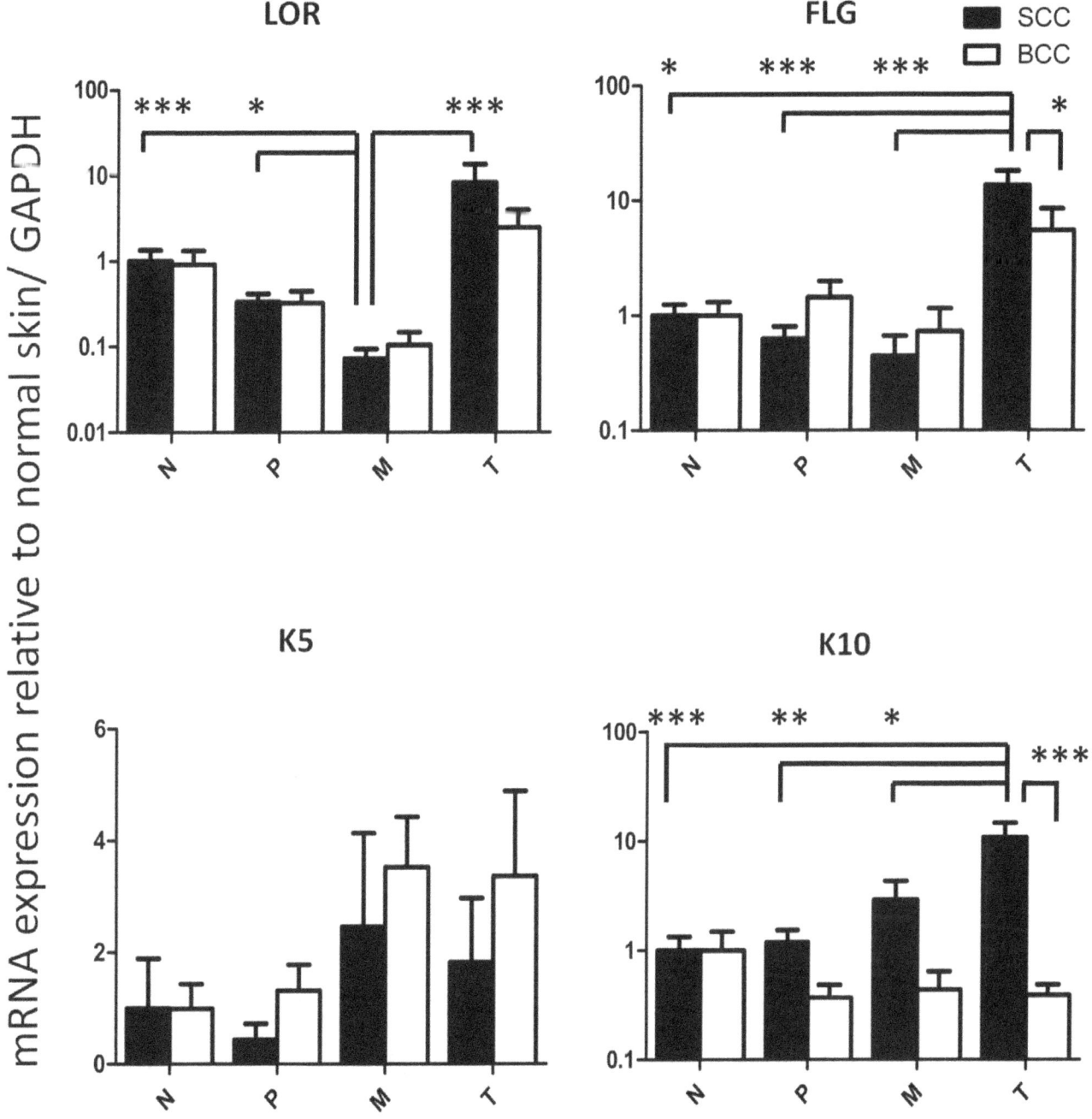

Figure 2. Distinct mRNA expression of differentiation genes in non-melanoma skin cancer. mRNA expression of differentiation gene loricrin (LOR), filaggrin (FLG), keratin 5 (K5) and keratin 10 (K10) in the tumor center (T), tumor margin (M), peritumoral tissue (P) and distant normal skin (N) in cutaneous squamous cell carcinoma (SCC, black bars) and basal cell carcinoma (BCC, white bars). Relative mRNA expression to glyceraldehyde 3-phosphate dehydrogenase (GAPDH) and normalized to normal skin is shown. Depicted are mean ± SEM values. *$p<0.05$, **$p<0.01$, ***$p<0.001$ by Kruskal-Wallis test with Dunn's post-test for comparison between N, P, M and T and by Mann Whitney U test for comparison between SCC and BCC in each group. N = 28 SCC and 19 BCC.

the immunocompromised host, these may partially explain the natural progression of NMSC.

Although full coverage of all molecules that participate in innate immunity would involve transcriptional profiling of several thousand gene products, and would be best approached by micro-array analysis [27] or RNASeq [28], the approach of real-time PCR analysis used here is the most quantitative and is commonly used for validation of high-throughput transcriptional

profiling results. Sample selection from each patient involved the tumor itself, peritumoral tissue and normal skin. Since each tissue specimen represented a heterogenous collection of cell types, our evaluation is limited by the inability to attribute the mRNA measured to specific resident cells, the malignancy itself, or recruited cell types. However, the data obtained reflected expected expression patterns for the tumor. For example, cutaneous SCC typically retains characteristics of squamous differentiation [29],

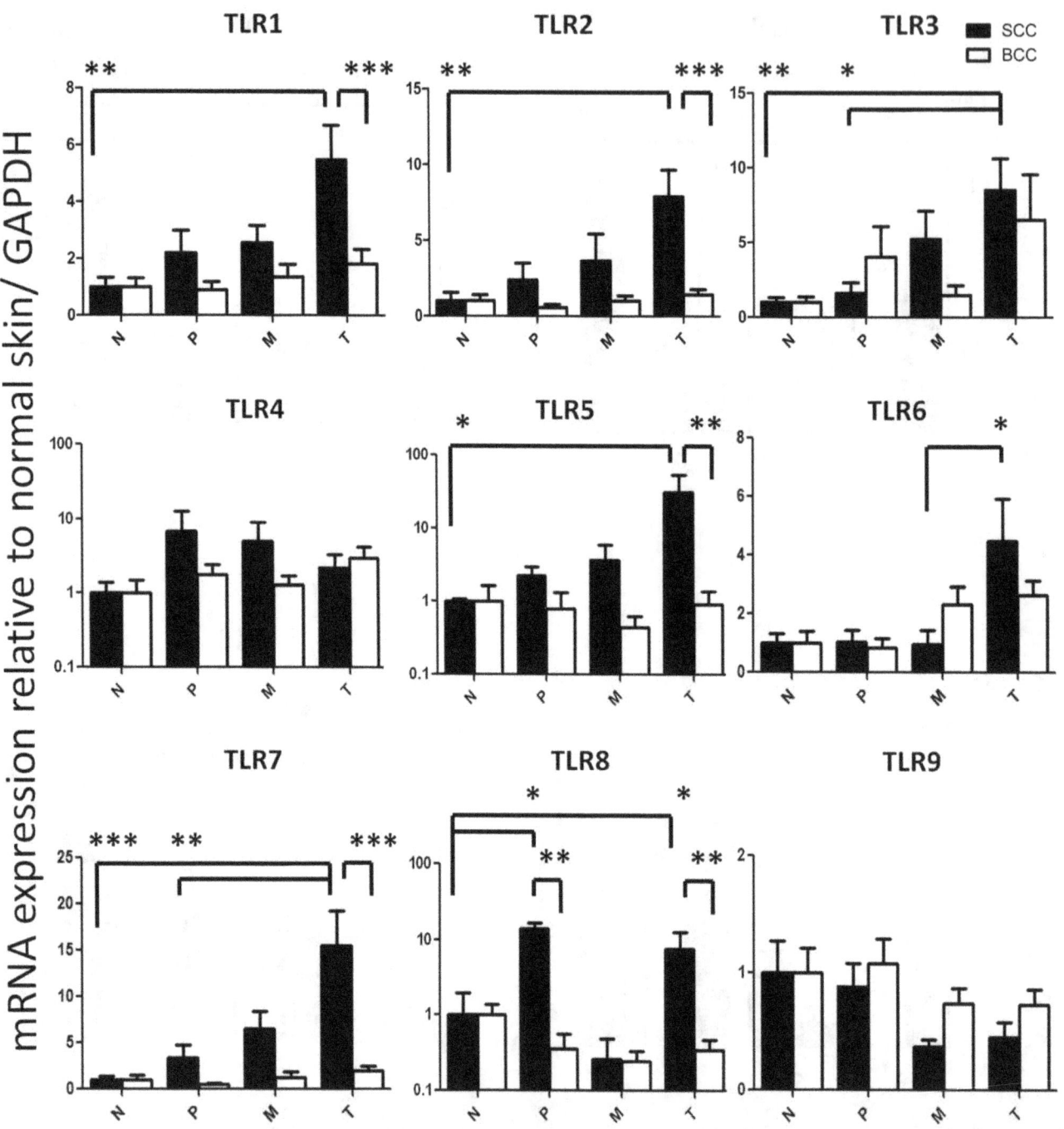

Figure 3. Distinct expression of toll like receptor genes in non-melanoma skin cancer. mRNA expression of toll like receptor genes 1–9 (TLR1-9) in the tumor center (T), tumor margin (M), peritumoral tissue (P) and distant normal skin (N) in cutaneous squamous cell carcinoma (SCC, black bars) and basal cell carcinoma (BCC, white bars). Relative mRNA expression to glyceraldehyde 3-phosphate dehydrogenase (GAPDH) and normalized to normal skin is shown. Depicted are mean ± SEM values. *p<0.05, **p<0.01, ***p<0.001 by Kruskal-Wallis test with Dunn's post-test for comparison between N, P, M and T and by Mann Whitney U test for comparison between SCC and BCC in each group. N = 28 SCC and 19 BCC.

and we found elevated filaggrin and keratin 10 gene expression in the SCC tissue of the tumor center. Expression was not only higher than in normal skin but also higher than in the tumor margin and in BCC. These results underline substantial differences in differentiation between SCC, BCC and normal skin, and served to validate the samples selected.

Activation of TLRs can result in a wide variety of responses that include apoptosis, inflammatory and non-inflammatory reactions

(reviewed in [11]). TLRs are known to be expressed on a variety of murine and human cancer cells (reviewed in [30]). However, little information is available on TLR expression in SCC, and this has come mostly from cervical [31–32] or head and neck SCC [33–34], but not from cutaneous SCC. Our study showed significantly elevated expression of TLR1,2,3,5,6,7 and 8 in cutaneous SCC. For several TLRs a 5- to 10-fold induction was seen in SCC. Notable responses unique to SCC included TLR5 (responsible for

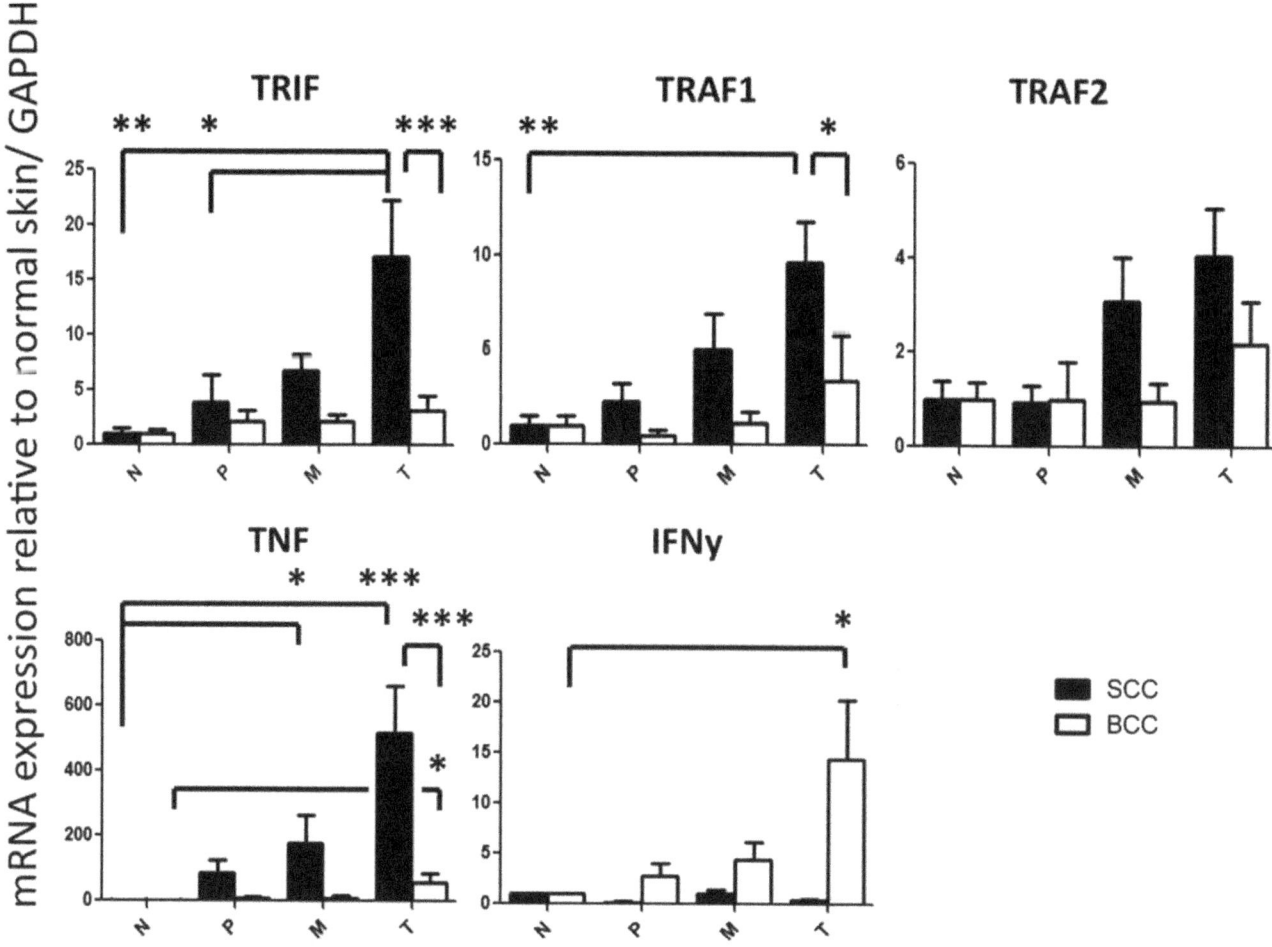

Figure 4. Distinct expression of innate immune receptor signaling molecules and cytokines in non-melanoma skin cancer. mRNA expression of TIR-domain-containing adaptor-inducing interferon-β (TRIF), TNF receptor-associated factors 1 and 2 (TRAF1 and 2), tumor necrosis factor (TNF) and interferon-γ (IFNγ) in the tumor center (T), tumor margin (M), peritumoral tissue (P) and distant normal skin (N) in cutaneous squamous cell carcinoma (SCC, black bars) and basal cell carcinoma (BCC, white bars). Relative mRNA expression to glyceraldehyde 3-phosphate dehydrogenase (GAPDH) and normalized to normal skin is shown. Depicted are mean ± SEM values. *p<0.05, **p<0.01, ***p<0.001 by Kruskal-Wallis test with Dunn's post-test for comparison between N, P, M and T and by Mann Whitney U test for comparison between SCC and BCC in each group. N = 28 SCC and 19 BCC.

recognition of flagellin), TLR7 (the target of imiquimod), and TLR8, which along with TLR7, can recognize RNA. The TLR8 response was particularly interesting as it also included an induction in the peri-tumoral region. We also observed high TLR2 expression in SCC which could be a characteristic of SCC or a result of a defective skin barrier in SCC. In this way the increase is comparable to the TLR2 upregulation seen in skin wounds [35]. Equally remarkable was the relatively little change in innate immune gene expression seen in BCC. This may be a pertinent negative response given that some TLR induction would be expected from damaged skin. To define a potential functional role of TLR overexpression in cutaneous SCC, further functional studies are needed.

TRIF and TRAF are downstream signaling molecules of TLR activation and their expression correlated with increased TLR expression in SCC. Similarly, the cytokine response was highest in SCC and correlated with increased TLR expression and signaling. However, in BCC TNF was significantly elevated compared to normal skin despite a lesser TLR response. Increased IFNγ was seen only in BCC. This underlines fundamental differences of innate immune receptor signaling and cytokine expression in BCC

and SCC and likely reflects both the local expression of these molecules and expression in recruited inflammatory cells.

Because of the action of AMPs to alter cell growth and differentiation [36], their expression may be highly relevant in cancer. This association has been directly demonstrated for cathelicidin, where in mouse tumor models a lack of cathelicidin resulted in much more rapid tumor growth [21]. In the present study we found increased hBD1, hBD2, hBD3 and psoriasin in SCC compared to normal skin, but no increase in cathelicidin. Previously, enhanced hBD2 expression was also reported for oral SCC tumor cells and intratumoral vascular endothelia [29,37–38]. Furthermore, previous studies reported increased hBD3 in *in-situ* and invasive oral SCC, correlating with specific macrophage recruitment to the lesion site [20,39]. In contrast, the expression of AMPs in BCCs was much different than SCC. We found a significant decrease of hBD1 expression in the invading tumor margin of BCC but not in the tumor center. A decrease in hBD1 was previously reported in BCC [40]. The functional significance of altered hBD expression in cancer is unclear at present. However, treatment of head and neck SCC (HNSCC) cell lines

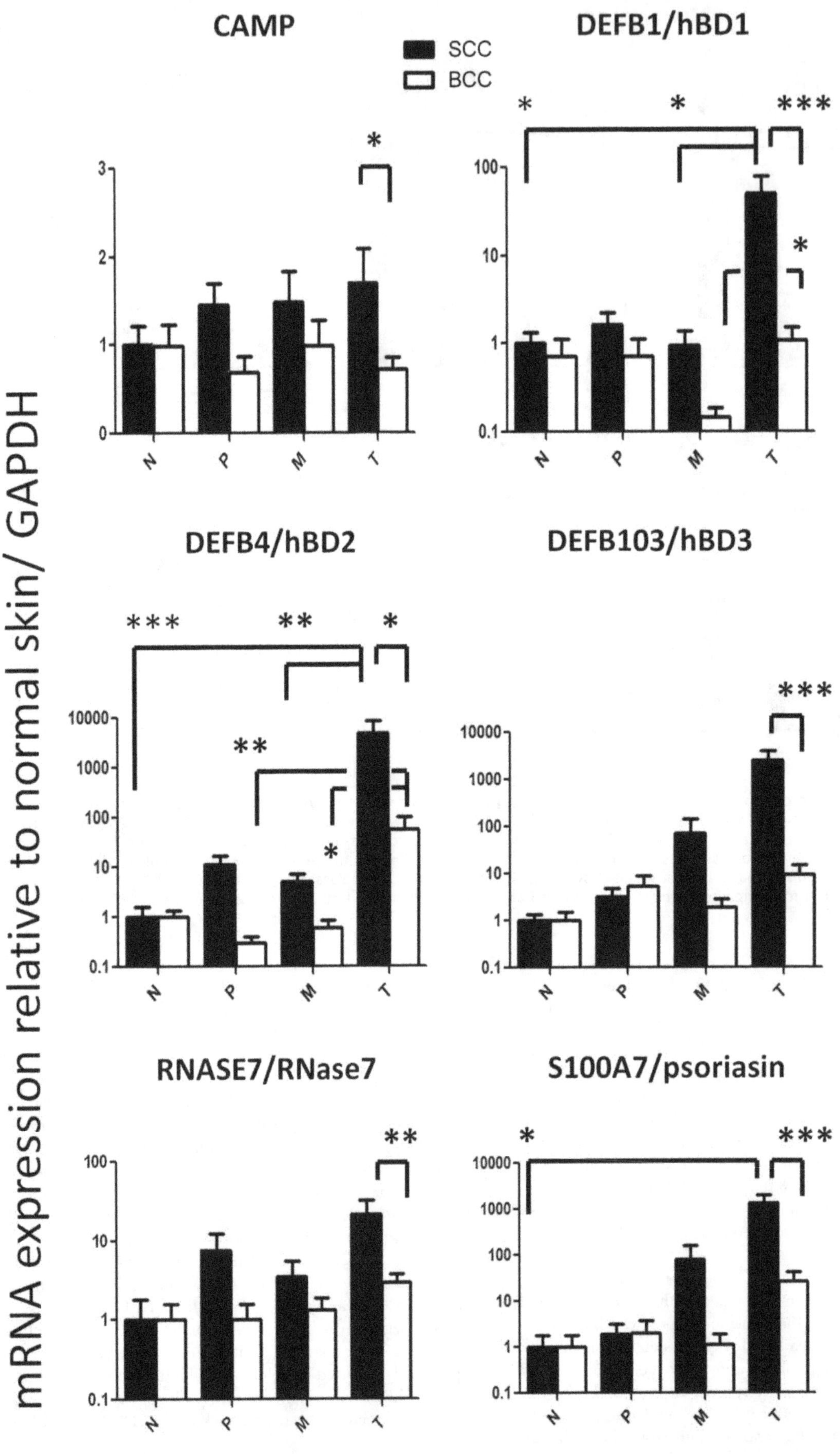

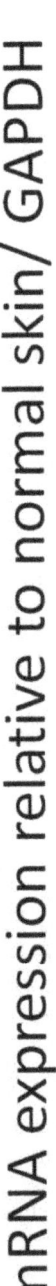

Figure 5. Distinct expression of antimicrobial peptides in non-melanoma skin cancer. mRNA expression of cathelicidin antimicrobial peptide (*CAMP*), human β-defensins 1–3 (hBD1–3, genes *DEFB1*, *DEFB4* and *DEFB103*), RNase 7 (*RNASE7*) and psoriasisin (S100A7) in the tumor center (T), tumor margin (M), peritumoral tissue (P) and distant normal skin (N) in cutaneous squamous cell carcinoma (SCC, black bars) and basal cell carcinoma (BCC, white bars). Relative mRNA expression to glyceraldehyde 3-phosphate dehydrogenase (GAPDH) and normalized to normal skin is shown. Depicted are mean ± SEM values. *p<0.05, **p<0.01, ***p<0.001 by Kruskal-Wallis test with Dunn's post-test for comparison between N, P, M and T and by Mann Whitney U test for comparison between SCC and BCC in each group. N = 17 SCC from immunocompetent patients (ICP) and 19 BCC.

with hBD3 improved resistance against cis platin, indicating that higher hBD expression may enhance tumor survival [41].

Psoriasin (S100A7) represents a much different type of molecule than the hBDs or cathelicidin and warrents separate discussion. Psoriasin is a much larger protein, is found in much greater abundance in skin, and has different antimicrobial activity

(reviewed in [25]). It also does not appear to be expressed by bone marrow derived cells as is the case with many antimicrobial peptides. Rather, psoriasin is expressed primarily in a variety of epithelia. The functions of psoriasin in immunity are thus less clear although it has been associated with resistance to skin surface colonization by *E. coli* [24]. A previous study described elevated

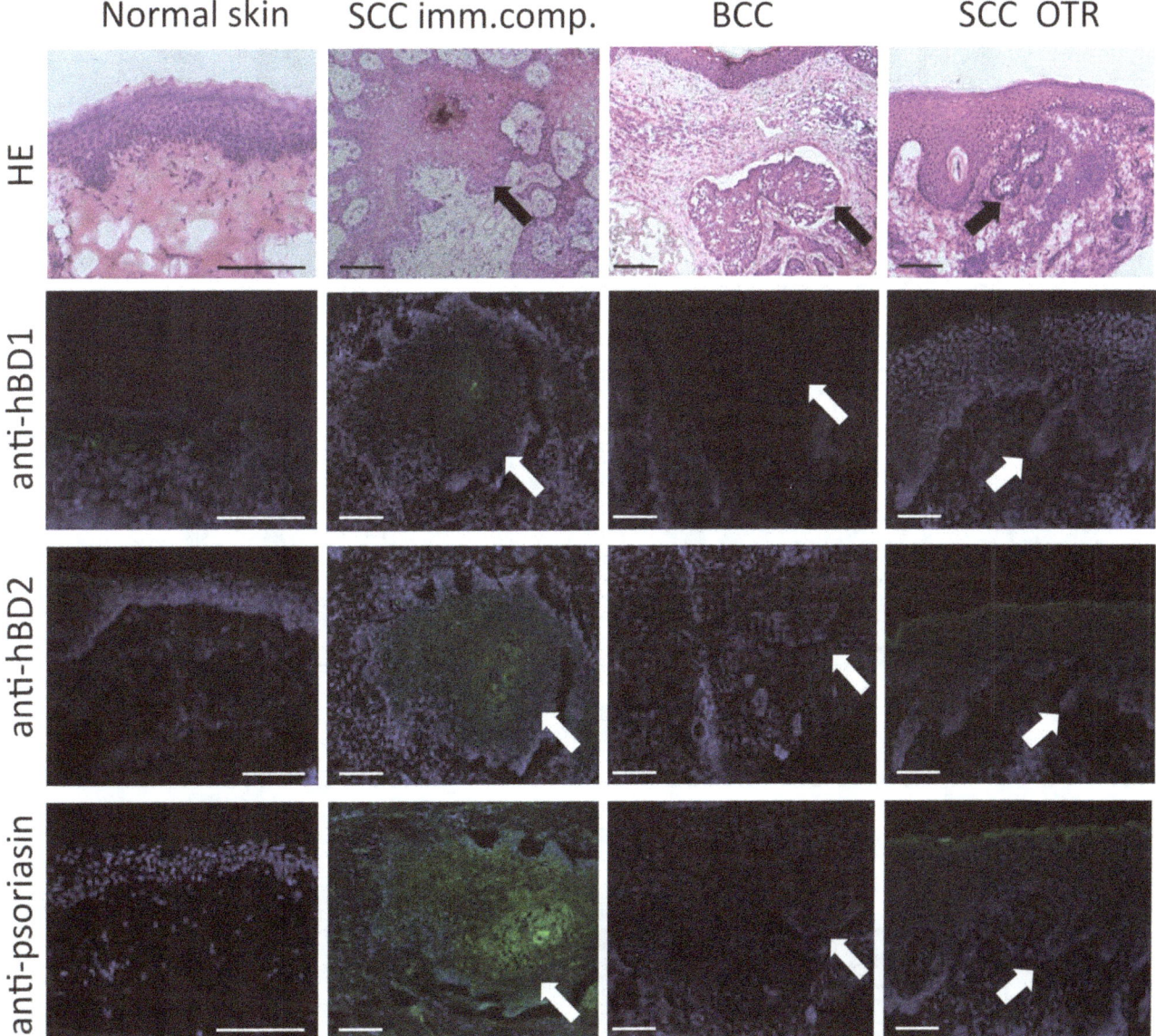

Figure 6. Distinct protein expression of the antimicrobial peptides hBD1, hBD2 and psoriasin in squamous cell carcinoma of immunocompetent patients and organ transplant recipients. Protein expression of the antimicrobial peptides hBD1, hBD2 and psoriasin as detected by immunofluorescence staining (green) in normal skin, basal cell carcinoma (BCC) and squamous cell carcinomas in immunocompetent patients (SCC imm.comp.) and organ transplant recipients (SCC OTR). Nuclei were visualized with 4′-6-diamidino-2-phenylindole (DAPI, blue). The top row shows hematoxylin and eosin (HE) staining of the same skin samples. Arrows point at groups of tumor cells. Bar = 100 μm. Data are representative of five samples each.

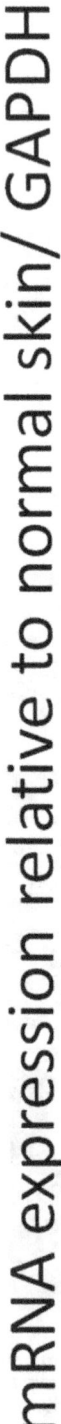

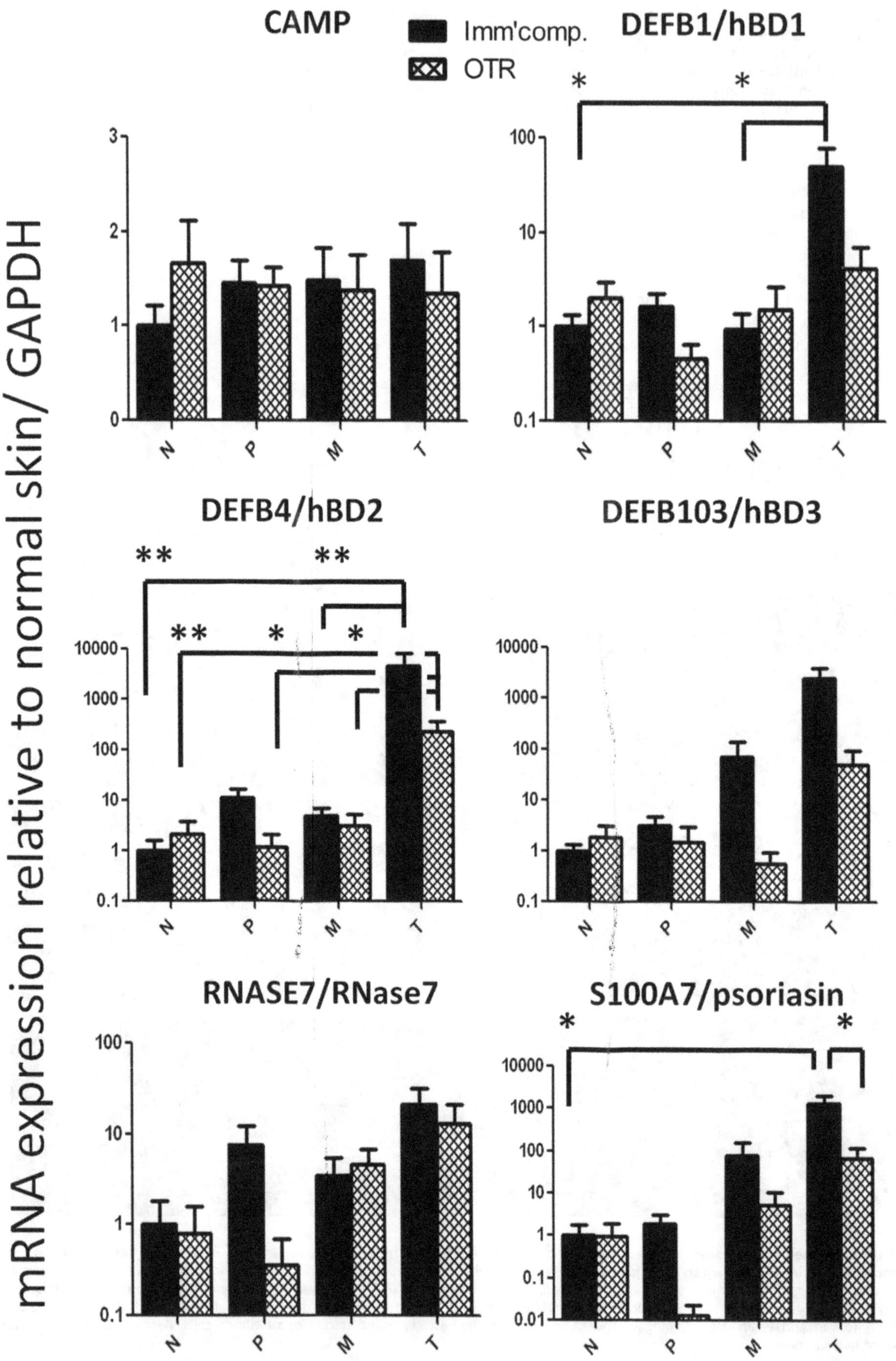
CAMP
Imm'comp.
OTR
DEFB1/hBD1
DEFB4/hBD2
DEFB103/hBD3
RNASE7/RNase7
S100A7/psoriasin
mRNA expression relative to normal skin/ GAPDH
N
P
M
T

Figure 7. Distinct expression of antimicrobial peptides in squamous cell carcinoma of organ transplant recipients. mRNA expression of cathelicidin antimicrobial peptide (*CAMP*), human β-defensins 1–3 (hBD1-3, genes *DEFB1*, *DEFB4* and *DEFB103*), RNase 7 (*RNASE7*) and psoriasisin (*S100A7*) in the tumor center (T), tumor margin (M), peritumoral tissue (P) and distant normal skin (N) in cutaneous squamous cell carcinoma (SCC) of immunocompetent (Imm'comp., black bars) and immunosuppressed patients (OTR = organ transplant recipients, cross-hatched bars). Relative mRNA expression to glyceraldehyde 3-phosphate dehydrogenase (GAPDH) and normalized to normal skin is shown. Depicted are mean ± SEM values. *p<0.05, **p<0.01, ***p<0.001 by Kruskal-Wallis test with Dunn's post-test for comparison between N, P, M and T and by Mann Whitney U test for comparison between immunocompetent and immunosuppressed patients in each group. N = 17 SCC from immunocompetent patients (ICP) and 11 SCC from organ transplant recipients (OTR).

psoriasin mRNA expression in *in-situ* and invasive SCC [42], and thus agreed with our results. Psoriasin overexpression has also been reported for other tumors such as breast cancer [43], where persistent expression in invasive tumor areas was associated with poorer prognosis [44–46]. Upregulation of psoriasin at transcriptional and protein level was recently also reported for early oral SCC [19]. Psoriasin can bind αvβ6-integrin to promote invasive behavior in oral SCC cells [47]. Therefore, as was discussed for TLRs and their signaling intermediates, the current findings validate the need for further study of the functional relevance of these antimicrobial peptides and proteins.

Immunocompromised patients such as organ transplant recipients (OTRs) have a 60- to 100-fold increased risk for SCC [4], however the exact mechanisms for how immunosuppressive drugs increase the risk for more frequent and more aggressive SCCs are still largely unknown. Long-term immunosuppressive drug treatment in OTR was recently shown to alter the composition of the SCC peritumoral inflammatory infiltrate. Reduced proportions of CD3+, CD8+, and CD14+ (monocytes), FOXP3+ (regulatory T cells) and 123+ (plasmacytoid dendritic cells) cells but more CD138+ plasma cells in SCC of OTR compared to immunocompetent patients have been reported [48–49]. Most OTRs are treated with several immunosuppressive drugs simultaneously, making it difficult to elucidate the exact mechanisms how an immunosuppressant contributes to the increased SCC risk.

To investigate if drug-induced immunosuppression altered innate immune gene expression, we included 11 SCC from OTRs for comparison with SCC from immunocompetent patients. All patients in our study were on a treatment regimen with corticosteroids and the mTOR inhibitor rapamycin for at least a year before tumor diagnosis and excision. In epidemiological studies, switching from an immunosuppressive therapy with calcineurin inhibitors to the mTOR-inhibitor sirolimus was effective to reduce skin carcinogenesis in renal transplant patients by 50% [50]. In our study, comparison of expression of all innate immune genes revealed that in contrast to immunocompetent patients, SCC in OTR had lower hBD1 and psoriasin expression, but the abundance of expression of other genes measured was similar to SCC from immunocompetent patients. It would be of interest to determine if the lower expression of hBD1 and psoriasin might be functionally relevant and related to the worse outcome in these patients.

In summary, this study clearly shows that the expression of several genes involved in the innate immune response is different in SCC than normal tissues. There are many possible reasons why skin tumors showed elevated expression of these innate immune genes. Tumor infiltrating immune cells such as CD4+, CD8+ and FOXP3+ T-cells and macrophages secrete soluble effector molecules such as interferons, IL-6 and TNF, and some of these can directly influence innate immune gene expression in keratinocytes (reviewed in [12]). The higher degree of differentiation in SCC compared to BCC or normal basal keratinocytes might be another reason for overexpression of some innate immune genes, since highly differentiated keratinocytes showed enhanced expression of human β-defensins 2 and 3 [51]. A third driver of innate immune gene expression in SCC could be a defective skin barrier in these tumors. Skin SCCs often rupture and form wounds. Previous studies in non-malignant, sterile wounding experiments showed a strong induction of TLR2 and antimicrobial peptides in the wound edge [35]. Furthermore, uncontrolled growth of tumor cells and tissue necrosis lead to release of molecules such as cellular DNA, heat shock proteins and fibrinogen, all of which are danger signals that can activate TLRs and their downstream signaling and effector molecules [52–53]. However, even though these mechanisms might be responsible for part of the profile of innate immune gene expression which we found in our study, they provide only an incomplete explanation. Moreover, we believe that expression of some of these innate immune genes is tumor-intrinsic and independent from the tumor environment. Further studies are needed to better understand the exact mechanisms that lead to this distinct innate immune gene expression.

The approach of sampling tissue from the tumor margin and periphery distinguished expression of some genes of interest and provides an example of how basic research might be integrated in well established standardized clinical surgical procedures such as Mohs surgery. Furthermore, it would be a mistake to overlook the remarkably low response seen in BCC for some gene products. The expression (or lack of expression) of unique elements of the innate immune system provides clues to development of the next generation of targeted immune therapy for NMSC.

Materials and Methods

Patients

The study was designed to include 10 – 20 specimens each from SCC in immunocompetent patients, from SCC in organ transplant recipients and from basal cell carcinomas. Following approval by the Human Research Protection Program at the University of California, San Diego (IRB ref. # 071032), and upon receiving written informed consent prior to biopsy, skin specimens from subsequent patients undergoing Mohs surgery for non-melanoma skin cancer at the Division of Dermatology, University of California, San Diego, from December 2009 to June 2010 were collected. The only inclusion criterion was the tumor diagnosis. There were no exclusion criteria. None of the patients in this study was pregnant or had other underlying skin disorders in the areas from which skin samples were obtained. Storage and use of all tissues included in the work presented here was carried out in accordance with the Helsinki declaration. 37 patients were included. 19 patients had a basal cell carcinoma (BCC) and 28 squamous cell carcinoma (SCC). Because immunosuppressed patients such as organ transplant recipients (OTR) have a 60–100-fold greater risk for SCCs this study was designed to include 11 SCCs from OTRs for comparison with 17 SCC from immunocompetent patients (ICP). In the BCC patient group, 68.4% were men, and mean age was 67.1±3.9 years (± SEM). In the SCC ICP group, 76.5% were men and mean age was 74.3±2.7 years. In the SCC OTR group, 81.8% were men. As expected and published before [4,54], OTRs in this study developed SCC significantly earlier than ICPs (at 49.2±2.2 y, p<0.001) (**Figure 1A,B**). Transplanted organs were as follows: 8 kidneys, 1 liver and 2 hearts. Time since transplantation was ranging from 8 to 31 years. The current immunosuppressive regimens for at least one year before Mohs surgery were rapamycin & prednisone.

Collection of Human Skin Specimens

Mohs microscopically controlled surgery of these skin tumors was performed as described before [55]. During the course of Mohs surgery, 2x2x2 mm³ specimens were collected from the center of the tumor (T), from the margin of the tumor (M) consisting of tumor cells and non-tumor cells, from the peritumoral region (P) in close proximity to the tumor but without any tumor cells, and from normal skin (N) in far distance from the tumor, used to reconstruct the skin defect after complete tumor excision (**Figure 1C**). This approach allowed comparison of not only tumor tissue with normal skin in the same patients but also with the peritumoral microenvironment and with the invading tumor edge.

Quantitative Real-time PCR (qPCR)

Total RNA was isolated using TRIzol reagent (Invitrogen, Carlsbad, CA) and 1 µg RNA was reverse transcribed using iScript (BioRad, Hercules, CA). Expression of the cathelicidin gene (*CAMP*) was evaluated using the FAM-CAGAGGATTGT-GACTTCA-MGB probe with primers 5′-CTTCAC-CAGCCCGTCCTTC-3′ and 5′-CCAGGACGACACAG-CAGTCA-3′. Taqman gene expression assays detecting human loricrin (Hs01894962_s1), filaggrin (Hs00856927_g1), keratin 5 (Hs00361185_m1), keratin 10 (Hs00196158_m1), TLR1-9 (Hs00413978_m1, Hs00610101_m1, Hs01551078_m1, Hs00152937_m1, Hs01019558_m1, Hs00271977_s1, Hs00607866_m1, Hs00370913_s1), TRIF (Hs00706140_s1), TRAF1 (Hs01090170_m1) TRAF2 (Hs00184186_m1), TNFα (Hs00174128_m1), IFNγ (Hs00989291_m1), human β-defensins 1-3 (Hs00608345_m1, Hs00823638_m1, Hs00218678_m1), RN-Ase7 (Hs00261482_m1) and S100A7 (Hs00161488_m1) were purchased from Applied Biosystems (ABI, Foster City, CA). Gene expression was normalized against GAPDH. For GAPDH expression a VIC CATCCATGACCACCCCTGGCCAAG-MGB probe with primers 5′-CTTAGCACCCCTGGCCAAG-3′ and 5′-TGGTCATGAGTCCTTCCACG-3′ was used. RT-qPCR was run on a 7300 Real Time PCR System (ABI). The ΔΔCt method was used to calculate relative expression normalized to normal skin.

Immunostaining

For immunohistofluorescence, frozen sections (6 µm) were fixed with 4% paraformaldehyde, blocked with 3% BSA in phosphate-buffered saline (PBS), and incubated with mouse monoclonal anti-psoriasin antibody (47C1068, sc-52948, Santa Cruz Biotechnology), rabbit anti-hBD1 (FL-68, sc-20797, Santa Cruz) or anti-hBD2 antibody (FL-64, sc-20798, Santa Cruz). Normal mouse IgG (sc-3877, Santa Cruz) and rabbit pre-immune serum were used as negative controls (**Figure S1**). After washing with PBS, FITC-conjugated goat anti-mouse IgG (Sigma-Aldrich) or FITC-conjugated goat anti-rabbit IgG (Jackson Immuno Research Laboratories, West Grove, PA) was used as second antibody. Sections were mounted in ProLong Gold Anti-Fade reagent with 4′-6-diamidino-2-pheny-lindole (Molecular Probes/Invitrogen, Eugene, OR). Images were obtained using an Olympus BX41 fluorescent microscope (Scientific Instrument Company, Temecula, CA).

Statistical Analysis

Statistical analysis was performed using GraphPad Prism software v5.0 (GraphPad Software Inc., La Jolla). The means and standard errors of the mean (SEM) were calculated for each data set. Data were analyzed by analysis of variance (ANOVA) or the Kruskal-Wallis test with post-tests when appropriate, Mann-Whitney U test and unpaired t test. P-values < 0.05 were considered significant.

Acknowledgments

The authors thank Cuong Nguyen for assistance with experiments and Lars E. French for scientific advice.

Author Contributions

Performed the experiments: BM. Analyzed the data: BM RLG. Contributed reagents/materials/analysis tools: BM SJ MG JG TH. Wrote the paper: BM RLG.

References

1. Lomas A, Leonardi-Bee J, Bath-Hextall F (2012) A Systematic Review of worldwide incidence of Non-melanoma skin cancer. Br J Dermatol.
2. Jemal A, Siegel R, Ward E, Hao Y, Xu J, et al. (2009) Cancer statistics, 2009. CA Cancer J Clin 59: 225–249.
3. Rogers HW, Weinstock MA, Harris AR, Hinckley MR, Feldman SR, et al. (2010) Incidence estimate of nonmelanoma skin cancer in the United States, 2006. Arch Dermatol 146: 283–287.
4. Berg D, Otley CC (2002) Skin cancer in organ transplant recipients: Epidemiology, pathogenesis, and management. J Am Acad Dermatol 47: 1–17; quiz 18–20.
5. Norval M (2001) Effects of solar radiation on the human immune system. J Photochem Photobiol B 63: 28–40.
6. O'Dell BL, Jessen RT, Becker LE, Jackson RT, Smith EB (1980) Diminished immune response in sun-damaged skin. Arch Dermatol 116: 559–561.
7. Dunn GP, Bruce AT, Ikeda H, Old LJ, Schreiber RD (2002) Cancer immunoediting: from immunosurveillance to tumor escape. Nat Immunol 3: 991–998.
8. Schreiber RD, Old LJ, Smyth MJ (2011) Cancer immunoediting: integrating immunity's roles in cancer suppression and promotion. Science 331: 1565–1570.
9. Coley WB (1991) The treatment of malignant tumors by repeated inoculations of erysipelas. With a report of ten original cases. 1893. Clin Orthop Relat Res: 3–11.
10. Starnes CO (1992) Coley's toxins in perspective. Nature 357: 11–12.
11. Lai Y, Gallo RL (2008) Toll-like receptors in skin infections and inflammatory diseases. Infect Disord Drug Targets 8: 144–155.
12. Lai Y, Gallo RL (2009) AMPed up immunity: how antimicrobial peptides have multiple roles in immune defense. Trends Immunol 30: 131–141.
13. Ong PY, Ohtake T, Brandt C, Strickland I, Boguniewicz M, et al. (2002) Endogenous antimicrobial peptides and skin infections in atopic dermatitis. N Engl J Med 347: 1151–1160.
14. Schauber J, Gallo RL (2009) Antimicrobial peptides and the skin immune defense system. J Allergy Clin Immunol 124: R13–18.
15. Zanetti M (2005) The role of cathelicidins in the innate host defenses of mammals. Curr Issues Mol Biol 7: 179–196.

16. Dorschner RA, Pestonjamasp VK, Tamakuwala S, Ohtake T, Rudisill J, et al. (2001) Cutaneous injury induces the release of cathelicidin anti-microbial peptides active against group A Streptococcus. J Invest Dermatol 117: 91–97.

17. Nizet V, Ohtake T, Lauth X, Trowbridge J, Rudisill J, et al. (2001) Innate antimicrobial peptide protects the skin from invasive bacterial infection. Nature 414: 454–457.

18. Koczulla R, von Degenfeld G, Kupatt C, Krotz F, Zahler S, et al. (2003) An angiogenic role for the human peptide antibiotic LL-37/hCAP-18. J Clin Invest 111: 1665–1672.

19. Kesting MR, Sudhoff H, Hasler RJ, Nieberler M, Pautke C, et al. (2009) Psoriasin (S100A7) up-regulation in oral squamous cell carcinoma and its relation to clinicopathologic features. Oral Oncol 45: 731–736.

20. Yoshimoto T, Yamaai T, Mizukawa N, Sawaki K, Nakano M, et al. (2003) Different expression patterns of beta-defensins in human squamous cell carcinomas. Anticancer Res 23: 4629–4633.

21. Buchau AS, Morizane S, Trowbridge J, Schauber J, Kotol P, et al. (2010) The host defense peptide cathelicidin is required for NK cell-mediated suppression of tumor growth. J Immunol 184: 369–378.

22. Wagstaff AJ, Perry CM (2007) Topical imiquimod: a review of its use in the management of anogenital warts, actinic keratoses, basal cell carcinoma and other skin lesions. Drugs 67: 2187–2210.

23. Braff MH, Bardan A, Nizet V, Gallo RL (2005) Cutaneous defense mechanisms by antimicrobial peptides. J Invest Dermatol 125: 9–13.

24. Glaser R, Harder J, Lange H, Bartels J, Christophers E, et al. (2005) Antimicrobial psoriasin (S100A7) protects human skin from Escherichia coli infection. Nat Immunol 6: 57–64.

25. Glaser R, Koten B, Wittersheim M, Harder J (2011) Psoriasin: key molecule of the cutaneous barrier? J Dtsch Dermatol Ges 9: 897–902.

26. Kisich KO, Howell MD, Boguniewicz M, Heizer HR, Watson NU, et al. (2007) The constitutive capacity of human keratinocytes to kill Staphylococcus aureus is dependent on beta-defensin 3. J Invest Dermatol 127: 2368–2380.

27. Pollack JR, Perou CM, Alizadeh AA, Eisen MB, Pergamenschikov A, et al. (1999) Genome-wide analysis of DNA copy-number changes using cDNA microarrays. Nat Genet 23: 41–46.

28. Wang Z, Gerstein M, Snyder M (2009) RNA-Seq: a revolutionary tool for transcriptomics. Nat Rev Genet 10: 57–63.

29. Hudson LG, Gale JM, Padilla RS, Pickett G, Alexander BE, et al. (2010) Microarray analysis of cutaneous squamous cell carcinomas reveals enhanced expression of epidermal differentiation complex genes. Mol Carcinog 49: 619–629.

30. Huang B, Zhao J, Unkeless JC, Feng ZH, Xiong H (2008) TLR signaling by tumor and immune cells: a double-edged sword. Oncogene 27: 218–224.

31. Kelly MG, Alvero AB, Chen R, Silasi DA, Abrahams VM, et al. (2006) TLR-4 signaling promotes tumor growth and paclitaxel chemoresistance in ovarian cancer. Cancer Res 66: 3859–3868.

32. Lee JW, Choi JJ, Seo ES, Kim MJ, Kim WY, et al. (2007) Increased toll-like receptor 9 expression in cervical neoplasia. Mol Carcinog 46: 941–947.

33. Szczepanski M, Stelmachowska M, Stryczynski L, Golusinski W, Samara H, et al. (2007) Assessment of expression of toll-like receptors 2, 3 and 4 in laryngeal carcinoma. Eur Arch Otorhinolaryngol 264: 525–530.

34. Vahle AK, Kerem A, Ozturk E, Bankfalvi A, Lang S, et al. (2012) Optimization of an orthotopic murine model of head and neck squamous cell carcinoma in fully immunocompetent mice–role of toll-like-receptor 4 expressed on host cells. Cancer Lett 317: 199–206.

35. Schauber J, Dorschner RA, Coda AB, Buchau AS, Liu PT, et al. (2007) Injury enhances TLR2 function and antimicrobial peptide expression through a vitamin D-dependent mechanism. J Clin Invest 117: 803–811.

36. Frye M, Bargon J, Gropp R (2001) Expression of human beta-defensin-1 promotes differentiation of keratinocytes. J Mol Med (Berl) 79: 275–282.

37. Kawsar HI, Ghosh SK, Hirsch SA, Koon HB, Weinberg A, et al. (2010) Expression of human beta-defensin-2 in intratumoral vascular endothelium and in endothelial cells induced by transforming growth factor beta. Peptides 31: 195–201.

38. Sawaki K, Mizukawa N, Yamaai T, Yoshimoto T, Nakano M, et al. (2002) High concentration of beta-defensin-2 in oral squamous cell carcinoma. Anticancer Res 22: 2103–2107.

39. Jin G, Kawsar HI, Hirsch SA, Zeng C, Jia X, et al. (2010) An antimicrobial peptide regulates tumor-associated macrophage trafficking via the chemokine receptor CCR2, a model for tumorigenesis. PLoS One 5: e10993.

40. Gambichler T, Skrygan M, Huyn J, Bechara FG, Sand M, et al. (2006) Pattern of mRNA expression of beta-defensins in basal cell carcinoma. BMC Cancer 6: 163.

41. Mburu YK, Abe K, Ferris LK, Sarkar SN, Ferris RL (2011) Human beta-defensin 3 promotes NF-kappaB-mediated CCR7 expression and anti-apoptotic signals in squamous cell carcinoma of the head and neck. Carcinogenesis 32: 168–174.

42. Moubayed N, Weichenthal M, Harder J, Wandel E, Sticherling M, et al. (2007) Psoriasin (S100A7) is significantly up-regulated in human epithelial skin tumours. J Cancer Res Clin Oncol 133: 253–261.

43. Wolf R, Voscopoulos C, Winston J, Dharamsi A, Goldsmith P, et al. (2009) Highly homologous hS100A15 and hS100A7 proteins are distinctly expressed in normal breast tissue and breast cancer. Cancer Lett 277: 101–107.

44. Al-Haddad S, Zhang Z, Leygue E, Snell L, Huang A, et al. (1999) Psoriasin (S100A7) expression and invasive breast cancer. Am J Pathol 155: 2057–2066.

45. Emberley ED, Alowami S, Snell L, Murphy LC, Watson PH (2004) S100A7 (psoriasin) expression is associated with aggressive features and alteration of Jab1 in ductal carcinoma in situ of the breast. Breast Cancer Res 6: R308–315.

46. Leygue E, Snell L, Hiller T, Dotzlaw H, Hole K, et al. (1996) Differential expression of psoriasin messenger RNA between in situ and invasive human breast carcinoma. Cancer Res 56: 4606–4609.

47. Morgan MR, Jazayeri M, Ramsay AG, Thomas GJ, Boulanger MJ, et al. (2011) Psoriasin (S100A7) associates with integrin beta6 subunit and is required for alphavbeta6-dependent carcinoma cell invasion. Oncogene 30: 1422–1435.

48. Krynitz B, Lundh Rozell B, Lindelof B (2010) Differences in the peritumoral inflammatory skin infiltrate between squamous cell carcinomas in organ transplant recipients and immunocompetent patients. Acta Derm Venereol 90: 379–385.

49. Muhleisen B, Petrov I, Gachter T, Kurrer M, Scharer L, et al. (2009) Progression of cutaneous squamous cell carcinoma in immunosuppressed patients is associated with reduced CD123+ and FOXP3+ cells in the perineoplastic inflammatory infiltrate. Histopathology 55: 67–76.

50. Mathew T, Kreis H, Friend P (2004) Two-year incidence of malignancy in sirolimus-treated renal transplant recipients: results from five multicenter studies. Clin Transplant 18: 446–449.

51. Liu AY, Destoumieux D, Wong AV, Park CH, Valore EV, et al. (2002) Human beta-defensin-2 production in keratinocytes is regulated by interleukin-1, bacteria, and the state of differentiation. J Invest Dermatol 118: 275–281.

52. Asea A, Rehli M, Kabingu E, Boch JA, Bare O, et al. (2002) Novel signal transduction pathway utilized by extracellular HSP70: role of toll-like receptor (TLR) 2 and TLR4. J Biol Chem 277: 15028–15034.

53. Kuhns DB, Priel DA, Gallin JI (2007) Induction of human monocyte interleukin (IL)-8 by fibrinogen through the toll-like receptor pathway. Inflammation 30: 178–188.

54. Euvrard S, Kanitakis J, Claudy A (2003) Skin cancers after organ transplantation. N Engl J Med 348: 1681–1691.

55. Cumberland L, Dana A, Liegeois N (2009) Mohs micrographic surgery for the management of nonmelanoma skin cancers. Facial Plast Surg Clin North Am 17: 325–335.

9

Inhibition of Nuclear Factor-κB Activation in Pancreatic β-Cells has a Protective Effect on Allogeneic Pancreatic Islet Graft Survival

Roy Eldor[1], Roy Abel[1], Dror Sever[1], Gad Sadoun[1], Amnon Peled[2], Ronit Sionov[3], Danielle Melloul[1]*

1 Department of Endocrinology, Hadassah University Hospital, Jerusalem, Israel, **2** Goldyne Savad Institute of Gene Therapy, Hadassah University Hospital, Jerusalem, Israel, **3** Department of Biochemistry and Molecular Biology, IMRIC, Hebrew University-Hadassah Medical School, Jerusalem, Israel

Abstract

Pancreatic islet transplantation, a treatment for type 1 diabetes, has met significant challenges, as a substantial fraction of the islet mass fails to engraft, partly due to death by apoptosis in the peri- and post-transplantation periods. Previous evidence has suggested that NF-κB activation is involved in cytokine-mediated β-cell apoptosis and regulates the expression of pro-inflammatory and chemokine genes. We therefore sought to explore the effects of β-cell-specific inhibition of NF-κB activation as a means of cytoprotection in an allogeneic model of islet transplantation. To this end, we used islets isolated from the ToI-β transgenic mouse, where NF-κB signalling can specifically and conditionally be inhibited in β-cells by expressing an inducible and non-degradable form of IκBα regulated by the tet-on system. Our results show that β-cell-specific blockade of NF-κB led to a prolonged islet graft survival, with a relative higher preservation of the engrafted endocrine tissue and reduced inflammation. Importantly, a longer delay in allograft rejection was achieved when mice were systemically treated with the proteasome inhibitor, Bortezomib. Our findings emphasize the contribution of NF-κB activation in the allograft rejection process, and suggest an involvement of the CXCL10/IP-10 chemokine. Furthermore, we suggest a potential, readily available therapeutic agent that may temper this process.

Editor: Kathrin Maedler, University of Bremen, Germany

Funding: This work was supported by grants from the Juvenile Diabetes Research Foundation (1-2007-60), and European Union (STREP Savebeta, contract n° 036903) in the Framework Programme 6 and the Israel Ministry of Health. The funders had no role in study design, data collection and analysis, decision to publish, or preparation of the manuscript.

Competing Interests: The authors have declared that no competing interests exist.

* E-mail: daniellem@ekmd.huji.ac.il

Introduction

Although the past decade has witnessed substantial developments in the field of islet transplantation [1], only a fraction of grafted islets survives. The reduction in β-cell mass in the immediate post-transplantation period appears to be due to hypoxia, nutrient deprivation and inflammation at the site of implantation [2], [3]. A variety of approaches have been explored to prevent the apoptotic destruction of islets in the experimental setting and, while promising data has been generated *in vitro*, demonstration of an *in vivo* benefit to islet graft survival has been more elusive (reviewed in [2], [4]). Such attempts have included genetic manipulation of the donor islets with anti-inflammatory and antiapoptotic genes such as Bcl-2 [5], [6], X-linked inhibitor of apoptosis protein (XIAP) [6-9] and the suppressor of cytokine signalling 1 (SOCS1) [10], as well as the overexpression of the antiapoptotic A20, which preserved functional islet β-cell mass [11]. Pre-treatment of islets with the caspase inhibitors zDEVD-FMK [12], EP1013 [13] or V5 [14] also improved islet survival.

Since inflammation is a primary contributor to graft loss, inhibiting the pro-inflammatory activity of cytokines could eventually prevent the loss of functional islet grafts. Since the NF-κB/Rel family of transcription factors regulates biological processes ranging from apoptosis to inflammation and innate immunity, attempts have been made to block NF-κB activation in models of islet cell transplantation. In models of syngeneic islet transplantation, pretreatment of donor islets with the NF-κB inhibitor dehydroxymethylepoxyquinomicin (DHMEQ) [15], conditional β-cell inhibition of NF-κB improved hepatic intra-portal engraftments [16], and transplantation of TLR4−/− deficient islets [17] each improved graft survival with reduced islet NF-κB activation. Prolonged graft survival was also observed in an allogeneic model of islet transplantation, but when c-Rel null mice (a lymphoid-predominant member of the NF-κB/Rel family) were used as recipients [18].

To further study the role of NF-κB *in vivo*, we have generated a transgenic mouse model, the ToIβ [19], [20], in which NF-κB activation is specifically and conditionally (±doxycycline/Dox) inhibited in β-cells. We previously showed that these mice were more resistant to MLDS-induced diabetes when the NF-κB pathway was inhibited [19]. Using this model, we present in this study further evidence that NF-κB blockade prolonged islet survival in an allotransplantation model, with increased preservation of the engrafted islets under the kidney capsule, and suggest the involvement of the chemokine CXCL10/IP-10 in this process.

Research Design and Methods

ToI-β Transgenic Mice

The generated ToI-β transgenic mouse model was previously described [19]. It carries the nondegradable IκBα and luciferase genes (ΔNIκBα-luciferase), regulated by a tetracycline-responsive element, and the reverse tetracycline transactivator (rtTA) under the control of the rat insulin II promoter (RIP7-rtTA). The mouse was generated by cross-breeding two transgenic mouse lines, one carrying the ΔNIκBα-Luciferase genes in an in-house agouti strain of C57B/6:H2^b X BALB/c:H2^d backgrounds, and the other RIP7-rtTA in a predominantly C3H:H2^k background. The transgenic mouse was then inbred for over 20 generations to produce the ToI-β inbred strain. The transgenes were activated *in vivo* by administering 2 mg/ml of doxycycline (Dox; Taro, Israel) in the drinking water. All animals were maintained in a specific pathogen-free research animal facility, and the experiments were approved by the Hebrew University Institutional Animal Care and Use Committee and conducted in accordance with local ethical guidelines.

Isolation and Culture of Mouse Pancreatic Islets

ToI-β mouse islets were isolated and cultured as previously described [19], in the presence or absence of mouse recombinant cytokines IL-1β (50 U/ml) and INF-γ (1,000 U/ml) that were purchased from R&D Systems Inc. (Minneapolis, MN, USA).

Medium Nitrite-concentration Measurement

ToI-β isolated islets were preincubated for 24 h with Bortezomib (BZB) (100 nM, LC laboratories, Woburn, MA, USA) [21] before the cytokines were added for an additional 48 h. Medium (100 µl) from the islet cultures containing 200 islets/ml were added to an equal volume of Greiss reagent, as previously described [19].

Islet Transplantation

Prior to transplantation, 10-week-old recipient mice were rendered diabetic by a single intra-peritoneal injection of streptozocin (250 mg/kg) (Sigma, St Louis, MO, USA), reaching consecutive glycemic values of >360 mg/dl: Control 441.9+/−37.6 mg/dl; Dox 417+/−29.2 mg/dl; BZB 427.25+/−30.1 mg/dl.

Mice were anesthetized with isoflurane (Nicholas Piramal India Ltd, Mumbai, India) and 500 islets were transplanted under the kidney capsule [8], [14], [22]. In the allogeneic experiments, SJL (H2^s) mice were used as recipients since they do not share any of the MHC H2 haplotypes of the original double-transgenic ToI-β. In syngeneic islet transplantations, donor and recipient Tol-β inbred mice were from the same litter. The postoperative follow-up was conducted by daily measurements of blood glucose levels using an Accu-Check Performa glucose meter (Roche, Mannheim, Germany). Islet grafts were considered functional when the measurements of non-fasting blood glucose were below 200 mg/dl for at least 5 consecutive days after transplantation, whereas graft rejection was defined as a return to hyperglycemia when consecutive glycemic levels were higher than 200 mg/dl. In another set of transplantations, 1 mg/kg of the proteasome inhibitor Bortezomib was injected intraperitoneally twice weekly [21] until graft rejection.

For histological analysis of relative endocrine/graft area, the kidneys containing grafted islets of untreated and Dox-treated recipients were retrieved on day 7 post-transplantation, then paraffin-embedded and sectioned longitudinally at a thickness of 5 µm to encompass as much of the graft as possible. Sections were conventionally stained with hematoxylin-eosin and photographed at a 10X magnification with identical exposure times, using an Olympus BX41 microscope and the Olympus DP71 camera. The processed images were combined to create a whole picture of the graft while omitting the kidney tissue and then analyzed using the software ImageJ (Freeware, NIH, Bethesda, MD, USA). A standardized point-counting grid was superimposed on the reconstituted engrafted picture and the number of intersections containing endocrine tissue was compared to the total graft area (i.e., the total number of grid points hitting the structure of interest being counted). The grid technique has been often used to measure beta cell mass in a similar fashion [23], [24]. Immunohistochemistry of insulin was performed using Histostain Plus Broad Spectrum (Invitrogen, Frederick, MD), according to manufacturer instructions, on the graft-bearing kidneys sections. Guinea pig anti-insulin serum (Linco, Seaford, DE) or anti-mouse IP-10 antibody (R&D systems, Minneapolis, MN, USA) were used as primary antibodies followed by incubation with the secondary antibodies HRP-conjugated rabbit anti-guinea pig or HRP-streptavidin, respectively ((Zymed, San Francisco, CA, USA).

For gene expression analysis, the syngeneic grafts were retrieved 24 h post-transplantation and mRNA levels were assessed by real-time PCR using the primers listed in Supplementary Material. The results presented solely include those obtained from the grafts containing less than 5% of kidney tissue contamination as determined by the levels of the transcripts of novel kidney gene (NKT) in the retrieved islets.

Data Presentation and Statistical Analysis

The data are presented as the mean ± SEM. Statistical analysis of medium nitrite concentration, average graft survival and relative endocrine/total graft area was performed using the paired Student's *t*-test. Post-transplantation graft survival was assessed by Kaplan-Meier analysis and comparison of survival curves by logrank test using MedCalc 12.3.0.0. In all tests, $p < 0.05$ was considered statistically significant.

Results

Temporal Inhibition of NF-κB Activation in Pancreatic β-cells Improves Allogeneic Islet Graft Survival

To determine the role of NF-κB activation in islet graft rejection, 500 isolated islets from ToI-β mouse donors were transplanted into the diabetic allogeneic recipient SJL mouse strain. The SJL (H2^s) was chosen as it does not share any of the MHC H2 haplotypes of the original double-transgenic ToI-β mouse line (H2^b; H2^d; H2^k). Transplantation of untreated ToI-β islets (control) resulted in a swift recovery of normoglycemia, which was maintained for an average of 13.9 days before graft failure (FIG. 1A, Control; n = 10). Similar results were obtained when donors, recipients and islet grafts were exposed to Dox in the drinking water and in the culture media a few days prior to transplantation (data not shown). However, a modest but significant delay in graft failure of 4.5 days was achieved when Dox was introduced to the drinking water of recipient mice 24 hours after the transplantation (FIG. 1A, Dox; average days to rejection: 18.4; n = 9; $p = 0.004$ Dox *vs* Control).

Systemic Proteasome Inhibition Prolongs Allogeneic Islet Graft Survival

One of the major problems with employing genetically modified strategies or using viral vectors for transfection is the difficulty in expressing genes in primary islets. For possible future clinical use, we propose as a proof of concept the use of the known proteasome

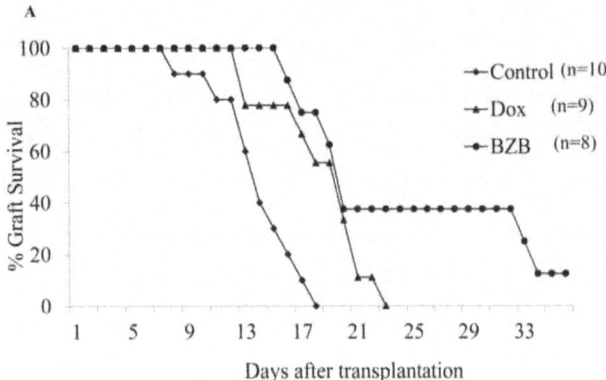

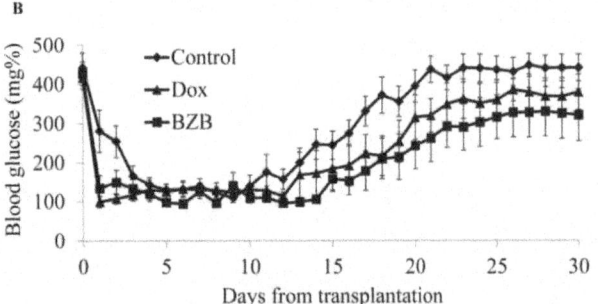

Figure 1. Survival of ToI-β pancreatic islet grafts in allogenic SJL- mice. 500 ToI-β islets were transplanted under the kidney capsule of allogeneic SJL mice. Rejection/graft survival was determined by tail blood glucose measurements. Graft rejection was defined as consecutive measurements of glycemia >200 mg/dl. (**A**) Untreated control mice (diamonds, n = 10); mice that were exposed to Dox 24 hours after transplantation (triangles, n = 9); and mice that were exposed to Bortezomib 24 hours after transplantation (circles, n = 8). Statistical analysis was done by Kaplan-Meier estimation and comparison of survival curves by the MedCalc logrank test. p = 0.004 Dox vs control, p = 0.001 BZB vs control. (**B**) Blood glucose of ToI-β islet grafts in untreated SJL control mice (black diamonds); mice exposed to Dox (triangles) and mice treated with Bortezomib (BZB, squares). Blood glucose areas under the curve (AUC) were smaller in treated vs untreated recipient mice: Dox vs. Control p = 0.025, BZB vs Control p = 0.01.

inhibitor Bortezomib (BZB) [21]. We initially tested its effect in vitro, exposing ToI-β islets to a combination of IL-1β+IFN-γ cytokines for 48 h and measuring nitrite secretion into the media. FIG. 2 demonstrates a reduction in cytokine-induced NO secretion with Bortezomib. Interestingly, a reduction of about 50% in cytokine-stimulated NO secretion was observed when NF-κB activation was inhibited, whether by using Bortezomib or by activation of the endogenous super-repressor IκB transgene in Dox-treated ToI-β islets (as previously demonstrated in Eldor et al [19]).

Similar allogeneic transplantation experiments were conducted in which the ToI-β islets were transplanted into diabetic allogeneic recipient SJL mice, which were injected with Bortezomib 24 h post-transplantation. FIG. 1A clearly shows that BZB led to a delay in graft rejection greater than that displayed in the Dox-treated model (BZB; average day of rejection: 26.5; n = 8; *p* = 0.001 BZB vs Control). The benefit of Dox- or Bortezomib-treatment was demonstrated by the decrease in blood glucose levels compared with untreated controls (FIG. 1B). When the glucose area under the curve (AUC) was calculated, treated mice had a significantly lower AUC compared with control animals (Dox vs. Control *p* = 0.025, BZB vs Control *p* = 0.01).

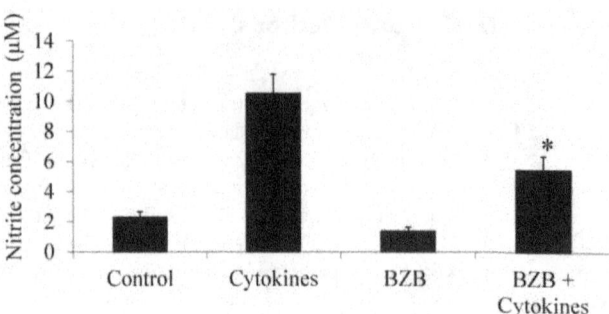

Figure 2. Medium nitrite levels secreted from islets exposed in vitro to IL-1β (50 units/ml) and IFN-γ (1,000 units/ml) for 48 h in the presence or absence of Bortezomib (BZB- 100 nM). Nitrite data are pooled from two separate experiments incorporating 5–6 repeats of each treatment, presented as the mean ± SEM. *p value = 0.023 for BZB+Cytokines vs Cytokines.

Post-transplantation NF-κB Inhibition Leads to Preservation of Endocrine Mass in the Islet Graft

To further study the role of NF-κB in the islet transplantation model, we sought to determine the relative endocrine vs total graft area. Measurements were taken 7 d post-transplantation, a point at which grafts were still fully functional, as evidenced by normoglycemia measured at this point and yet, sufficient time had elapsed for the development of an immune rejection response [25], FIG. 3 depicts a grid estimate of the relative area of endocrine tissue as a percentage of the total graft area in grafts retrieved from untreated mice (Control), and from mice exposed to Dox or BZB beginning 1 day post-operation. Since the mice were transplanted with the exact same number of 500 islets, this may be considered a rough estimate of the remaining β-cell/endocrine mass in the graft. There was greater preservation of the relative endocrine area in the Dox- and BZB-treated mice vs control mice (*p* = 0.033 Dox vs control; *p* = 0.0001 BZB vs control; n = 3), which correlated with a better preservation of islet graft structure and of insulin positive cells.

Potential Role of IP-10/CXCL10 in NF-κB-mediated Early Protection and Delay in Islet Graft Rejection

In an attempt to further elucidate the effect of NF-κB in the peri-transplantation period, we set out to analyze the expression of putative NF-κB target genes in Dox-treated and untreated grafts. To this end, syngeneic transplantation experiments were performed and the islet transplants were retrieved 24 h after transplantation, at a time of minimal inflammatory cell infiltration. Surprisingly, only IP-10/CXCL10 expression was significantly reduced by the β-cell specific inhibition of NF-κB (FIG. 4A; p = 0.03 Dox vs control; n = 5). However, no NF-κB-dependent changes were noted in the expression of genes previously shown to be stimulated by NF-κB activation *in vitro*, including iNOS, MCP-1 and NF-κB-mediated antiapoptotic genes such as A20 and XIAP (FIG. 4B–4F). In all grafts retrieved, expression of the kidney tissue-specific NKT (novel kidney transcript) gene was measured to assess the degree of kidney contamination. Only grafts with less than 5% kidney contamination are presented.

To confirm the effect of NF-κB blockade, or that of BZB on CXCL10/IP-10 expression, immunohistochemical staining of graft sections of kidneys collected 7 d post-transplantation from normoglycemic recipient mice, was performed. As shown in FIG. 5, CXCL10/IP-10 cytoplasmic staining was markedly

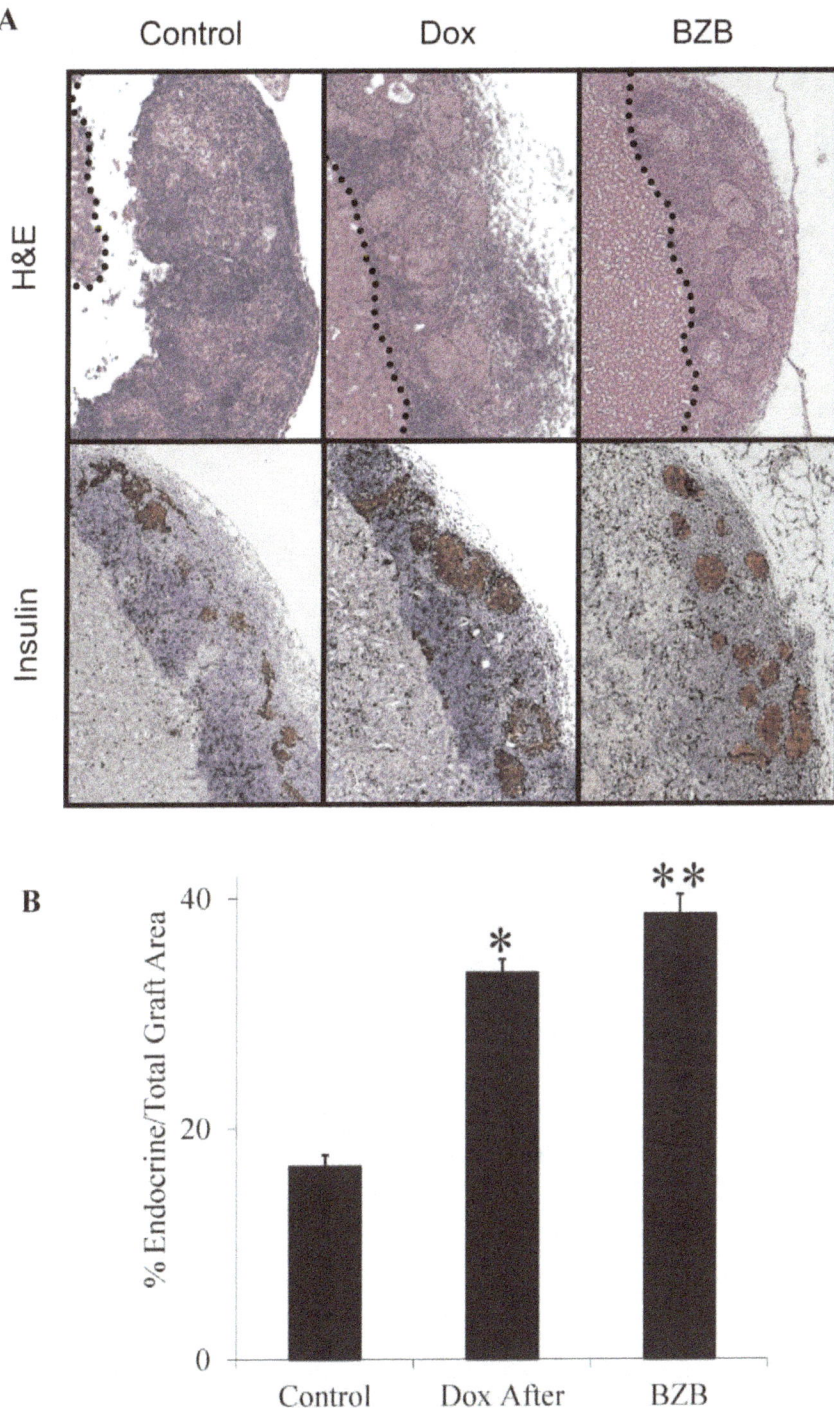

Figure 3. Inhibition of NF-κB activation is associated with an increased endocrine/total graft area ratio in the islet graft. A. The recipient graft-bearing kidneys from normoglycemic untreated mice, and Dox- or Bortezomib (BZB)-treated animals were removed 7 days after allogeneic transplantation, fixed in formaldehyde, thin-sliced and stained with hematoxylin/eosin solution. The border between the kidney and the graft is marked (Upper panel). Paraffin sections were stained for insulin (Lower panel). **B.** Using a fixed grid, the percentage of endocrine area was calculated from the total graft area. Results are the average of at least five non-consecutive sections incorporating the whole graft area. *p = 0.033 Dox *vs* control; **p = 0.0001 BZB *vs* control n = 3.

decreased in both islet grafts originated from Dox- or BZB- treated recipients when compared with untreated animals.

Thus NF-κB mediated IP-10 expression may be involved both during engraftment and, at later stages in attracting inflammatory cells. These results highlight that the NF-κB-mediated activation

of IP-10 could be a potential immediate target chemokine for islet graft survival and function in the peri-transplantation period.

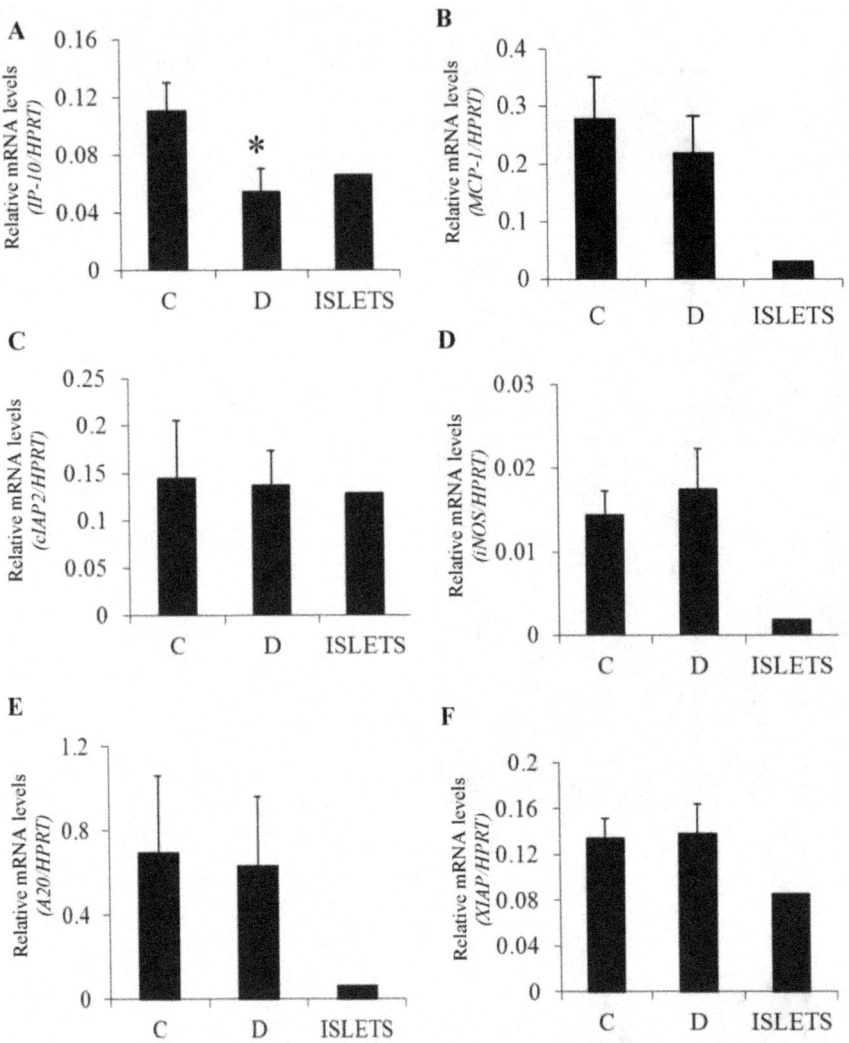

Figure 4. Real-time PCR analysis of NF-κB target genes in islet grafts 24 hours after transplantation. CXCL-10/IP-10 (*p = 0.03 Dox *vs* control) (**A**), MCP-1 (**B**), cIAP2 (**C**), iNOS (**D**), A20 (**E**) and XIAP (**F**). mRNA was extracted from Tol-β islet grafts retrieved from the kidney capsule 24 hours after syngeneic transplantation. Prior to transplantation, islet grafts were exposed to Dox in the culture media for 48 hours (D) or untreated controls (C). The right columns represent relative gene expression in isolated, untreated islets (ISLETS). Results are shown as fold induction normalized to HPRT values. Only retrieved grafts with less than 5% kidney contamination were included in the study, as assessed by expression of the kidney tissue-specific NKT (novel kidney transcript) gene. Results are the mean ± SEM of three to five independent experiments.

Discussion

The aim of our study was to investigate and test a strategy to induce cytoprotection following allogeneic islet transplantation. The current results demonstrate a delay in islet graft rejection when the NF-κB pathway was specifically inhibited in β-cells after transplantation. These results concur with preservation of the endocrine graft area (*vs* immune infiltrate) in Dox-treated *vs* untreated control mice as observed 7 d after transplantation, suggesting that NF-κB activation in β-cells could play a role in immune-mediated early islet graft rejection.

To explore a possible therapeutic option, the proteasome inhibitor Bortezomib was administered to recipient animals following islet transplantation. The systemic treatment resulted in further prolonged islet allograft survival, with histological preservation of the endocrine area. These results are in accordance with a recent report demonstrating a delay in porcine islet graft rejection transplanted into athymic nu/nu mice after a single injection of the IKK-β inhibitor, BMS-345541 [26]. In fact,

pharmacological inhibitors of the proteasome not only inhibit the activation of NF-κB in islet cells, but they also affect the function and survival of immune cells leading to reduced inflammatory manifestations in several models of immune-mediated disorders [27]. Bortezomib is currently approved for therapeutic use in multiple myeloma, with relatively low toxicity, and can therefore potentially be used as an immune modulator in the islet post-transplant period.

The transcription factor NF-κB has been shown to regulate the expression of numerous genes that play important roles in cellular stress responses, cell growth, survival and apoptosis [28-30]. Numerous reports, including our own, have shown that sustained activation of NF-κB is an important cellular signal in initiating the cascade of events culminating in β-cell death [31-38]. Transfection of an NF-κB "superrepressor" gene into MIN-6 insulinoma cell lines, human CM and NES2Y β cell lines, INS-1E cells, purified rat islet β cells, and human and mouse islets led to their protection from cytokine-induced, NF-κB-mediated apoptosis *in vitro* [32],

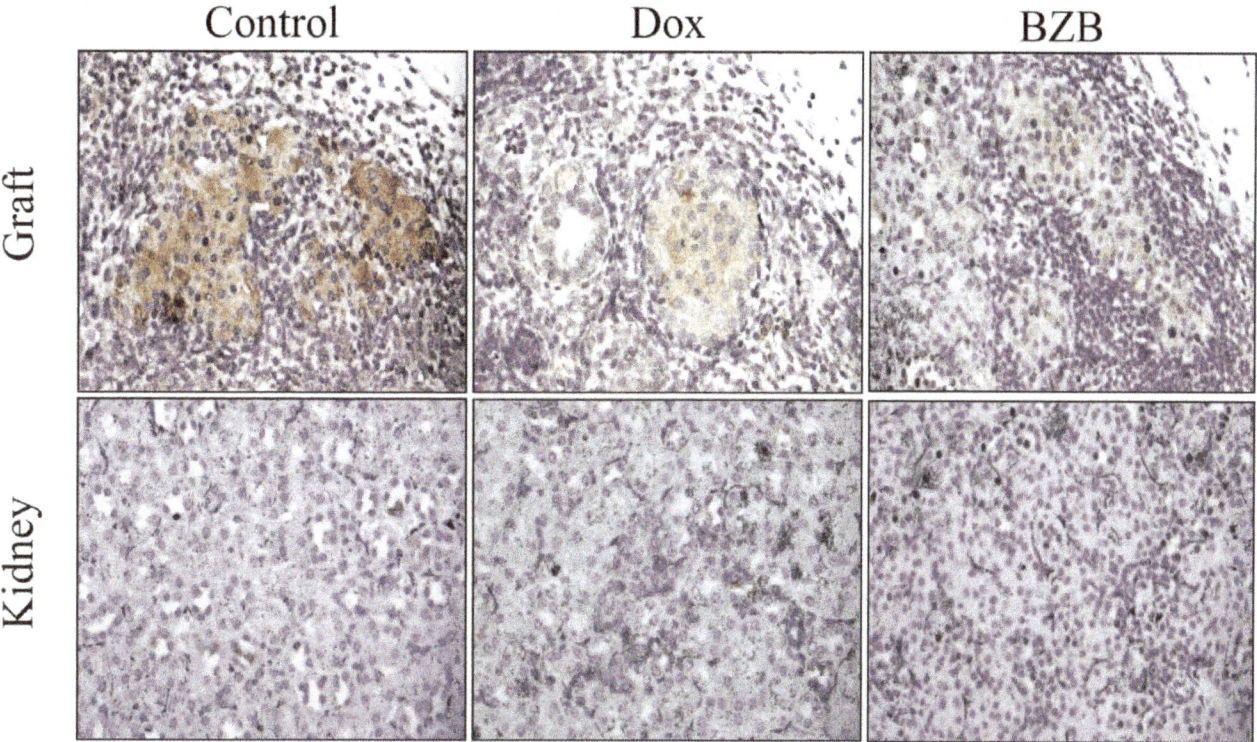

Figure 5. Decreased IP-10 in doxycycline- or Bortezomib-treated islet grafts. Representative anti-CXCL10/IP-10 stained graft-bearing kidney sections from normoglycemic untreated mice (control), Dox- or Bortezomib (BZB)-treated animals, 7 days after allogeneic transplantation (Upper panel- Graft). As noted in control the cytoplasmic IP-10 staining is more intense in control islets than in Dox- or Bortezomib-treated mice. The lower panel represents IP-10 staining of kidney sections of the corresponding graft adjacent areas.

[39], [40]. Similar results were obtained when NF-κB inhibition was achieved through transduction of human and mouse islets by a cationic peptide transduction domain. This in turn mediates delivery of a peptide inhibitor of IκB kinase [derived from IKKβ (NBD; Nemo-binding domain)], and completely blocks the detrimental effects of IL-1β on islet function and viability [41].

Nevertheless, a few several reports have challenged these observations by demonstrating a possible anti-apoptotic effect of NF-κB activation in certain experimental settings. In a model of overexpression of cFLIP [the cellular FLICE (FADD-like IL-1 beta-converting enzyme)-inhibitory protein] in β-TC-Tet cells, cytokine-dependent apoptosis was prevented concomitantly with increasing basal and IL-1β-mediated transcriptional activity of NF-κB [42]. In another model, siRNA-mediated gene silencing of NF-κB in INS-1E cells led to reduced iNOS and NF-κB gene expression but did not prevent cytokine-induced apoptosis [43]. Furthermore, exposure of β-cells to the tyrosine kinase inhibitor imatinib mesylate was associated with NF-κB activation and reduced β-cell apoptosis. The anti-apoptotic effect disappeared in the presence of an NF-κB inhibitor [44]. Additional observations indicated that stimulation of NF-κB protects β-cells from TNF-α-mediated apoptosis [45]. At low concentrations of IL-1β, and following exposure for a limited period of time, NF-κB activation by the cytokine increases β-cell replication and decreases apoptosis [46]. Finally, it has been suggested that transient and moderate laminin-5-rich extracellular-matrix activation of NF-κB may be essential to maintaining proper β-cell glucose-stimulated insulin secretion [47]. A possible reason for inconsistency may be the result of a more rapid, marked, and non-oscillatory activation of

NF-κB in β-cells exposed to cytokines as opposed to other cell types (e.g., fibroblasts) [39].

It is thus reasonable to postulate that, under physiological circumstances, the cytokine produced locally by islet cells, including β-cells, by activating NF-κB may play a role in maintenance of β-cell mass and survival [48]. However, under pathophysiological conditions, activation of NF-κB induces the expression of genes whose products can lead to β-cell apoptosis.

We further analyzed the expression of a selected set of putative NF-κB target genes in Dox-treated and untreated mice 24 h after transplantation in a syngeneic islet transplantation model. Surprisingly, only IP-10/CXCL10 expression was significantly reduced by β-cell-specific NF-κB inhibition, though this is consistent with the robust NF-κB-dependent increase in IP-10 secretion we previously found in ToI-β islets exposed to inflammatory cytokines [19]. A growing body of evidence has shown that there is an association between the levels of the chemokine IP-10/CXCL10 in various tissues and the inflammatory/immune processes occurring during organ transplantation [49]. Importantly, IP-10 was recently detected in the insulin-producing cells in islets of recent-onset T1D patients, and its receptor CXCR3 was associated with the infiltrating T cells in the islet area [50]. Similarly, neutralizing IP-10 antibodies suppressed the occurrence of cyclophosphamide-induced diabetes in NOD mice [51]. In this model, IP-10 expression was first being detected in β-cells in the peri-insulitis stage, and the levels gradually increased as the degree of insulitis progressed to the stage of intra-islet insulitis. Similar observations were made in the present study using ToI-β islet allografts, where a correlation was noticed between the IP-10 staining intensity in the islet grafts and the blockade of NF-κB pathway i.e. treated *vs* untreated mice (data not shown). Finally, in an allogeneic model of pancreatic islet transplantation, CXCR3−/− recipients or post-transplantation administration of anti-IP-10 antibodies inhibited T-cell trafficking to the graft site and prolonged islet survival [25]. Interestingly, this extended period of islet survival was similar to that observed in our experimental model, in which the NF-κB pathway was specifically inhibited in β-cells. These results suggest that IP-10 may be a potential contributor to the NF-κB-mediated inflammatory/immune mechanism.

In conclusion, we present evidence for a beneficial therapeutic effect of NF-κB inhibition in islet transplantation, and suggest NF-κB-mediated IP-10 expression as an early activated chemokine, involved in islet graft survival and function in the post-transplantation period.

Author Contributions

Conceived and designed the experiments: RE RA DM. Performed the experiments: RE RA DS GS RS. Analyzed the data: RE DS RA RS DM. Contributed reagents/materials/analysis tools: AP DM. Wrote the paper: RE DM.

References

1. Barton FB, Rickels MR, Alejandro R, Hering BJ, Wease S, et al. (2012) Improvement in outcomes of clinical islet transplantation: 1999–2010. Diabetes Care 35: 1436–1445.
2. Emamaullee JA, Shapiro AM (2006) Interventional strategies to prevent beta-cell apoptosis in islet transplantation. Diabetes 55: 1907–1914.
3. Matsumoto S, Noguchi H, Yonekawa Y, Okitsu T, Iwanaga Y, et al. (2006) Pancreatic islet transplantation for treating diabetes. Expert Opin Biol Ther 6: 23–37.
4. Robertson RP (2010) Update on transplanting beta cells for reversing type 1 diabetes. Endocrinol Metab Clin North Am 39: 655–667.
5. Contreras JL, Bilbao G, Smyth CA, Jiang XL, Eckhoff DE, et al. (2001) Cytoprotection of pancreatic islets before and soon after transplantation by gene transfer of the anti-apoptotic Bcl-2 gene. Transplantation 71: 1015–1023.
6. Emamaullee JA, Rajotte RV, Liston P, Korneluk RG, Lakey JR, et al. (2005) XIAP overexpression in human islets prevents early posttransplant apoptosis and reduces the islet mass needed to treat diabetes. Diabetes 54: 2541–2548.
7. Emamaullee J, Liston P, Korneluk RG, Shapiro AM, Elliott JF (2005) XIAP overexpression in islet beta-cells enhances engraftment and minimizes hypoxia-reperfusion injury. Am J Transplant 5: 1297–1305.
8. Plesner A, Liston P, Tan R, Korneluk RG, Verchere CB (2005) The X-linked inhibitor of apoptosis protein enhances survival of murine islet allografts. Diabetes 54: 2533–2540.
9. Plesner A, Soukhatcheva G, Korneluk RG, Verchere CB (2010) XIAP inhibition of beta-cell apoptosis reduces the number of islets required to restore euglycemia in a syngeneic islet transplantation model. Islets 2: 18–23.
10. Qin J, Jiao Y, Chen X, Zhou S, Liang C, et al. (2009) Overexpression of suppressor of cytokine signaling 1 in islet grafts results in anti-apoptotic effects and prolongs graft survival. Life Sci 84: 810–816.
11. Grey ST, Longo C, Shukri T, Patel VI, Csizmadia E, et al. (2003) Genetic engineering of a suboptimal islet graft with A20 preserves beta cell mass and function. J Immunol 170: 6250–6256.
12. Emamaullee JA, Stanton L, Schur C, Shapiro AM (2007) Caspase inhibitor therapy enhances marginal mass islet graft survival and preserves long-term function in islet transplantation. Diabetes 56: 1289–1298.
13. Emamaullee JA, Davis J, Pawlick R, Toso C, Merani S, et al. (2008) The caspase selective inhibitor EP1013 augments human islet graft function and longevity in marginal mass islet transplantation in mice. Diabetes 57: 1556–1566.
14. Rivas-Carrillo JD, Soto-Gutierrez A, Navarro-Alvarez N, Noguchi H, Okitsu T, et al. (2007) Cell-permeable pentapeptide V5 inhibits apoptosis and enhances insulin secretion, allowing experimental single-donor islet transplantation in mice. Diabetes 56: 1259–1267.
15. Takahashi T, Matsumoto S, Matsushita M, Kamachi H, Tsuruga Y, et al. (2010) Donor pretreatment with DHMEQ improves islet transplantation. J Surg Res 163: e23–34.
16. Rink JS, Chen X, Zhang X, Kaufman DB (2012) Conditional and specific inhibition of NF-kappaB in mouse pancreatic beta cells prevents cytokine-induced deleterious effects and improves islet survival posttransplant. Surgery 151: 330–339.
17. Gao Q, Ma LL, Gao X, Yan W, Williams P, et al. (2010) TLR4 mediates early graft failure after intraportal islet transplantation. Am J Transplant 10: 1588–1596.
18. Yang H, Thomas D, Boffa DJ, Ding R, Li B, et al. (2002) Enforced c-REL deficiency prolongs survival of islet allografts1. Transplantation 74: 291–298.
19. Eldor R, Yeffet A, Baum K, Doviner V, Amar D, et al. (2006) Conditional and specific NF-kappaB blockade protects pancreatic beta cells from diabetogenic agents. Proc Natl Acad Sci U S A 103: 5072–5077.
20. Eldor R, Baum K, Abel R, Sever D, Melloul D (2009) The ToI-beta transgenic mouse: a model to study the specific role of NF-kappaB in beta-cells. Diabetes Res Clin Pract 86 Suppl 1: S7–14.
21. Poff JA, Allen CT, Traughber B, Colunga A, Xie J, et al. (2008) Pulsed high-intensity focused ultrasound enhances apoptosis and growth inhibition of squamous cell carcinoma xenografts with proteasome inhibitor bortezomib. Radiology 248: 485–491.
22. Goldberg A, Parolini M, Chin BY, Czismadia E, Otterbein LE, et al. (2007) Toll-like receptor 4 suppression leads to islet allograft survival. Faseb J 21: 2840–2848.
23. Bock T, Pakkenberg B, Buschard K (2003) Increased islet volume but unchanged islet number in ob/ob mice. Diabetes 52: 1716–1722.
24. Jelsing J, Vrang N, van Witteloostuijn SB, Mark M, Klein T (2012) The DPP4 inhibitor linagliptin delays the onset of diabetes and preserves beta-cell mass in non-obese diabetic mice. J Endocrinol 214: 381–387.
25. Baker MS, Chen X, Rotramel AR, Nelson JJ, Lu B, et al. (2003) Genetic deletion of chemokine receptor CXCR3 or antibody blockade of its ligand IP-10 modulates posttransplantation graft-site lymphocytic infiltrates and prolongs functional graft survival in pancreatic islet allograft recipients. Surgery 134: 126–133.
26. Chen C, Moreno R, Samikannu B, Bretzel RG, Schmitz ML, et al. (2010) Improved Intraportal Islet Transplantation Outcome by Systemic IKK-beta Inhibition: NF-kappaB Activity in Pancreatic Islets Depends on Oxygen Availability. Am J Transplant 11: 215–224.
27. Nencioni A, Grunebach F, Patrone F, Ballestrero A, Brossart P (2006) The proteasome and its inhibitors in immune regulation and immune disorders. Crit Rev Immunol 26: 487–498.
28. Karin M, Ben-Neriah Y (2000) Phosphorylation meets ubiquitination: the control of NF-[kappa]B activity. Annu Rev Immunol 18: 621–663.
29. Karin M, Lin A (2002) NF-kappaB at the crossroads of life and death. Nat Immunol 3: 221–227.
30. Perkins ND (2007) Integrating cell-signalling pathways with NF-kappaB and IKK function. Nat Rev Mol Cell Biol 8: 49–62.
31. Giannoukakis N, Rudert WA, Trucco M, Robbins PD (2000) Protection of human islets from the effects of interleukin-1beta by adenoviral gene transfer of an Ikappa B repressor. J Biol Chem 275: 36509–36513.
32. Baker MS, Chen X, Cao XC, Kaufman DB (2001) Expression of a dominant negative inhibitor of NF-kappaB protects MIN6 beta-cells from cytokine-induced apoptosis. J Surg Res 97: 117–122.
33. Eizirik DL, Mandrup-Poulsen T (2001) A choice of death–the signal-transduction of immune-mediated beta-cell apoptosis. Diabetologia 44: 2115–2133.
34. Heimberg H, Heremans Y, Jobin C, Leemans R, Cardozo AK, et al. (2001) Inhibition of cytokine-induced NF-kappaB activation by adenovirus- mediated expression of a NF-kappaB super-repressor prevents beta-cell apoptosis. Diabetes 50: 2219–2224.
35. Mandrup-Poulsen T (2003) Apoptotic signal transduction pathways in diabetes. Biochem Pharmacol 66: 1433–1440.
36. Melloul D (2008) Role of NF-kappaB in beta-cell death. Biochem Soc Trans 36: 334–339.
37. Ortis F, Pirot P, Naamane N, Kreins AY, Rasschaert J, et al. (2008) Induction of nuclear factor-kappaB and its downstream genes by TNF-alpha and IL-1beta has a pro-apoptotic role in pancreatic beta cells. Diabetologia 51: 1213–1225.
38. Zhao Y, Krishnamurthy B, Mollah ZU, Kay TW, Thomas HE (2011) NF-kappaB in Type 1 Diabetes. Inflamm Allergy Drug Targets 10: 208–217.
39. Ortis F, Cardozo AK, Crispim D, Storling J, Mandrup-Poulsen T, et al. (2006) Cytokine-induced proapoptotic gene expression in insulin-producing cells is related to rapid, sustained, and nonoscillatory nuclear factor-kappaB activation. Mol Endocrinol 20: 1867–1879.
40. Ou D, Wang X, Metzger DL, Robbins M, Huang J, et al. (2005) Regulation of TNF-related apoptosis-inducing ligand-mediated death-signal pathway in human beta cells by Fas-associated death domain and nuclear factor kappaB. Hum Immunol 66: 799–809.
41. Rehman KK, Bertera S, Bottino R, Balamurugan AN, Mai JC, et al. (2003) Protection of islets by in situ peptide-mediated transduction of the Ikappa B kinase inhibitor Nemo-binding domain peptide. J Biol Chem 278: 9862–9868.
42. Cottet S, Dupraz P, Hamburger F, Dolci W, Jaquet M, et al. (2002) cFLIP protein prevents tumor necrosis factor-alpha-mediated induction of caspase-8-dependent apoptosis in insulin-secreting betaTc-Tet cells. Diabetes 51: 1805–1814.
43. De Paula D, Bentley MV, Mahato RI (2007) Effect of iNOS and NF-kappaB gene silencing on beta-cell survival and function. J Drug Target 15: 358–369.

44. Hagerkvist R, Sandler S, Mokhtari D, Welsh N (2007) Amelioration of diabetes by imatinib mesylate (Gleevec): role of beta-cell NF-kappaB activation and anti-apoptotic preconditioning. Faseb J 21: 618–628.

45. Chang I, Kim S, Kim JY, Cho N, Kim YH, et al. (2003) Nuclear factor kappaB protects pancreatic beta-cells from tumor necrosis factor-alpha-mediated apoptosis. Diabetes 52: 1169–1175.

46. Maedler K, Schumann DM, Sauter N, Ellingsgaard H, Bosco D, et al. (2006) Low concentration of interleukin-1beta induces FLICE-inhibitory protein-mediated beta-cell proliferation in human pancreatic islets. Diabetes 55: 2713–2722.

47. Hammar EB, Irminger JC, Rickenbach K, Parnaud G, Ribaux P, et al. (2005) Activation of NF-kappaB by extracellular matrix is involved in spreading and glucose-stimulated insulin secretion of pancreatic beta cells. J Biol Chem 280: 30630–30637.

48. Donath MY, Boni-Schnetzler M, Ellingsgaard H, Halban PA, Ehses JA (2010) Cytokine production by islets in health and diabetes: cellular origin, regulation and function. Trends Endocrinol Metab 21: 261–267.

49. Romagnani P, Crescioli C (2012) CXCL10: A candidate biomarker in transplantation. Clin Chim Acta 413: 1364–1373.

50. Uno S, Imagawa A, Saisho K, Okita K, Iwahashi H, et al. (2012) Expression of chemokines, CXC chemokine ligand 10 (CXCL10) and CXCR3 in the inflamed islets of patients with recent-onset autoimmune type 1 diabetes. Endocr J 57: 991–996.

51. Morimoto J, Yoneyama H, Shimada A, Shigihara T, Yamada S, et al. (2004) CXC chemokine ligand 10 neutralization suppresses the occurrence of diabetes in nonobese diabetic mice through enhanced beta cell proliferation without affecting insulitis. J Immunol 173: 7017–7024.

10

Value of the First Post-Transplant Biopsy for Predicting Long-Term Cardiac Allograft Vasculopathy (CAV) and Graft Failure in Heart Transplant Patients

Carlos A. Labarrere[1]*, John R. Woods[2], James W. Hardin[3], Gonzalo L. Campana[1], Miguel A. Ortiz[1], Beate R. Jaeger[4], Lee Ann Baldridge[5], Douglas E. Pitts[6], Philip C. Kirlin[7]

1 Experimental Pathology, Methodist Research Institute, Indiana University Health Methodist Hospital, Indianapolis, Indiana, United States of America, 2 Outcomes Research, Methodist Research Institute, Indiana University Health Methodist Hospital, Indianapolis, Indiana, United States of America, 3 Epidemiology and Biostatistics, University of South Carolina, Columbia, South Carolina, United States of America, 4 Dr. Stein und Kollegen, Mönchengladbach, Germany, 5 Department of Pathology and Laboratory Medicine, Indiana University School of Medicine, Indianapolis, Indiana, United States of America, 6 St Vincent Medical Group, St Vincent Hospital, Indianapolis, Indiana, United States of America, 7 Transplant Center, Indiana University Health Methodist Hospital, Indianapolis, Indiana, United States of America

Abstract

Background: Cardiac allograft vasculopathy (CAV) is the principal cause of long-term graft failure following heart transplantation. Early identification of patients at risk of CAV is essential to target invasive follow-up procedures more effectively and to establish appropriate therapies. We evaluated the prognostic value of the first heart biopsy (median: 9 days post-transplant) versus all biopsies obtained within the first three months for the prediction of CAV and graft failure due to CAV.

Methods and Findings: In a prospective cohort study, we developed multivariate regression models evaluating markers of atherothrombosis (fibrin, antithrombin and tissue plasminogen activator [tPA]) and endothelial activation (intercellular adhesion molecule-1) in serial biopsies obtained during the first three months post-transplantation from 172 patients (median follow-up = 6.3 years; min = 0.37 years; max = 16.3 years). Presence of fibrin was the dominant predictor in first-biopsy models (Odds Ratio [OR] for one- and 10-year graft failure due to CAV = 38.70, p = 0.002, 95% CI = 4.00–374.77; and 3.99, p = 0.005, 95% CI = 1.53–10.40) and loss of tPA was predominant in three-month models (OR for one- and 10-year graft failure due to CAV = 1.81, p = 0.025, 95% CI = 1.08–3.03; and 1.31, p = 0.001, 95% CI = 1.12–1.55). First-biopsy and three-month models had similar predictive and discriminative accuracy and were comparable in their capacities to correctly classify patient outcomes, with the exception of 10-year graft failure due to CAV in which the three-month model was more predictive. Both models had particularly high negative predictive values (e.g., First-biopsy vs. three-month models: 99% vs. 100% at 1-year and 96% vs. 95% at 10-years).

Conclusions: Patients with absence of fibrin in the first biopsy and persistence of normal tPA in subsequent biopsies rarely develop CAV or graft failure during the next 10 years and potentially could be monitored less invasively. Presence of early risk markers in the transplanted heart may be secondary to ischemia/reperfusion injury, a potentially modifiable factor.

Editor: Lucienne Chatenoud, Université Paris Descartes, France

Funding: The study was supported by the Showalter Foundation and the Methodist Research Institute. The funders had no involvement in the design and conduct of the study; collection, management, analysis, and interpretation of the data; or preparation, review, or approval of the manuscript.

Competing Interests: The authors have declared that no competing interests exist.

* E-mail: clabarrere@iuhealth.org

Introduction

Modern immunosuppressive regimens have reduced the incidence of acute rejection and extended early survival following heart transplantation but have done little to reduce the incidence of cardiac allograft vasculopathy (CAV), the principal long-term cause of graft failure. CAV, an aggressive form of atherosclerosis that develops within months to a few years after transplantation, accounts for 30% of all deaths [1]. Because heart transplant patients lack premonitory symptoms, CAV first presents clinically as a silent myocardial infarction, severe arrhythmia, or sudden death. Thus, research has focused on identifying early predictors of CAV onset and progression.

The Invasive Monitoring Attenuation through Gene Expression (IMAGE) trial recently showed that patients at low risk of rejection can be monitored safely with noninvasive gene-expression profiling [2]. It might be possible to devise a similar noninvasive strategy to monitor CAV, provided that low-risk patients could be reliably identified. We recently showed that absence of atherothrombotic risk markers in the first three months post-transplantation identifies patients that rarely develop CAV, suggesting that they might be candidates for less invasive monitoring [3]. This finding led us to study the predictive value of the *first* biopsy, obtained 7–12 days post-transplant. Thus, the aim of this study was to determine whether very early data from a single biopsy are sufficient to identify low-risk patients. Our analysis showed that patients with absence of fibrin in the first biopsy rarely develop CAV or graft failure during the next 10 years. Furthermore, the high negative predictive value of the first-biopsy was comparable to that of multiple biopsies obtained over three-months, implying that patients with negative findings in the first biopsy potentially could be monitored less invasively, thereby, avoiding the risk and expense of multiple heart biopsy procedures.

Materials and Methods

Patients

Consecutive adult heart-transplant recipients transplanted from August 1989 to August 2004 and followed prospectively until September 2010, were candidates for study. Patients (n = 172) were included if they survived at least three months post-transplantation, had serial endomyocardial biopsies performed in the first three months, and had their coronary arteries examined angiographically and/or histopathologically for CAV at annual follow-ups. Of 241 candidates, 29 patients were excluded because they had missing three-month biopsy data, either because they died prior to three months (n = 14) or because they were transplanted at another institution (n = 15); 38 survived three-months but were excluded because they had incomplete biopsy data; and two survived but were excluded because of missing follow-up coronary evaluations. The study protocol was approved by the Indiana University local Institutional Review Board and all subjects signed a consent form.

Clinical management

All patients received triple-drug immunosuppression [4]. Rejection grades 2R-3R [5] were treated with steroids plus rabbit antithymocyte globulin or OKT3 monoclonal antibody. Higher dose immunosuppressants and clinical treatment strategies were used at the physician's discretion without knowledge of immuno-histochemical data regarding markers of atherothrombosis and endothelial activation.

Baseline (time-zero) endomyocardial biopsies were performed on all of the 172 donor hearts at the time of transplantation but before reperfusion. Additional biopsies were performed serially during the first three months after transplantation, with the first post-transplant biopsy obtained within a median 9 days of transplantation.

Cytomegalovirus disease was defined during follow-up by clinical symptoms and by cytopathologic-tissue culture evidence of invasion. Cytomegalovirus prophylaxis with gancyclovir was used in seronegative recipients of seropositive donors.

Outcome Criteria

CAV was evaluated in side-by-side comparisons of identical projections of serial angiograms performed annually (Mean: 5.25 ± 1.0/patient) and diagnosed by evidence of coronary artery narrowing or luminal irregularities either in left main or any primary or branch vessels. CAV was considered severe if left main stenosis was >70%, if two or more primary vessels had stenoses >70%, or if branch stenoses were >70% in all three systems [6]. Presence and severity of CAV were determined by consensus of two experienced angiographers unaware of immunohistochemical biopsy results. In recipients who died before their first annual angiogram, coronary arteries were examined histopathologically and severe CAV was identified using similar criteria to those described for angiographic evaluation. Graft failure due to CAV was defined as: (a) death associated with CAV-related cardiac allograft dysfunction, or (b) need for a second transplant due to severe CAV.

Immunohistochemistry studies

Endomyocardial biopsies were tested immunohistochemically for fibrin (NYBT2G1, Accurate, Westbury, NY; a-Fib Beta, American Diagnostica, Stamford, CT); tissue plasminogen activator (tPA, ESP-1, American Diagnostica); antithrombin (A0296, DAKO, Carpinteria, CA) and intercellular adhesion molecule-1 (ICAM-1, LB-2, Santa Cruz Biotechnology, Santa Cruz, CA).

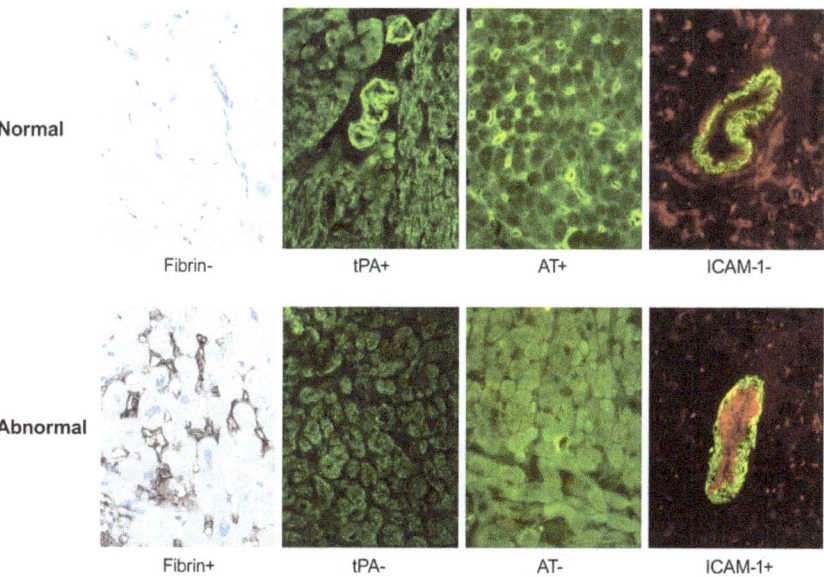

Figure 1. Immunohistochemical characteristics of a thrombotic/activated microvasculature. Normal hearts (top row) have absence of fibrin (Fib−), presence of microvascular antithrombin (AT+) and tissue plasminogen activator (tPA+) and absence of arterial endothelial ICAM-1 (ICAM-1−). Abnormal thrombotic and activated hearts (bottom row) are characterized by presence of fibrin (Fib+), loss of microvascular antithrombin (AT−) and tissue plasminogen activator (tPA−) and expression of arterial endothelial ICAM-1 (ICAM-1+). Original magnification ×640.

Affinity-purified, fluorochrome-labeled or peroxidase-labeled polymer conjugated anti-mouse or fluorochrome-labeled anti-rabbit F(ab')$_2$ fragments served as secondary antibodies (Molecular Probes, Eugene, OR and Protos ImmunoResearch, Burlingame, CA). Arteries were identified with fluorescein-labeled mouse monoclonal antibody to human smooth muscle α-actin (1A4, Sigma-Aldrich, St Louis, MO).

For immunofluorescence studies, tissue samples were embedded in optimum cutting temperature compound (Miles, Elkhart, IN), snap-frozen in liquid nitrogen and stored at −75°C. Cryostat sections (4 μm) were air-dried overnight without fixation, and immunostained. Rhodamine-conjugated anti-mouse and Alexa Fluor 488 anti-rabbit or anti-mouse were used as secondary antibodies.

For immunoperoxidase studies, slides from paraffin blocks were antigen-retrieved using DAKO Target Retrieval solution (pH 6.0) to expose antigens masked by formalin. Endogenous biotin was blocked with avidin/biotin blocking system (DAKO) and endogenous peroxidase with 3% hydrogen peroxide. Fibrin antibody was applied for 60 minutes at room temperature. Slides were developed using DAKO's EnVision+ Dual Link, HRP kit for mouse primary antibodies in a DAKO Autostainer. Immunohistochemical data were evaluated by two investigators unaware of clinical outcome.

Coding of biopsy markers

Immunohistochemical data were scored as described by Labarrere et al [3]. As illustrated in Figure 1 (top row), normal hearts have absence of fibrin (Fib−), presence of microvascular antithrombin (AT+) and tPA (tPA+) and absence of arterial endothelial ICAM-1 (ICAM-1). Thrombotic and activated hearts, shown in Figure 1 (bottom row), have myocardial fibrin deposits in capillaries and cardiomyocytes (Fib+), loss of microvascular antithrombin (AT−), loss of arteriolar tPA (tPA−) and expression of arterial endothelial ICAM-1 (ICAM-1+). For predictive models that used data from only the first biopsy, each of these signs was scored either 0, if normal, or 1, if abnormal. For models that used all biopsies obtained during the first three months, we calculated the *proportion* of abnormal signs for each marker (e.g., if a patient had four biopsies and three had fibrin deposits, the marker for fibrin was scored: Fib+ = 3/4 = .75 for that patient). Proportions were re-scaled by a factor of 10 so that regression coefficients could be interpreted as a 10% change in the proportion of abnormal biopsies, a change in approximately one biopsy from normal to abnormal for the typical patient. Four predictors were tested representing the presence or absence of abnormality in the four markers (Fib+, AT−, tPA−, ICAM-1+).

Statistical model

Univariate logistic regression models were estimated using each biomarker in turn as the sole predictor in the equation. Multivariate stepwise models were then developed in two stages. In stage-one, statistically significant biomarkers were identified by stepwise backward elimination to establish base models. In stage-two, clinical and laboratory covariates shown in Table 1, that were found to be significantly associated with outcome in initial bivariate analyses were forced into the base models. Because time-zero biopsies revealed normal immunohistochemical markers in all cases and exhibited no between-patient variation, they were not considered as potential predictors in any of the regression models.

Table 1. Summary of demographic and clinical variables (Patients: n = 172).

VARIABLE	VALUE				
Donor:					
Age, mean years (±SD)	28.8			(±11.2)	
Sex (percent male)	78.5				
Recipient:					
Age, mean years (±SD)	48.7			(±10.2)	
Sex (percent male)	66.9				
Race (percent white)	89.5				
Body mass index (kg/m²), mean (±SD)	26.5			(±5.0)	
Diabetics (%)	40.1				
Insulin dependent diabetics (%)	31.4				
Reason for transplantation:					
Coronary artery disease (%)	45.9				
Cardiomyopathy (%)	47.1				
Other (%)	7.0				
Ischemic time (minutes), mean (±SD)	156.8			(±56.6)	
Smokers after transplantation (%)	7.6				
Hypertensives (%)	89.0				
Cholesterol (mmol/l):					
Total cholesterol, mean (±SD)	5.4			(±1.0)	
LDL-C, mean (±SD)	2.6			(±0.8)	
HDL-C, mean (±SD)	1.2			(±0.4)	
Number of HLA mismatches:	0	1	2	3	4
A/B (%)	0	5.8	16.3	47.1	30.8
DR (%)	7.00	39.0	54.0		
Creatinine >123.8 μmol/l (%)	58.1				
Ejection fraction, mean (%) (±SD)	54.3			(±7.4)	
2R-3R rejections (1st 3-mos), mean (±SD)	0.2			(±0.4)	
Biopsies (1st 3-months), mean (±SD)	5.2			(±1.0)	
CMV infections (% positive)	12.8				
Cell Panel Reactive Antibodies >0% (%)	8.1				
Treatment:					
Prednisone (%)	100.0				
Cyclosporine (%)	94.2				
Azathioprine (%)	68.0				
Mycophenolate mofetil (%)	65.7				
Tacrolimus (%)	11.0				
Sirolimus (%)	7.0				
Statins (%)	77.9				
Calcium Channel Blockers (%)	77.9				
ACE Inhibitors/ARBs (%)	43.0				

All data based on entire sample of 172 patients. Abbreviations: SD: Standard Deviation; LDL-C: low density lipoprotein cholesterol; HDL-C: high density lipoprotein cholesterol; CMV: cytomegalovirus; ACE: Angiotensin-Converting Enzyme; ARB: Angiotensin Receptor Blockers.

Table 2. Univariate logistic regression models using information from the first post-transplant biopsy (N = 172 patients).[a]

Model	CAV:	One-Year Risk (31 cases)[b]			Five-Year Risk (85 cases)			Ten-Year Risk (106 cases)		
		C	OR	CI	C	OR	CI	C	OR	CI
1	Fibrin	0.64	3.21	1.46–7.07	0.67	5.39	2.64–11.0	0.67	5.83	2.54–13.4
2	AT	0.64	3.30	1.45–7.50	0.67	4.36	2.29–8.29	0.70	5.68	2.77–11.7
3	tPA	0.63	2.89	0.98–4.79	0.67	4.77	2.44–9.34	0.68	5.60	2.58–12.1
4	ICAM-1	0.59	2.17	1.32–6.36	0.63	3.88	1.90–7.93	0.62	3.76	1.68–8.41
	Severe CAV:	One-Year Risk (10 cases)			Five-Year Risk (36 cases)			Ten-Year Risk (58 cases)		
		C	OR	CI	C	OR	CI	C	OR	CI
5	Fibrin	0.75	8.96	1.84–43.7	0.67	4.05	1.87–8.79	0.67	4.38	2.22–8.66
6	AT	0.68	5.26	1.08–25.5	0.66	3.96	1.76–8.91	0.62	2.66	1.39–5.12
7	tPA	0.67	4.07	1.01–16.4	0.65	3.58	1.65–7.75	0.70	5.49	2.76–10.9
8	ICAM-1	0.50	1.02	0.25–4.10	0.62	2.86	1.33–6.17	0.61	2.67	1.35–5.29
	Failure Due To CAV:	One-Year Risk (7 cases)			Five-Year Risk (18 cases)			Ten-Year Risk (31 cases)		
		C	OR	CI	C	OR	CI	C	OR	CI
9	Fibrin	0.77	13.04	1.53–111	0.75	8.75	2.73–28.0	0.67	4.14	1.84–9.32
10	AT	0.71	7.75	0.91–65.8	0.71	7.22	2.01–26.0	0.62	2.60	1.16–5.84
11	tPA	0.67	4.26	0.80–22.6	0.69	3.95	1.68–14.6	0.64	3.17	1.42–7.07
12	ICAM-1	0.51	0.95	0.18–5.05	0.64	3.45	1.27–9.33	0.61	2.73	1.23–6.08

Abbreviations: C: C-Statistic (Area under the ROC curve); OR: Odds Ratio; CI: Confidence Intervals; AT: Antithrombin; tPA: tissue Plasminogen Activator; ICAM-1: Intercellular Adhesion Molecule-1.
[a]Each model uses one biomarker as the single predictor of CAV, severe CAV and failure due to CAV at one-, five-, and ten-years post-transplant.
[b]Numbers in parentheses (cases) represent the cumulative number of patients experiencing the indicated event at each follow-up interval.

Model cross-validation

Using the method of Austin and Tu [7], regression models were re-estimated for 200 bootstrap [8] samples drawn with replacement from the original data. Bootstrap re-estimation of model parameters is equivalent to performing multiple split-sample validation estimates and provides assessments of model performance without sacrificing sample size [9]. Statistically significant biomarkers identified in stage one and covariates that were found to be univariately associated with outcomes were included in final multivariate models if those variables were retained in ≥60% of the 200 bootstrapped models. A total of $3 \times 3 \times 2 = 18$ models were derived to predict one-, five-, and 10-year odds of CAV, severe CAV and graft failure due to CAV using markers from either the first biopsy only, or from all biopsies available at three months.

The Youden Index calculated from receiver operating characteristic (ROC) curves were used to identify optimum cut-off values for the models [10]. Model performance was quantified by evaluating sensitivity, specificity, and predictive accuracy. The C-statistic (area under the ROC curve) was used to quantify discriminative accuracy [11]. Models were further evaluated by comparing the overall percentages of patients correctly classified.

Predicted values from ten-year models were stratified into three groupings: (1) LOW RISK (lower 25% of risk distribution); (2) MODERATE RISK (middle 50%) and (3) HIGH RISK (upper 25%) and separate Kaplan-Meier curves were constructed for these risk groups.

Results

Demographic and clinical characteristics of the patient population assessed at three months post-transplant are shown in Table 1. Time-zero biopsies performed at the time of transplant but before reperfusion all showed the characteristics of a thromboresistant microvasculature (as illustrated in Figure 1, top row). Because these baseline biopsies were all normal and exhibited no variation they were not considered further in regression models.

When evaluated in univariate regression models (Table 2), individual markers from the first biopsy were statistically significant and possessed good predictive value in most cases (C-statistics: 0.50 to 0.77; odds ratios [ORs]: 0.95 to 13.04). The presence of fibrin emerged as the most common univariate predictor in first-biopsy models. This is in contrast with previous analyses which showed that loss of tPA was the predominant predictor in three-month models [3].

In final multivariate models (Tables 3, 4 and 5), presence of fibrin with or without ICAM-1 expression was the most common statistically significant predictor in first-biopsy models, and loss of tPA was the dominant predictor in three-month models. Once the odds associated with these markers were accounted for, none of the other markers were able to explain additional odds.

The odds ratio (OR) in first-biopsy models represents the multiplicative increase in risk associated with the presence of an abnormal marker. In three-month models the OR is the

Table 3. Final multivariate logistic regression models using first-biopsy-only or three-month biopsy data to predict CAV, severe CAV, and graft failure due to CAV at one year post-transplant.

ONE-YEAR RISK of OUTCOME					
CAV:					
Using 1st biopsy, only:			**Using all biopsies available at 3 months:**		
Predictor Variable	**OR**	**CI**	**Predictor Variable**	**OR**	**CI**
Antithrombin	3.30	1.45–7.50	tPA	1.36	1.18–1.57
			Ischemic time	0.99	0.99–1.00
SEVERE CAV:					
Using 1st biopsy, only:			**Using all biopsies available at 3 months:**		
Predictor Variable	**OR**	**CI**	**Predictor Variable**	**OR**	**CI**
Fibrin	30.68	3.91–240.6	tPA	2.22	1.29–3.83
ICAM-1	0.08	0.01–0.60	Ischemic time	0.98	0.96–1.00
Statins	0.05	0.01–0.29	Statins	0.02	0.00–0.17
GRAFT FAILURE DUE TO CAV:					
Using 1st biopsy, only:			**Using all biopsies available at 3 months:**		
Predictor Variable	**OR**	**CI**	**Predictor Variable**	**OR**	**CI**
Fibrin	38.70	4.00–374.8	tPA	1.81	1.08–3.03
ICAM-1	0.13	0.02–0.82			

Abbreviations: OR: Odds Ratio; CI: 95% confidence interval for the OR; tPA: Tissue Plasminogen Activator; ICAM-1: Intercellular Adhesion Molecule-1.
Models on the left use information from the first biopsy only. Models on the right use information from all biopsies available in the first three months post-transplantation.

multiplicative increase in risk associated with a 10% increase in the proportion of abnormal biopsy results (equivalent to approximately one biopsy result over the first three months). As an example, the three-month model predicting graft failure due to CAV at 10 years, which shows an OR for tPA of 1.31 (Table 5), indicates that the 10-year odds of graft failure increases by a factor of 1.31 with each 10% increase in the proportion of biopsies showing loss of tPA in the first three months. A 20% increase in biopsies showing loss of tPA (equivalent to approximately two biopsy results in the first three months) increases the 10-year odds by $1.31 \times 1.31 = 1.7161$.

Performance characteristics for all models are summarized in Table 6. Considering positive and negative outcomes together, first-biopsy and three-month models showed similar capacities to classify patients correctly. The one exception was for 10-year predictions of graft failure due to CAV where the three-month model correctly classified a significantly higher percentage of patients (87%) compared to the first-biopsy model (76%).

Positive predictive values for both first-biopsy and three-month models tended to be low, with the lowest values associated with one-year predictions. By contrast, negative predictive values were high for both sets of models. For example, in first-biopsy models patients with no evidence of fibrin deposition had a 99% chance of avoiding graft failure due to CAV at one year, and continued to have a 98% and 96% chance of being risk-free at five- and 10-years (Table 6). Similarly, patients showing sustained levels of microvascular tPA over the next three-months had a 100% chance of avoiding graft failure due to CAV at one year, and continued to have a 99% and 95% chance of being risk-free at five- and 10-years, respectively. *Thus, the earliest information available from a single biopsy is sufficient to identify a subgroup of patients with very low odds of long-term (10-year) graft failure due to CAV.*

Kaplan-Meier curves using risk-stratified predictive values from 10-year regression models (Figure 2) showed significant time-to-event differences by the log-rank test for CAV (p = .001), severe CAV (p = .001), and failure due to CAV (p = .001) for both first-biopsy and three-month models. Thus, first-biopsy models are similar to three-month models not only in their predictions of adverse event incidence, but also in their predictions of *time* to event.

Discussion

Prediction models using information derived from a single endomyocardial biopsy obtained within a median 9 days post-transplant accurately identified heart transplant patients with *substantially* reduced risk of developing long-term CAV and graft failure.

The high negative predictive accuracies of our models have important clinical implications. First, models that used only the first biopsy had negative predictive values comparable to models that used all biopsies available at three months, confirming our hypothesis that a single early biopsy is sufficient to identify patients with very low risk of long-term (10-year) graft failure due to CAV. This finding implies that it may be possible to reduce the number of follow-up biopsies and coronary angiographies for low-risk patients, provided there is continued absence of symptoms or signs of rejection. Moreover, multiple biopsies during the first three months may be *unnecessary* in patients with no evidence of fibrin deposits in the first biopsy. Of course, patients that are not identified as low-risk would still need to be followed with definitive monitoring. A potential strategy would be to follow low-risk patients non-invasively with gene expression profiling, as has been suggested for the monitoring of patients with low risk for rejection

Table 4. Final multivariate logistic regression models using first-biopsy-only or three-month biopsy data to predict CAV, severe CAV, and graft failure due to CAV at five years post-transplant.

FIVE-YEAR RISK of OUTCOME

CAV:

Using 1st biopsy, only:			Using all biopsies available at 3 months:		
Predictor Variable	OR	CI	Predictor Variable	OR	CI
Antithrombin	5.34	2.69–10.58	tPA	1.41	1.26–1.58
HLA-AB Mismatch	0.33	0.14–0.75	Recipient Sex (Male)	2.34	1.05–5.19
			HLA-AB Mismatch	0.37	0.15–0.88

SEVERE CAV:

Using 1st biopsy, only:			Using all biopsies available at 3 months:		
Predictor Variable	OR	CI	Predictor Variable	OR	CI
Fibrin	4.13	1.77–9.68	tPA	1.45	1.23–1.71
MMF Regimen	0.36	0.15–0.84	MMF Regimen	0.45	0.18–1.11
Recipient Sex (Male)	2.22	0.84–5.90	Recipient Sex (Male)	4.17	1.41–12.31
HLA-AB Mismatch	0.41	0.16–1.06	HLA-AB Mismatch	0.33	0.11–0.95
Statins	0.36	0.15–5.90	Statins	0.27	0.10–0.73

GRAFT FAILURE DUE TO CAV:

Using 1st biopsy, only:			Using all biopsies available at 3 months:		
Predictor Variable	OR	CI	Predictor Variable	OR	CI
Fibrin	9.33	2.34–37.12	tPA	1.73	1.22–2.45
MMF Regimen	0.08	0.02–0.35	MMF Regimen	0.11	0.02–0.49
Statins	0.10	0.03–0.38	Statins	0.06	0.01–0.27

Abbreviations: OR: Odds Ratio; CI: 95% confidence interval for the OR; tPA: Tissue Plasminogen Activator; HLA: Human Leukocyte Antigen; MMF: Mycophenolate Mofetil. Models on the left use information from the first biopsy only. Models on the right use information from all biopsies available in the first three months post-transplantation.

[2], while continuing to follow all other patients using conventional monitoring protocols. In doing so, the complications and costs associated with invasive heart biopsies would be reduced and limited resources could be freed up for more intensive follow-up of higher-risk patients.

The *positive predictive accuracies* of our models were not as strong as the negative predictive accuracies, suggesting that it is harder to identify high-risk than low-risk patients. A likely explanation is that patients with evolving disease are eventually identified and treated preventively during the 10-year follow-up interval, thereby reducing the odds initially predicted based on prior three-month data.

Absence of myocardial fibrin in the first biopsy and persistence of microvascular tPA in all biopsies obtained during the first three months emerged as the best *independent* predictors in most multivariate models, suggesting that the underlying biological process upon which statistical prediction is based evolves over time during the first three months following transplantation. We conclude that early absence of microthrombosis and continued persistence of an intact fibrinolytic system are indicative of a protective phenotype against long-term CAV and allograft failure.

Lack of antithrombin typifies a system that is failing to prevent microvascular fibrin deposits. Thus, it is reasonable that loss of antithrombin in the first-biopsy model would turn out to be the best early predictor of CAV, and that the subsequent unchecked accumulation of microvascular fibrin, secondary to the loss of antithrombin, would be the best early predictor of *severe* CAV and

graft failure due to CAV. If microvascular fibrin continues to be deposited due to the failure of antithrombin to prevent it, the patient will still retain some capacity to remove it as long as there is a sustained presence of tPA. However, if there is also loss of tPA, fibrinolytic capacity will be diminished, fibrin deposition will continue unabated, and the patient's status will worsen. Thus, it is reasonable that three-month models would pinpoint loss of tPA as the single best independent predictor of long-term CAV and graft failure.

In first-biopsy models it is noteworthy that ICAM-1 expression, a marker of endothelial activation, appears with fibrin as a co-predictor of severe CAV and graft failure at one year, indicating that endothelial activation in the presence of microvascular fibrin further heightens the odds of very early and very serious CAV. This is consistent with observations from a transient cerebral artery occlusion model showing that concomitant reduction of both ICAM-1 expression and microvascular fibrin significantly reduced brain injury and improved post-ischemic blood flow [12].

The importance of early microthrombosis, reduced fibrinolysis and microvascular arterial endothelial activation for CAV and graft failure has been previously demonstrated [4,6,13,14,15,16,17,18]. Until now, however, the *sequence* in which these markers emerge during the immediate post-transplant period has not been well described and the prognostic significance of the information contained in the first biopsy has been underappreciated.

Table 5. Final multivariate logistic regression models using first-biopsy-only or three-month biopsy data to predict CAV, severe CAV, and graft failure due to CAV at ten years post-transplant.

TEN-YEAR RISK of OUTCOME

CAV:

Using 1st biopsy, only:			Using all biopsies available at 3 months:		
Predictor Variable	OR	CI	Predictor Variable	OR	CI
Antithrombin	8.73	3.81–20.04	Antithrombin	1.47	1.29–1.68
MMF Regimen	0.37	0.16–0.84	MMF Regimen	0.49	0.21–1.12
Recipient Sex (Male)	2.01	0.93–4.37	Recipient Sex (Male)	2.55	1.12–5.80
HLA-AB Mismatch	0.41	0.17–0.99	HLA-AB Mismatch	0.48	0.19–1.21
Statins	2.12	0.85–5.30	Rejections (1st 3 mo)	0.40	0.13–1.21

SEVERE CAV:

Using 1st biopsy, only:			Using all biopsies available at 3 months:		
Predictor Variable	OR	CI	Predictor Variable	OR	CI
Fibrin	1.62	0.57–4.59	tPA	1.36	1.21–1.54
tPA	5.86	2.02–17.00	Recipient Sex (Male)	3.53	1.51–8.73
MMF Regimen	0.43	0.20–0.92	HLA-AB Mismatch	0.22	0.09–0.53
HLA-AB Mismatch	2.72	1.14–6.47	Ischemic time	0.99	0.99–1.00
Statins	0.22	0.09–0.54			

GRAFT FAILURE DUE TO CAV:

Using 1st biopsy, only:			Using all biopsies available at 3 months:		
Predictor Variable	OR	CI	Predictor Variable	OR	CI
Fibrin	3.99	1.53–10.40	tPA	1.31	1.12–1.55
MMF Regimen	0.12	0.04–0.32	MMF Regimen	0.15	0.06–0.41
Statins	0.21	0.08–0.55	Recipient Sex (Male)	2.77	0.88–8.77
			Statins	0.17	0.06–0.47

Abbreviations: OR: Odds Ratio; CI: 95% confidence interval for the OR; tPA: Tissue Plasminogen Activator; HLA: Human Leukocyte Antigen; MMF: Mycophenolate Mofetil. Models on the left use information from the first biopsy only. Models on the right use information from all biopsies available in the first three months post-transplantation.

The very early appearance of myocardial fibrin suggests that ischemia-reperfusion (I/R) may be a trigger of coagulation activation. The absence of a prothrombotic microvasculature in all time-zero biopsies performed at the time of transplant *and before reperfusion* further confirms that this phenotype developed after the graft was placed into the recipient. These findings rule out the possibility that our risk predictors are a consequence of brain trauma to the donor or damage to the donor heart occurring during the harvesting procedure. Likewise, they increase the likelihood that abnormal markers detected in time-one biopsies are related to I/R occurring immediately after transplantation. I/R appear to damage endothelium by reducing anticoagulation, increasing thrombogenicity and promoting vascular inflammation and microthrombus formation leading to microinfarctions. Mass-berg et al [19] observed massive ICAM-1-mediated microvascular fibrinogen deposition and platelet adhesion as early as ten minutes after reperfusion in an intestinal I/R model. Furthermore, I/R induce production of reactive oxygen species, promoting endo-thelial dysfunction and upregulation of ICAM-1 and P-selectin [20]. Interestingly, the fibrin-derived peptide $B\beta_{15-42}$ (FX06) was shown to significantly attenuate I/R injury in a heart transplant model with extended cold ischemia by reducing infiltrating leukocytes [21]. Pathophysiologically, I/R probably promotes

endothelial dysfunction and CAV by inducing platelet adhesion, growth factor release, major histocompatibility class I and II antigen upregulation, donor antigen release, and by promoting adhesion molecule expression and smooth muscle cell proliferation [22,23].

Considering the emergence of antibody-mediated rejection (AMR) as a model of microcirculation injury and endothelial activation [24,25] and its potential as a predictor of long-term outcome [26,27], it is relevant to briefly discuss the relationship of I/R with respect to AMR and our own findings [28]. Revelo et al [29] recently showed that the combination of complement components, HLA-DR and fibrin defines AMR in patients at risk for allograft loss from cardiovascular causes and they recognized fibrin as being particularly important for defining severe AMR with a high likelihood of poor patient outcome. I/R may facilitate endothelial susceptibility to a recipient's antibody response leading to further endothelial injury caused by AMR. Since complement and antibody-mediated damage leads to vascular endothelial injury with sometimes puzzling histologic consequences, the additional evaluation of fibrin and HLA-DR over time could help define persistent AMR in the presence of endothelial injury and loss. A hypothesis worth testing is whether patients that develop a prothrombotic microvasculature immediately following transplan-

Table 6. Performance characteristics for first-biopsy (First) and three-month (All) biopsy models.[a]

	CAV						SEVERE CAV						GRAFT FAILURE DUE TO CAV					
	At 1 Year		At 5 Years		At 10 Years		At 1 Year		At 5 Years		At 10 Years		At 1 Year		At 5 Years		At 10 Years	
Measure	First	All	First	All	First	All	First	All	First	All	First	All	First	All	First	All	First	All
C (ROC Area)[b]	0.64	0.76	0.72	0.79	0.78	0.81	0.89	0.95	0.77	0.84	0.80	0.78	0.84	0.84	0.92	0.95	0.86	0.88
Sensitivity	0.69	0.81	0.79	0.78	0.62	0.76	0.90	1.00	0.74	0.83	0.74	0.82	0.86	1.00	0.83	0.94	0.87	0.77
Specificity	0.60	0.68	0.58	0.70	0.83	0.75	0.78	0.78	0.72	0.78	0.72	0.70	0.68	0.61	0.85	0.82	0.74	0.89
PPV	0.28	0.37	0.65	0.72	0.86	0.85	0.20	0.22	0.41	0.49	0.57	0.57	0.10	0.10	0.39	0.39	0.43	0.60
NPV	0.89	0.94	0.74	0.76	0.55	0.64	0.99	1.00	0.92	0.95	0.85	0.89	0.99	1.00	0.98	0.99	0.96	0.95
Cutoff Value[c]	0.11	0.21	0.27	0.44	0.68	0.58	0.01	0.03	0.17	0.22	0.31	0.30	0.01	0.02	0.04	0.05	0.12	0.23
Pct Correct[d]	0.62	0.70	0.69	0.74	0.70	0.75	0.79	0.79	0.72	0.79	0.73	0.74	0.69	0.63	0.85	0.83	0.76	0.87[e]
Prevalence[f]	0.19		0.50		0.63		0.06		0.20		0.33		0.04		0.10		0.18	

Abbreviations: PPV: positive predictive value; NPV: negative predictive value.
[a]First-biopsy (First) and three-month (All) models show similar discriminative and predictive accuracy, particularly with respect to the prediction of severe CAV and graft failure. Negative predictive values (NPV) are particularly high for both first-biopsy and three-month models, indicating that it is possible, using only information from the first biopsy, to identify a patient subgroup at substantially reduced risk of developing long-term CAV or graft failure.
[b]C: C-statistics: A measure of the area under the receiver operating characteristic (ROC) curve. Equivalently, it is the proportion of all case versus non-case pairs that were correctly classified by the model.
[c]Cutoff value: The expected value from the logistic regression model that serves as the threshold for predicting the event in question. Patients with expected values that exceed the cutoff are predicted to experience the event.
[d]Pct Correct is the percent correctly classified by the model and includes both positive and negative classifications.
[e]Three-month model (All) is significantly better (p<.02) than the first-biopsy model (First) in classifying failure due to CAV at 10 years.
[f]Prevalence: the proportion of patients that experienced the indicated event by the indicated time point.

tation are also more prone to develop AMR. We are at present evaluating C4d and CD68 within the grafts to establish the relationship of those antibody reactivities to the pro- or anti-coagulant status of the microvasculature.

From a prognostic perspective, it is important to ascertain how much predictive information is actually added by incorporating a new marker into the best current model, since new markers may contain little or no additional information not already conveyed by existing factors optimally combined [30]. For this reason, the predictive accuracy of AMR-related factors should be judged by comparing the best current model, with and without the AMR-related factors included, using an overall indicator of model discrimination such as the area under the ROC curve as the criteria for judging the degree of improvement [31,32]. Since we have shown here that our models have excellent *negative* predictive accuracy, it would be especially important to know whether the *positive* predictive accuracy of our models could be significantly improved by adding AMR-related factors.

Our data suggest that graft failure may depend upon the extent of very early post-transplant microvascular damage and the capacity of the transplanted heart to remove microthrombi through active fibrinolysis. Thus, therapies designed to de-escalate hypercoagulability may be most effective if applied during the pre- to peri- and early post-operative periods.

Our study has strengths and weaknesses. Weaknesses include the utilization of angiography rather than intravascular ultrasound [33] and the lack of baseline angiograms at the time of transplantation. From a statistical point of view, our prediction models ultimately need to be tested in other populations by other investigators working in other settings in order to evaluate their generalizability. However, our models did undergo cross-validation on repeated bootstrap samples. Cross-validation produces estimates of a model's likely performance on future data and greatly reduces the likelihood of spurious variable selection that is

often the most important source of bias arising from stepwise regression on a single sample [9]. Strengths include the relatively large number of transplant patients, the long multi-year follow-up, and the availability of a large immunohistochemical heart-biopsy database.

The most important clinical message that emerges from our data is that first-biopsy models are comparable to three-month models as evidenced by their similar capacities to classify patients correctly and to single out patients at low risk of CAV and graft failure. The only exception was the superior performance of the three-month model to correctly classify patients with respect to 10-year graft failure due to CAV. The high negative predictive accuracies associated with both, first-biopsy and three-month models are especially noteworthy. Absence of a prothrombotic microvasculature, even when observed as early as 9 days post-transplant in a single biopsy, identifies patients that rarely develop CAV and graft failure. These very low-risk patients are unlikely to derive benefit from further invasive monitoring. Since repeated heart biopsy procedures are both risky and expensive, our findings have implications for both patients and payers. Of course, patients that do not fall within this low-risk group should continue to be followed under standard protocols using more definitive (invasive) monitoring.

Although our findings show that it is possible, using markers that are available within days of the transplant procedure, to identify a subgroup of patients that almost never develops long-term CAV or graft failure, they do not show what the impact on patient outcomes would be if physicians used our prediction models as a clinical tool to manage their transplant patients. Clinical impact can only be demonstrated in a prospective outcome trial in which some patients are randomly assigned to receive usual care and others to a protocol that uses our models to guide treatment decisions.

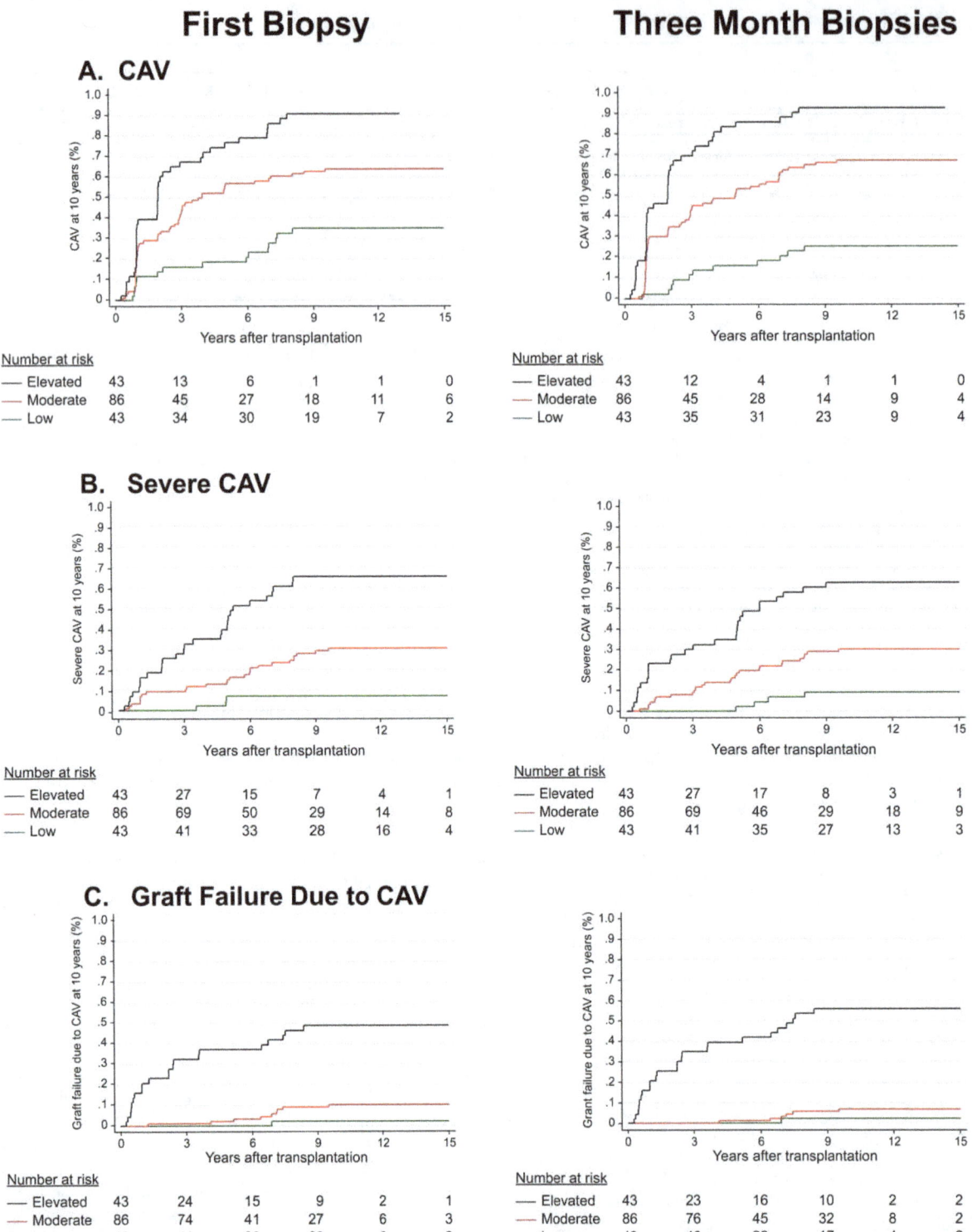

Figure 2. Kaplan-Meier curves using 10-year regression models. Kaplan-Meier curves of risk-stratified groupings derived from first-biopsy versus three-month biopsy models showing time to (a) CAV, (b) severe CAV, and (c) failure due to CAV. Risk groupings were formed from the distributions of the predictive probabilities from 10-year logistic regression models (low risk=lower 25%, moderate risk=middle 50%, and high risk=upper 25%).

Acknowledgments

We thank Roula Antonopoulos for excellent immunohistochemical studies, all members of the Indiana University Health Heart Transplant team for their help and support, and Elaine Bammerlin for artwork and editing of the manuscript.

Author Contributions

Conceived and designed the experiments: CL JW JH BJ. Performed the experiments: CL GC MO LB. Analyzed the data: CL JW JH. Wrote the paper: CL. Contributed to the writing of the manuscript: CL JW JH BJ. Collected data for the study: GC DP PK. Enrolled patients: DP PK. Clinic management where study conducted: DP PK. ICMJE criteria for authorship read and met: CL JW JH BJ GC MO LB DP PK. Agree with manuscript results and conclusions: CL JW JH BJ GC MO LB DP PK.

References

1. Mehra MR (2006) Contemporary concepts in prevention and treatment of cardiac allograft vasculopathy. Am J Transplant 6: 1248–1256.
2. Pham MX, Teuteberg JJ, Kfoury AG, Starling RC, Deng MC, et al. (2010) Gene-expression profiling for rejection surveillance after cardiac transplantation. N Engl J Med 362: 1890–1900.
3. Labarrere CA, Woods JR, Hardin JW, Campana GL, Ortiz MA, et al. (2011) Early Prediction of Cardiac Allograft Vasculopathy and Heart Transplant Failure. Am J Transplant 11: 528–535.
4. Labarrere CA, Lee JB, Nelson DR, Al-Hassani M, Miller SJ, et al. (2002) C-reactive protein, arterial endothelial activation and development of transplant coronary artery disease: a prospective study. Lancet 360: 1462–1467.
5. Stewart S, Winters GL, Fishbein MC, Tazelaar HD, Kobashigawa J, et al. (2005) Revision of the 1990 working formulation for the standardization of nomenclature in the diagnosis of heart rejection. J Heart Lung Transplant 24: 1710–1720.
6. Labarrere CA, Torry RJ, Nelson DR, Miller SJ, Pitts DE, et al. (2001) Vascular antithrombin and clinical outcome in heart transplant patients. Am J Cardiol 87: 425–431.
7. Austin PC, Tu JV (2004) Boostrap Methods for Developing Predictive Models. Am Stat 58: 131–137.
8. Efron B (1979) Bootstrap methods: Another look at the jackknife. Ann Stat 7: 1–26.
9. Harrell FE, Jr. (2001) Regression Modeling Strategies: with applications to linear models, logistic regression, and survival analysis. New York: Springer. pp 87–103.
10. Schisterman EF, Perkins NJ, Liu A, Bondell H (2005) Optimal cut-point and its corresponding Youden Index to discriminate individuals using pooled blood samples. Epidemiology 16: 73–81.
11. Hanley JA, McNeil BJ (1982) The meaning and use of the area under a receiver operating characteristic (ROC) curve. Radiology 143: 29–36.
12. Shibata M, Kumar SR, Amar A, Fernandez JA, Hofman F, et al. (2001) Anti-inflammatory, antithrombotic, and neuroprotective effects of activated protein C in a murine model of focal ischemic stroke. Circulation 103: 1799–1805.
13. Labarrere CA, Pitts D, Nelson DR, Faulk WP (1995) Vascular tissue plasminogen activator and the development of coronary artery disease in heart-transplant recipients. N Engl J Med 333: 1111–1116.
14. Labarrere CA, Nelson DR, Cox CJ, Pitts D, Kirlin P, et al. (2000) Cardiac-specific troponin I levels and risk of coronary artery disease and graft failure following heart transplantation. JAMA 284: 457–464.
15. Yen MH, Pilkington G, Starling RC, Ratliff NB, McCarthy PM, et al. (2002) Increased tissue factor expression predicts development of cardiac allograft vasculopathy. Circulation 106: 1379–1383.
16. Labarrere CA, Nelson DR, Miller SJ, Nieto JM, Conner JA, et al. (2000) Value of serum-soluble intercellular adhesion molecule-1 for the noninvasive risk assessment of transplant coronary artery disease, posttransplant ischemic events, and cardiac graft failure. Circulation 102: 1549–1555.
17. Labarrere CA, Nelson DR, Faulk WP (1997) Endothelial activation and development of coronary artery disease in transplanted human hearts. JAMA 278: 1169–1175.
18. Stork S, Behr TM, Birk M, Uberfuhr P, Klauss V, et al. (2006) Assessment of cardiac allograft vasculopathy late after heart transplantation: when is coronary angiography necessary? J Heart Lung Transplant 25: 1103–1108.
19. Massberg S, Enders G, de Melo Matos FC, Domschke Tomic LI, Leiderer R, et al. (1999) Fibrinogen deposition at the postischemic vessel wall promotes platelet adhesion during ischemia-reperfusion in vivo. Blood 94: 3829–3838.
20. Rao DA, Pober JS (2008) Endothelial injury, alarmins, and allograft rejection. Crit Rev Immunol 28: 229–248.
21. Wiedemann D, Schneeberger S, Friedl P, Zacharowski K, Wick N, et al. (2010) The fibrin-derived peptide $B\beta_{15-42}$ significantly attenuates ischemia-reperfusion injury in a cardiac transplant model. Transplantation 89: 824–829.
22. Rahmani M, Cruz RP, Granville DJ, McManus BM (2006) Allograft vasculopathy versus atherosclerosis. Circ Res 99: 801–815.
23. Valantine HA (2003) Cardiac allograft vasculopathy: Central role of endothelial injury leading to transplant "atheroma". Transplantation 76: 891–899.
24. Mengel M, Sis B, Kim D, Chang J, Famulski KS, et al. (2010) The molecular phenotype of heart transplant biopsies: relationship to histopathological and clinical variables. Am J Transplant 10: 2105–2115.
25. Sis B, Halloran PF (2010) Endothelial transcripts uncover a previously unknown phenotype: C4d-negative antibody-mediated rejection. Curr Opin Organ Transplant 15: 42–48.
26. Wu GW, Kobashigawa JA, Fishbein MC, Patel JK, Kittleson MM, et al. (2009) Asymptomatic antibody-mediated rejection after heart transplantation predicts poor outcomes. J Heart Lung Transplant 28: 417–422.
27. Kfoury AG, Hammond MEH, Snow GL, Drakos SG, Stehlik J, et al. (2009) Cardiovascular mortality among heart transplant recipients with asymptomatic antibody-mediated or stable mixed cellular and antibody-mediated rejection. J Heart Lung Transplant 28: 781–784.
28. Labarrere CA, Jaeger BR (2012) Biomarkers of heart transplant rejection: the good, the bad, and the ugly! Transl Res 159: 238–251.
29. Revelo MP, Stehlik J, Miller D, Snow GL, Everitt MD, et al. (2011) Antibody testing for cardiac antibody-mediated rejection: which panel correlates best with cardiovascular death? J Heart Lung Transplant 30: 144–150.
30. Begg CB, Cramer LD, Venkatraman ES, Rosai J (2000) Comparing tumor staging and grading systems: A case study and a review of the issues, using thymoma as a model. Stat Med 19: 1997–2014.
31. Pencina MJ, D'Agostino RB, Sr, D'Agostino RB, Jr., Vasan RS (2008) Evaluating the added predictive ability of a new marker: from area under the ROC curve to reclassification and beyond. Stat Med 27: 157–172.
32. Tzoulaki I, Liberopoulos G, Ioannidis JPA (2009) Assessment of claims of improved prediction beyond the Framingham risk score. JAMA 302: 2345–2352.
33. Schmauss D, Weis M (2008) Cardiac allograft vasculopathy: recent developments. Circulation 117: 2131–2141.

11

Tolerogenic Function of Dimeric Forms of HLA-G Recombinant Proteins: A Comparative Study *In Vivo*

Benoit Favier[1,2◗], Kiave-Yune HoWangYin[1,2,3◗], Juan Wu[4◗], Julien Caumartin[1,2], Marina Daouya[1,2], Anatolij Horuzsko[4], Edgardo D. Carosella[1,2], Joel LeMaoult[1,2]*

1 CEA-I2BM-Service de Recherches en Hemato-Immunologie, Paris, France, 2 Institut Universitaire d'Hematologie, Hopital Saint Louis, Paris, France, 3 Biology and Biotechnology Ph.D. Program, University Paris 7, Paris, France, 4 Center for Molecular Chaperone/Radiobiology and Cancer Virology, Georgia Health Science University, Augusta, Georgia, United States of America

Abstract

HLA-G is a natural tolerogenic molecule involved in the best example of tolerance to foreign tissues there is: the maternal-fetal tolerance. The further involvement of HLA-G in the tolerance of allogeneic transplants has also been demonstrated and some of its mechanisms of action have been elucidated. For these reasons, therapeutic HLA-G molecules for tolerance induction in transplantation are actively investigated. In the present study, we studied the tolerogenic functions of three different HLA-G recombinant proteins: HLA-G heavy chain fused to β2-microglobulin (B2M), HLA-G heavy chain fused to B2M and to the Fc portion of an immunoglobulin, and HLA-G alpha-1 domain either fused to the Fc part of an immunoglobulin or as a synthetic peptide. Our results demonstrate the tolerogenic function of B2M-HLA-G fusion proteins, and especially of B2M-HLA-G5, which were capable of significantly delaying allogeneic skin graft rejection in a murine *in vivo* transplantation model. The results from our studies suggest that HLA-G recombinant proteins are relevant candidates for tolerance induction in human transplantation.

Editor: Jacques Zimmer, Centre de Recherche Public de la Santé (CRP-Santé), Luxembourg

Funding: This work was supported by Commissariat a l'Energie Atomique, by the Agence de la Biomedecine, in part by HLA-G Technologies (to A.H.), and by National Institute of Health grant R56 AI055923 (to A.H.). No additional external funding received for this study. The funders had no role in study design, data collection and analysis, decision to publish, or preparation of the manuscript.

Competing Interests: The commercial source HLA-G Technologies has partially funded this study by contributing to the expenses of *in vivo* experiments. They did not take any part in study design, data collection and analysis, decision to publish, or preparation of the manuscript.

* E-mail: Joel.LeMaoult@cea.fr

◗ These authors contributed equally to this work.

Introduction

Since the first successful kidney allo-transplantation in human beings in 1952, the development of treatments limiting acute allograft rejection has been the purpose of intense investigations. Even though the discovery of immunosuppressive molecules such as Cyclosporin A dramatically reduced acute allograft rejection cases, their action on chronic allograft rejection is not optimal. Moreover, besides their lack of efficiency on chronic allograft rejection, these immunosuppressive treatments have side effects including high susceptibility to infections, and renal and neural toxicity.

Among the biological molecules involved in the induction of tolerance that have been characterized over the past years, the non-classical HLA class I Human Leukocyte Antigen G molecule (HLA-G) has unique features that make it an ideal candidate for the development of new therapies in transplantation.

HLA-G (reviewed in [1,2]) is characterized by seven isoforms which derive from the alternative splicing of a unique primary transcript, by a very low amount of polymorphism, and by an expression which is restricted to fetal trophoblast cells, adult epithelial thymic cells, cornea, erythroid and endothelial cell precursors, and pancreatic islets. HLA-G may also be pathologically expressed by (i) non-rejected allografts [3,4], (ii) lesion-infiltrating antigen presenting cells (APC) during inflammatory diseases [5,6],

and (iii) tumor tissues and their tumor infiltrating APC [7–11]. HLA-G is further expressed by (iv) monocytes in multiple sclerosis [12], and by (v) monocytes and T cells in viral infections [13–15].

HLA-G is a potent tolerogenic molecule that strongly inhibits the function of immune cells. Indeed, HLA-G inhibits NK cell and cytotoxic T lymphocyte cytolytic activity [16,17], CD4$^+$ T cell alloproliferative responses [18], T cell and NK cell ongoing proliferation [18–20], and dendritic cell maturation [21,22]. Furthermore, HLA-G was shown to induce regulatory T cells [18,23]. HLA-G mediates its functions by interacting with three inhibitory receptors: ILT2 (CD85j/LILRB1) which is expressed by B cells, some T cells, some NK cells and all monocytes/dendritic cells [24], ILT4 (CD85d/LILRB2) which is expressed by myeloid cells [25], and KIR2DL4 (CD158d) [26] which is expressed by some peripheral and decidual NK cells.

The efficiency of the HLA-G binding to its receptors and the delivery of potent inhibitory signals have been shown to depend on HLA-G dimerization [27]. Biochemical studies indicate that HLA-G dimerization occurs through disulfide-bond formation between unique cysteine residues localized in position 42 of the HLA-G alpha-1 domain (C42). Point mutation of C42 in Serine, which leads to the exclusive expression of HLA-G monomers demonstrated that HLA-G dimers, but not HLA-G monomers, carry HLA-G tolerogenic function [27,28].

The expression of HLA-G dimers has been reported in trophoblast cells, where it confers protection against the mother's immune system. This mechanism of natural tolerance in a semi-allogeneic context has led to investigate the potential role of HLA-G in transplanted patients (reviewed in [2]). To date, clinical studies have demonstrated that HLA-G expression may be induced in some heart, kidney, liver/kidney, lung, pancreas, and kidney/pancreas transplanted patients. Statistical analyses indicate that the presence of HLA-G in plasma and biopsies of transplanted patients correlates with a decreased number of acute rejection episodes and with no chronic rejection, as first described for heart transplants [3,29].

The direct role of HLA-G in transplantation *in vivo* was evidenced by skin allotransplantation in HLA-G transgenic mice or in wild-type mice pre-treated with HLA-G tetramer-coated beads. In both experiments the presence of HLA-G significantly delayed skin allograft rejection [30,31].

For these reasons, and also because it already contributes to the best example of successful tolerance there is: the maternal-fetal tolerance, therapeutic HLA-G molecules for transplantation are actively investigated. Yet, the use of HLA-G molecules as therapeutic agents faces several hurdles, among which the problems of structure and stability. Indeed, HLA-G is a trimolecular complex composed of a heavy chain of 3 globular domains non-covalently associated with the β2-microglobulin (B2M) and a peptide which is active only as a multimer.

Here, we evaluated (i) the tolerogenic function of two types of HLA-G homodimers (C42-C42 dimers *vs* Fc-Fc dimers), (ii) whether the alpha-1 domain of HLA-G which is common to all HLA-G isoforms could carry a tolerogenic function by itself as it was originally postulated, and (iii) whether the trimolecular complex that constitutes HLA-G could be stabilized by fusing B2M to HLA-G heavy chain while retaining its tolerogenic properties.

Our results demonstrate the tolerogenic function of all investigated dimeric forms of HLA-G recombinant proteins *in vitro* and *in vivo*, and especially that of the B2M-HLA-G5 dimers *in vivo*, but do not fully support a tolerogenic function for the alpha-1 domain of HLA-G in human beings, even dimeric.

Materials and Methods

Engineering of HLA-G fusion proteins

B2M-HLA-G1s-Fc (β2-microglobulin fused to the extra-cellular part of HLA-G1 and to the Fc part of a human IgG). The sequence coding for the human β2-microglobulin (B2M) was amplified by PCR with the primers B2M_Sig_Mlu-I_Sph-I_F and B2M-Link-a1_R (Table 1). The B2M_Link-a1_R primer, which is reverse complementary to the B2M coding sequence, is constituted

of three parts: B2M 3′ sequence excluding the stop codon, fused to a sequence coding for a (GGGGS)×2 linker, fused to the reverse complementary sequence of the HLA-G alpha-1 domain 5′ end.

In parallel, the cDNA sequence corresponding to the α1 through α3 domains of HLA-G1 was amplified by PCR with primers HLA-G-a1_Mlu_Sph_F and HLA-G-a3_Xho_Sal_R (Table 1). This removed the HLA-G peptide leader sequence and the stop codon. The PCR fragments corresponding to B2M and the α1-α2-α3 domains of HLA-G were then digested with the Eag-I restriction enzyme, purified, and ligated together. Mlu-I and Xho-I were then used to insert the obtained B2M_α1-α2-α3 fusion sequence (B2M-HLA-G1s) into a PGEMT/easy vector (Promega). The restriction enzymes Age-I and Xho-I were used to transfer the B2M-HLA-G1s sequence to the pFUSE-hFc1 (InVivogen, Toulouse, France) in order to fuse B2M-HLA-G1s to the Fc part of a human IgG.

B2M-HLA-G5 (β2-microglobulin fused to the HLA-G5 heavy chain). To generate B2M fused to the heavy chain of the HLA-G5 isoform, the pFUSE-B2M-HLA-G1s-Fc plasmid described above was used as template and amplified with B2M_sig_TOPO_F and a3_i4_Xho_Stop_R (Table 1). a3_i4_Xho_Stop_R contains the HLA-G intron 4 sequence that replaces the transmembrane and intracellular and domains of HLA-G1 in HLA-G5. The PCR fragment was then ligated into the pcDNA 3.1 D/V.5-His-Topo vector (Invitrogen) using 3.1 Directional TOPO® Expression Kit (Invitrogen).

Alpha1-Fc (HLA-G alpha-1 domain fused to the Fc part of a murine IgG). The cDNA sequence of HLA-G alpha-1 domain was amplified by PCR using the primers EcoRI_a1_F and EcoRV_a1_R (Table 1). The EcoRI and EcoRV restriction enzymes were used to insert the HLA-G alpha-1 coding sequence into the pFUSE-mFc2 vector (Invivogen), fusing it to the secretion sequence of IL-2 and a mouse IgG Fc fragment.

Alpha1_peptide (synthetic peptide corresponding to the HLA-G alpha-1 domain). The peptide corresponding to the alpha-1 domain of HLA-G was synthesized by Jerini, Berlin, Germany.

Figure 1 is a schematic representation of the generated proteins and peptides.

Cell culture and proteins production

For production of HLA-G fusion proteins, the HeLa human cell line (ATCC) was transfected by the various plasmids using the Lipofectamine™ 2000 transfection reagent (Invitrogen) and kept at 37°C, 5% CO_2 in DMEM (Dulbco's Modified EagleMedium GIBCO) GlutaMAX™ supplemented with 10% fetal calf serum (GIBCO) and the appropriate selective antibiotics. For B2M-HLA-G1s-Fc and Alpha1-Fc, zeocin™ was used at a concentration of 500 µg/mL. For B2M-HLA-G5, geneticin was used at a concentration of 1 mg/mL.

Table 1. Primers used for fusion protein generation.

B2M_Sig_Mlu-I_Sph-I_F	5′ CGTCGCATGCACGCGTCGATGTCTCGCTCCGTGGCC 3′
B2M-Link-a1_R	5′ TCATGGAGTGGGAGCCGGATCCGCCACCTCCGGATCCGCCACCTCCGGATCCGCCACCTCCCATGTCTCGATCCCACTT 3′
HLA-G-a1_Mlu_Sph_F	5′ ACTGGCATGCACGCGTCGGGCTTCCACTCCATGA 3′
HLA-G-a3_Xho_Sal_R	5′ TATGGTCGACCTCGAGCGCAGCTGCCTTCCATCTCAGCATGAG 3′
B2M_sig_TOPO_F	5′ CACCATGTCTCGCTCCGTGGCC 3′
a3_i4_Xho_Stop_R	5′ ATCTTAACTCGAGAGGTCTTCAGAGAGGCTCCTGCTTTCC>TAACAGACATGATGCCTCCATCTCCCTCCTTACTCCATCTCAGCATGAG 3′
EcoRI_a1_F	5′ AAAGAATTCGGGCTCCCACTCCATGAGGT 3′
EcoRV_a1_R	5′ AAAGATATCCCACTGGCCTCGCTCTGGTTG 3′

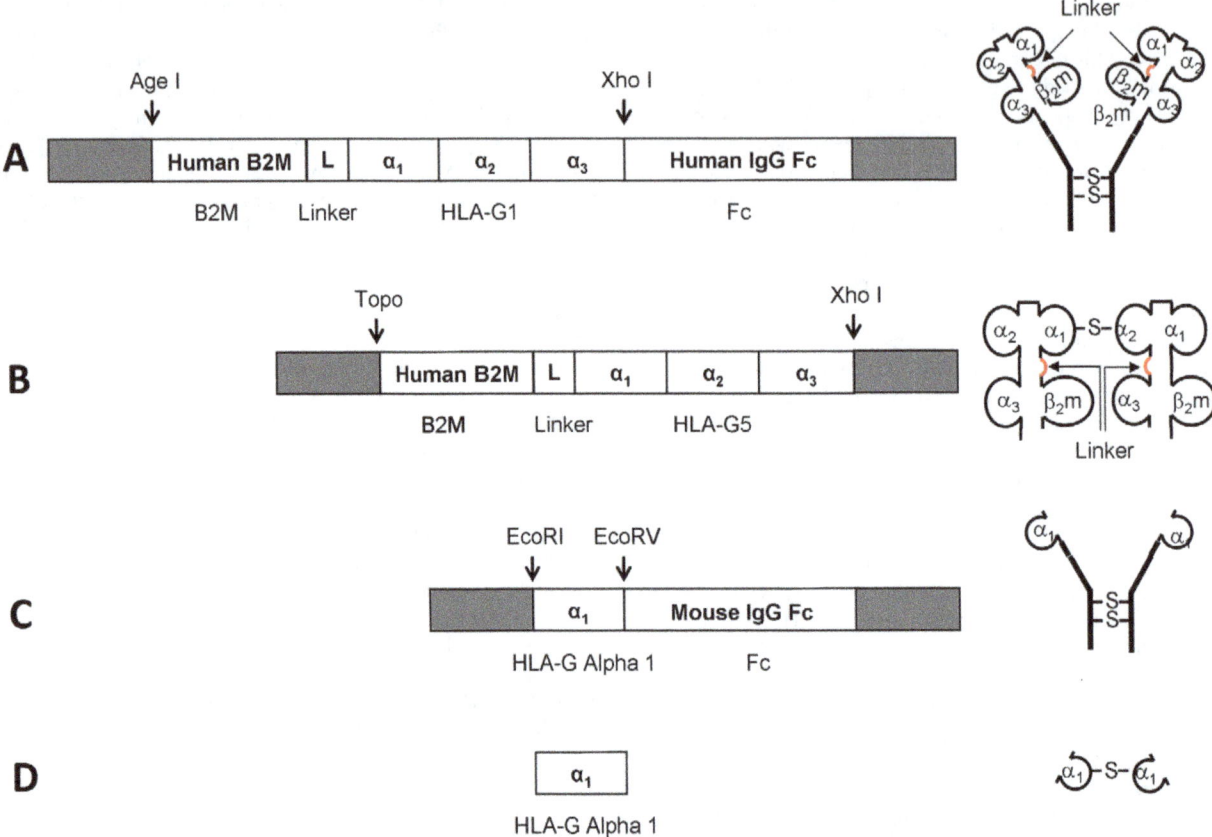

Figure 1. Schematic representation of the generated proteins and their coding sequences. (A) B2M-HLA-G1s-Fc, (B) B2M-HLA-G5, (C) Alpha1-Fc, (D) Alpha1_peptide. Arrows indicate the linker between beta-2-microglobulin and HLA-G alpha-1 domain.

For the collection of fusion protein-containing culture supernatants, cells were harvested after 48 hours. Supernatants were filtered through 0.2 μM filter (Millipore) and then used as is, or stored at −20°C.

HLA-G-specific ELISA

HLA-G-specific ELISAs were performed on cell culture supernatants using Mem-G/09 (Exbio, Praha) as capture antibody and anti-B2m as detection antibody as described [32]. Purified HLA-G5 was used as standard protein. Samples were run as duplicates and represented as mean+/−SEM.

Western-blot analysis

Immunoprecipitation. HLA-G-Fc proteins were immunoprecipitated from cell culture supernatants using Protein G sepharose beads (GE Healthcare). B2M-HLA-G5 fusion proteins were immunoprecipitated from supernantants using anti-HLA-G5-coated Protein G sepharose beads (clone 5A6, Exbio, Praha). Supernatants of non-transfected cells were used as negative controls. Immunoprecipitates were then washed three times with 1×PBS and the proteins were eluted by incubation in Laemmli buffer under reducing or non-reducing conditions, and boiled before loading.

Western blots. Samples were loaded on polyacrylamide SDS-PAGE gels and transferred onto Hybond nitrocellulose membranes (Amersham Pharmacia Biosciences). Following blocking with 5% non-fat milk in TBS/0,2% Tween 20, membranes were incubated overnight with anti-HLA-G antibody (clone 4H84, Exbio, Praha),

and revealed using HorseRadish peroxydase-conjugated goat anti-mouse secondary antibody. Membranes were revealed with the ECL+ detection system (Amersham Pharmacia Biosciences).

ILT2 NFAT-GFP reporter cell assay

NFAT-GFP reporter cells expressing the ILT2-PILRβ chimera were described previously [22]. The cell-surface expression of ILT2-PILRβ chimera was monitored by FACS staining with PE-Cy5-conjugated ILT2-specific mAb (clone GHI/75, BD Biosciences). In this system, GFP expression can be induced only upon proper ILT2 receptor binding.

Mice

C57BL/6 and B6.C-H-2^bm12 (bm12) mice were purchased from Jackson Laboratory. ILT4-transgenic mice have been described in [21]. The use of animals for this work was approved by the animal care committee of the Medical College of Georgia.

In vivo allograft experiments

The *in vivo* experimental procedures were approved by the animal care committee of the Medical College of Georgia (approval ID: BR08-06-070) and the experiments were conducted in accordance with institutional guidelines for animal care and use.

For B2M-HLA-G1s-Fc and alpha1-Fc fusion proteins, 1×10^8 sulfate latex beads 4%w/v 5 μm (Invitrogen) were coated with 20 μg/ml AffiniPure anti-human IgG Fc fragment or Goat Anti-mouse, respectively (Jackson ImmunoResearch) for 2 hours at 37°C followed by a 2-hour incubation with BSA (2 mg/ml). After washing, the beads were incubated with 0.5 µg/ml of HLA-G/Fc fusion proteins at 4°C for 16 hours. Subsequently, the beads were washed twice with PBS. 5 ml of HLA-G-Fc fusion proteins (1 µg/ml) were used for 5×10^6 sulfate latex beads. As a negative control, sulfate latex beads were prepared in an identical manner except that PBS or HeLa mock supernatant was used rather than supernatants containing HLA-G-Fc fusion proteins.

For B2M-HLA-G5, beads were generated by grafting the anti-HLA-G5 antibody 5A6 (Exbio, Praha) on beads prior to incubation in B2M-HLA-G5-containing culture media.

For alpha1_peptide, beads were generated by direct coating onto latex beads.

Sulfate latex beads (5×10^6) were injected intraperitoneally on the day before skin grafting. Specific pathogen-free C57BL/6 mice and ILT4-transgenic mice (both H-2b, 8–10 weeks of age) were used as skin graft recipients throughout the study. Recipient mice received HLA-G-coupled latex beads, donor skin was from MHC class II-disparate B6.CH-2bm12 (bm12, H-2b) mice. Allogeneic skin grafts were performed by standard methods. Briefly, skin (1.0 cm^2) from the tail of donor mice (12–14 weeks old) was grafted onto the flank of recipient, anesthetized mice. The graft was covered with gauze and plaster, which were removed on day 10. Grafts were scored daily until rejection (defined as 80% of grafted tissue becoming necrotic and reduced in size). All skin grafting survival data were tested by Kaplan Meier Survival Analysis.

Results

Structural validation of the HLA-G recombinant proteins

We first investigated the conformation of the recombinant proteins, focussing primarily on their monomeric/multimeric status, and then on the conformation of the B2M-HLA-G fusion proteins.

To investigate the monomeric/multimeric status of the engineered proteins, these were immuno-precipitated using protein G-Sepharose beads either directly (for Fc-containing proteins), or after binding to anti-HLA-G5 mAb (for B2M-HLAG5). No immunoprecipitation was required for alpha1_peptide. Proteins and peptide were then analyzed by electrophoresis on non-reducing gels. Figure 2A shows that Fc fusion proteins were present only as dimers, and that B2M-HLA-G5 and alpha1_peptide also efficiently formed multimers, even if some monomeric structures remained. Thus, all generated proteins and peptide were capable of forming dimers and/or multimers and found mainly as such.

We next investigated whether the B2M-HLA-G5 and B2M-HLA-G1s-Fc fusion proteins were properly folded. For this, we took advantage of the existence of an ELISA assay based on the conformational anti-HLA-G antibody MEM-G/09 which recognizes only HLA-G folded in combination with B2M. We performed conformational ELISA on supernatants which contained similar amounts of B2M-HLA-G1s-Fc, B2M-HLA-G5, using purified HLA-G5 protein as standard. Figure 2C shows these similar amounts of B2M-HLA-G1s-Fc, B2M-HLA-G5, and HLA-G5 control protein, were detected by conformational ELISA with similar efficiency. This means that the (GSSS)×2 spacer linking B2M and HLA-G heavy chain did not alter the B2M:HLA-G conformation. These results are in agreement with a previous study on a similarly produced B2M-HLA-A2 fusion protein [33]. The absence of conformational antibodies for the alpha-1 domain of HLA-G prevented a similar investigation for the alpha1-Fc construct.

Thus, B2M-HLA-G5, B2M-HLA-G1s-Fc, and alpha1-Fc were dimerized, properly folded (B2M-HLA-G5 and B2M-HLA-G1s-Fc), and thus, potentially capable of being functional.

In vitro binding to ILT2

In vitro, the inhibitory effect of HLA-G is mainly due to its interaction with ILT2, as shown by HLA-G:ILT2 interaction blocking experiments [20]. Furthermore, it was reported that ILT2 binds primarily to dimers of B2M-associated HLA-G molecules, but not to monomers [22,34]. Thus, we investigated the capability of B2M-HLA-G5 and B2M-HLA-G1s-Fc proteins to bind and activate ILT2. For this, we used an ILT2 NFAT-GFP reporter cell assay in which HLA-G binding to, and activation of ILT2 leads to GFP expression [22]. The results in Figure 3 show that B2M-HLA-G5 and B2M-HLA-G1s-Fc molecules induced GFP expression, i.e. ILT2 activation. Thus, these two molecules had the potential of being functional. Alpha1-Fc and alpha1_peptide were not investigated, since it is known that ILT2 does not bind HLA-G through its alpha-1 but through its alpha-3 domain [35].

In vivo function of recombinant HLA-G molecules

HLA-G promotes skin allograft survival in mice [30]. This has been demonstrated by immunization of wild type and ILT4-transgenic graft recipients mice with recombinant HLA-G 24 hours prior to skin grafting [21,31]. In these experiments, HLA-G was provided as recombinant soluble HLA-G1 produced in bacteria, refolded with B2M, and then tetramerized prior to be coated onto latex beads. In the current study, HLA-G was provided as B2M-HLA-G5 bound to anti HLA-G5-coated beads (5A6 mAb), B2M-HLA-G1s-Fc bound to anti-Fc-coated beads, alpha1-Fc bound to anti-Fc-coated beads, and alpha1_peptide covalently bound to beads (B2M-HLA-G5 beads, B2M-HLA-G1s-Fc beads, alpha1-Fc beads, and alpha1_peptide beads, respectively). Control beads were mAb-coated beads alone (no HLA-G) or non-coated beads (control for alpha1_peptide beads).

The results obtained in the case of a MHC class II-disparate B6.C-H-2^{bm12} (bm12) to C57BL/6 allogeneic skin transplantation are shown in Figure 4A. Immunization of the recipient with mAb-coated control beads prior to transplantation had no effect on allograft survival, ruling out any effect of the beads or animal manipulation on the results (not shown). However, all recombinant HLA-G proteins proved to be tolerogenic. B2M-HLA-G5 beads were the most efficient and increased the median graft survival time from 18 to 29 days (n = 9, p = 0.0001). By comparison, B2M-HLAG1s-Fc beads were less efficient but still increased the median graft survival time from 18 to 23 days (n = 8, p = 0.055). Alpha1-Fc beads prolonged skin allograft median survival time, from 18 to 29 days (n = 10, p = 0.001), but by comparison, alpha1_peptide-coated beads were less efficient, increasing the median graft survival from 20.5 to 22 days only (n = 9, p = 0.0081). These results demonstrate an inhibitory effect observed in vivo for all fusion proteins and for alpha1_peptide. It is surprising that B2M-HLA-G5 was more efficient than B2M-HLA-G1s-Fc, since these two molecular constructs have the same B2M-HLA-G sequence. It is even more surprising to observe a tolerogenic effect of alpha1-Fc molecules and alpha1_peptide. Indeed, it is known that HLA-G-induced increased survival of skin allograft time is mediated through PIR-B [31], which shares sequence similarities with ILT molecules, and in particular with ILT4. However, ILT4 binds HLA-G through its alpha-3 domain, but does not recognize its alpha-1 domain [36].

Thus, to investigate this issue, we evaluated the tolerogenic function of B2M-HLA-G5 and alpha1-Fc recombinant proteins using ILT4-transgenic mice as skin allograft recipients. B2M-HLA-G5 and Alpha1-Fc were chosen because they were the two most efficient B2M-HLA-G and alpha1 structures.

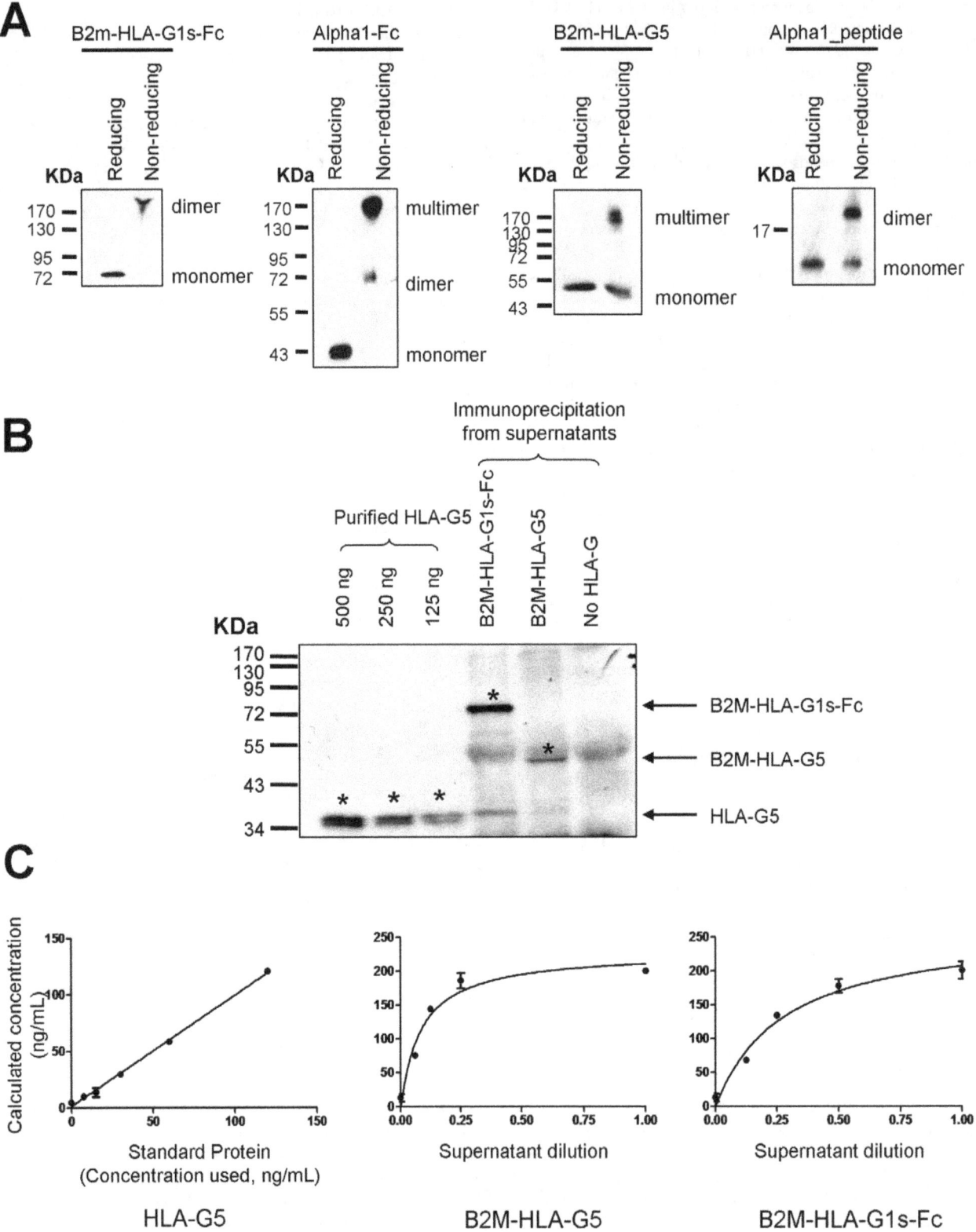

Figure 2. Monomeric/multimeric status and conformation of recombinant proteins. *A Monomeric/multimeric status of recombinant proteins.* Western blot analysis of recombinant proteins immunoprecipitated from supernatants of HeLa B2M-HLA-G1s-Fc, HeLa Alpha1-Fc, HeLa B2M-HLA-G5, and of alpha1_peptide. *B Quantification of B2M-HLA-G5 and B2M-HLA-G1s-Fc proteins.* Western blot analysis of recombinant B2M-HLA-G5 and B2M-HLA-G1s-Fc proteins immunoprecipitated from cell culture supernatants. Purified HLA-G5 recombinant protein was used as quantification standard. *C Conformation of B2M-HLA-G5 and B2M-HLA-G1s-Fc proteins.* Recombinant HLA-G5 protein was used as a standard in HLA-G-specific ELISA. Curves represent the concentration of the proteins properly folded into the supernatant according to the dilution.

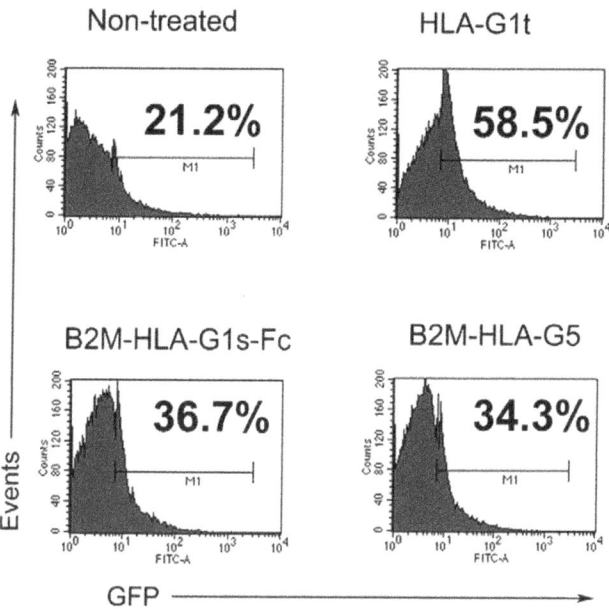

Figure 3. ILT2-mediated signaling by B2M-HLA-G5 and B2M-HLA-G1s-Fc proteins. NFAT-GFP reporter cells expressing the ILT2-PILRβ chimera were stimulated for 16 h with 1.5 μg/ml of the indicated HLA-G recombinant proteins. Non-treated reporter cells were used as negative control, and tetrameric complexes of HLA-G1 (HLA-G1t, [31]) were used as positive control. GFP expression on reporter cells was analyzed by flow cytometry. Numbers indicate the percentage of GFP-positive cells. Data shown are from one of four independent experiments.

Figure 4B shows that in this configuration, B2M-HLA-G5 retained its tolerogenic function, increasing the median graft survival time from 17 to 24.5 days (n = 8, p = 0.0004), whereas alpha1-Fc did not (n = 10, p = 0.039).

Discussion

In this work, we investigated the tolerogenic properties of HLA-G recombinant proteins. These were B2M-HLA-G heavy chain fusions and HLA-G alpha-1 domains dimerized either through an Fc fragment, or naturally through a C42-C42 disulfide bond. Of note, because of the presence of B2M and the linker in our constructs, the cysteines involved in HLA-G homodimerization were no longer in position 42, but for the sake of clarity, we kept calling C42 the cysteines of the HLA-G alpha-1 domain that are responsible for homodimerization.

Our first aim was to evaluate the tolerogenic function of two types of single-chain B2M-HLA-G homodimers. In this study, we showed that all generated proteins and peptide were multimerized. Furthermore, B2M-HLA-G fusions were properly folded and could bind and activate the ILT2 receptor. These data also showed that with respect to binding to and signaling through ILT receptors, dimerization through C42-C42 disulfide bonding or Fc did not seem to matter. This seemed to be confirmed by *in vivo* data, which showed that both dimer types were functional. Yet, B2M-HLA-G5 was more efficient than B2M-HLA-G1s-Fc, and alpha1-Fc was more efficient than alpha1_peptide *in vivo*. It is possible that Fc-dimers and natural dimers might not be structurally identical: whereas dimers formed via C42-C42 bonds are likely to closely resemble "natural" HLA-G dimers, dimers formed via Fc might not. As

far as HLA-G structure is concerned, B2M-HLA-G1s-Fc dimers might actually be two HLA-G monomers next to each other rather than "real" HLA-G dimers, although additional dimerization through the C42 residues of HLA-G molecules cannot be ruled out and might happen through the C42 of B2M-HLA-G1s-Fc HLA-G portions located within the same homodimer or not. The same hypothesis can be made for alpha1 constructs: alpha1_peptides may only dimerize through C42-C42 disulfide bridging, whereas alpha1-Fc proteins may multimerize further. Our data seem to indicate that for B2M-HLA-G structures, natural multimers are more efficient than Fc-multimers (B2M-HLA-G structures), and that multimers are more efficient than dimers (alpha1 structures). Whether this will hold true when soluble HLA-G multimers and not bead-bound multimers are used is currently under investigation.

It was reported that all isoforms of HLA-G have immunosuppressive functions [16], including HLA-G3 which extracellular part is constituted of the alpha-1 domain only and which was shown to block the functions of NK cells and CTLs. The other goal of this study was to determine if tolerance induction *in vivo* could be induced by the alpha-1 domain of HLA-G only. For this purpose, alpha1-Fc molecules and a synthetic peptide of HLA-G alpha-1 domain were produced. Alpha1-Fc molecules multimerized, whereas alpha1_peptide molecules dimerized. Interestingly, *in vivo* data showed that the alpha-1 domain of HLA-G prolonged the survival of allo-transplanted skin in mice. This was especially true of alpha1-Fc molecules. Once again, this was unexpected because HLA-G-induced tolerance in mice is mediated through HLA-G binding to PIR-B. This receptor shares sequence similarity with the human ILT family of molecules, and particularly with ILT4 which is known to bind HLA-G alpha-3 domain. One explanation for this could be that when it is not part of the HLA-G1:B2M:peptide complex, the HLA-G alpha-1 domain adopts a conformation that allows it to bind to PIR-B, in which case it might also bind ILT molecules. One other explanation could be that HLA-G alpha-1 domain cross-reacts with inhibitory molecules other than PIR-B, such as murine KIRs for instance. In order to discriminate between these two hypotheses, we tested B2M-HLA-G5 and alpha1-Fc in skin transplantation experiments in which the recipient was an ILT4-transgenic mouse. In these experiments, B2M-HLA-G5 retained its tolerogenic capability, whereas alpha1-Fc almost lost it all. It remains unclear why alpha1-Fc was less tolerogenic in ILT4-transgenic mice than in wild type mice, given that their background was identical, although one can hypothesize that ILT4 may have behaved as a dominant positive PIR-B homologue, thus functionally replacing it. Regardless of the reason, these data clearly show that alpha1-Fc was unable to function through ILT4, whereas B2M-HLA-G5 could. Thus, the originally observed tolerogenic function of alpha1-Fc *in vivo* was most likely due to a specific interaction with PIRB that does not happen with ILT4, or to a cross-reaction with a murine receptor other than PIR-B, indicating that HLA-G alpha1 multimers may function through other receptors than ILT molecules. KIR2DL4, a HLA-G specific receptor which is supposed to bind the alpha-1 domain of HLA-G was not present in our system (no shown) and was also ruled out. Consequently, the mechanism by which HLA-G alpha1 multimers function remains unknown for lack of a receptor, which weakens its position as a candidate tolerogenic molecule to be used in human beings.

Nevertheless, it remains that the alpha-1 domain of HLA-G is present on all HLA-G isoforms. In the light of the data gathered, we propose that one of the main functions of the alpha-1 domain

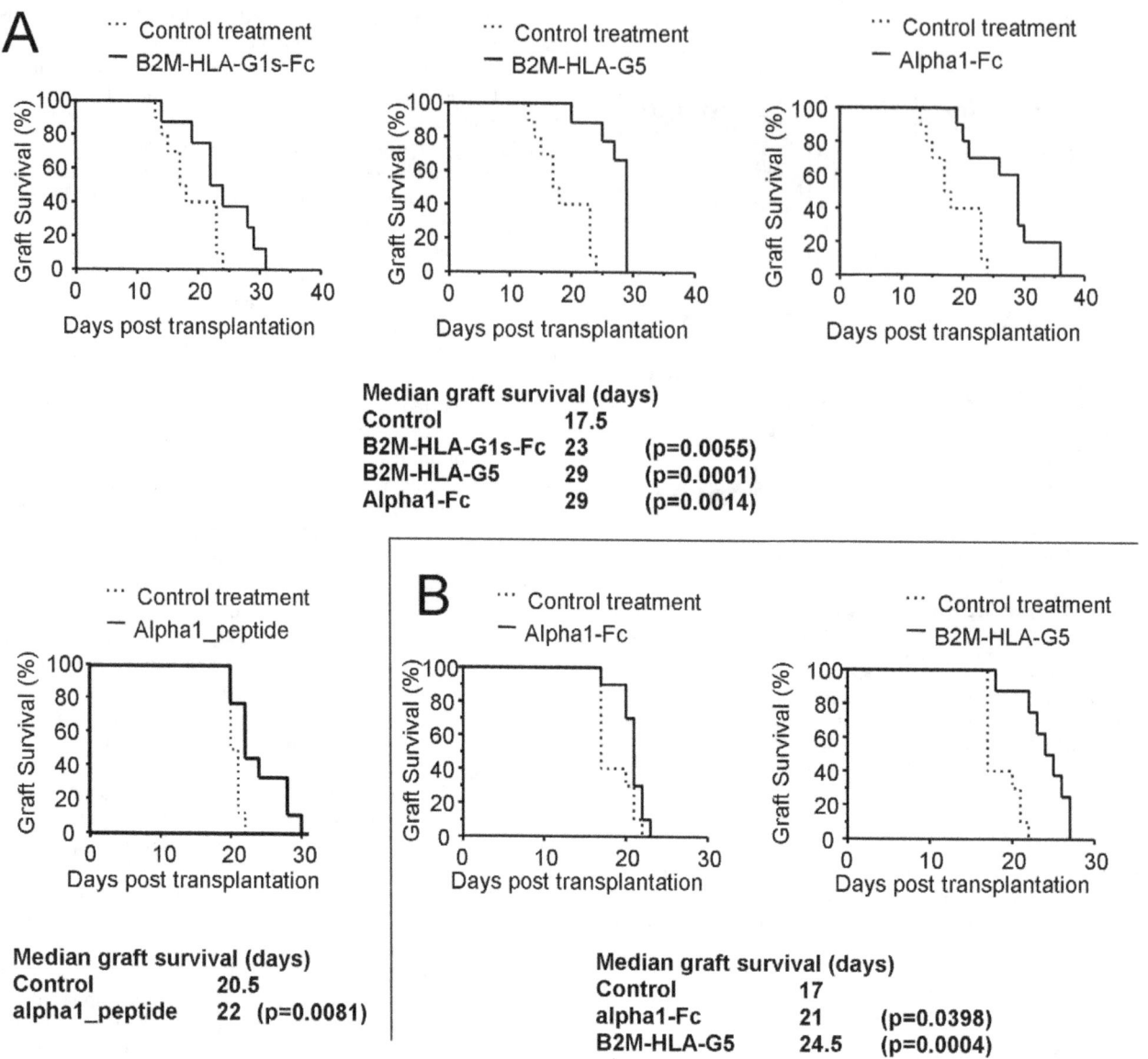

Figure 4. Tolerogenic function of HLA-G fusion proteins and peptide. A. C57BL/6 mice strongly recognize the MHC class II-disparate mutant bm12 mouse that carries the I-Abm12 alloantigen. The capability of HLA-G-coated beads to delay rejection was evaluated. Control treatment (dotted lines): beads coated with mAb but without HLA-G proteins. Results are expressed as Median of graft survival time. Kaplan-Meier curves representing graft survival are shown for each HLA-G protein/peptide for controls (plain lines). Associated values are indicated as a table underneath the curves. **B.** The same experiments were performed using ILT4-transgernic mice as skin graft recipients, and for Alpha1-Fc and B2M-HLA-G5. **Tables**: Median survival of transplant, number of animals, and significance are indicated below the corresponding survival graphs.

of HLA-G may not be to participate directly in immune inhibition, but to induce dimerization, which is required for ILT binding and for proper function. In this context, it seems that the most stable and active forms of HLA-G might indeed be B2M-associated HLA-G1/-G5, or, as an alternative possibility, HLA-G2/-G6 dimers, containing only the alpha-3 domain required for ILT binding and the alpha-1 domain necessary for dimerization.

In this study, we have demonstrated the tolerogenic properties of artificial single-chain B2M:HLA-G dimers *in vivo* in the context of allogeneic skin transplantation. *In vivo* tolerization was achieved according to a protocol developed with refolded B2M:HLA-G tetramer-coated beads. Apparently, the B2M-HLA-G structures presented here did not perform better than refolded ones.

However, it has to be noted that tolerization was obtained by a single injection of HLA-G-coated beads, which is an impressive tolerogenic effect. The advantage of dimerized B2M-HLA-G single-chains over refolded HLA-G tetramers might come from increased stability, which would allow for a longer tolerogenic effect and better prospects for use as soluble molecules rather than coated on beads. The suitability of these constructs for tolerance induction, as well as their *in vivo* stability are currently under investigation.

Author Contributions

Conceived and designed the experiments: JL BF K-YH AH EDC. Performed the experiments: BF K-YH JC MD JW. Analyzed the data: JL AH EDC BF K-YH JW. Wrote the paper: JL AH K-YH BF.

References

1. Carosella ED, Favier B, Rouas-Freiss N, Moreau P, LeMaoult J (2008) Beyond the increasing complexity of the immunomodulatory HLA-G molecule. Blood 111: 4862–4870.

2. Carosella ED, Moreau P, LeMaoult J, Rouas-Freiss N (2008) HLA-G: from biology to clinical benefits. Trends Immunol 29: 125–132.

3. Lila N, Carpentier A, Amrein C, Khalil-Daher I, Dausset J, et al. (2000) Implication of HLA-G molecule in heart-graft acceptance. Lancet 355: 2138.

4. Rouas-Freiss N, LeMaoult J, Moreau P, Dausset J, Carosella ED (2003) HLA-G in transplantation: a relevant molecule for inhibition of graft rejection? Am J Transplant 3: 11–16.

5. Wiendl H, Behrens L, Maier S, Johnson MA, Weiss EH, et al. (2000) Muscle fibers in inflammatory myopathies and cultured myoblasts express the nonclassical major histocompatibility antigen HLA-G. Ann Neurol 48: 679–684.

6. Aractingi S, Briand N, Le Danff C, Viguier M, Bachelez H, et al. (2001) HLA-G and NK receptor are expressed in psoriatic skin: a possible pathway for regulating infiltrating T cells? Am J Pathol 159: 71–77.

7. Paul P, Rouas-Freiss N, Khalil-Daher I, Moreau P, Riteau B, et al. (1998) HLA-G expression in melanoma: a way for tumor cells to escape from immunosurveillance. Proc Natl Acad Sci USA 95: 4510–4515.

8. Pangault C, Le Friec G, Caulet-Maugendre S, Lena H, Amiot L, et al. (2002) Lung macrophages and dendritic cells express HLA-G molecules in pulmonary diseases. Hum Immunol 63: 83–90.

9. Morandi F, Levreri I, Bocca P, Galleni B, Raffaghello L, et al. (2007) Human Neuroblastoma Cells Trigger an Immunosuppressive Program in Monocytes by Stimulating Soluble HLA-G Release. Cancer Res 67: 6433–6441.

10. Nuckel H, Rebmann V, Durig J, Duhrsen U, Grosse-Wilde H (2005) HLA-G expression is associated with an unfavorable outcome and immunodeficiency in chronic lymphocytic leukemia. Blood 105: 1694–1698.

11. Kren L, Muckovaa K, Lzicarovab E, Sovac M, Vybihalc V, et al. (2010) Production of immune-modulatory nonclassical molecules HLA-G and HLA-E by tumor infiltrating ameboid microglia/macrophages in glioblastomas: A role in innate immunity? Journal of Neuroimmunology 220: 131–135.

12. Mitsdoerffer M, Schreiner B, Kieseier BC, Neuhaus O, Dichgans J, et al. (2005) Monocyte-derived HLA-G acts as a strong inhibitor of autologous CD4 T cell activation and is upregulated by interferon-beta in vitro and in vivo: rationale for the therapy of multiple sclerosis. J Neuroimmunol 159: 155–164.

13. Lozano JM, Gonzalez R, Kindelan JM, Rouas-Freiss N, Caballos R, et al. (2002) Monocytes and T lymphocytes in HIV-1-positive patients express HLA-G molecule. Aids 16: 347–351.

14. Chen H-X, Chen B-G, Shi W-W, Zhen R, Xu D-P, et al. (2010) Induction of cell surface HLA-G expression in pandemic H1N1 2009 and seasonal H1N1 influenza virus infected patients. Human Immunology In Press, Accepted Manuscript.

15. Huang J, Burke P, Yang Y, Seiss K, Beamon J, et al. (2010) Soluble HLA-G Inhibits Myeloid Dendritic Cell Function in HIV-1 Infection by Interacting with Leukocyte Immunoglobulin-Like Receptor B2. J Virol 84: 10784–10791.

16. Riteau B, Rouas-Freiss N, Menier C, Paul P, Dausset J, et al. (2001) HLA-G2, -G3, and -G4 isoforms expressed as nonmature cell surface glycoproteins inhibit NK and antigen-specific CTL cytolysis. J Immunol 166: 5018–5026.

17. Rouas-Freiss N, Marchal RE, Kirszenbaum M, Dausset J, Carosella ED (1997) The alpha1 domain of HLA-G1 and HLA-G2 inhibits cytotoxicity induced by natural killer cells: is HLA-G the public ligand for natural killer cell inhibitory receptors? Proc Natl Acad Sci USA 94: 5249–5254.

18. LeMaoult J, Krawice-Radanne I, Dausset J, Carosella ED (2004) HLA-G1-expressing antigen-presenting cells induce immunosuppressive CD4+ T cells. Proc Natl Acad Sci USA 101: 7064–7069.

19. Bahri R, Hirsch F, Josse A, Rouas-Freiss N, Bidere N, et al. (2006) Soluble HLA-G Inhibits Cell Cycle Progression in Human Alloreactive T Lymphocytes. J Immunol 176: 1331–1339.

20. Caumartin J, Favier B, Daouya M, Guillard C, Moreau P, et al. (2007) Trogocytosis-based generation of suppressive NK cells. EMBO J 26: 1423–1433.

21. Ristich V, Liang S, Zhang W, Wu J, Horuzsko A (2005) Tolerization of dendritic cells by HLA-G. Eur J Immunol 35: 1133–1142.

22. Liang S, Ristich V, Arase H, Dausset J, Carosella ED, et al. (2008) Modulation of dendritic cell differentiation by HLA-G and ILT4 requires the IL-6–STAT3 signaling pathway. Proc Natl Acad Sci U S A 105: 8357–8362.

23. Gregori S, Tomasoni D, Pacciani V, Scirpoli M, Battaglia M, et al. (2010) Differentiation of type 1 T regulatory cells (Tr1) by tolerogenic DC-10 requires the IL-10-dependent ILT4/HLA-G pathway. Blood 116: 935–944.

24. Colonna M, Navarro F, Bellon T, Llano M, Garcia P, et al. (1997) A common inhibitory receptor for major histocompatibility complex class I molecules on human lymphoid and myelomonocytic cells. J Exp Med 186: 1809–1818.

25. Colonna M, Samaridis J, Cella M, Angman L, Allen RL, et al. (1998) Human myelomonocytic cells express an inhibitory receptor for classical and nonclassical MHC class I molecules. J Immunol 160: 3096–3100.

26. Rajagopalan S, Long EO (1999) A Human Histocompatibility Leukocyte Antigen (HLA)-G-specific Receptor Expressed on All Natural Killer Cells. J Exp Med 189: 1093–1100.

27. Gonen-Gross T, Achdout H, Gazit R, Hanna J, Mizrahi S, et al. (2003) Complexes of HLA-G protein on the cell surface are important for leukocyte Ig-like receptor-1 function. J Immunol 171: 1343–1351.

28. Boyson JE, Erskine R, Whitman MC, Chiu M, Lau JM, et al. (2002) Disulfide bond-mediated dimerization of HLA-G on the cell surface. Proc Natl Acad Sci USA 99: 16180–16185.

29. Lila N, Amrein C, Guillemain R, Chevalier P, Latremouille C, et al. (2002) Human leukocyte antigen-G expression after heart transplantation is associated with a reduced incidence of rejection. Circulation 105: 1949–1954.

30. Horuzsko A, Lenfant F, Munn DH, Mellor AL (2001) Maturation of antigen-presenting cells is compromised in HLA-G transgenic mice. Int Immunol 13: 385–394.

31. Liang S, Baibakov B, Horuzsko A (2002) HLA-G inhibits the functions of murine dendritic cells via the PIR-B immune inhibitory receptor. Eur J Immunol 32: 2418–2426.

32. Rebmann V, LeMaoult J, Rouas-Freiss N, Carosella ED, Grosse-Wilde H (2005) Report of the Wet Workshop for Quantification of Soluble HLA-G in Essen, 2004. Human Immunology 66: 853–863.

33. Greten TF, Korangy F, Neumann G, Wedemeyer H, Schlote K, et al. (2002) Peptide-[beta]2-microglobulin-MHC fusion molecules bind antigen-specific T cells and can be used for multivalent MHC-Ig complexes. Journal of Immunological Methods 271: 125–135.

34. Shiroishi M, Kuroki K, Ose T, Rasubala L, Shiratori I, et al. (2006) Efficient Leukocyte Ig-like Receptor Signaling and Crystal Structure of Disulfide-linked HLA-G Dimer. J Biol Chem 281: 10439–10447.

35. Shiroishi M, Tsumoto K, Amano K, Shirakihara Y, Colonna M, et al. (2003) Human inhibitory receptors Ig-like transcript 2 (ILT2) and ILT4 compete with CD8 for MHC class I binding and bind preferentially to HLA-G. Proc Natl Acad Sci USA 100: 8856–8861.

36. Shiroishi M, Kuroki K, Rasubala L, Tsumoto K, Kumagai I, et al. (2006) Structural basis for recognition of the nonclassical MHC molecule HLA-G by the leukocyte Ig-like receptor B2 (LILRB2/LIR2/ILT4/CD85d). PNAS 103: 16412–16417.

Transplantation of Oligodendrocyte Precursor Cells Improves Locomotion Deficits in Rats with Spinal Cord Irradiation Injury

Yan Sun[1♦]*, Chong-Chong Xu[1♦], Jin Li[2], Xi-Yin Guan[3], Lu Gao[1], Li-Xiang Ma[1], Rui-Xi Li[1], Yu-Wen Peng[1]*, Guo-Pei Zhu[3]*

1 Department of Anatomy, Histology and Embryology, Shanghai Medical College, Fudan University, Shanghai, China, 2 Institutes of Biomedical Sciences, Fudan University, Shanghai, China, 3 Department of Radiation Oncology, Shanghai Cancer Hospital, Fudan University, Shanghai, China

Abstract

Demyelination contributes to the functional impairment of irradiation injured spinal cord. One potential therapeutic strategy involves replacing the myelin-forming cells. Here, we asked whether transplantation of $Olig2^+$-GFP^+-oligodendrocyte precursor cells (OPCs), which are derived from Olig2-GFP-mouse embryonic stem cells (mESCs), could enhance remyelination and functional recovery after spinal cord irradiation injury. We differentiated Olig2-GFP-mESCs into purified $Olig2^+$-GFP^+-OPCs and transplanted them into the rats' cervical 4–5 dorsal spinal cord level at 4 months after irradiation injury. Eight weeks after transplantation, the $Olig2^+$-GFP^+-OPCs survived and integrated into the injured spinal cord. Immunofluorescence analysis showed that the grafted $Olig2^+$-GFP^+-OPCs primarily differentiated into adenomatous polyposis coli (APC^+) oligodendrocytes (54.6±10.5%). The staining with luxol fast blue, hematoxylin & eosin (LFB/H&E) and electron microscopy demonstrated that the engrafted $Olig2^+$-GFP^+-OPCs attenuated the demyelination resulted from the irradiation. More importantly, the recovery of forelimb locomotor function was enhanced in animals receiving grafts of $Olig2^+$-GFP^+-OPCs. We concluded that OPC transplantation is a feasible therapy to repair the irradiated lesions in the central nervous system (CNS).

Editor: Brahim Nait-Oumesmar, Université Pierre et Marie Curie-Paris6, INSERM, CNRS, France

Funding: This study was supported the by the National Natural Science Foundation of China (No. 30770637, 30901615 and 81201029). The funders had no role in study design, data collection and analysis, decision to publish, or preparation of the manuscript.

Competing Interests: The authors have declared that no competing interests exist.

* E-mail: antica@gmail.com (GPZ); ywpeng@fudan.edu.cn (YWP)

♦ These authors contributed equally to this work.

Introduction

The spinal cord is one of the important dose-limiting normal tissues in clinical radiotherapy. Excessive doses of radiation to the spinal cord result in radiation injury, which is a rare but serious complication of radiotherapy for cancer [1,2]. The pathophysiology involved in irradiation-induced spinal cord injury is demyelination caused by death of oligodendrocytes [3,4]. Reduction in the number of oligodendrocytes was observed as early as 24 hours after X-ray irradiation [5,6]. There is a persistent decline in the number of OPCs from two weeks to three months after X-ray irradiation [7,8]. Remyelination often fails because of primary deficiency in the precursor cells, failure of precursor cells' recruitment, or incompetence of differentiation and maturation of precursor cells [9]. Persistent demyelination may result in further axonal loss. Such changes could be associated with permanent motor and sensory deficits [10], which become fatal if the damage occurs at the upper cervical level [11]. There are currently no therapeutic approaches that promote remyelination available in a clinical setting.

Cell therapy offers an attractive option as grafted cells may replace the lost ones as well as provide neurotrophic benefits to surrounding tissue [9,12]. To date, primary cultured adult neural stem cells, Schwann cells and olfactory ensheathing cells have been transplanted into the radiation-injured spinal cord [13,14,15,16,17]. However, these cells have limited capacity in producing oligodendrocytes, the primary cell type that is damaged in radiation injury. Oligodendrocyte precursor cells (OPCs), which can be isolated from brain tissues [18,19], offer an alternative source. Nevertheless, they need to be derived from brain tissues. Embryonic stem cells (ESCs) may become a suitable candidate because they are genetically normal, pluripotent, and capable of indefinite replication, and they can be differentiated to all the cell types in the body, including OPCs [20,21,22]. Although the induced differentiation of ESCs is a well-developed approach, there are still problems, especially the purity of target cells [23]. Therefore, it is important to develop strategies for the directed differentiation of ESCs into specialized functional cell types and/or purification of the target cells *in vitro* before transplantation.

In the present study, we employed a mESCs line that carries a GFP reporter in the locus of Olig2, a transcription factor that is critical for OPCs development [24]. Following transplantation of $Olig2^+$-GFP^+-OPCs into the spinal cord of rat that underwent irradiation injury, the grafted OPCs survived, differentiated to myelinating oligodendrocytes and improved locomotor function of the injured rats.

Materials and Methods

Ethics Statement

This study was carried out in strict accordance with the recommendations in the Guide for the Care and Use of Laboratory Animals of the National Institutes of Health. The protocol was approved by the Committee on the Ethics of Animal Experiments of Fudan University (Permit Number: SCXK 2009-0019). All efforts were made to minimize suffering.

Irradiation Injury of the Spinal Cord

Female Wistar adult rats (180–200 g, Slrc Laboratory Animal, China) were anesthetized by an intraperitoneal injection of 7.5 mg/kg ketamine, 60 mg/kg xylazine and immobilized during irradiation. The rats' cervical spinal cords were irradiated using a 6 Mev Electron Beam Linear Accelerator (Elekta AB, Stockholm, Sweden). A 22 Gy radiation dose was delivered to a 2 cm×2 cm radiation field, maintaining cervical 4–5 as the center of the electron-irradiated zone. Radiographs were taken before and after X-irradiation to confirm that all the animals were in the same position. After irradiation, the animals were given subcutaneous saline (5 ml) and housed in a 25°C warm room.

Derivation of Olig2⁺-GFP⁺-OPCs from Olig2-GFP-mESCs

Olig2-GFP-mESCs were the gift of Dr. Su-Chun Zhang (University of Wisconsin, USA) and have been previously described [25]. Olig2-GFP-mESCs were differentiated according to a modified protocol [25]. Briefly, mESCs were trypsinized and placed onto low attachment flasks (Greiner, Germany) in a neural differentiation medium containing DMEM/F12, N2 supplement, leukemia inhibitory factor (LIF), nonessential amino acids, L-glutamine, 2-mercaptoethanol and 10% knockout serum replacement (all from Invitrogen, Carlsbad, CA, USA). Under this condition for 2 days, mESCs formed small aggregates. Retinoic acid (RA, 0.5 µM, Sigma, St Louis, MO, USA) and Purmorphamine (Pur, 0.5 µM, Calbiochem, San Diego, CA, USA) were added at days 2–6 to induce neural progenitors. The aggregates were cultured in suspension in the neural differentiation medium with bFGF (20 ng/ml, R&D systems) and heparin (2 µg/ml, Sigma) for another 6 days. On day 12, the differentiated aggregates were dissociated with trypsin-EDTA (0.05%, Gibco) and plated onto flasks coated with Matrigel in modified Bottenstein-Sato medium. The modified Bottenstein-Sato medium contained insulin (10 µg/ml), BSA (100 µg/ml), human transferrin (100 µg/ml), progesterone (60 µg/ml), sodium selenite (40 µg/ml), N-acetyl-cysteine (60 µg/ml), putrescine (16 µg/ml), biotin (10 ng/ml) and cAMP (5 µM) (all reagents from Sigma). T3 (40 ng/ml, Sigma), PDGF-AA (10 ng/ml) and NT3 (5 ng/ml) (all from R&D systems) were added to promote the proliferation of the OPCs.

For immunofluorescence, dissociated spheres (2×10^4 cells/µl) were plated on coverslips coated with poly-L-lysine and human laminin (Sigma).

For fluorescence activated cell sorting (FACS), cells were harvested at day 12, gently dissociated to single cells and washed with a FACS buffer (PBS, 1%N2, 200 mM L-glutamine, 55 mM β-ME, 50 ng/ml NAC). Cells were analyzed by a Becton Dickinson FACSCaliber with CellQuest Pro (BD Biosciences, San Diego, CA, USA).

For transplantation, FACS-sorted Olig2⁺-GFP⁺-OPCs were resuspended in a fresh culture medium and cultured for 2 days. At day 14, cells were dissociated with accutase (Invitrogen) and prepared at approximately 100,000 cells/µl in artificial cerebrospinal fluid (aCSF). Trypan blue exclusion testing indicated that this preparation consisted of 95% viable cells at time of transplantation.

Cell Transplantation

Transplantation was performed as described [26]. The animals were immunosuppressed using cyclosporine A (10 mg/kg/d, s.c; Novartis Pharma Schweiz AG, Switzerland) 1 day prior to transplantation and then every day for the duration of the study. Cell transplantation occurred 4 months after irradiation surgery. The animals were anesthetized as above, and the spinal cord was exposed by laminectomy at the cervical 4–5 vertebral level. After immobilization of the spinal cord, a 10 µl Hamilton syringe (Hamilton, Reno, NV) was lowered into the spinal cord using a stereotactic manipulator arm. Cell suspension (2 µl) was injected into two sites along the midline at a depth of 1.2 mm, 4 mm cranial and 4 mm caudal to the lesion epicenter, at a rate of 1.0 µl/min. The needle was removed after 5 min. The animals in which the injected solution was observed to exit from the needle track during injection or after withdrawal of the needle were omitted from the experiment. Animals receiving the same surgery and injection of 2 µl aCSF solution (without cells) were served as controls.

Histology

For the histological analysis, the animals were deeply anesthetized with an overdose of 3% pentobarbitone and perfused with 0.9% saline following by 4% ice-cold paraformaldehyde prepared with phosphate buffer (0.1 M, pH7.4). The spinal cord was divided into eight 1 mm blocks that extended 4 mm cranial to and 4 mm caudal to the injury epicenter. Alternate blocks were processed to produce cryostat sections. Some of the cryostat sections were stained with LFB/H&E to examine general morphology and the extent of demyelination. Some of the cryostat sections were used for immunofluorescent analysis of grafted cells.

To quantify the demyelination of injured spinal cord, we used Image J (http://rsbweb.nih.gov/ij/index.html) to measure the relative optical density of the dorsal funiculus from all groups. A pre-defined region of interest was selected to encompass the dorsal funiculus. Color images were acquired at the same exposure level, coverted to 8-bit gray scale, and the mean density calculated from the threshold pixels excluding the background. Density was analyzed in four regions of the dorsal funiculus per section. Eight sections per spinal cord were analyzed. There were six animals in each group.

Immunofluorescence

Immunostaining was performed on cultured cells or cryosectioned spinal cord using standard protocols [27]. Primary antibodies used in present study included mouse anti-Oct4 (1:2000, Santa Cruz Biotechnology, Santa Cruz, CA), goat anti-Sox2 (1:1000, R&D Systems), rabbit anti-NG2 (1:500, Chemicon International Inc, Temecula, CA, USA), rabbit anti-O4 (1:50, Santa Cruz), rabbit anti-PDGFRα (1:500, Santa Cruz), rabbit anti-MBP (1:500, Abcam, Cambridge, MA), goat anti-GFP (1:200; Abcam), mouse anti-APC (1:1000; Abcam), mouse anti-p75 (1:1000; Chemicon), rabbit anti-GFAP (1:500; Chemicon), and mouse anti-NF (1:2000; Chemicon). Coverslip cultures or spinal cord sections were incubated in a blocking buffer (10% donkey serum and 0.2% Triton X-100 in phosphate buffer saline) for 60 min at room temperature before being incubated in the primary antibodies overnight at 4°C. Fluorescently conjugated secondary antibodies were used to reveal the binding of primary antibodies (1:2000, Invitrogen) and nuclei were stained with 4,6-dianidina-2-phenylindole (DAPI) (0.1 µg/ml, Sigma). The immu-

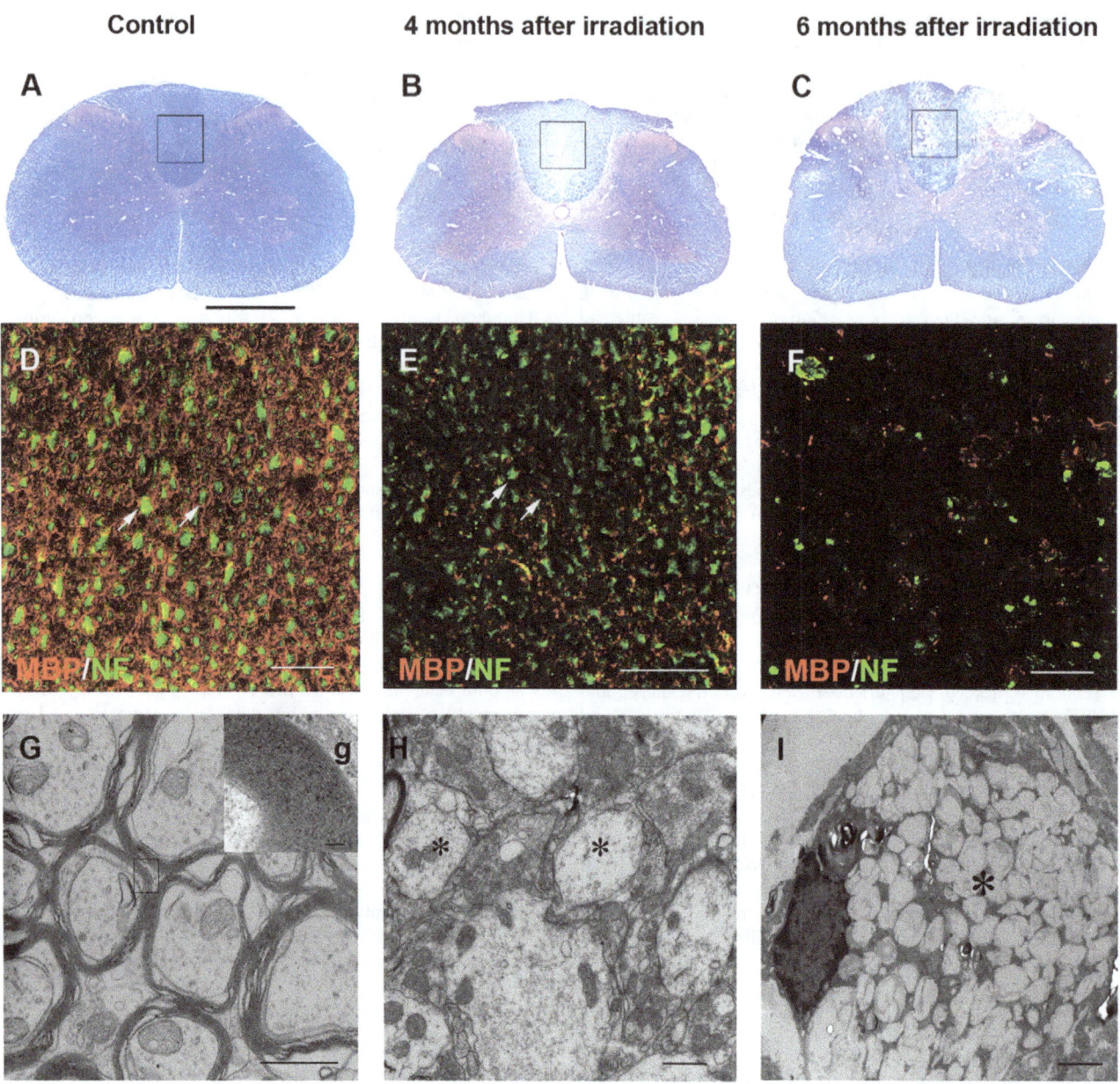

Figure 1. Radiation-induced demyelination in the dorsal funiculus of cervical spinal cord. (A) LFB/H&E staining showed normal spinal cord without irradiation. (B) Four months after irradiation, there was a focal demyelinated zone in the dorsal funiculus. (C) Six months following injury, focal necrosis was seen in the dorsal funiculus. (D) Immunostaining for MBP and NF, enlargement of framed area in A, depicted that non-irradiated myelin surrounding the axons (arrows). (E) Four months after irradiation, most of the axons lost myelin (arrows). (F) At six months, axons began to show necrosis. (G) Electron microscopy confirmed the normal structure of myelin. g, Higher magnification of the tissue in the box in G, indicated the compact myelin sheath. (H) Four months after irradiation, most of axons remained demyelinated (asterisk). (I) Six months following damage, axons necrosis was found (asterisk). Bar, 200 μm (A–C); bar, 50 μm (D–F); bar, 1 μm (G, H); bar, 100 nm (g); bar, 2 μm (I).

nofluorescent samples were visualized using a Nikon-Eclipse TE 2000-S fluorescence microscope (Nikon Instruments, Sterling Heights, MI, USA) or a Leica TCS-SP5 laser-scanning confocal microscope (Leica, Germany).

To quantify the differentiation pattern *in vitro*, the percentage of immunopositive cells was determined by dividing the total number of immunopositive cells by the total number of GFP/DAPI positive cells in each imaging field and then averaging the result from three fields per marker. These fixed fields were randomly selected from biological replicates using "Image J".

To assess the differentiation of grafted $Olig2^+$-GFP^+-OPCs in the injured spinal cord, four coronal sections, 200 μm apart, were taken spanning the lesion epicenter. The percentage of engrafted OPCs that co-expressed NG2, APC, MBP, p75 and GFAP was quantified for the grafted animals.

Electron Microscopy

For electron microscopic processing, the animals were sacrificed by aortic perfusion with isotonic, heparinized saline followed with 4% paraformaldehyde and 1% glutaraldehyde in 0.1 M phosphate buffer. The fixed spinal cords were washed in 0.1 M phosphate

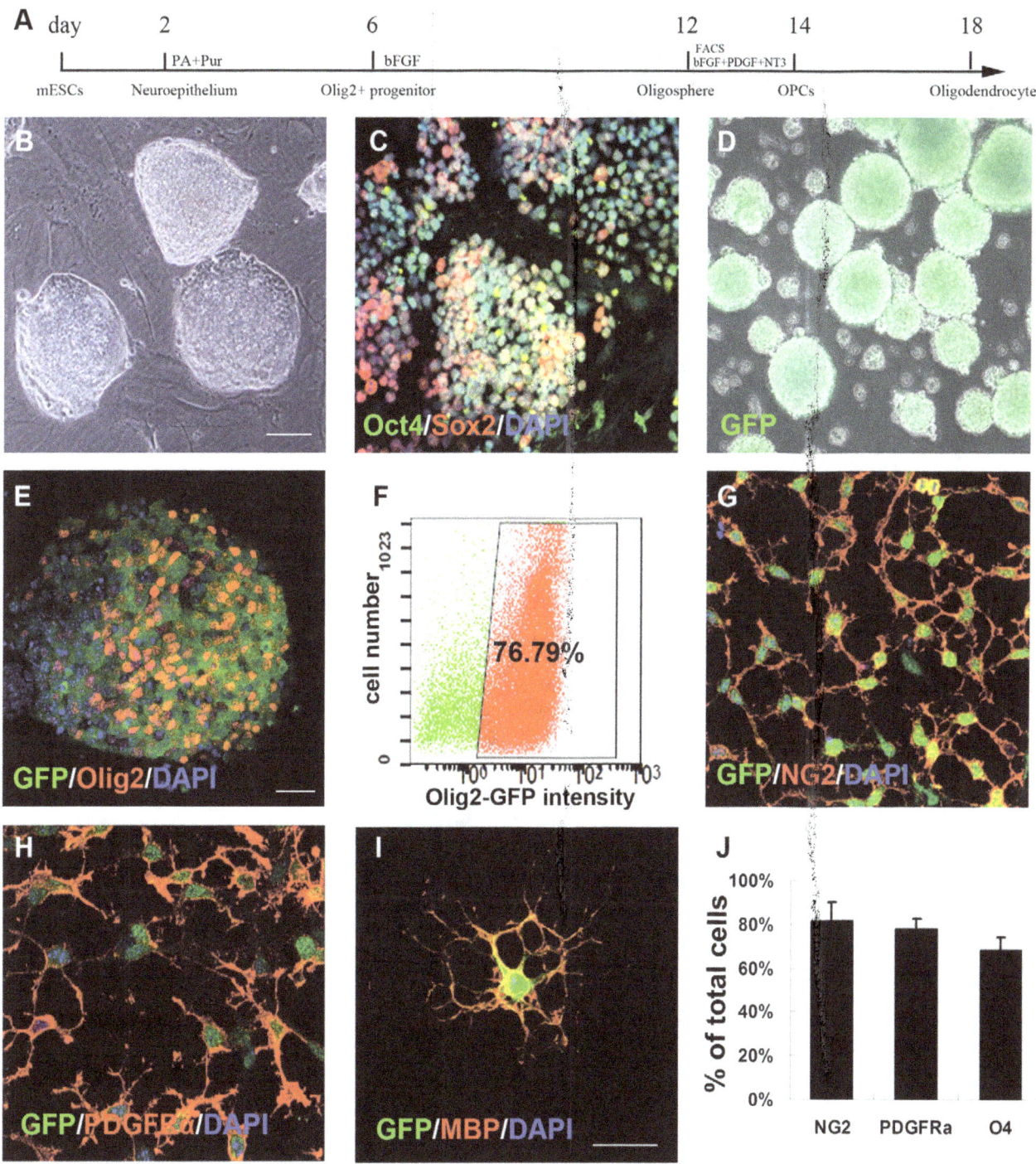

Figure 2. *In vitro* differentiation of Olig2-GFP-mouse mESCs into Olig2$^+$-GFP$^+$- OPCs. (A) Schematic procedure for differentiation of Olig2-GFP-mESCs into Olig2$^+$-GFP$^+$-OPCs. (B) Phase contrast photograph of mESCs colonies on mouse embryonic fibroblast. (C) mESCs remained undifferentiated and stained positive for Oct4/Sox2. (D) Phase contrast photograph of Olig2$^+$-GFP$^+$ spheres at day 12. (E) GFP$^+$ spheres expressed Olig2. (F) At day 12, the percentage of GFP$^+$ cells was 76.79%$\pm$1.35%, sorted by FACS method. At day 14, all purified OPCs expressed GFP as well as the OPC markers NG2 (G) and PDGFRα (H). At day 18, plated cells adopted a typical oligodendrocyte morphology characterized by multiple branches and expressed GFP and MBP (I). (J) Quantification of immunostaining: 81.69$\pm$8.16% of cells expressed NG2, 78$\pm$4.31% of cells expressed PDGFRα, and 68.47$\pm$5.59% of cells expressed O4. Data in J are expressed as the mean$\pm$SEM, n=3 independent experiments, 6 total replicates. Bar, 200 μm (B–D); bar, 50 μm (E–H); bar, 30 μm (I).

buffer and embedded in 3% agar. Transverse sections (40 μm thick) were obtained on a vibrotome (Leica, VT1000S, Nussloch, Germany) and mounted onto slides. The sections were washed in PB and subjected to an additional fixation in 2% OsO$_4$ in

phosphate buffer for 2 h at room temperature. After sequential dehydration in increasing concentrations of ethanol (50–100%) and pure acetone, the sections were embedded in Epon 812. Ultrathin sections (80 nm) obtained using an ultramicrotome (UI-

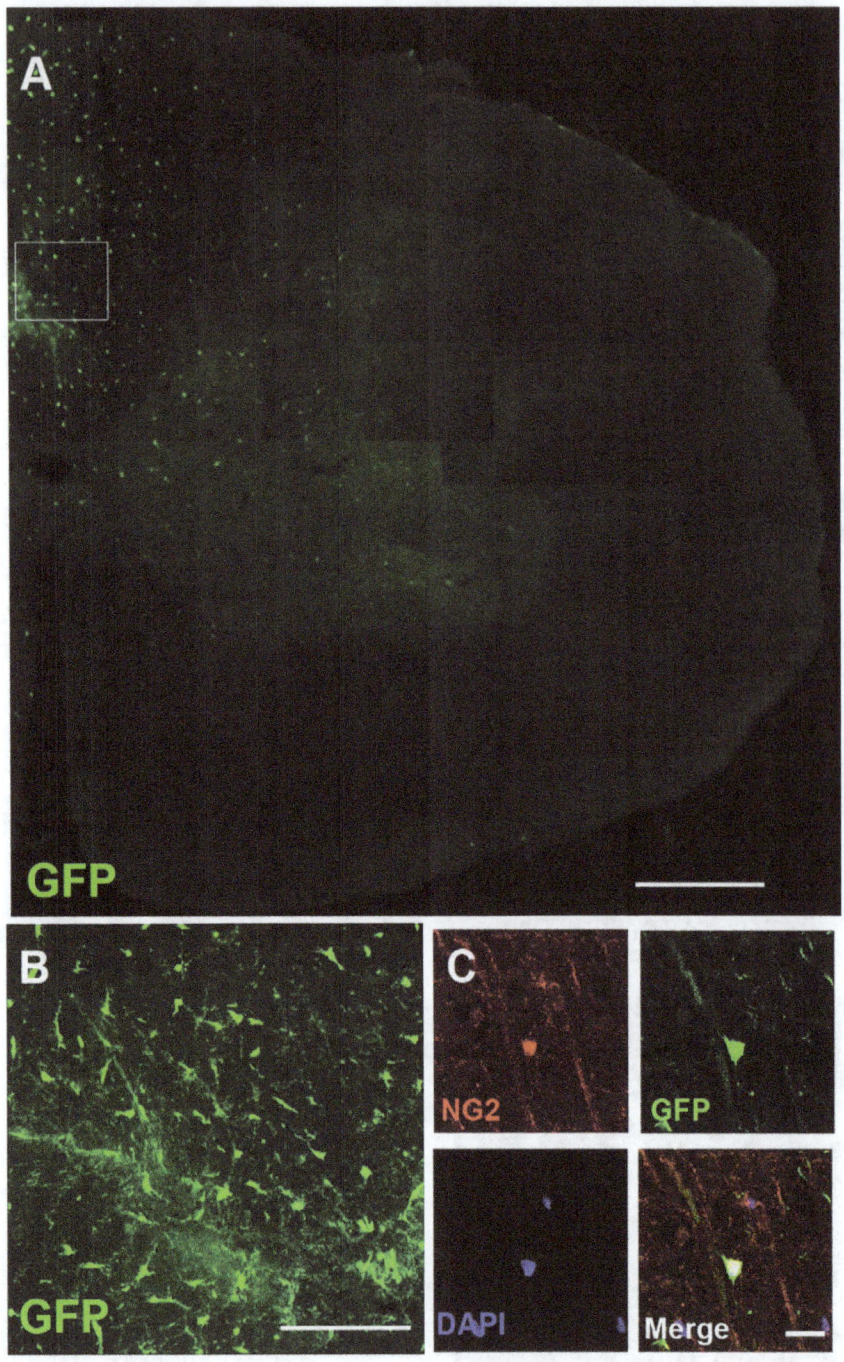

Figure 3. Distribution and morphology of Olig2$^+$-GFP$^+$-OPCs in irradiated spinal cord at four weeks after transplantation. (A) GFP$^+$ cells were observed and distributed in the damaged spinal cord. (B) At higher magnification of the boxed area from (A), the GFP$^+$ cells exhibited typical bipolar OPC morphology. (C) Many grafted Olig2$^+$-GFP$^+$-OPCs co-expressed the OPCs marker NG2. Bar, 250 µm (A); bar, 100 µm (B); bar, 20 µm (C).

tracut E, Reicher-Jung, NY, USA) were stained with uranyl acetate and lead citrate, examined and photographed under a transmission electron microscope (Philips CM120, Amsterdam Netherlands).

Behavioral Assessments

The clinical degree of weakness was graded according to a scale developed by Ushio et al. [28,29]: grade 0 = normal; grade 1 = forelimb instability seen only when the animal jumps or runs;

grade 2 = mild weakness, but able to run; grade 3 = moderate weakness, able to walk but not run; grade 4 = marked weakness, attempts to walk; grade 5 = severe weakness, purposeless movements of legs or complete paraplegia. All rats were allowed to live for 8 weeks after transplantation.

Statistical Analysis

All data are reported as Mean±SEM. Repeated measures ANOVA followed by the Tukey-Kramer test was used for

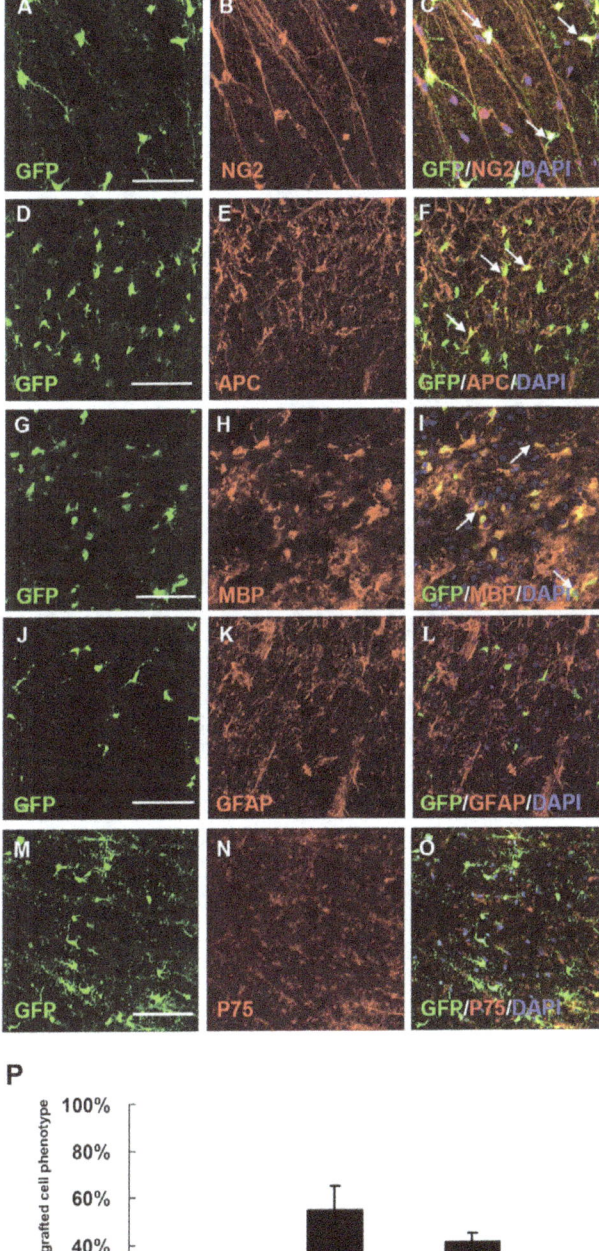

Figure 4. Olig2⁺-GFP⁺-OPCs primarily differentiate along the oligodendrocyte lineage. At eight weeks after transplantation, a certain number of grafted GFP⁺ cells still expressed NG2 (A–C, arrows) and most of the grafted GFP⁺ cells became APC-positive mature oligodendrocytes (D–F, arrows). Double staining for GFP and MBP in cross-sections further confirmed that GFP-immunoreactive rings were composed of MBP⁺ myelin (G–I, arrows). The grafted GFP⁺ cells did not co-expressed GFAP (J–L) or P75 (M–O). (P) Quantification of GFP⁺ cell populations in the spinal cord. Data are expressed as the mean number of cells/spinal cord±SEM (n = 6). GFP⁺ cells expressed NG2 (15.1±5.53%), APC (54.6±10.5%) and MBP (40.5±3.8%). Bar, 50 μm (A–C); bar, 35 μm (D–O).

comparison of clinical grade scores at each time point. The difference between the two was compared using Student's tests. Statistical analysis was performed using SPSS 16.0. Differences were considered to be statistically significant at $p<0.05$.

Results

Demyelination Induced by Irradiation

Non-irradiated animals (n = 6) did not show any evidence of demyelination (Fig. 1A, D and G). Even though there was no histological evidence of demyelination observed from 1 to 3-month after irradiation, 80% of the animals (n = 60) developed a focally demyelinated zone in the dorsal funiculus from the fourth month, as shown by LFB/H&E staining (Fig. 1B). This was confirmed by immunostaining for myelin basic protein (MBP) and neurofilament (NF), showing the presence of many axons but sharply reduced MBP staining (Fig. 1E). Electron microscopy showed many viable demyelinated axons in the dorsal funiculus (Fig. 1H). Six months after irradiation, focal areas of necrosis were apparent in the white matter (Fig. 1C), with MBP loss and axonal degeneration (Fig. 1F). Axon necrosis was also found by electron microscopy (Fig. 1I).

The clinical degree of weakness was consistent with the histological changes. The mean interval between irradiation and manifestation of the first neurological symptoms (grade 1 = fore-limb instability seen only when the animal jumps or runs) was 112±14 days. Four months after irradiation, the animals (n = 12) that did not manifest neurological symptoms (grade 0 = normal) were omitted from the experiment.

Generation and Purification of Olig2⁺-GFP⁺-OPCs from mESCs

We used an established mESCs line (Olig2-GFP-mESCs) in which GFP was knocked into the locus of Olig2, a transcription factor expressed by ventral spinal cord progenitors [24]. In order to identify and purify OPCs, we used a modified protocol established in the Zhang Lab to differentiate mESCs into OPCs [25] (Fig. 2A). The Olig2-GFP-mESCs, expanding as discrete colonies on mouse embryonic fibroblast (Fig. 2B) and expressing Oct4/Sox2 (Fig. 2C), were detached from mouse embryonic fibroblasts to initiate differentiation and grown as free floating embryoid bodies (EB) for 2 days in the medium before being treated with RA (0.5 μM) and Pur (0.5 μM). At day 6, GFP⁺ spheres began to appear and by day 12 almost all the spheres were green (Fig. 2D). FACS analysis, confirmed by confocal microscopy, indicated that 76.79± 1.35% of the total differentiated cells expressed Olig2 and GFP (Fig. 2E, F). To further purify the OPCs, we used FACS based on GFP expression. FACS isolated cells were plated in the presence of FGF2, PDGF-AA and NT3. The majority of GFP cells expressed NG2 (81.69±8.16%) (Fig. 2G, J), PDGFRα (78±4.31%) (Fig. 2H, J) and O4 (68.47±5.59%) (Fig. 2J). Further differentiation of the OPCs for 6 days resulted in generation of highly branched oligodendrocytes, as indicated by positive staining for MBP (Fig. 2I).

Survival and Migration of Transplanted OPCs within the Spinal Cord

A total of 24 injured animals received transplantation of Olig2⁺-GFP⁺-OPCs 4 months after irradiation. Four weeks after transplantation, grafted cells revealed by GFP, were found in the spinal cord of all transplanted animals. The animals (n = 24) without cell transplantation did not exhibit such labeling. The GFP-expressing cells were mainly distributed in the dorsal funiculus with a small number of cells migrating into the gray matter (Fig. 3A). At a higher magnification, the GFP⁺ cells

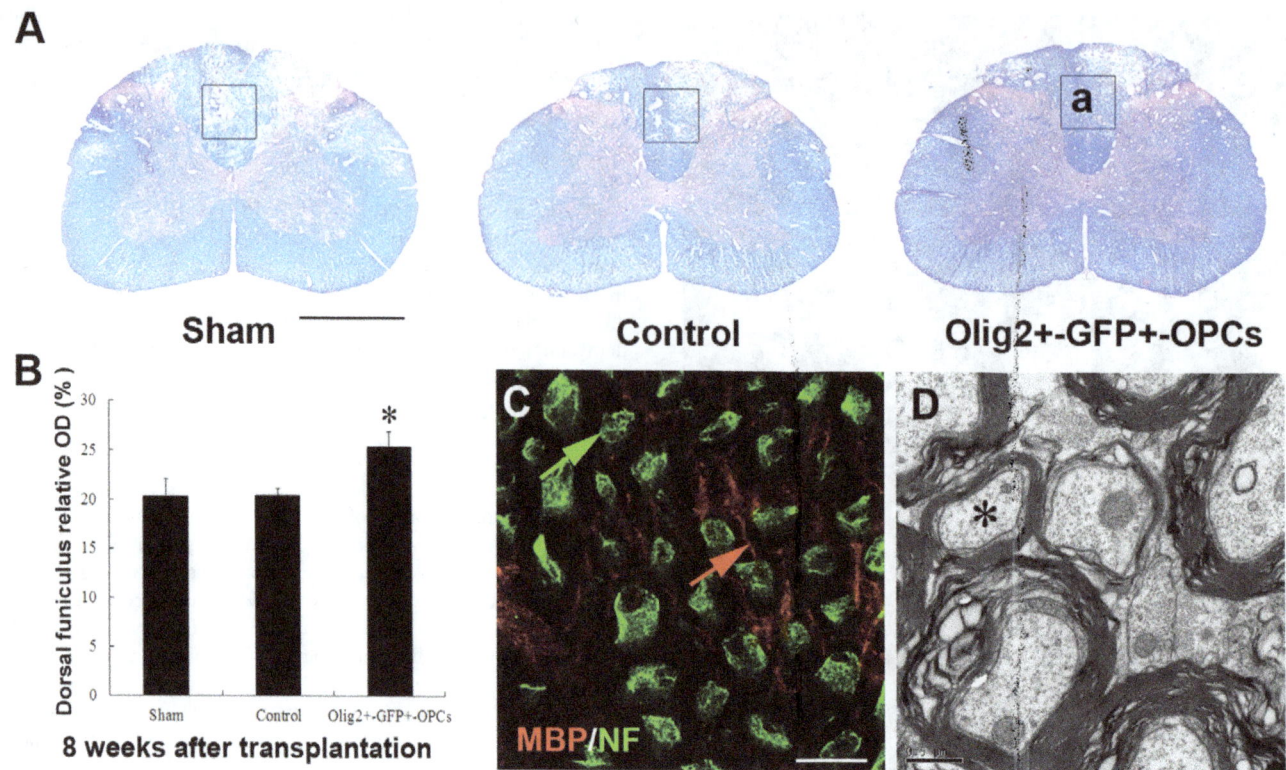

Figure 5. Transplantation of Olig2⁺-GFP⁺-OPCs results in a delayed demyelination and cavitation. (A) LFB/H&E staining showed smaller cystic cavitations in the transplanted cord than those in the sham and the control group in the dorsal funiculus. (B) Optical densities of dorsal funiculus in spinal cord was significantly increased in rats grafted with Olig2⁺-GFP⁺-OPCs, as compared to the sham and the control group (*$p < 0.05$, n = 12). (C) Enlargement of framed area in part a, illustrated immunostaining of MBP and NF, showing axons (green arrow) with or without myelin (red arrow). (D) Electron microscopy confirmed the structure of axons (asterisk). Bar, 200 μm (A); bar, 35 μm (C); bar, 0.5 μm (D).

adopted a typical OPCs morphology, as characterized by bipolar branches (Fig. 3B), and expressed the OPCs marker NG2 (which marks undifferentiated OPCs) (Fig. 3C), indicating that these grafted cells retain the OPCs identity.

Transplanted OPCs Primarily Differentiate into Oligodendrocytes

Eight weeks after transplantation, 15.1±5.53% of the GFP positive cells were double labeled with NG2, a specific protein for precursor cells (Fig. 4A–C, arrows). Around 54.6±10.5% of GFP⁺ cells expressed APC (Fig. 4D–F, arrows), indicating that the majority of grafted OPCs differentiated into mature oligodendrocytes. About 40.5±3.8% of the grafted cells also expressed MBP, a major constitute of myelin (Fig. 4G–I, arrows). Although several previous studies [30,31] showed that adult OPCs differentiated into Schwann cells after transplantation into the chemically demyelinated spinal cord, our transplanted OPCs did not express p75 (Fig. 4M–O). Other studies suggest that the microenvironment in the injured spinal cord induces grafted neural stem cells to differentiate primarily into astrocytes [14,32]. In the present study, the transplanted OPCs did not differentiate into astrocytes marked by GFAP (Fig. 4J–L). In summation, the staining results revealed that Olig2⁺-GFP⁺-OPCs mostly differentiate into mature oligodendrocytes in the injured spinal cord. Over the course of the experiment, tumors, teratomas, or non-neuronal tissue formation were not observed in the transplant recipients.

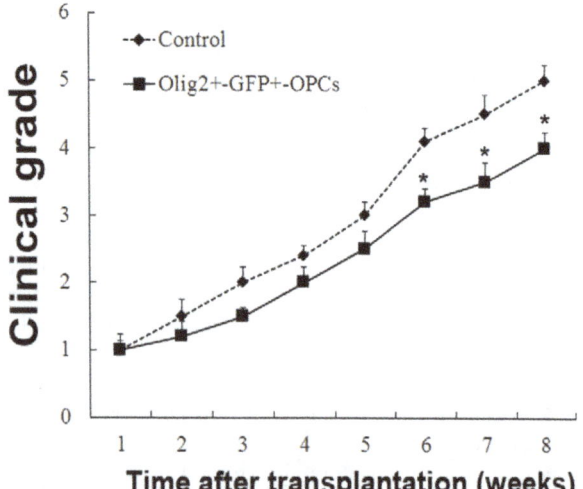

Figure 6. Forelimb locomotion is improved after transplantation of Olig2⁺-GFP⁺-OPCs. Locomotion function, as defined using the clinical grade score, was significantly reduced in Olig2⁺-GFP⁺-OPCs grafted animals at six to eight weeks after transplantation, as compared to the control group (*$p < 0.05$, n = 12).

OPCs Transplantation Attenuated Demyelination after Radiation

Eight weeks after transplantation, irradiated spinal cord exhibited obvious demyelination and cavitation (Fig. 5A). However, the degree of demyelination was significantly decreased by OPCs transplantation as compared to the sham and the control group (Fig. 5B). Immunostainning for MBP and NF indicated numerous clusters of axons that maintained integrity (Fig. 5C). Electron microscopic analysis showed myelinated axons (Fig. 5D).

OPCs Grafts Alleviated the Deterioration of Neurologic Function Following Injury

To determine whether transplantation of OPCs improved recovery of function after injury, locomotion was assessed by using the clinical scoring. Six to eight weeks after transplantation, Olig2$^+$-GFP$^+$-OPCs grafted animals exhibited significantly lower clinical scores as compared to the control group (Fig. 6) (all $p<0.05$). The behavioral results showed that transplantation of Olig2$^+$-GFP$^+$-OPCs significantly improved forelimb functions.

Discussion

In this study, we have directed mESCs to a purified population of OPCs based on the GFP expression in the Olig2 locus, which differentiate into oligodendrocytes *in vitro* and *in vivo*. More importantly, the oligodendrocytes derived from the Olig2$^+$-GFP$^+$-OPCs express MBP, an essential component of myelin sheath, which corresponds to correction of locomotion deficits in rats with irradiation injury of spinal cord. These results raise the prospect of cell-based therapy as a potential treatment for irradiation spinal cord injury.

Cell transplantation has been attempted for the radiation injured spinal cord. Adult rat neural stem cells differentiate predominantly into Schwann-like cells and generated peripheral myelin after transplantation into the irradiation injured spinal cord [14]. Olfactory ensheathing cells appear to migrate within X-irradiated area, they behave similarly as Schwann cells, which survive poorly and are unable to migrate significant distances when transplanted into either intact or X-irradiated spinal cords [16,33]. OPCs are extremely motile and can differentiate into oligodendrocytes and produce myelin [34,35]. Differentiation of oligodendrocytes from mESCs was explored by Billon and colleagues [36]. One of the greatest challenges facing ESCs research is the derivation of high purity target cells from pluripotent ESCs [23]. In the present study, we employed a mESCs line that carries a GFP reporter in the Olig2 locus. The modified differentiation protocol that we used is unique in that it generates highly enriched OPCs. FACS sorting resulted in an enriched population of OPCs ($76.79\pm1.35\%$) (Fig. 2F). This provided us with a novel tool to investigate the ability of these cells to remyelinate demyelinated regions of irradiation spinal cord injury and determine whether remyelination confers functional benefit.

Most irradiation injury models are made using 40 Gy of X-irradiation which creates acute demyelination in the spinal cord [13,14,16,37,38]. However, the latent period of spinal cord irradiation in human has been reported to vary from 4 months to 4 years after cervical or thoracic irradiation [39]. In experimental animals, irradiation of the spinal cord leads to white matter necrosis within 3–8 months [3]. In the present study, we have used the dosage of 22 Gy to mimic the delayed demyelination of the spinal cord irradiation injury. The demyelination latent period was about 112 ± 14 days, while the white matter necrosis and paralysis that occurred within 6 months of radiation exposure. Therefore, our model is similar to the clinical pathology changes of spinal cord irradiation injury.

Promoting remyelination is an important strategy to treat spinal cord injury. Chronic demyelination predisposes axons to degeneration [40], an irreversible event that is thought to be the major cause of progressive functional decline [41]. Previous studies observed cells with the capacity to myelinate following spinal cord injury [32,34,35,42,43,44,45]. The functional behavioral improvement is correlated with the capacity of the transplanted cells to integrate, differentiate, and myelinate axons at sufficient number [9,46,47]. In our study, we have found that transplanted cells migrate to the injured region and approximately 40% of them differentiate into mature oligodendrocytes expressing MBP. More importantly, immunostaining and electron microscopy analysis reveal the presence of many axons in the areas with Olig2$^+$-GFP$^+$-OPCs transplantation, suggesting the protection of axonal integrity by transplanted cells. Further study is needed by immunoelectron microscopy to prove remyelination occurred by transplanted cells.

The increased recovery in the transplantation group may also be explained by mechanisms other than remyelination. CNS neurons require multiple signals for optical survival and maturation, and continued oligodendrocyte-derived signals are necessary to maintain neuronal integrity [48]. In addition to their role in myelinating axons, oligodendrocytes release soluble factors, including insulin-like growth factor (IGF-1), glial-derived neurotrophic factor (GDNF) and brain-derived neurotrophic factor (BDNF), that promote neuronal survival, maintain axonal structure, and support synaptic plasticity in surviving axons [49,50,51,52]. The expression and release of trophic factors offer a platform by which oligodendrocytes interact with neurons to form and maintain functional neural circuits in the injured spinal cord. Therefore, neural protection may be another mechanism by which grafted OPCs promote functional recovery.

Acknowledgments

We are grateful to Ya-Ling Huang and Guo-Ping Zhang (Institutes of Biomedical Sciences, Fudan University) for their technical assistance.

Author Contributions

Conceived and designed the experiments: YWP GPZ. Performed the experiments: YS CCX JL XYG. Analyzed the data: YS CCX JL XYG LG LXM RXL. Contributed reagents/materials/analysis tools: YWP. Wrote the paper: YS CCX GPZ.

References

1. Fowler JF, Bentzen SM, Bond SJ, Ang KK, van der Kogel AJ, et al. (2000) Clinical radiation doses for spinal cord: the 1998 international questionnaire. Radiother Oncol 55: 295–300.

2. Bijl HP, van Luijk P, Coppes RP, Schippers JM, Konings AW, et al. (2003) Unexpected changes of rat cervical spinal cord tolerance caused by inhomogeneous dose distributions. Int J Radiat Oncol Biol Phys 57: 274–281.

3. Okada S, Okeda R (2001) Pathology of radiation myelopathy. Neuropathology 21: 247–265.

4. Wong CS, Van der Kogel AJ (2004) Mechanisms of radiation injury to the central nervous system: implications for neuroprotection. Mol Interv 4: 273–284.

5. Li YQ, Jay V, Wong CS (1996) Oligodendrocytes in the adult rat spinal cord undergo radiation-induced apoptosis. Cancer Res 56: 5417–5422.

6. Atkinson S, Li YQ, Wong CS (2003) Changes in oligodendrocytes and myelin gene expression after radiation in the rodent spinal cord. Int J Radiat Oncol Biol Phys 57: 1093–1100.

7. Chari DM, Huang WL, Blakemore WF (2003) Dysfunctional oligodendrocyte progenitor cell (OPC) populations may inhibit repopulation of OPC depleted tissue. Journal of Neuroscience Research 73: 787–793.

8. Hopewell JW, van der Kogel AJ (1999) Pathophysiological mechanisms leading to the development of late radiation-induced damage to the central nervous system. Front Radiat Ther Oncol 33: 265–275.

9. Franklin RJ, Ffrench-Constant C (2008) Remyelination in the CNS: from biology to therapy. Nat Rev Neurosci 9: 839–855.

10. Schultheiss TE, Kun LE, Ang KK, Stephens LC (1995) Radiation response of the central nervous system. Int J Radiat Oncol Biol Phys 31: 1093–1112.

11. Schultheiss TE, Stephens LC, Peters LJ (1986) Survival in radiation myelopathy. Int J Radiat Oncol Biol Phys 12: 1765–1769.

12. Franklin RJ, Kotter MR (2008) The biology of CNS remyelination: the key to therapeutic advances. J Neurol 255 Suppl 1: 19–25.

13. Rezvani M, Birds DA, Hodges H, Hopewell JW, Milledew K, et al. (2001) Modification of radiation myelopathy by the transplantation of neural stem cells in the rat. Radiat Res 156: 408–412.

14. Mothe AJ, Tator CH (2008) Transplanted neural stem/progenitor cells generate myelinating oligodendrocytes and Schwann cells in spinal cord demyelination and dysmyelination. Exp Neurol 213: 176–190.

15. Chari DM, Gilson JM, Franklin RJM, Blakemore WF (2006) Oligodendrocyte progenitor cell (OPC) transplantation is unlikely to offer a means of preventing X-irradiation induced damage in the CNS. Experimental Neurology 198: 145–153.

16. Lankford KL, Sasaki M, Radtke C, Kocsis JD (2008) Olfactory ensheathing cells exhibit unique migratory, phagocytic, and myelinating properties in the X-irradiated spinal cord not shared by Schwann cells. Glia 56: 1664–1678.

17. Monje ML, Mizumatsu S, Fike JR, Palmer TD (2002) Irradiation induces neural precursor-cell dysfunction. Nat Med 8: 955–962.

18. Zhang SC, Lundberg C, Lipsitz D, O'Connor LT, Duncan ID (1998) Generation of oligodendroglial progenitors from neural stem cells. J Neurocytol 27: 475–489.

19. Avellana-Adalid V, Nait-Oumesmar B, Lachapelle F, Baron-Van Evercooren A (1996) Expansion of rat oligodendrocyte progenitors into proliferative "oligospheres" that retain differentiation potential. J Neurosci Res 45: 558–570.

20. Bain G, Kitchens D, Yao M, Huettner JE, Gottlieb DI (1995) Embryonic stem cells express neuronal properties in vitro. Dev Biol 168: 342–357.

21. Okabe S, Forsberg-Nilsson K, Spiro AC, Segal M, McKay RD (1996) Development of neuronal precursor cells and functional postmitotic neurons from embryonic stem cells in vitro. Mech Dev 59: 89–102.

22. Brustle O, Jones KN, Learish RD, Karram K, Choudhary K, et al. (1999) Embryonic stem cell-derived glial precursors: a source of myelinating transplants. Science 285: 754–756.

23. Evans M (2011) Discovering pluripotency: 30 years of mouse embryonic stem cells. Nat Rev Mol Cell Biol 12: 680–686.

24. Zhou Q, Choi G, Anderson DJ (2001) The bHLH transcription factor Olig2 promotes oligodendrocyte differentiation in collaboration with Nkx2.2. Neuron 31: 791–807.

25. Du ZW, Li XJ, Nguyen GD, Zhang SC (2006) Induced expression of Olig2 is sufficient for oligodendrocyte specification but not for motoneuron specification and astrocyte repression. Molecular and Cellular Neuroscience 33: 371–380.

26. Sharp J, Frame J, Siegenthaler M, Nistor G, Keirstead HS (2010) Human embryonic stem cell-derived oligodendrocyte progenitor cell transplants improve recovery after cervical spinal cord injury. Stem Cells 28: 152–163.

27. Zhang SC, Wernig M, Duncan ID, Brustle O, Thomson JA (2001) In vitro differentiation of transplantable neural precursors from human embryonic stem cells. Nat Biotechnol 19: 1129–1133.

28. Ushio Y, Posner R, Posner JB, Shapiro WR (1977) Experimental spinal cord compression by epidural neoplasm. Neurology 27: 422–429.

29. Delattre JY, Rosenblum MK, Thaler HT, Mandell L, Shapiro WR, et al. (1988) A model of radiation myelopathy in the rat. Pathology, regional capillary permeability changes and treatment with dexamethasone. Brain 111 (Pt 6): 1319–1336.

30. Talbott JF, Cao Q, Enzmann GU, Benton RL, Achim V, et al. (2006) Schwann cell-like differentiation by adult oligodendrocyte precursor cells following engraftment into the demyelinated spinal cord is BMP-dependent. Glia 54: 147–159.

31. Cao Q, He Q, Wang Y, Cheng X, Howard RM, et al. Transplantation of ciliary neurotrophic factor-expressing adult oligodendrocyte precursor cells promotes remyelination and functional recovery after spinal cord injury. J Neurosci 30: 2989–3001.

32. Hofstetter CP, Holmstrom NA, Lilja JA, Schweinhardt P, Hao J, et al. (2005) Allodynia limits the usefulness of intraspinal neural stem cell grafts; directed differentiation improves outcome. Nat Neurosci 8: 346–353.

33. Iwashita Y, Fawcett JW, Crang AJ, Franklin RJ, Blakemore WF (2000) Schwann cells transplanted into normal and X-irradiated adult white matter do not migrate extensively and show poor long-term survival. Exp Neurol 164: 292–302.

34. Keirstead HS, Nistor G, Bernal G, Totoiu M, Cloutier F, et al. (2005) Human embryonic stem cell-derived oligodendrocyte progenitor cell transplants remyelinate and restore locomotion after spinal cord injury. J Neurosci 25: 4694–4705.

35. Cao Q, He Q, Wang Y, Cheng X, Howard RM, et al. (2010) Transplantation of ciliary neurotrophic factor-expressing adult oligodendrocyte precursor cells promotes remyelination and functional recovery after spinal cord injury. J Neurosci 30: 2989–3001.

36. Billon N, Jolicoeur C, Ying QL, Smith A, Raff M (2002) Normal timing of oligodendrocyte development from genetically engineered, lineage-selectable mouse ES cells. J Cell Sci 115: 3657–3665.

37. Franklin RJ, Bayley SA, Blakemore WF (1996) Transplanted CG4 cells (an oligodendrocyte progenitor cell line) survive, migrate, and contribute to repair of areas of demyelination in X-irradiated and damaged spinal cord but not in normal spinal cord. Exp Neurol 137: 263–276.

38. Jeffery ND, Crang AJ, O'Leary M T, Hodge SJ, Blakemore WF (1999) Behavioural consequences of oligodendrocyte progenitor cell transplantation into experimental demyelinating lesions in the rat spinal cord. Eur J Neurosci 11: 1508–1514.

39. Schultheiss TE, Stephens LC (1992) Invited review: permanent radiation myelopathy. Br J Radiol 65: 737–753.

40. Nave KA, Trapp BD (2008) Axon-glial signaling and the glial support of axon function. Annu Rev Neurosci 31: 535–561.

41. Trapp BD, Nave KA (2008) Multiple sclerosis: an immune or neurodegenerative disorder? Annu Rev Neurosci 31: 247–269.

42. Cummings BJ, Uchida N, Tamaki SJ, Salazar DL, Hooshmand M, et al. (2005) Human neural stem cells differentiate and promote locomotor recovery in spinal cord-injured mice. Proc Natl Acad Sci U S A 102: 14069–14074.

43. Karimi-Abdolrezaee S, Eftekharpour E, Fehlings MG (2004) Temporal and spatial patterns of Kv1.1 and Kv1.2 protein and gene expression in spinal cord white matter after acute and chronic spinal cord injury in rats: implications for axonal pathophysiology after neurotrauma. Eur J Neurosci 19: 577–589.

44. Mitsui T, Shumsky JS, Lepore AC, Murray M, Fischer I (2005) Transplantation of neuronal and glial restricted precursors into contused spinal cord improves bladder and motor functions, decreases thermal hypersensitivity, and modifies intraspinal circuitry. J Neurosci 25: 9624–9636.

45. Cao Q, Zhang YP, Iannotti C, DeVries WH, Xu XM, et al. (2005) Functional and electrophysiological changes after graded traumatic spinal cord injury in adult rat. Exp Neurol 191 Suppl 1: S3–S16.

46. Bruce CC, Zhao C, Franklin RJ (2010) Remyelination - An effective means of neuroprotection. Horm Behav 57: 56–62.

47. Jadasz JJ, Aigner L, Rivera FJ, Kury P (2012) The remyelination Philosopher's Stone: stem and progenitor cell therapies for multiple sclerosis. Cell Tissue Res.

48. Goldberg JL, Barres BA (2000) The relationship between neuronal survival and regeneration. Annu Rev Neurosci 23: 579–612.

49. Wilkins A, Majed H, Layfield R, Compston A, Chandran S (2003) Oligodendrocytes promote neuronal survival and axonal length by distinct intracellular mechanisms: a novel role for oligodendrocyte-derived glial cell line-derived neurotrophic factor. J Neurosci 23: 4967–4974.

50. Du Y, Dreyfus CF (2002) Oligodendrocytes as providers of growth factors. Journal of Neuroscience Research 68: 647–654.

51. Dai X, Lercher LD, Clinton PM, Du Y, Livingston DL, et al. (2003) The trophic role of oligodendrocytes in the basal forebrain. J Neurosci 23: 5846–5853.

52. Maier IC, Schwab ME (2006) Sprouting, regeneration and circuit formation in the injured spinal cord: factors and activity. Philos Trans R Soc Lond B Biol Sci 361: 1611–1634.

13

The Prevalence of Immunologic Injury in Renal Allograft Recipients with *De Novo* Proteinuria

Qiquan Sun*, Song Jiang, Xue Li, Xianghua Huang, Kenan Xie, Dongrui Cheng, Jinsong Chen, Shuming Ji, Jiqiu Wen, Mingchao Zhang, Caihong Zeng, Zhihong Liu

Research Institute of Nephrology, Jinling Hospital, Nanjing University School of Medicine, Nanjing, China

Abstract

Post-transplant proteinuria is a common complication after renal transplantation; it is associated with reduced graft and recipient survival. However, the prevalence of histological causes has been reported with considerable variation. A clinico-pathological re-evaluation of post-transplant proteinuria is necessary, especially after dismissal of the term "chronic allograft nephropathy," which had been considered to be an important cause of proteinuria. Moreover, urinary protein can promote interstitial inflammation in native kidney, whether this occurs in renal allograft remains unknown. Factors that affect the graft outcome in patients with proteinuria also remain unclear. Here we collected 98 cases of renal allograft recipients who developed proteinuria after transplant, histological features were characterized using Banff scoring system. Cox proportional hazard regression models were used for graft survival predictors. We found that transplant glomerulopathy was the leading (40.8%) cause of post-transplant proteinuria. Immunological causes, including transplant glomerulopathy, acute rejection, and chronic rejection accounted for the majority of all pathological causes of proteinuria. Nevertheless, almost all patients that developed proteinuria had immunological lesions in the graft, especially for interstitial inflammation. Intraglomerular C3 deposition was unexpectedly correlated with the severity of proteinuria. Moreover, the severity of interstitial inflammation was an independent risk factor for graft loss, while high level of hemoglobin was a protective factor for graft survival. This study revealed a predominance of immunological parameters in renal allografts with post-transplant proteinuria. These parameters not only correlate with the severity of proteinuria, but also with the outcome of the graft.

Editor: Michael Zimmerman, University of Colorado School of Medicine, United States of America

Funding: This study was supported by a grant from the General Program of National Natural Science Foundation of China (No. 81070593, No. 30600572), and a grant from 333 Talent Training Program of Jiangsu Province, China. The funders had no role in study design, data collection and analysis, decision to publish, or preparation of the manuscript.

Competing Interests: The authors have declared that no competing interests exist.

* E-mail: sunqiquan@hotmail.com

Introduction

Post-transplant proteinuria is a common complication after renal transplantation. It is found in 25% of renal allograft recipients at 6 months [1], and nearly 50% at 1 year after transplantation [2]. The development of proteinuria is associated with reduced graft survival, independent of other risk factors, including glomerular pathology, graft function, and acute rejection [2,3]. If urine protein is at the level of nephrotic syndrome, half of the patients will lose their graft within 2 years [4]. Even low-grade proteinuria is correlated with decreased graft survival [5,6]. Nevertheless, proteinuria is also an independent risk factor for both cardiovascular and non-cardiovascular death [7,8]. As a result, post-transplant proteinuria is becoming a significant barrier to both renal allograft and recipient survival.

The pathogenesis of proteinuria is complex. It can originate from both the native kidney and the allograft [9,10], and may be caused by both glomerular damage and interstitial/tubular injury. Although this has been known for some time [11,12], the overall clinico-histological features of patients with post-transplant proteinuria are far from clarified. The prevalence of histological causes reported by different centers has been quite different [1,2,4,8,12]. "Chronic allograft nephropathy," which has been defunct as a term since 2005 [13] had also been counted as an important cause of proteinuria [2,4,9]. Urine protein can promote interstitial inflammation [14] in patients with kidney diseases, however, whether post-transplant proteinuria shares the same mechanism in inducing allograft injury need to be clarified. Moreover, factors that affect the graft outcome in patients with proteinuria also remain unclear. Thus, a clinico-pathological reevaluation of post-transplant proteinuria under the current Banff classification is necessary.

This study was performed to evaluate the overall clinical features and histological spectrum of post-transplant proteinuria. We unexpectedly revealed a high prevalence of immunological parameters in these patients, and moreover, these factors were correlated with the severity and outcome of the grafts. These findings question current strategies of managing post-transplant proteinuria.

Materials and Methods

Patients

Patients were selected from renal transplant recipients developing proteinuria from Jan. 2005 to Dec. 2008 at the Research Institute of Nephrology, Jinling Hospital, Nanjing University School of Medicine. Proteinuria is defined as urine protein over 0.4 g/d measured in 24-h collections by colorimetric methods.

Inclusion criteria were as follows: (1) renal transplant recipients, (2) *de novo* proteinuria >0.4 g/d, (3) aged 18–60 years old, (4) having received baseline renal biopsies and index renal biopsy when proteinuria emerged, and (5) under follow-up for no less than 1 year. Patients who received sirolimus treatment were excluded because the incidence of proteinuria depends on the proportion of patients receiving this medicine. Patients in whom proteinuria emerged immediately after transplantation and declined over time were also excluded as this may have been related to the native kidney and have less influence on long-term graft survival.

Patients were followed at our institution, and all patients had a thorough evaluation once per week during the first 3 months, then once every 2 weeks until 6 months, monthly till the end of the first year, and bi-monthly thereafter. Data were recorded using a web-based recording system. Proteinuria was screened by urine test strips cassette with the URISYS 2400 urinalysis analyzer (Roche Diagnostics GmbH, Mannheim, Germany) at each visit, and by 24-h collection at every 6 months, or whenever the screening test was positive. The urine protein level was measured in 24-h collections by colorimetric methods. Urine n-acetyl-β-glucosaminidase (β-NAG) [15] and retinol binding protein (RBP) [16,17] were used to evaluate the tubular injury. Graft function was evaluated with estimated glomerular filtration rate (eGFR).

HLA-I, II antibody detection and lymphocytotoxic crossmatch

IgG anti-HLA class I and class II antibodies in serum samples were detected by flow cytometric analysis using the methods described by Pei et al [18]. Sera with >10% reactivity for HLA class I and/or II were considered positive for the presence of anti-HLA antibodies. HLA-I, II antibodies were monitored pre- and post-transplant, and whenever a renal biopsy was performed. Pre-transplant screening for donor-specific alloantibodies was also performed through complement-dependent lymphocytotoxicity methods using the National Institutes of Health technique with undiluted complement (without wash).

Renal allograft pathology

Baseline biopsies were performed in all allografts to exclude any ongoing disease in the transplanted kidney. Diagnostic biopsies were performed whenever proteinuria emerged. Two needle biopsy cores were obtained from each renal allograft for morphological study, which were then divided into two parts: one for formalin fixation and one for quick-freezing. Hematoxylin and eosin, periodic acid Schiff, methenamine-silver, and Masson staining were routinely used on the formalin-fixed tissue. Fresh frozen tissue was analyzed by immunofluorescence microscopy using a conventional panel of antibodies against IgG, IgM, IgA, C3, C4, C1q, and C4d. Ultrastructural study were routinely studied using electron microscopy (EM) for all the samples. Since 2007, polyomavirus-associated nephropathy was routinely screened using the anti-SV-40 large T antigen antibody on all the biopsies. Histological features were scored using the latest Banff scoring criteria [13,19,20,21] and CADI scoring [22]. All biopsies contained at least ten glomerular and two arterial sections. The pathology lesions are sorted into acute rejection, chronic rejection, TG, IF/TA, and de novo or recurrent glomerular diseases, such as IgA nephropathy, membranous nephropathy (MN), and focal segmental glomerulosclerosis (FSGS). The definition of the diagnosis terms were listed in table 1. Twenty protocol biopsy samples taken over one year post transplantation were randomized selected as controls.

Initial immunosuppression

Two primary immunosuppressive protocols were used in the course of this study: cyclosporine A (CsA), mycophenolate mofetil (MMF) and steroids or tacrolimus, MMF, and steroids. The main immunosuppressive protocols were CsA+MMF+steroid during June 2004 to June 2006, and tacrolimus+MMF+steroid since July 2006. AZA instead of MMF was also used before 2000. Induction therapy with daclizumab or basiliximab could also be used. The maintenance doses of tacrolimus and CsA were adjusted to target specific trough levels: 6–12 ng/mL during the first 6 months, 4–8 ng/mL thereafter for tacrolimus, and 150–250 ng/mL during the first 6 months and 100–200 ng/mL thereafter for CsA.

Management of Proteinuria

Patients were given angiotensin-converting enzyme inhibitors and/or angiotensin receptor blockers when proteinuria occurred. For patients developing TG, the dose of MMF was increased to 1.5 g/d if the current dose was lower than 1.5 g/d. Additional immunoadsorption was used too if there were high levels of HLA class-I or II antibodies.

Statistics

Descriptive statistical values are expressed as means±SD. Analyses were performed using the SPSS software (ver. 15.0; SPSS, Chicago, IL, USA). A t-test was used for comparing means and a chi-squared test was used for testing the significance of categorical variables. Survival curves were estimated using the Kaplan-Meier method, and differences were evaluated by the log-rank test. Cox proportional hazard regression models were used to adjust for the potential confounding effects of variables with statistical differences between the groups to evaluate the association between predictor variables and graft survival. A p value of <0.05 was considered to indicate statistical significance.

Results

Baseline Characteristics

Ninety-eight renal transplant recipients who developed proteinuria were included; there were 77 males and 21 females, all were negative for HLA-I and II antibodies before transplantation. The emerging time of proteinuria was 4.19±2.96 years (ranged from 1months to 10 years) post transplant, and the biopsies were performed immediately after protein emerging. As to the primary diseases that caused renal failure, 3 were diabetic nephropathy, 3 were FSGS, 4 were IgAN, 2 were membranous nephropathy, 1 were HSPN and 1 were crescent nephritis. Two were polycystic kidney disease. As the surveillance of kidney disease was not performed in China, the majority of patients were found to be at end stage renal failure with not native renal biopsies available. Baseline characteristics are listed in Table 2. The mean level of proteinuria was 2.2±2.0 g/d. A total of 34.7% of patients also showed different degrees of hematuria.

When the biopsies were performed, 41 patients used tacrolimus+MMF+steroid as immunosuppressive protocols and 46 patients were on CsA+MMF+steroid. There were no differences between the two groups on baseline characteristics such as age, gender, emerging time of proteinuria, etc. The degree of proteinuria were similar (2.11±1.76 vs 2.28±1.06 g/d, p = 0.700). The other eleven patients received CsA+Aza+steroid as immunosuppressive protocols. In addition, those patients were randomized matched with 20 recipients who received protocol biopsies 6 months after the transplant surgery. There were no differences in recipients' age, gender, baseline immunosuppres-

Table 1. Definition of the diagnosis terms.

Term	Abbreviation	Definition
Transplant glomerulopathy	TG	Pathological featured duplication of the GBMs [21], and excluding other conditions that might result in similar histological changes, confirmed by EM.
Chronic rejection	CR	Including chronic active antibody-mediated rejection, chronic active T-cell mediated rejection [19], TG was excluded considering its high prevalence and unique histological feature.
Acute rejection	AR	Including acute antibody-mediated rejection, acute T-cell mediated rejection [19]
IgA nephropathy	IgAN	Dominant or codominant staining with IgA in glomeruli by immunofluorescence or immunoperoxidase [38], excluding TG.
Tubular atrophy and interstitial fibrosis	TA/IF	Interstitial fibrosis and tubular atrophy, with no evidence of any above specific etiology [19]

sant, and post-transplant complications between the control group and patients with proteinuria.

Characteristics of patients with different degrees of proteinuria

Compared with control group, post-transplant proteinuria was correlated with higher level of serum creatinine (2.86 ± 2.36 vs 1.06 ± 0.32 mg/dL, $p < 0.05$), cholesterol (5.48 ± 2.01 vs 3.72 ± 0.72 mmol/L, $p < 0.05$), triglyceride (1.56 ± 0.68 vs 1.10 ± 0.36, $p < 0.05$), and lower level of serum albumin (34.6 ± 5.4 vs 41.8 ± 4.6, $p < 0.05$).

In native kidney diseases, >3.5 g/d usually is defined as nephritic range proteinuria, while <1 g/d usually is tubulointerstitial non-neprotic proteinuria. We divide the patients into 3 groups based on the level of urine protein: urine protein >3.5 g/d, 1–3.5 g/d, and <1 g/d. There was no difference between groups in patient age or gender. The onset time was significantly later in patients with high levels (>3.5 g/d) of proteinuria compared with patients with low levels (<1.0 g/d) of proteinuria (3.45 ± 2.85 vs 5.80 ± 3.01 years, $p < 0.05$). Higher levels of proteinuria were correlated with lower serum albumin, higher levels of blood lipid, and urinary NAG (u/g.cr; Figure 1).

TG was the leading cause of overall post-transplant proteinuria; it accounted for 41% of proteinuria in all ranges, followed by

IgAN for 16%, chronic rejection (TG excluded) for 12%, and acute rejection for 11% (Figure 2A).

For proteinuria below 1.0 g/d, TG was still the leading cause. While acute rejection was the second most important cause of proteinuria, it accounted for 25% of this subgroup, followed by chronic rejection (14%). Only one (3%) patient in this group was diagnosed as having IgAN (Figure 2B). For proteinuria between 1–3.5 g/d, TG was also the most important lesion in histology; however, the incidence of acute rejection decreased to 4.9%, while the incidence of IgAN increased to 24.4% (Figure 2C). In the group of proteinuria over 3.5 g/d, TG accounted for 47.6% of all causes, and IgAN accounted for 19%, while no patient was diagnosed as having acute rejection (Figure 2D).

Characteristics of patients with different pathologies

We compared the clinical characteristics of six major causes of proteinuria (Table 3). TG was the latest lesion that could cause proteinuria, with a diagnosis time of 5.21 ± 2.71 years post-transplant, followed by IgAN and chronic rejection. Acute rejection was the earliest lesion, occurring at 1.20 ± 1.31 years post-transplant, which was significantly earlier than TG ($p < 0.05$).

Patients in the TG group had a higher level of de novo HLA class I and class II antibodies, especially for class II antibodies. More than 40% patients with TG were positive for HLA class II antibodies (over 10% in PRA). The acute rejection group had a higher level of HLA class I antibodies, but the difference was not statistically significant. Hematuria could be found in TG, IgAN, and acute rejection, but seldom in chronic rejection, TA/IF, or FSGS groups.

TG could cause different ranges of proteinuria, whereas in IgAN group, most patients (93.4%) had proteinuria over 1 g/d, compared with 18.2% ($p < 0.05$) in the acute rejection group. Half of the patients in the FSGS group had proteinuria over 3.5 g/d.

With respect to graft function, all patients in the acute rejection and chronic rejection groups, and 92.5% in the TG group had impaired graft function, while nearly half of the patients in the IgAN group had normal graft function. Post-transplant proteinuria in different groups correlated with different incidences of hypoproteinemia and hyperlipidemia. Compared with the acute rejection group, the TG and IgAN groups had significantly higher incidences of hypoproteinemia ($p < 0.05$). The acute rejection group had the lowest serum lipid levels among the six groups.

Prevalence of immunological parameters in histology

Regardless of histological diagnosis, we found that almost all patients (95.9%) with proteinuria suffered from one or more kinds

Table 2. Baseline characteristics of patients that developed post-transplant proteinuria.

Parameter	Value
N	98
Gender (male/female)	77 (78.6%)/21 (21.4%)
Age (years)	$40.6 \pm 11.8/47.5 \pm 10.0$
Onset of proteinuria (years post transplantation)	4.19 ± 2.96
Peritoneal/hemodialysis before transplantation	3/95 (3.1%/96.9%)
Post-transplant complications	
Diabetes	10(10.2%)
Hepatitis	15(15.3%)
Pneumonia infection	14(14.3%)
Acute rejection	20(20.4%)

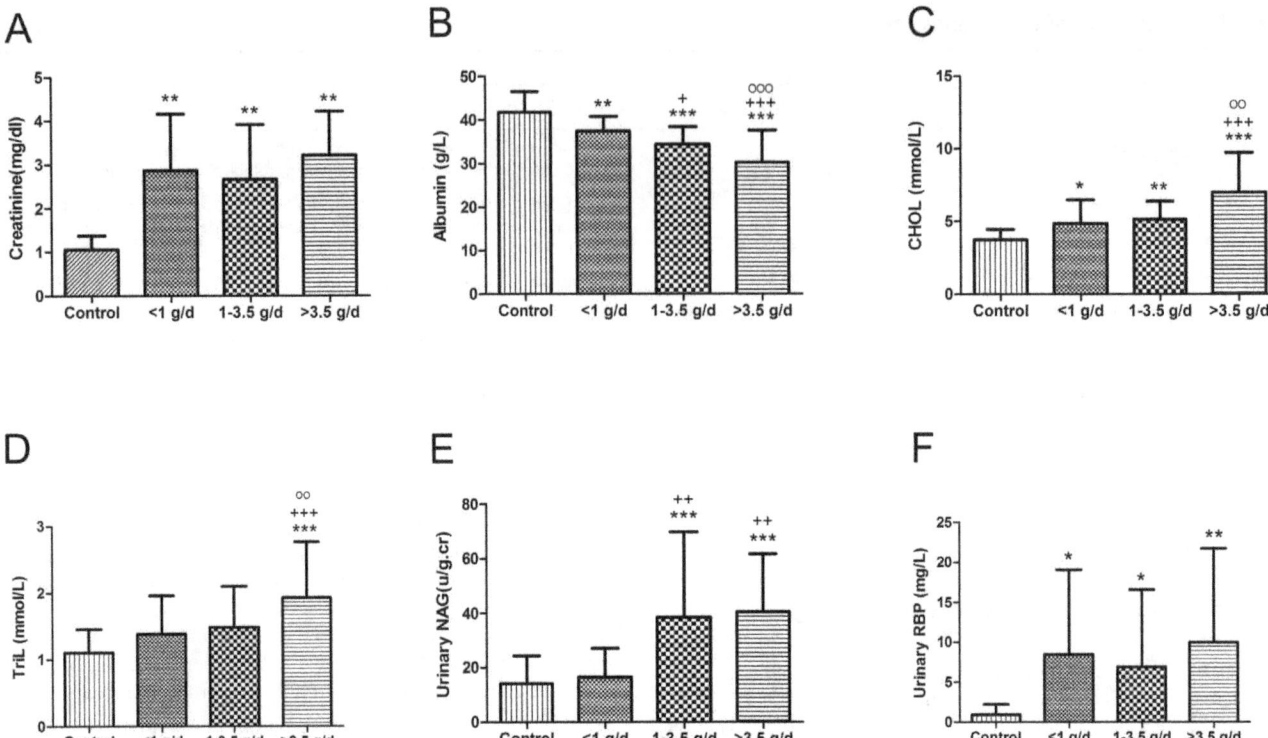

Figure 1. Characteristics of patients with different ranges of proteinuria. *, P<0.05 compared with control group; **, P<0.01 compared with control group; ***, P<0.001 compared with control group. +, P<0.05 compared with urinary protein<1 g/d group; ++, P<0.01 compared with urinary protein<1 g/d group; +++, P<0.001 compared with urinary protein<1 g/d group. O, P<0.05 compared with urinary protein 1–3.5 g/d group; OO, P<0.01 compared with urinary protein 1–3.5 g/d group; OOO, P<0.001 compared with urinary protein 1–3.5 g/d group.

of immunological lesions, as detected by histology. Among those lesions, interstitial inflammation was the most common and could be found in 95.9% patients with proteinuria, followed by glomerulitis in 70.4%, C4d deposition in peritubular capillaries in 53.1%, tubulitis in 46.9%, and intimal arteritis in 14.3%. As a typical lesion of TG, glomerular double contours could be detected in 43.9% patients. Only four patients (4.1%) were negative for all immunological lesions. The incidences of above lesions were significantly higher than the matched group of graft receiving protocol biopsies (Figure 3). Looking into the causes of proteinuria, there was high prevalence of interstitial inflammation in each group. TG group has a higher incidence of tubular atrophy than acute rejection group and a higher incidence of C4d deposition comparing with IgAN (table 4).

Factors correlated with the grade of urine protein

We also attempted to study the grade of urine protein using clinical and histological features. We found that the quantity of urine protein was strongly correlated with the incidence of intraglomerular C3 deposition (r = 0.293, p = 0.007), degree of tubular atrophy (Ct, r = 0.289, p = 0.008), glomerular sclerosis (Cg, r = 0.238, p = 0.009), and interstitial fibrosis (Ci, r = 0.227, p = 0.038). In contrast, it did not correlate with patient age, gender, degree of interstitial inflammation, C4d deposition, or graft function at diagnosis.

Prognostic factors for graft survival

TG had a poor graft survival at 5-years post-diagnosis with 32.6%, similar to the outcome of IF/TA and non-TG chronic rejection. The 5-year graft survival in the acute rejection group was 46.8%. IgAN had the best 5-year graft survival of 71.1% in this cohort (Figure 4).

We performed a Cox regression analysis, which included clinical factors such as age, gender, onset time of proteinuria, hematuria, NAG, serum creatinine, albumin, as well the diagnosis. Univariable analyses revealed that eGFR, range of proteinuria, degree of interstitial inflammation, score of vascular lesions, and degree of tubular atrophy were all risk factors for early graft loss. In contrast, level of serum hemoglobin and albumin, the diagnosis of IgAN were associated with graft survival. However, multivariate analyses revealed that only the degrees of interstitial inflammation (Figure 5A) and tubular atrophy (Figure 5B) were independent risk factors of graft loss, while levels of serum hemoglobin (Figure 5C) were independent protection factors for graft survival (Table 5).

Although C4d deposition could be detected in 52 (53.1%) patients (39 diffuse, 13 focal), we did not find correlation between C4d deposition and graft outcome. Although TG group seemed to be correlated with a poor graft survival, univariate analyses didn't show TG is independent risk factor for graft loss.

Discussion

This study outlined clinicopathological features of *de novo* post-transplant proteinuria under modern immunosuppressive protocols and the current Banff classification system. We revealed a predominance of immunological parameters in patients developing *de novo* proteinuria after transplantation. Immunological causes, including TG, acute rejection, and chronic rejection, accounted for 64.3% of all causes; indeed, almost all patients who developed proteinuria had histological immunological lesions in the graft, especially interstitial inflammation. Moreover, intraglo-

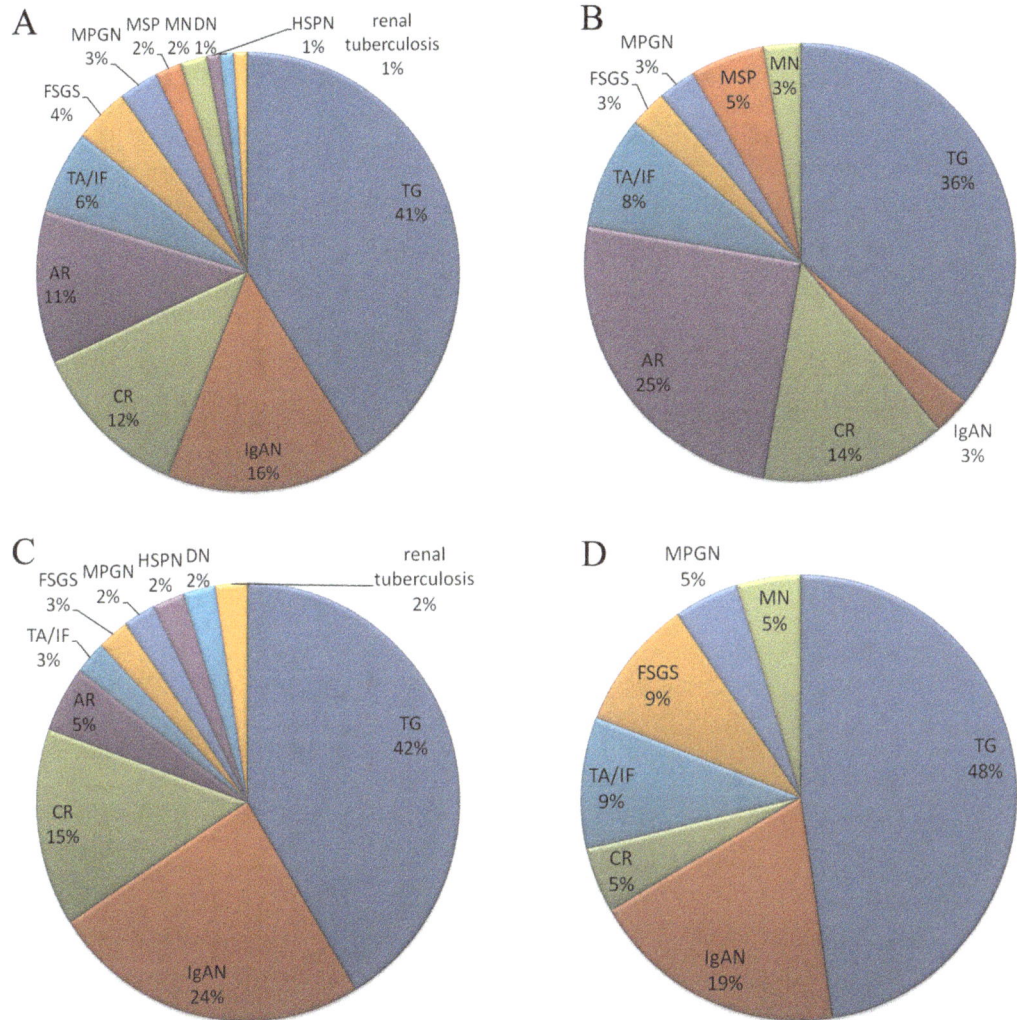

Figure 2. Histological causes of post-transplant proteinuria. Figures shows histological causes of proteinuria in all patients (1A), urine protein <1 g/d (1B), between 1–3.5 g/d (1C), and over 3.5 g/d (1D). TG was the leading cause of overall post-transplant proteinuria and each subgroup, followed by IgAN, chronic rejection (TG excluded), and acute rejection. For proteinuria below 1.0 g/d, acute rejection was the second most important cause of proteinuria, accounting for 25% in this subgroup; only one (3%) patient was diagnosed as having IgAN. For proteinuria between 1–3.5 g/d, the incidence of acute rejection decreased to 4.9%, while the incidence of IgAN increased to 24.4%. In proteinuria over 3.5 g/d, IgAN accounted for 19%, and no patient was diagnosed as having acute rejection. TG, transplant glomerulopathy; IgAN, IgA nephropathy; AR, acute rejection; CR, chronic rejection; TA/IF, tubular atrophy and interstitial fibrosis; FSGS, Focal segmental glomerulosclerosis; MPGN, Membranoproliferative glomerulonephritis; HSPN, Henoch-Schönlein purpura nephritis; DN, diabetic nephropathy; MSP, mesangial proliferative glomerulonephritis; MN, Membranous nephropathy.

merular C3 deposition correlated with the grade of proteinuria, and the severity of interstitial inflammation was an independent risk factor for graft loss. These data suggest the involvement of immunological factors in graft dysfunction.

Immunological causes, including TG, acute rejection, and chronic rejection, account for the majority of post-transplant proteinuria. Among them, TG was the leading cause, accounting for 41% of proteinuria, covering different ranges of urine protein, and 42.5% of them were accompanied by hematuria. TG is regarded as a form of late antibody-mediated rejection, however, as it has featured glomerular damage differing to chronic rejection, we list it separately in this study. As reported [23], the TG group had a higher level of HLA class I and class II antibodies, especially class II antibodies. Patients with proteinuria caused by TG had a poor outcome, with only 32.6% 5-year graft survival. The high incidence and poor outcome of TG might account for the poor

graft outcome of post-transplant proteinuria. It is noteworthy that the onset of proteinuria was at 5 years after transplantation in this group. This may explain why a recent study based on biopsies performed at 1-year post transplantation showed only a low incidence of TG [2]. However, TG was also the leading cause of graft loss in that group.

Another immunological entity, acute rejection, is an important cause of early post-transplant proteinuria and is related to poor graft survival. Proteinuria caused by acute rejection is characterized by early (within 1 year) occurrence and low levels (<1 g/d). It was rarely accompanied by hypoalbuminemia and lower levels of serum CHOL. This is likely due to the acute tubular damage caused by rejection, because a raised NAG level had been observed in this group. Although proteinuria caused by acute rejection is not as heavy as IgAN, the outcome is much worse. Our study was consistent with data reported by Halimi *et al.* [24], in

Table 3. Characteristics of patients with different histologies.

	TG	IgAN	CR	AR	TA/IF	FSGS
	(n=40)	(n=15)	(n=12)	(n=11)	(n=6)	(n=4)
Basic Characteristics						
Age (years)	44.7±12.3	40.9±8.1	37.8±1.8	36.4±11.6	44.3±12.6	36.8±7.9
Gender (male%)	31 (77.5%)	13 (86.7%)	8 (66.7%)	8 (72.7%)	5 (83.3%)	3 (75.0%)
Diagnosis time (years post Tx)	5.21±2.71	4.61±2.82	4.56±3.30	1.20±1.31[a]	3.99±3.66	2.58±2.10
Urine examination						
Upro (g/24 h)	2.30±1.94	2.42±1.27	1.73±2.09	1.06±0.91[b]	2.98±3.52	3.25±2.34
<1 g/24 h	13 (32.5%)	1 (6.7%)[c]	5 (41.7%)	9 (81.8%)[d]	3 (50.0%)	1 (25.0%)
1–3.5 g/24 h	17 (42.5%)	10 (66.7%)	6 (50.0%)	2 (18.2%)[b]	2 (33.3%)	1 (25.0%)
>3.5 g/24 h	10 (25%)	4 (26.7%)	1 (8.3%)	0 (0)[e]	1 (16.7%)	2 (50.0%)
Hematuria	17 (42.5%)	8 (53.3%)	1 (8.3%)	3 (27.3%)	0 (0)[f]	0 (0)
NAG (u/g.cr)	29.5±20.7	24.8±11.2	25.9±7.0	35.5±36.9	22.0±18.3	33.5±25.3
RBP (mg/L)	6.03±8.28	1.6±2.2	18.2±13.1[g]	7.4±9.4	13.0±16.0	6.9±8.9
Blood examination						
Albumin (g/L)	33.4±5.6	35.0±4.9[#]	36.3±4.8	38.0±2.5[#]	34.8±5.4	37.0±4.1
≥35 g/L	18 (45%)	8 (53.3%)	8 (66.7%)	10 (90.9%)[h]	2 (33.3%)	3 (75.0%)
<35 g/L	22 (55%)	7 (46.7%)	4 (33.3%)	1 (9.1%)[h]	4 (66.7%)	1 (25.0%)
Scr (mg/dL)	2.69±1.67	2.14±2.82[b]	2.44±1.16	4.21±2.59	4.29±5.10	4.50±3.29
<1.24 mg/dL	3 (7.5%)	7 (46.7%)[i]	0 (0)	0 (0)	1 (12.7%)	0 (0)
≥1.24 mg/dL	37 (92.5%)	8 (53.3%)	12 (100%)	11 (100%)	5 (83.3%)	4 (100%)
CHOL (mmol/L)	5.37±1.66	5.40±1.40	5.39±1.38	4.88±2.50	5.94±2.27	5.96±1.10
TriG (mmol/L)	1.58±0.72	1.40±0.45	1.50±0.75	1.35±0.46	1.48±0.28	2.20±0.95[j]
HLA-I antibodies	12.6±17.6	3.93±1.83	2.49±2.08	18.2±26.5	0.7	1.2
HLA II antibodies	23.62±27.91	4.29±3.47	2.44±1.21	7.76±9.64	1.3	0.3
Hemoglobin	9.67±2.44	11.67±2.31[k]	10.19±2.22	9.48±2.55	10.33±3.31	11.0±4.06
>12 g/L	6 (15.0%)	8 (53.3%)	3 (25.0%)	1 (9.1%)	1 (16.7%)	1 (25.0%)
9–12 g/L	16 (40.0%)	5 (33.3%)	7 (58.3%)	5 (45.5%)	2 (33.3%)	2 (50.0%)
6–9 g/L	15 (37.5%)	2 (13.3%)	2 (16.7%)	4 (36.4%)	3 (50%)	1 (25.0%)
<6 g/L	3 (8.1%)	0 (0)	0 (0)	1 (9.1%)	0 (0)	0 (0)

TG: transplant glomerulopathy; IgAN: IgA nephropathy; CR, chronic rejection; AR, acute rejection; TA/IF: tubular atrophy and interstitial fibrosis; Tx, transplantation; Upro, urine protein; NAG, n-Acetyl-β-glucosaminidase; RBP, retinol binding protein; SCr, serum creatinine; CHOL, cholesterol; TriL, Triglyceride.
[a], $P<0.01$, AR vs. TG, IgAN, CR;
[b], $P<0.05$, IgAN vs. AR group;
[c], $p<0.05$, IgAN vs. AR, CR, and TA/IF;
[d], $P<0.05$, AR vs. IgAN, FSGS and TG;
[e], $p<0.05$, AR vs. FSGS;
[f], $P<0.05$, TA/IF vs. TG and IgAN;
[g], $P<0.05$, CR vs. TG, IgAN;
[h], $P<0.05$, AR vs. TG, IgAN, TA/IF;
[i], $P<0.05$, IgAN vs. TG, CR, AR;
[j], $P<0.05$, IgAN vs. FSGS, AR;
[k], $P<0.05$, IgAN vs. TG, AR.

which the incidence of early (within 3 months after transplantation) lower grade proteinuria and graft outcomes correlated with episodes of acute rejection. Unfortunately, they did not perform surveillance biopsies in their study, so it is unclear whether there were other coexisting lesions in those grafts.

Our data reveal a high prevalence of immunological lesions in the histology of renal allografts with *de novo* proteinuria. Regardless of histological cause, almost all patients who developed proteinuria had interstitial inflammation in the graft, which is much higher than in the grafts without urine protein. Although it is difficult to clarify the cause and consequence of inflammation, it is possible

that urinary protein itself could stimulate interstitial inflammation. In native kidney, it is well known that protein overload can stimulate proximal tubular cells to synthesize chemokines, which may contribute to the chronic tubulointerstitial inflammation [14]. Our data suggest that this pathway maybe also exist in renal allograft recipients, even in the era of modern immunosuppressants. Anyway, this hypothesis needs to be further proved.

Never the less, interstitial inflammation was strongly correlated with graft outcome. Our data reveal that many factors correlated with graft outcome, including graft function (measured with eGFR), grade of proteinuria, scores of interstitial inflammation,

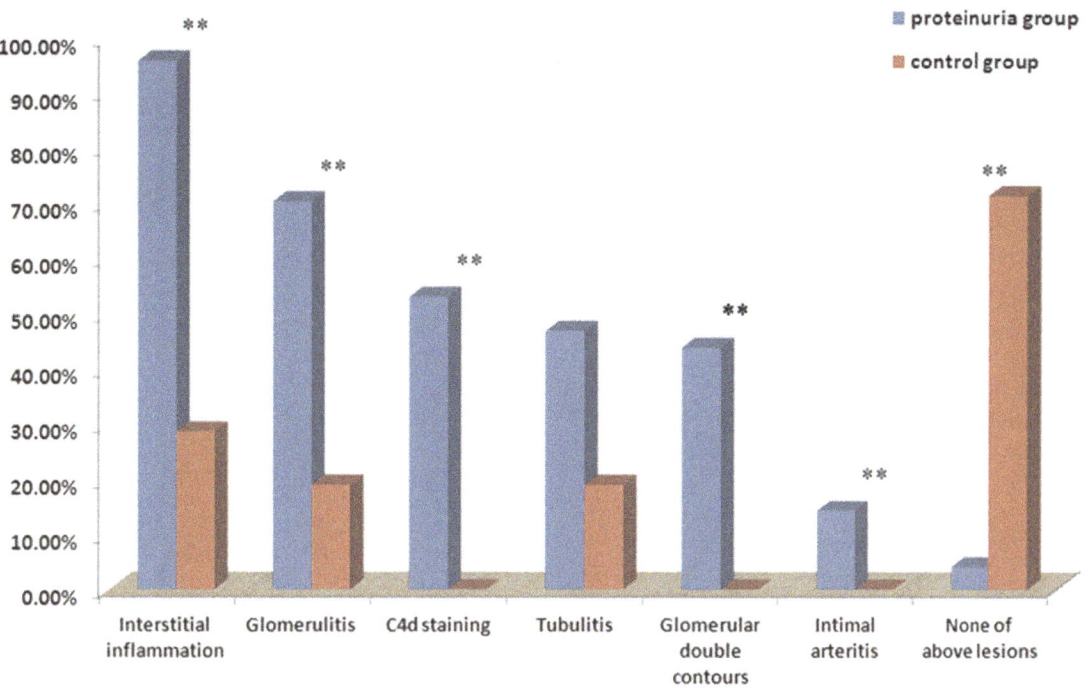

Figure 3. Prevalence of histological lesions related to immune activity. Most (95.9%) of the patients with proteinuria had at least one kind of immunological lesion, based on histology. Interstitial inflammation was the most common lesion, which could be detected in 95.9% patients with proteinuria, followed by glomerulitis in 70.4%, C4d deposition in peritubular capillaries in 53.1%, tubulitis in 46.9%, and intimal arteritis in 14.3%. While in the control group, only few recipients have immunological lesion. *, p<0.05 comparing with control group; **, p<0.001 comparing with control group.

Table 4. Histologic findings of patients with different histologies.

	TG	IgAN	CR	AR	TA/IF	FSGS
	(*n*= 40)	(*n*= 15)	(*n*= 12)	(*n*= 11)	(*n*= 6)	(*n*= 4)
Interstitial inflammation, n (%)	37 (92.5%)	12 (80.0%)	11 (91.7%)	11 (100.0%)	5 (83.3%)	3 (75.0%)
Glomerulitis, n (%)	33 (82.5%)	11 (73.3%)	9 (75.0%)	9 (81.8%)	2 (33.3%)	3 (75.0%)
Tubulitis, n (%)	18 (45.0%)	6 (40.0%)	7 (58.3%)	10 (90.9%)	2 (33.3%)	2 (50.0%)
Tubular atrophy, n (%)	36 (90.0%)*	14 (93.3%)	10 (83.3%)	5 (45.5%)	5 (83.3%)	3 (75.0%)
Interstitial infiltrate, n (%)	37 (92.5%)	12 (80.0%)	11 (91.7%)	11 (100%)	5 (83.3%)	3 (75.0%)
Plasma cell infiltrate, n (%)	19 (47.5%)	4 (26.7%)	7 (58.3%)	5 (45.5%)	2 (33.3%)	0 (0)
Interstitial fibrosis, n (%)	33 (82.5%)	9 (60.0%)	12 (100.0%)	7 (63.6%)	4 (66.7%)	2 (50.0%)
C4d deposition	28 (70.0%)#	4 (26.7%)	8 (66.7%)	7(63.6%)	1 (16.7%)	1 (25.0%)
Diffuse	22 (55.0%)#	2 (13.3%)	5 (41.7%)	3 (27.3%)	0 (0)	0 (0)
Focal	6 (15.0%)	2 (13.3%)	3 (25.0%)	4(36.4%)	1 (16.7%)	1 (25.0%)
Negative	12 (30.0%)#	11 (73.3%)	4 (33.3%)	4 (36.4%)	5 (83.3%)	3 (75.0%)
Intraglomerular C3 deposition, n (%)	22 (55.0%)*	13 (86.7%)	5 (41.7%)	1 (9.1%)	3 (50.0%)	2 (50.0%)
Diffuse	7 (17.5%)#*	10 (66.7%)	1 (8.3%)	1 (9.1%)	2 (33.3%)	2 (50.0%)
Focal	15 (37.5%)*	3 (20.0%)	4 (33.3%)	0 (0)	1 (16.7%)	0 (0)
Negative	18 (45.0%)*	2 (13.3%)	7 (58.3%)	10 (90.9%)	3 (50.0%)	2 (50.0%)
Intimal arteritis, n (%)	3 (7.5%)	0 (0)	1 (8.3%)	2(18.2%)	0 (0)	1 (25.0%)
small vessel fibrinoid necrosis	3 (7.5%)	1 (6.7%)	1 (8.3%)	1 (9.1%)	0 (0)	0 (0)
Small vessel thrombi	3 (7.5%)	1 (6.7%)	0 (0)	1 (9.1%)	0 (0)	0 (0)

*, p<0.05 vs AR group;
#, p<0.05 vs IgAN group.

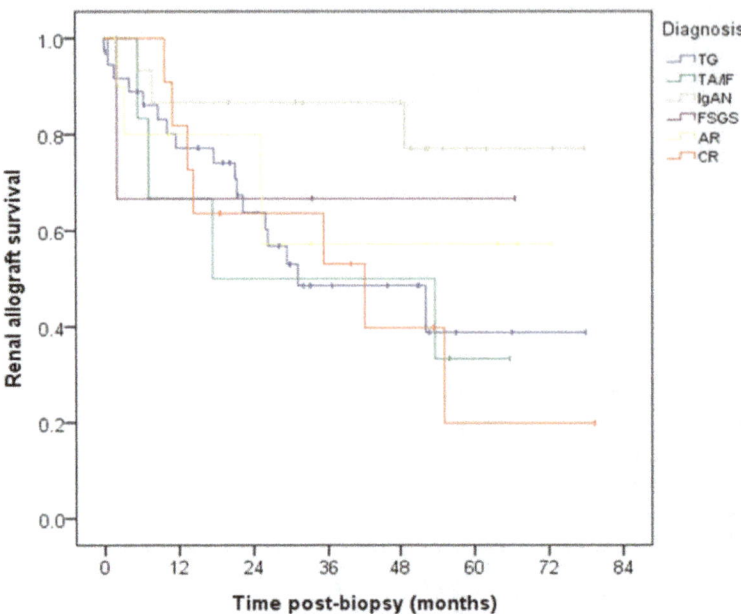

Diagnosis	One year survival rate	Three years survival rate	Five years survival rate
TG	70.4%	48.9%	32.6%
TA/IF	66.7%	50.0%	25.0%
IgAN	80%	71.1%	71.1%
FSGS	50%	50%	50%
AR	72.7%	46.8%	46.8%
No-TG-CR	63.6%	39.8%	26.5%

Figure 4. Graft survival for patients with different histological causes of proteinuria. IgAN has the best graft outcome, with a 5-year graft survival of 71.1%, while graft survival was very poor in patients with TG, TA/IF, and CR. TG, transplant glomerulopathy; IgAN, IgA nephropathy; AR, acute rejection; CR, chronic rejection; TA/IF, tubular atrophy and interstitial fibrosis; FSGS, Focal segmental glomerulosclerosis.

vascular lesions and tubular atrophy, level of serum hemoglobin, and albumin. However, only degrees of interstitial inflammation (Figure 5A) and tubular atrophy (Figure 5B) were independent risk factors of graft loss. In contrast, levels of serum hemoglobin (Figure 5C) were independent protective factors for graft survival. Among risk factors, interstitial inflammation had the highest hazard ratio. Although a high prevalence of C4d-deposition had been noticed in this cohort, we didn't find correlation between C4d deposition and graft outcome, which is consistent with data from Sis et al based on a population of TG [25].

For the first time, we report that hemoglobin is an independent protective factor for renal allograft survival in patients who develop *de novo* post-transplant proteinuria. Specifically, anemia is an independent risk factor for graft loss. The estimated graft survival was 44.5 months for patients without anemia, while it was only 22.1 months for patients with hemoglobin between 6–9 g/dL and 13.4 months for patients with hemoglobin levels below 6 g/dL (Figure 5C). This is another important finding that may impact clinical practice, because anemia is common in renal allograft recipients with proteinuria and usually is believed to be related with eGFR. This finding is consisted with data from a multicenter clinical trial that showed complete correction of anemia reduce the rate of progression of chronic allograft nephropathy. [26]

Evidence that the degree of interstitial inflammation and anemia correlates with graft survival brings into question the traditional management of proteinuria, which consists primarily of angiotensin-converting enzyme inhibitors and/or angiotensin receptor blockers as the first-line treatment. [27,28,29,30,31,32] Physicians may need to consider dealing with the underlying immunological activity and maintaining the hemoglobin at a higher level. A renal biopsy will still be necessary to assess the underlying histological causes to exclude non-immunological lesions, which may be more suitable for traditional management. Nevertheless, our data support the hypothesis that proteinuria-induced graft loss occurs via complex mechanisms other than the presence of glomerular disease [28].

Our study also revealed that another immunological lesion, intraglomerular C3 deposition, correlated with the grade of proteinuria. Cox regression analysis revealed that in addition to histological causes and onset time, proteinuria levels also correlated with intraglomerular C3 deposition, degree of allograft glomerulopathy, tubular atrophy, and interstitial fibrosis. However, it did not correlate with patient age, gender, degree of interstitial inflammation (i0–3), C4d deposition, or graft function at diagnosis. For the first time, we report that the degree of *de novo* post-transplant proteinuria correlated with the incidence of C3 deposition. C3 deposition in glomerulus is not rare in patients undergoing kidney diseases, and can even be detected in living donors during nephrectomy [33]. The significance of C3 deposition in the development of proteinuria remains to be clarified, although it has been reported that co-deposition of C3 with C4d is

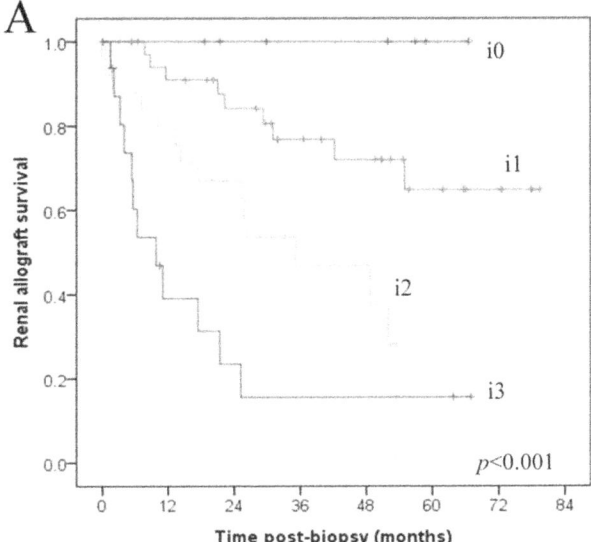

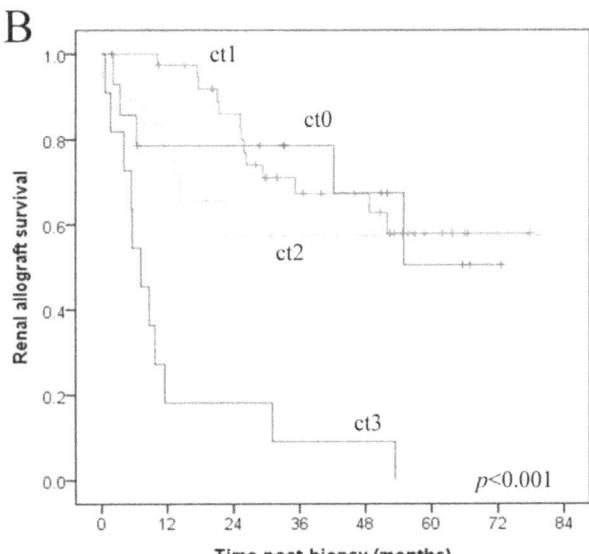

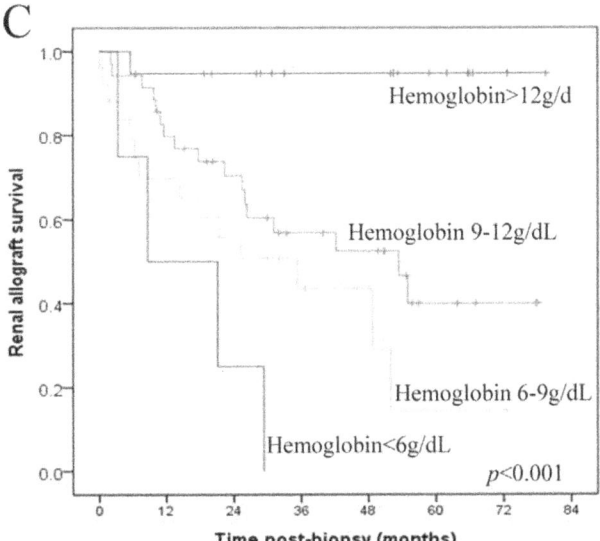

Figure 5. Risk factors correlated with the graft survival in patients with post-transplant proteinuria. Degrees of interstitial

inflammation (A) and renal tubular atrophy (B) and levels of hemoglobin (C) were strongly correlated with graft survival. i 0–3, mononuclear cell interstitial inflammation grade 0–3; ct 0–3, tubular atrophy grade 0–3. [21]

correlated with early graft loss [34]. We did not find a correlation between C3 deposition and graft survival in this cohort.

Because IgAN is the most common primary glomerulonephritis worldwide [35] and the recurrent rate is high after transplantation [36,37], it is not surprising that renal allograft IgAN was common in this cohort. Our data suggest that IgAN is one of the main causes of proteinuria over 1 g/d, and is a relatively benign lesion, which had the best 5-year graft survival in the current cohort. Univariation analysis also showed the diagnosis of IgAN is protecting factor for graft loss. IgAN in this group should be regarded as *de novo* or recurrent, because baseline biopsies had been performed to exclude disease derived from the donor. The high incidence of IgAN in this group might be partly due to its high prevalence in the general population [35]. Although the 5-year graft looks good in this group, additional attention should be paid to these recipients because longer term observation revealed decreased graft survival [36].

Moreover, our study revealed that different grades of proteinuria emerging at different times correlated with different histological findings, which could explain why a different prevalence of histological causes had been previously reported from different centers [1,2,4,8,12]. Low-grade (<1 g/d) proteinuria was mostly associated with interstitial and tubular damage, such as acute rejection, chronic rejection, and TA/IF. Glomerular damage is likely involved in the development of high-grade proteinuria. Our data support the hypothesis that early proteinuria is usually correlated with acute allograft damage, such as acute rejection. Based on these data, β-NAG and RBP are helpful factors in distinguishing acute and chronic lesions. Acute lesions typically manifest as higher levels of NAG and lower levels of RBP. In contrast, chronic lesions are correlated with lower NAG and higher RBP. Due to the exclusion of proteinuria emerging immediately after transplantation, no acute tubular necrosis cases were observed in this group. Overall, based on the above data, it is

Table 5. Independent risk factors and protective factors for transplantation kidney survival.

Variable	Univariate			Multivariate		
	HR	CI	P	HR	CI	P
Interstitial inflammation	2.772	1.859–4.134	<0.001	2.397	1.535–3.742	<0.001
Tubular atrophy	2.173	1.488–3.173	<0.001	2.270	1.546–3.334	<0.001
Serum hemoglobin	0.965	0.951–0.979	<0.001	0.971	0.953–0.990	0.003
Serum albumin	0.932	0.874–0.993	0.028			
eGFR	0.953	0.934–0.972	<0.001			
Urine protein	1.255	1.072–1.470	0.005			
Intimal arteritis	1.443	1.025–2.033	0.036			
IgA Nephropathy	0.294	0.090–0.961	0.043			

not surprising that studies focused on proteinuria occurring at different times and/or of different ranges would lead to different histological findings. This is why rare TG was reported in patients developing proteinuria 1-year after transplantation, [2] while rare acute rejection was reported in patients with post-transplant nephrotic syndrome. [4]

It is necessary to acknowledge the lack of native renal biopsies in most recipients prior to transplantation, which prevented us from making a diagnosis of recurrent or *de novo* renal disease. However, in this group, excluding IgAN, only 13.3% are likely to have *de novo* or recurrent glomerulonephritis. The conclusion we draw is not limited, because we did not focus on patients with *de novo* or recurrent renal disease.

Overall, our study revealed a predominance of immunological parameters in renal allografts with post-transplant proteinuria. These parameters not only correlate with the severity of proteinuria, but also with the outcome of the graft. These findings are important because they bring into question current strategies of managing post-transplant proteinuria. Specifically, patients might benefit from the introduction of anti-inflammatory treatments.

Acknowledgments

Part of this work was orally presented at the 2010 American Transplant Congress in San Diego, California, May 1–5, 2010.

Author Contributions

Conceived and designed the experiments: QS ZL. Performed the experiments: QS SJ XH DC JC SJ JW MZ. Analyzed the data: QS SJ KX XL. Contributed reagents/materials/analysis tools: MZ CZ. Wrote the paper: QS SJ.

References

1. Hohage H, Kleyer U, Bruckner D, August C, Zidek W, et al. (1997) Influence of proteinuria on long-term transplant survival in kidney transplant recipients. Nephron 75: 160–165.

2. Amer H, Fidler ME, Myslak M, Morales P, Kremers WK, et al. (2007) Proteinuria after kidney transplantation, relationship to allograft histology and survival. Am J Transplant 7: 2748–2756.

3. Einecke G, Reeve J, Sis B, Mengel M, Hidalgo L, et al. (2010) A molecular classifier for predicting future graft loss in late kidney transplant biopsies. J Clin Invest 120: 1862–1872.

4. Yakupoglu U, Baranowska-Daca E, Rosen D, Barrios R, Suki WN, et al. (2004) Post-transplant nephrotic syndrome: A comprehensive clinicopathologic study. Kidney Int 65: 2360–2370.

5. Halimi J-M, Laouad I, Buchler M, Al-Najjar A, Chatelet V, et al. (2005) Early Low-Grade Proteinuria: Causes, Short-Term Evolution and Long-Term Consequences in Renal Transplantation. American Journal of Transplantation 5: 2281–2288.

6. Cherukuri A, Welberry-Smith MP, Tattersall JE, Ahmad N, Newstead CG, et al. (2010) The clinical significance of early proteinuria after renal transplantation. Transplantation 89: 200–207.

7. Roodnat JI, Mulder PG, Rischen-Vos J, van Riemsdijk IC, van Gelder T, et al. (2001) Proteinuria after renal transplantation affects not only graft survival but also patient survival. Transplantation 72: 438–444.

8. Fernandez-Fresnedo G, Plaza JJ, Sanchez-Plumed J, Sanz-Guajardo A, Palomar-Fontanet R, et al. (2004) Proteinuria: a new marker of long-term graft and patient survival in kidney transplantation. Nephrol Dial Transplant 19 Suppl 3: iii47–51.

9. Myslak M, Amer H, Morales P, Fidler ME, Gloor JM, et al. (2006) Interpreting post-transplant proteinuria in patients with proteinuria pre-transplant. Am J Transplant 6: 1660–1665.

10. Morath C, Zeier M (2007) When should post-transplantation proteinuria be attributed to the renal allograft rather than to the native kidney? Nat Clin Pract Nephrol 3: 18–19.

11. Sethi K, First MR, Pesce AJ, Fidler JP, Pollak VE (1977) Proteinuria following renal transplantation. Nephron 18: 49–59.

12. First MR, Vaidya PN, Maryniak RK, Weiss MA, Munda R, et al. (1984) Proteinuria following transplantation. Correlation with histopathology and outcome. Transplantation 38: 607–612.

13. Solez K, Colvin RB, Racusen LC, Sis B, Halloran PF, et al. (2007) Banff '05 Meeting Report: differential diagnosis of chronic allograft injury and elimination of chronic allograft nephropathy ('CAN'). Am J Transplant 7: 518–526.

14. Eddy AA (2004) Proteinuria and interstitial injury. Nephrol Dial Transplant 19: 277–281.

15. Wiland P, Swierkot J, Szechinski J (1997) N-acetyl-beta-D-glucosaminidase urinary excretion as an early indicator of kidney dysfunction in rheumatoid arthritis patients on low-dose methotrexate treatment. Br J Rheumatol 36: 59–63.

16. Bernard AM, Vyskocil AA, Mahieu P, Lauwerys RR (1987) Assessment of urinary retinol-binding protein as an index of proximal tubular injury. Clin Chem 33: 775–779.

17. Kotanko P, Margreiter R, Pfaller W (2000) Urinary N-acetyl-beta-D-glucosaminidase and neopterin aid in the diagnosis of rejection and acute tubular necrosis in initially nonfunctioning kidney grafts. Nephron 84: 228–235.

18. Pei R, Wang G, Tarsitani C, Rojo S, Chen T, et al. (1998) Simultaneous HLA Class I and Class II antibodies screening with flow cytometry. Hum Immunol 59: 313–322.

19. Sis B, Mengel M, Haas M, Colvin RB, Halloran PF, et al. (2010) Banff '09 meeting report: antibody mediated graft deterioration and implementation of Banff working groups. Am J Transplant 10: 464–471.

20. Racusen LC, Colvin RB, Solez K, Mihatsch MJ, Halloran PF, et al. (2003) Antibody-mediated rejection criteria – an addition to the Banff 97 classification of renal allograft rejection. Am J Transplant 3: 708–714.

21. Racusen LC, Solez K, Colvin RB, Bonsib SM, Castro MC, et al. (1999) The Banff 97 working classification of renal allograft pathology. Kidney Int 55: 713–723.

22. Isoniemi HM, Krogerus L, von Willebrand E, Taskinen E, Ahonen J, et al. (1992) Histopathological findings in well-functioning, long-term renal allografts. Kidney Int 41: 155–160.

23. Issa N, Cosio FG, Gloor JM, Sethi S, Dean PG, et al. (2008) Transplant glomerulopathy: risk and prognosis related to anti-human leukocyte antigen class II antibody levels. Transplantation 86: 681–685.

24. Halimi JM, Laouad I, Buchler M, Al-Najjar A, Chatelet V, et al. (2005) Early low-grade proteinuria: causes, short-term evolution and long-term consequences in renal transplantation. Am J Transplant 5: 2281–2288.

25. Sis B, Campbell PM, Mueller T, Hunter C, Cockfield SM, et al. (2007) Transplant glomerulopathy, late antibody-mediated rejection and the ABCD tetrad in kidney allograft biopsies for cause. Am J Transplant 7: 1743–1752.

26. Choukroun G, Kamar N, Dussol B, Etienne I, Cassuto-Viguier E, et al. (2012) Correction of postkidney transplant anemia reduces progression of allograft nephropathy. J Am Soc Nephrol 23: 360–368.

27. Reichel H, Zeier M, Ritz E (2004) Proteinuria after renal transplantation: pathogenesis and management. Nephrol Dial Transplant 19: 301–305.

28. Amer H, Cosio FG (2009) Significance and management of proteinuria in kidney transplant recipients. J Am Soc Nephrol 20: 2490–2492.

29. Rell K, Linde J, Morzycka-Michalik M, Gaciong Z, Lao M (1993) Effect of enalapril on proteinuria after kidney transplantation. Transpl Int 6: 213–217.

30. Grekas D, Dioudis C, Kalevrosoglou I, Papoulidou F, Goutsaridis N, et al. (1995) Management of moderate to severe hypertension and proteinuria by nifedipine retard and perindopril after renal transplantation. Clin Nephrol 44: 299–302.

31. Navarro JF, Macia ML, Garcia J (1998) Control of severe proteinuria with losartan after renal transplantation. Am J Nephrol 18: 261–262.

32. Borchhardt K, Haas N, Yilmaz N, Oberbauer R, Schmidt A, et al. (1997) Low dose angiotensin converting enzyme inhibition and glomerular permselectivity in renal transplant recipients. Kidney Int 52: 1622–1625.

33. Sund S, Reisaeter AV, Scott H, Fauchald P, Bentdal O, et al. (1998) Morphological studies of baseline needle biopsies from living donor kidneys: light microscopic, immunohistochemical and ultrastructural findings. APMIS 106: 1017–1034.

34. Sund S, Hovig T, Reisaeter AV, Scott H, Bentdal O, et al. (2003) Complement activation in early protocol kidney graft biopsies after living-donor transplantation. Transplantation 75: 1204–1213.

35. Levy M, Berger J (1988) Worldwide perspective of IgA nephropathy. Am J Kidney Dis 12: 340–347.

36. Chandrakantan A, Ratanapanichkich P, Said M, Barker CV, Julian BA (2005) Recurrent IgA nephropathy after renal transplantation despite immunosuppressive regimens with mycophenolate mofetil. Nephrol Dial Transplant 20: 1214–1221.

37. Wang AY, Lai FM, Yu AW, Lam PK, Chow KM, et al. (2001) Recurrent IgA nephropathy in renal transplant allografts. Am J Kidney Dis 38: 588–596.

38. Roberts IS, Cook HT, Troyanov S, Alpers CE, Amore A, et al. (2009) The Oxford classification of IgA nephropathy: pathology definitions, correlations, and reproducibility. Kidney Int 76: 546–556.

14

Human Induced Pluripotent Stem Cells Differentiation into Oligodendrocyte Progenitors and Transplantation in a Rat Model of Optic Chiasm Demyelination

Alireza Pouya[1], **Leila Satarian**[1,2], **Sahar Kiani**[1], **Mohammad Javan**[1,2], **Hossein Baharvand**[1,3]*

1 Department of Stem Cells and Developmental Biology, Cell Science Research Center, Royan Institute for Stem Cell Biology and Technology, ACECR, Tehran, Iran, **2** Department of Physiology, Faculty of Medical Sciences, Tarbiat Modares University, Tehran, Iran, **3** Department of Developmental Biology, University of Science and Culture, ACECR, Tehran, Iran

Abstract

Background: This study aims to differentiate human induced pluripotent stem cells (hiPSCs) into oligodendrocyte precursors and assess their recovery potential in a demyelinated optic chiasm model in rats.

Methodology/Principal Findings: We generated a cell population of oligodendrocyte progenitors from hiPSCs by using embryoid body formation in a defined medium supplemented with a combination of factors, positive selection and mechanical enrichment. Real-time polymerase chain reaction and immunofluorescence analyses showed that stage-specific markers, Olig2, Sox10, NG2, PDGFRα, O4, A2B5, GalC, and MBP were expressed following the differentiation procedure, and enrichment of the oligodendrocyte lineage. These results are comparable with the expression of stage-specific markers in human embryonic stem cell-derived oligodendrocyte lineage cells. Transplantation of hiPSC-derived oligodendrocyte progenitors into the lysolecithin-induced demyelinated optic chiasm of the rat model resulted in recovery from symptoms, and integration and differentiation into oligodendrocytes were detected by immunohistofluorescence staining against PLP and MBP, and measurements of the visual evoked potentials.

Conclusions/Significance: These results showed that oligodendrocyte progenitors generated efficiently from hiPSCs can be used in future biomedical studies once safety issues have been overcome.

Editor: Mark P. Mattson, National Institute on Aging Intramural Research Program, United States of America

Funding: This study was funded by grants from the Royan Institute and the Iranian Council of Stem Cell Technology. The funders had no role in study design, data collection and analysis, decision to publish, or preparation of the manuscript.

Competing Interests: The authors have declared that no competing interests exist.

* E-mail: baharvand@royaninstitute.org

Introduction

Demyelinating diseases such as multiple sclerosis (MS) are characterized by damage to the myelin sheath surrounding neurons, causing impaired nerve impulses that lead to a constellation of neurological symptoms. Recent research on cell transplantation has yielded new insights into the novel possibilities of using stem cell-derived oligodendrocytes in graft-based remyelination therapy to restore action potential conduction. However, to date, an efficient and reliable cell source has not been introduced (for review, see [1]. The recent groundbreaking developments regarding induced pluripotent stem cells (iPSCs) generated from easily accessible somatic cells [2] appear to offer a nearly inexhaustible source of transplantable, autologous neural stem cells (for review, see [3,4]. Many studies have demonstrated that mouse and human iPSCs are highly morphologically, molecularly and phenotypically similar to their respective embryo-derived embryonic stem cell (ESC) counterparts [5,6]. The use of iPSCs also circumvents the ethical issue related to using ES cells and producing human disease models *in vitro* (for review, see [7].

Several studies have reported the functional maturation and neural and oligodendrocyte differentiation of ESCs *in vitro* as well as therapeutic use of ESCs in animal models of demyelinating diseases and remyelination after spinal cord injury [8–24]. These studies have suggested that ESC-derived oligodendrocyte progenitors (OPs) can potentially promote regeneration and reduce secondary degeneration by protecting and restoring axons.

To date, there have been two reports of differentiation of OPs from mouse iPSCs [25,26]. However, there is no report of differentiation of OPs from human iPSCs (hiPSCs) and their transplantation into a demyelinating animal model. Based on the similarity of hiPSCs and human ESCs (hESCs), we hypothesized that generation and maturation of OPs from hiPSCs *in vitro* could be achieved with the same protocol used with hESCs. Therefore, we applied a previously described protocol for differentiating hESCs into oligodendrocyte lineage cells [27] to hiPSCs. Additionally, following transplantation, we investigated the capacity of the hiPSC-derived OPs to improve demyelinated optic chiasm in a rat model, which had been induced by lysolecithin.

Results

Differentiation and characterization of hiPSCs and hESCs into OPs and oligodendrocytes

The differentiation procedure and the morphology of cells at different stages are illustrated in Figure 1. Selective oligodendrocyte differentiation from undifferentiated feeder-free hiPSCs (stage 1) was performed by forming EB and culturing the cells in a GRM/hESC medium containing 4 ng/ml bFGF at a 1:1 ratio. The EBs were then exposed to GRM in the presence of RA and EGF for nine days (stage 2). This exposure led to the appearance of a transparent sphere of cells (Figure 1, B type) and yellow

spheres of cells (Figure 1, A type) that contained oligodendrocyte-lineage cells. With the removal of RA and continuing the suspension cultures in GRM supplemented with EGF for 18 days, the size of the yellow spheres increased. At day 28, yellow-type free-floating spheres were plated on Matrigel. In the Matrigel cultures, cells migrated progressively outward from the spheres and were maintained and proliferated in the same medium. Cells were passaged (1:2) twice every seven days (day 42, stage 3). At this step, cells displayed immature oligodendrocyte bipolar and multipolar morphologies, which were similar to those of OPs. To evaluate the oligodendrocyte maturation potential of these cells, induction was used by removing EGF from the medium, and

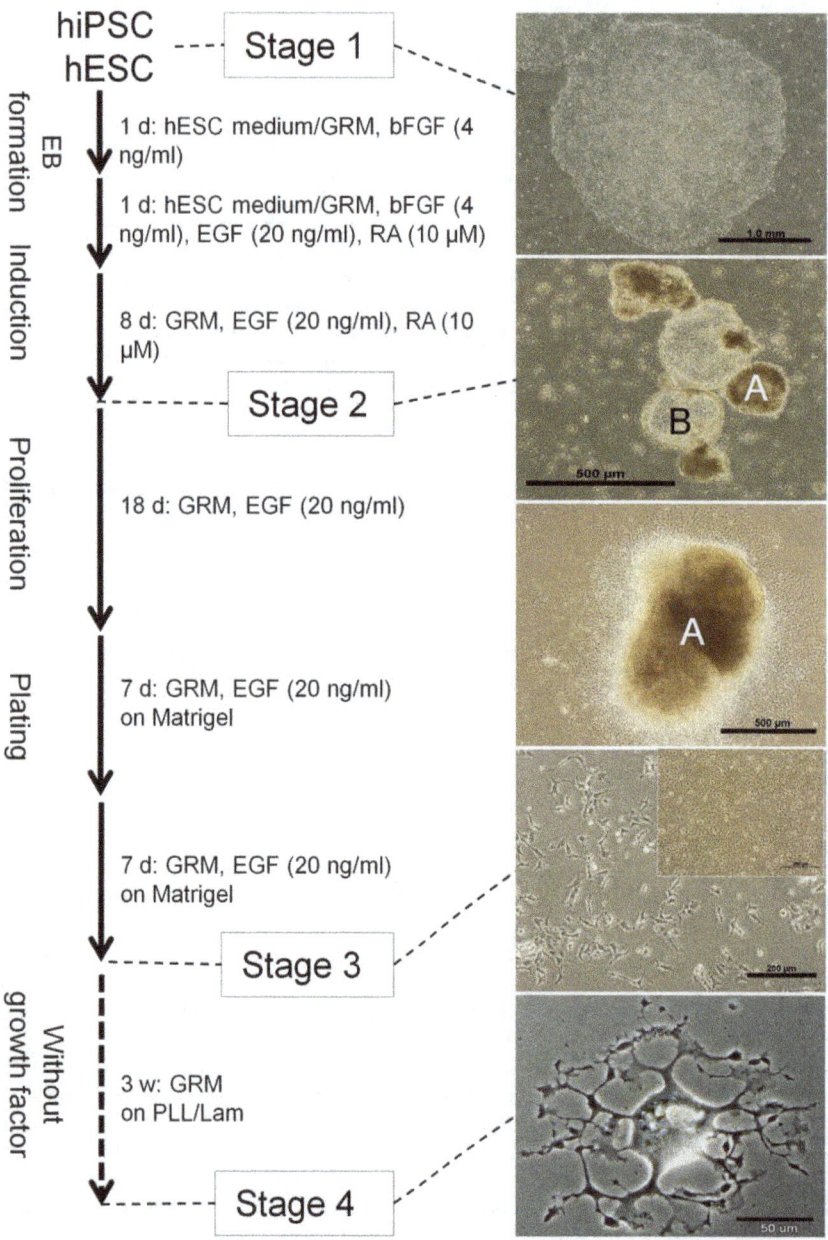

Figure 1. Differentiation protocol and cellular morphologies during oligodendroglial-lineage cell differentiation. hiPSCs (hiPSC1 and hiPSC8 lines) and hESCs (Royan H6 line) were differentiated to oligodendrocyte lineage cells during induction of neural-lineage cells with the preferential selection of oligodendroglial-lineage cells using media components. Morphologies of cells at the related stages are depicted. Two types of spheres were observed in stage 2: yellow spheres (A), which were plated on Matrigel for the subsequent stages, and transplant spheres (B), which were removed from cultures. The representative pictures showed hiPSC1 differentiation.

cells were replated at a low density (10,000 cells/cm^2) on a PLL/lam substrate for three weeks. After this treatment, plated cells adopted an oligodendroglial morphology characterized by multiple branches (stage 4). The same morphological results were observed for hESCs.

Cells were examined by qRT-PCR at different points of differentiation for expression of markers typical of oligodendrocyte development in hiPSCs and hESCs (Figure 2). *OCT4* and *SOX2*, markers of pluripotency, were down-regulated following induction. Additionally, we could not detect OCT4-positive cells by immunofluorescence staining at stages 3 and 4 in the hiPSC-derived OPs. Expression of the neural markers *PAX6* and *TUJ1* was up-regulated, and the expression of *TUJ1* decreased at stage 4 following additional maturation. The expression levels of *PDGFRα* and *OLIG2* (OPs markers) were up-regulated during OP induction (stages 2 and 3) and down-regulated after more differentiation (stage 4).

We evaluated the OPs (stage 3) and differentiated immature oligodendrocytes (stage 4) at the cellular level by immunofluorescence staining (Figure 3). Random field counting of immunoflu-

A: hiPSC1-derived cells

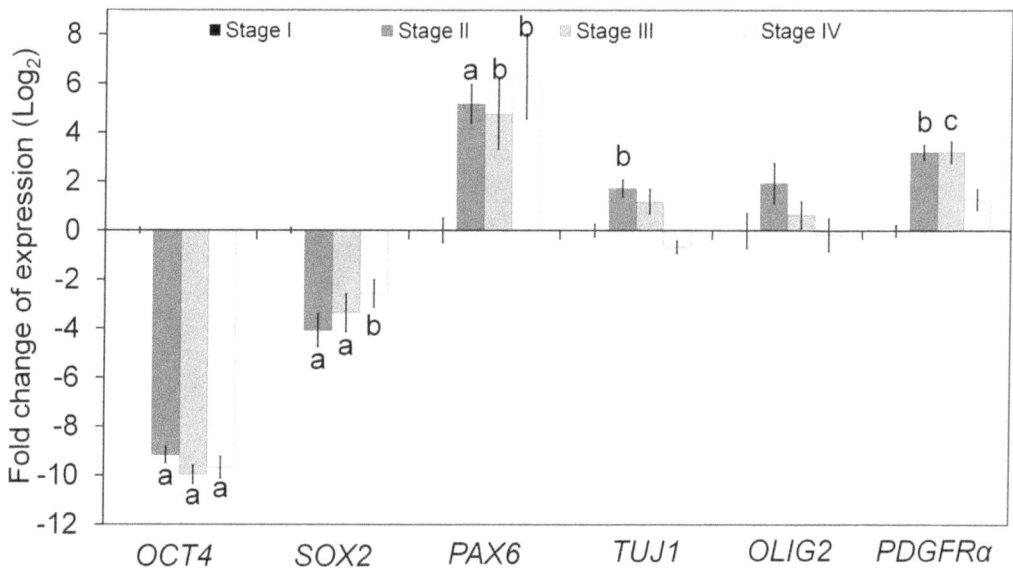

B: hESC (Royan H6 line)-derived

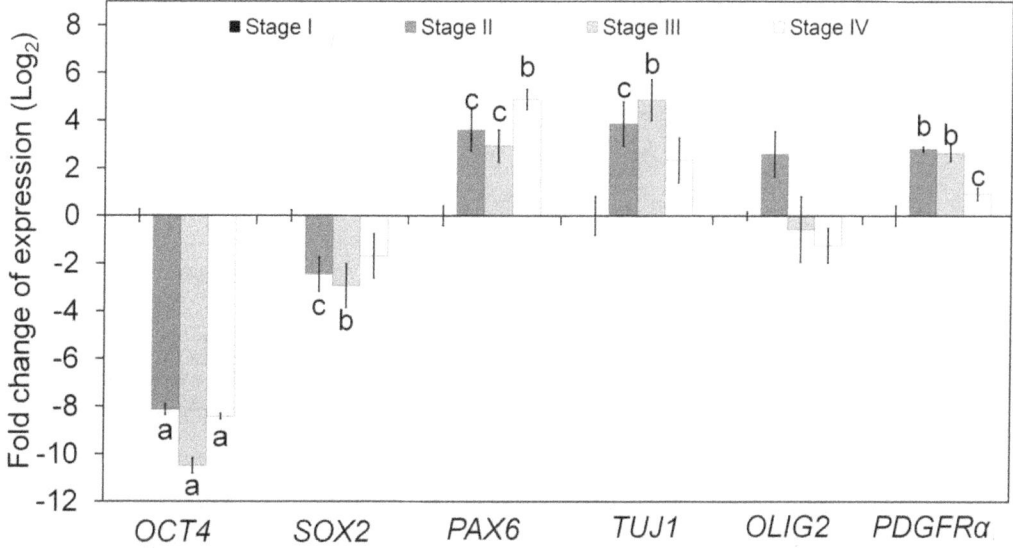

Figure 2. Relative gene expression using real-time PCR. Fold changes of expression were reported as log2. For real-time PCR, sampling was performed at four different stages during the differentiation protocol. Several primers were used for the pluripotent genes (Oct4 and Sox2), the neural lineage genes (Pax6 and Tuj1), and the oligodendrocyte lineage genes (Olig2 and PDGFRα). Expression of the pluripotent-specific genes decreased during the differentiation of hiPSC1(A) and hESC (Royan H6 line) (B) lines into oligodendrocytes when compared to stage 1. Expression levels of Pax6, Tuj1, and PDGFRα increased, but Tuj1 and PDGFRα expression decreased in stage 4. Gene expression levels at different hiPSCs and hESC-oligodendrocyte lineage cell stages relative to the levels in stage 1 approximate the gene expression levels of derived cells. c: p<0.05, b: p<0.01, a: p<0.001 vs. hiPSC1 or hESC stage; Error bar: SEM.

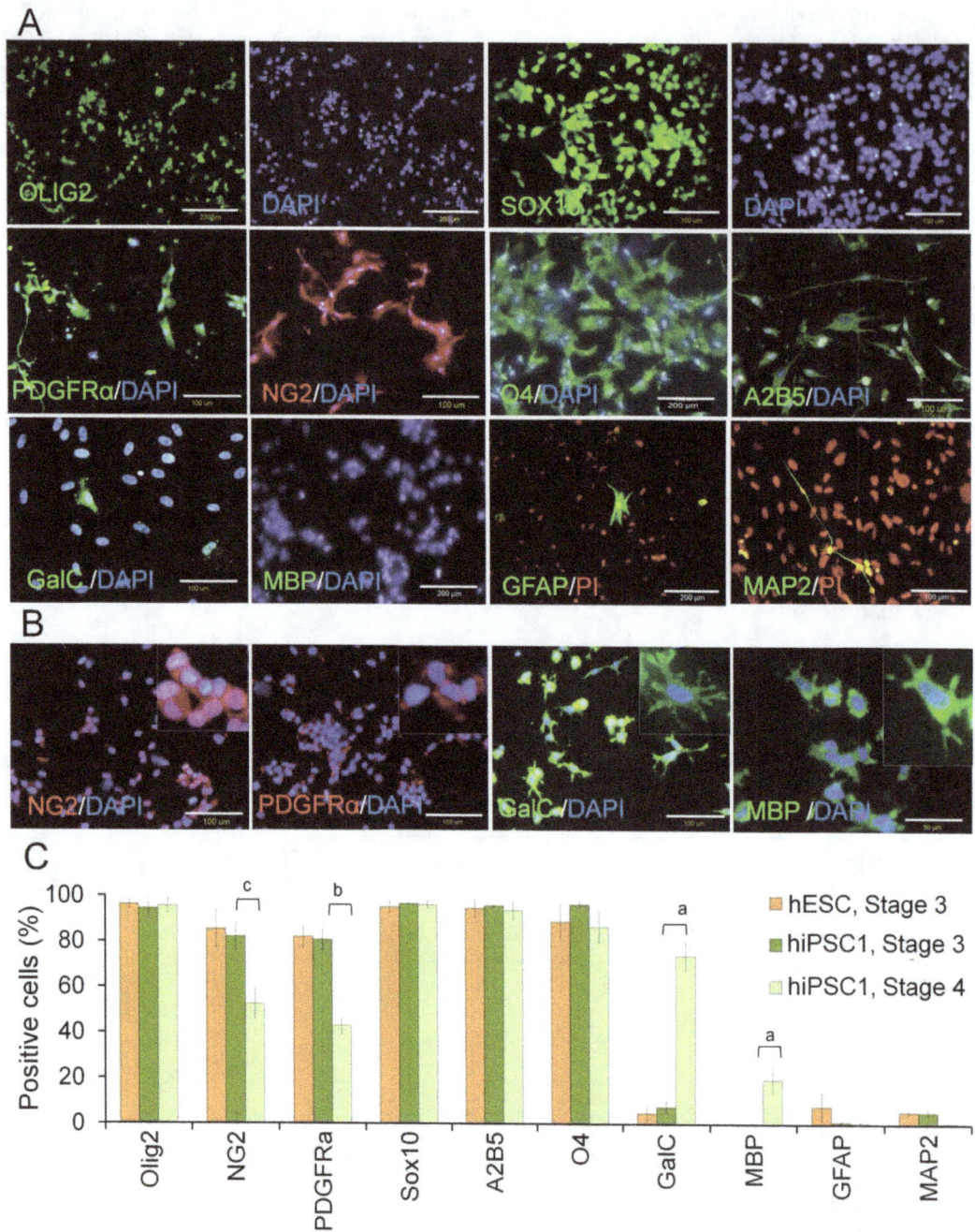

Figure 3. Immunofluorescence staining of differentiated oligodendrocyte lineage cells from hiPSCs and hESCs. (A) The representative pictures of Olig2, Sox10, PDGFRα, NG2, O4, A2B5, GalC, MBP, GFAP, and MAP2 expression in hiPSC1-derived OPs. Oligodendrocyte lineage markers exhibit high levels of expression in the OP stage, while the astrocyte cell protein GFAP and the neuronal protein MAP2 are minimally expressed (A). The removal of EGF from the hiPSC1-derived OPs medium results in down-regulation of NG2 and PDGFRα and up-regulation of GalC and MBP, as shown in (B). The percentage of positive cells at stage 3 and 4 for hiPSC1-derived oligodendrocyte lineage cells and hESC-derived OPs at stage 3 for some markers (C). (c) $p < 0.05$; (b) $p < 0.01$; (a) $p < 0.001$. Error bar: SEM.

orescence images showed that the majority of hiPSC-derived OPs (>90%) expressed related oligodendrocyte lineage markers (Figure 3) including OLIG2 (94.37±2.69%), SOX10 (96.61± 0.80%), A2B5 (95.74±0.22%) and O4 (96.46±1.21%). Immuno-fluorescence in hiPSC-derived OPs was also positive for NG2 (82.04±5.88%) and PDGFRα (80.72±4.43%). However, the number of cells positive for these OP markers significantly decreased to 52.41±6.55% ($p < 0.05$) and 42.87±3.19%

($p < 0.01$) in stage 4, respectively (Figure 3 B, C). The number of counted cells for each antibody has presented in Table S1. PDGFRα, A2B5 and NG2 are membrane epitopes typically expressed in OPs [40,41]. SOX10 is a member of the high-mobility group domain family of DNA binding proteins expressed within OPs, yet it is not expressed in neurons or astrocytes [42]. The Olig2 transcription factor is critical for oligodendrocyte and motor neuron differentiation [43].

After the final differentiation (stage 4), the expression of oligodendrocyte-specific genes such as MBP and GalC increased (GalC: $7.49 \pm 2.37\%$ to $73.75 \pm 5.97\%$, $p < 0.01$; MBP: $0.30 \pm 0.15\%$ to $19.51 \pm 5.56\%$, $p < 0.05$). MBP is localized to the major dense lines of myelin and confined to the interior of oligodendrocytes [44,45]. No significant differences were noted among the expressions of OLIG2, SOX10, O4, GFAP, and MAP2 in hiPSC-derived cells in stages 3 and 4 (Figure 3C). O4 is a surface antigen on immature and mature oligodendrocytes [46]. Importantly, the levels of the astrocyte marker GFAP and the neuronal marker MAP2 were the same before and after differentiation [GFAP ($1.07 \pm 0.42\%$) and MAP2 ($5.26 \pm 1.17\%$)] (Figure 3C). Therefore, the oligodendrocyte lineage was enriched relative to neurons or astrocytes. Additionally, this *in vitro* protocol for oligodendrocyte differentiation of hESCs resulted in efficient induction of oligodendrocytes and their progenitors from hiPSCs.

Similar results in expression were observed in hESCs (Royan H6 line, Figure 3C) and hiPSC8 in RNA and protein levels (Figures S1 and S2). Therefore, we continued our transplantation experiments with hiPSC1-derived OPs.

Transplantation into the optic chiasm rat model of demyelination

The amounts of demyelination and remyelination were histologically evaluated using Luxol fast blue myelin-specific staining one, five and nine weeks post-lesion. Extensive demyelination was demonstrated one week post-lesion (Figure 4A). Four and eight weeks after transplantation of hiPSC1-derived OPs an obvious remyelination was seen, while less remyelination was seen in control chiasms (Figure 4B and C).

Improvement in remyelination of the optic chiasm and nerves was functionally evaluated using VEP recording from the skull. Changes in the P1 wave-latency was assessed in the control, vehicle and cell transplanted animals (Figure 4D). While low levels of endogenous recovery of P1-latency were observed in the control and vehicle-treated animals eight weeks post-lesion, cell grafting reduced the elevated latency relative to the control by one week post-transplantation, and this reduction persisted until eight weeks post-transplantation.

Eight weeks after transplantation, tracing of DiI-labeled cells showed that the transplanted cells survived and integrated within the chiasm (Figure 5). Double labeling for DiI and PLP, MBP, GFAP, or MAP2 showed that the majority of the grafted cells were PLP+ and/or MBP+, which demonstrated differentiation of hiPSC1-derived OPs into mature oligodendrocytes *in vivo* and confirmed remyelination by the transplanted cells (Figure 5). Additionally, a few of the transplanted cells were GFAP+ or MAP2+, which indicated non-astroglial and non-neuronal differentiation of the grafted cells *in vivo*. DiI-unlabeled transplanted cells were used as negative control, eight weeks post-cell transplantation (Figure S3).

Additionally, we did not observe tumor, teratoma or non-neuronal tissue formation in the transplant recipients at four or eight weeks following hiPSC1-derived OPs transplantation.

Discussion

Several studies have demonstrated generation of oligodendrocyte lineage cells from hESCs with different efficiencies [14–23]. Based on these reports, we developed a protocol and applied it to differentiate hiPSC into an oligodendrocyte lineage. Our data showed that our protocol efficiently generated hiPSC-derived OPs *in vitro*. Additionally, the transplantation of these OPs seven days after lysolecithin induced demyelination to the optic chiasm of the rat models resulted in significant functional recovery compared to the control and vehicle groups.

The method used to differentiate hiPSCs toward an oligodendrocytic cell lineage was based on sequential induction at proper time intervals by introducing appropriate induction and growth factors. This method has previously been used to generate OPs from hESC (Hatch et al., 2009).

Our hiPSCs were induced into an oligodendrocyte lineage by EB formation following the plating of yellow spheres that were generated in the presence of RA in GRM. Bipolar and proliferating hiPSC-derived OPs appeared following migration of cells from yellow spheres and became complex ramified oligodendrocytes after growth factors were withdrawn. Thyroid hormone was needed to ensure oligodendrocyte survival and to initiate the differentiation of OPs into mature oligodendrocytes [47].

Moreover, our quantitative real-time PCR and immunostaining data has shown that hiPSCs share similarities in gene expression patterns with hESCs during differentiation to oligodendrocytes. The percentage of antigen-expressing cells measured by immunofluorescence staining exhibited no significant difference between hiPSC-derived OPs and hESC-derived OPs. OP specific markers such as OLIG2, A2B5, SOX10, NG2, PDGFRα, and O4 were expressed in the majority of cells. However, later oligodendrocyte markers, such as GalC and MBP, were expressed in few cells. Contamination with other neural lineage types was low, as few of the cells were positive for GFAP and MAP2 at the OP step. Additionally, the expression of pluripotent genes was strongly down-regulated. We continued to culture adherent hiPSC-derived OPs by trypsinization during several passages (results not shown) using a method similar to one previously described for expandable hESC-derived OPs [48]. These findings demonstrated that a population of pure hiPSC-derived OPs was generated in this study as well as a population of pure hESC-derived OPs.

Furthermore, developmental studies have demonstrated that GalC (70%) and MBP (20%) begin to express in both immature oligodendrocytes and mature oligodendrocytes [49,50]. These results indicate that hiPSC-derived OPs can differentiate into more mature oligodendrocytes, but our conditions were insufficient to achieve full maturation *in vitro*, which may require other parameters such as cell contact with other types of CNS cells.

This study has assessed the therapeutic effects of transplanted hiPSC-derived OPs in toxically-induced demyelination of the rat chiasm. The production of animal models with CNS white matter locally demyelinated by toxic materials such as lysolecithin provides a good tool for assessing the therapeutic effects of transplanted oligodendrocyte cells. Lysolecithin in applied concentration is toxic and particularly affects myelin-producing cells [51,52] and can therefore be used to produce local, acute demyelination in the CNS [34]. Cells were transplanted one week after and in the same manner as the lysolecithin injection. Our histology results demonstrated that demyelination occurred in the chiasm one week after the lysolecithin injection. Luxol fast blue staining of chiasm sections four and/or eight weeks after hiPSC-derived OPs transplantation showed increased staining and remyelinating axons. The engrafted OPs survived, migrated and integrated into the host tissue at week's post-cell transplantation. Functional changes to the optic nerve were recorded with VEP measurements. It was also shown that hiPSC-derived OPs promoted recovery in transplanted rats compared to vehicle-injected and control rats. This improvement was observed particularly in the first week after cell transplantation, which indicates the short-term effectiveness of this transplantation. Immunohistofluorescence analysis of the grafts indicated that the

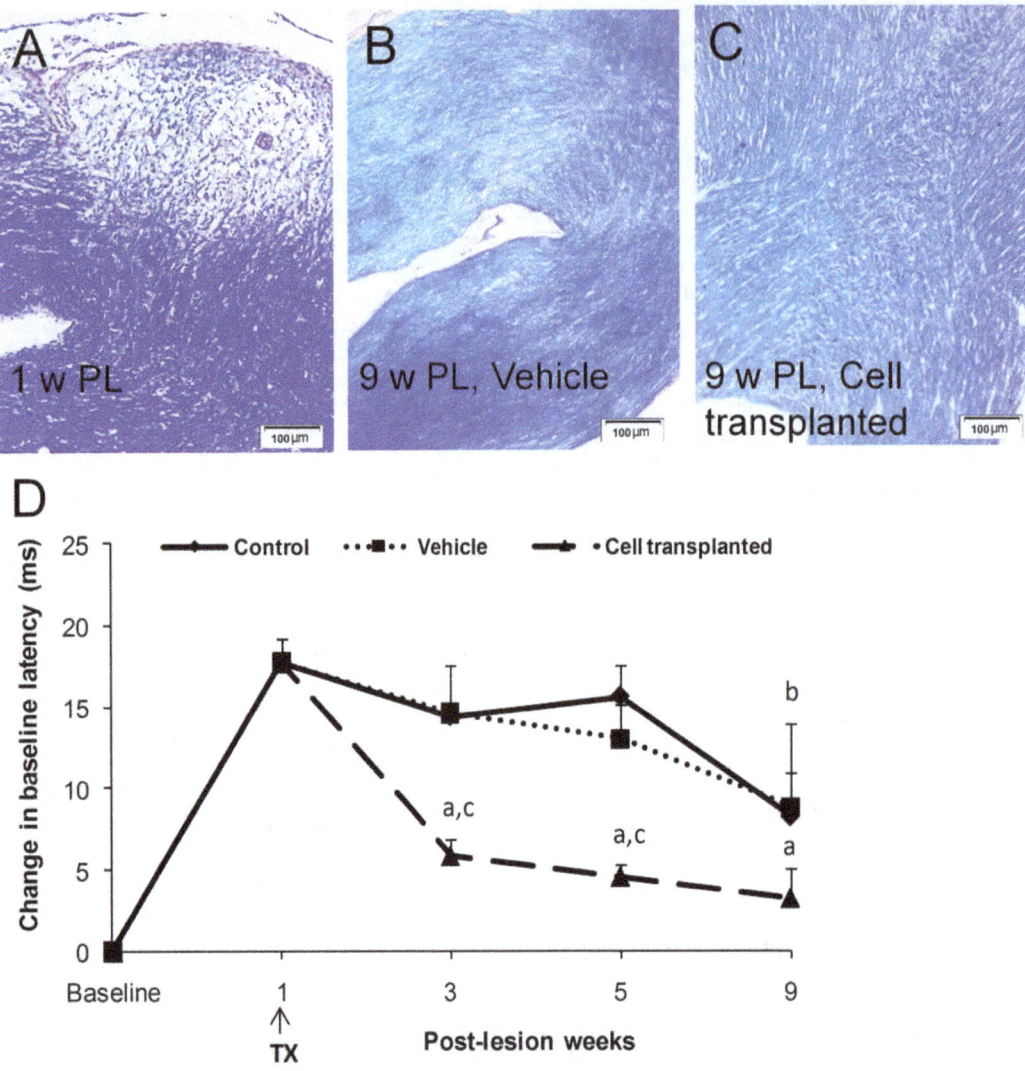

Figure 4. Histological and behavioral assessments following demyelinated chiasm injury and cell transplantation. (A) A longitudinal section of a demyelinated region stained with Luxol fast blue at the first week post-lesion. (B) Representative Luxol fast blue staining of chiasm sections nine weeks' post-lesion in vehicle group. (C) Myelin repair in the optic chiasm using Luxol fast blue in representative sections eight weeks post-transplantation with hiPSC1-derived OPs. (D) Functional evaluation of the optic apparatus using VEP recording in animal models. Changes in the baseline latency of the P1 wave following local injection of hiPSC1-derived OPs in the transplant group are shown along with those of the medium (vehicle) and control groups. The arrow shows the time of cell or medium injection. b: $p<0.01$ and a: $p<0.001$ vs. week 1, c: $p<0.01$ vs. vehicle treated and control groups in the same week. Error bar: SEM. Tx: transplantation. PL: post-lesion.

majority of the transplanted hiPSC-derived OPs expressed the MBP protein, demonstrating that OPs derived from hiPSCs completed differentiation after transplantation to the demyelinated chiasm. A few of the cells displayed the astrocyte marker, GFAP in the chiasm of the transplanted rats. It has been shown that transplanted hESC-derived OPs improve the recovery of spinal cord injury in demyelination models [14–22]. Recently, it was shown that mouse iPSC-OPs could also become functional remyelinating oligodendrocytes, as demonstrated *in vitro* by co-culture of these cells with neurons and *in vivo* after implantation in the demyelinated corpus callosum of cuprizone-treated mice [26]. Additionally, it was reported that axonal loss in eyes that received concurrent inflammatory activated OPs was lower than axonal loss in control eyes in a glaucoma model [53].

On the other hand, in addition to their differentiation into mature oligodendrocytes following transplantation, hiPSC-derived OPs may also have indirect effects on the host tissue through secretion of anti-inflammatory and tropic molecules. hESC-derived OPs have been shown to express several neurotrophic factors that result in neuronal survival and the regeneration of damaged neurons [16]. Also, the trophic effect of transplanted NPs enhanced myelin regeneration of the host OPs in a chronic cuprizone-induced demyelination model in aged mice [54]. Moreover, we could not identify OCT4-positive cells at the OP generation stage. We did not observe teratoma formation after eight weeks, indicating that no undifferentiated iPSCs were present after our oligodendrocyte differentiation procedure.

To our knowledge, this is the first report on the differentiation of hiPSCs into oligodendrocyte-lineage cells and their transplantation in an animal model. These hiPSC-derived OPs improved myelin repair in lysolecithin-induced demyelinated-rat optic chiasm which reveal the possible application of these patient specific cells in future regenerative biomedicine. However, several issues remain to be solved before hiPSC-derived cells can be safely applied in

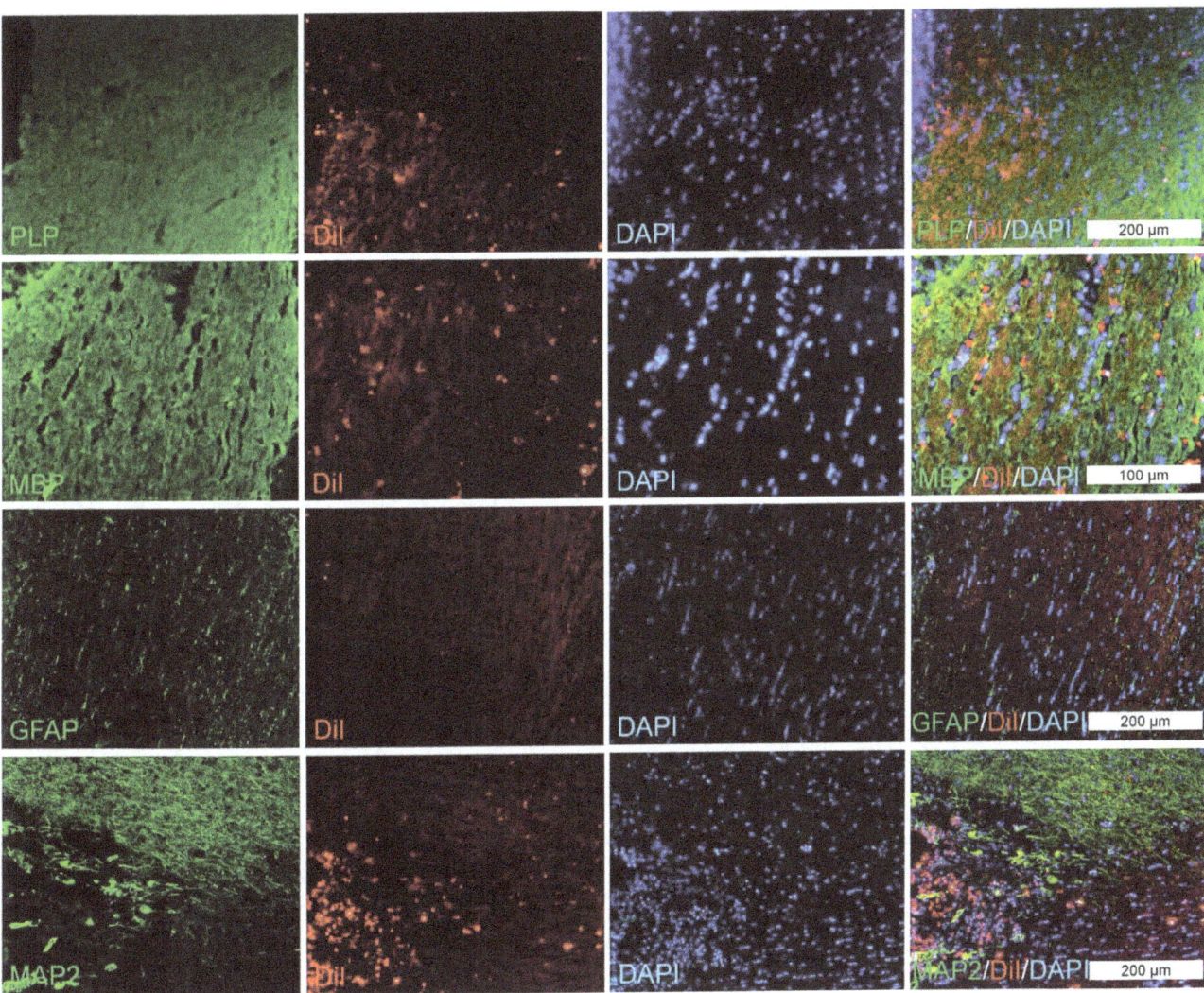

Figure 5. Immunofluorescence staining of transplanted cells. The hiPSC1-derived OPs were labeled with DiI before transplantation into chiasms and immunostained with antibodies against PLP, MBP, GFAP, or MAP2 eight weeks after transplantation. The majority of DiI-labeled cells showed PLP and/or MBP reactivity, and a few of them were GFAP+ and/or MAP2+.

clinical settings (for reviews, see [3,4]). For example, recently it has reported that transplantation of undifferentiated iPSCs which derived by either retroviral approach or a episomal approach showed T-cell-dependent immune response in recipient syngeneic mice due to the abnormal expression of antigens following genetic manipulation [55,56]. Improvements in the production of safe and non-immunogenic hiPSCs will increase the number of applications of iPSC derivatives.

Materials and Methods

Pluripotent stem cell culture and differentiation into oligodendrocyte lineage cells

The hiPSC line Royan hiPSC1 and hiPSC8 [28] at passages 29–47 was used in these experiments. Cells were expanded and passaged under feeder-free culture conditions in a hESC medium that contained 100 ng/ml basic fibroblast growth factor (bFGF, Royan Institute) using a previously described technique [29]. The medium was changed every other day until day 7. The differentiation procedure (outlined in Figure 1) was divided into four stages, as described in (Hatch et al., 2009). The hiPSC

colonies were exposed to an enzymatic mixture that contained 1 mg/ml collagenase IV (Invitrogen, 17104-019) and 2 mg/ml dispase (Invitrogen, 17105-041) for 7 min at 37°C. The enzymes were then removed, and the colonies were rinsed with Dulbecco's phosphate-buffered saline (D-PBS, Invitrogen, 14190-144). Cell clusters were scraped from the dish after the addition of hESC medium/glial restriction medium (GRM) at a 1:1 ratio and collected in low-attachment bacteriological dishes (Falcon, 351029). A total of 4 ng/ml bFGF was added to the culture media, and cells were then transferred to an incubator. The GRM consisted of DMEM/F12 (Invitrogen, 21331-020), 2% B27 supplement (Invitrogen, 17504-044), 2 mM L-glutamine (Invitrogen, 25030-024), 10 µg/ml insulin (Sigma-Aldrich, I1882), 10 µg/ml putrescine (Sigma-Aldrich, P6024), 63 ng/ml progesterone (Sigma-Aldrich, P6149), 50 ng/ml sodium selenite (Sigma-Aldrich, S9133), 50 µg/ml holo-transferrin (Sigma-Aldrich, T1408), and 40 ng/ml triiodothyronine (T3; Sigma-Aldrich, T6397). The following day, cell clusters were collected and transferred to hESC medium/GRM containing 4 ng/ml bFGF, 20 ng/ml human epidermal growth factor (EGF; Sigma-Aldrich, E9644) and 10 µM all-trans-retinoic acid (RA; Sigma-Aldrich, R2625). Over the next eight days, the medium was exchanged daily with GRM containing 20 ng/ml EGF and 10 μM RA. After eight days, RA was omitted from the media, and floating clusters were cultured for 18 days during which the medium was changed every other day. At day 28 of the differentiation protocol, yellow clusters were cultured on matrigel- (Sigma-Aldrich, E1270) coated 6 cm tissue culture dishes in the same medium. Clusters adhered to the dishes, and cells were dislodged one week later using 0.05% trypsin/EDTA (Invitrogen, 25300) for 3 min at 37°C. Trypsin was neutralized with DMEM/F12 containing 10% fetal bovine serum (FBS; Hyclone, SH30070) and centrifuged, and the cell pellet was resuspended in GRM plus 20 ng/ml EGF and reseeded on matrigel-coated dishes for seven days. Cells underwent weekly passaging.

OPs were more differentiated on poly-L-Lysine (Sigma-Aldrich, P4707)/laminin-coated plates (Sigma-Aldrich, L2020) (PLL/lam) in the absence of EGF over a three-week period. In some of the experiments, the Royan H6 hESC line [30] at passages 102–127 was used as a control group.

Real-time reverse transcription PCR

At each stage, cells were collected, and the total RNA was extracted using TRIzol reagent (Invitrogen, 15596-018). DNA was degraded with the use of the DNase I, RNase-free kit (Fermentas, EN0521), whereas RNA was protected using RiboLockTM RNase Inhibitor (Fermentas, E00381). cDNA was synthesized using a RevertAidTM H Minus First Strand cDNA Synthesis kit (Fermentas, K1632). Relative gene expression analysis was performed with real-time PCR. The expression of several genes, including POU5F1 (Oct4), Sox2, Pax-6, Tuj1, Olig2 PDGFRα and a housekeeping gene, β-actin, were analyzed at four stages of the oligodendrocyte differentiation procedure. Real-time PCR used specific primers (Table S2), a 96-well optical reaction plate and the 7500 Real Time PCR system (Applied Biosystems). In each PCR reaction, 1X Power SYBR® Green PCR Master Mix (ABI PRISM, 4368702) was mixed with 12 ng cDNA and specific primers in a total volume of 20 μl. Thermal conditions were the same for all genes, and the annealing temperature was 60°C.

The comparative Ct method, $2^{-\Delta\Delta Ct}$, was used for relative gene expression analysis [31]. All Ct values calculated from the target genes were normalized to β-actin and calibrated using calculations from the undifferentiated pluripotent cells from stage 1. In each experiment, there were at least three independent replicates of each stage, and each replicate included two identical samples.

Immunofluorescence staining

For immunofluorescence staining, cultured cells were washed with washing buffer (phosphate-buffered saline (PBS) with 0.05% tween-20 (Sigma-Aldrich, P7949), pH 7.4) and fixed with 4% paraformaldehyde (Sigma-Aldrich, P6148) in PBS for 10 min. If necessary, cells were then permeabilized with 0.5% Triton X-100 (Sigma-Aldrich, T8532) for 15 min. Cells were twice washed and blocked in 10% secondary antibody host serum in washing buffer for 30 min at 37°C. Cells were incubated overnight at 4°C with primary antibodies (Table S3) diluted in washing buffer. Cells were washed three times (5 min each) and then incubated with fluorescence-labeled secondary antibodies in washing buffer at room temperature and rinsed three times (5 min each). For negative controls, only the secondary antibody was used (results not shown). Either the fluorescent dye propidium iodide (PI; Fluka, 81845) or 4′,6-diamidino-2-phenylindole (DAPI; Sigma-Aldrich, D-8417) was used for staining nuclei.

Images were obtained on an Olympus IX71 fluorescence microscope with a DP72 digital camera and captured by analySIS

LS Starter version 3.2. For cell counting, 10 random images were prepared from different sites on each plate, and fluorescent-stained cells of each marker were counted in each image. The experiment was performed on at least three independent cell cultures for each antibody. The percentage of positive cells was determined as the ratio of positive cells to the total number of counted cells (stained with PI or DAPI) in each experiment.

Implantation of hiPSC-derived OPs in lysolecithin-induced demyelinated rat chiasm

To evaluate the capacity of hiPSC-derived OPs to restore myelination in vivo, cells were implanted in the demyelinated optic chiasm of lysolecithin-injected rat models.

Ethics statement. All animal use procedures were in strict accordance with the approval of the Royan Institutional Review Board and Institutional Ethical Committee under the approval ID of J/90/1397.

Animals. Adult male Sprague Dawley rats (240–280 g) were obtained from Razi Institute (Karaj, Iran). Rats were maintained in temperature-controlled rooms with a 12/12 h light/dark cycle and 50–55% humidity and had free access to food and water.

Preparation of cells for transplantation. For identification after transplantation, the cells were prelabeled with the plasma membrane marker, red fluorescence-CellTracker CM-DiI (chloromethyl benzyl-amide derivatives of 1,1-dioctadecyl-3,3,3′,3′ tetramethylindocarbocyanine perchlorate; Invitrogen, C7001), which allowed in vivo identification of grafted cells. Cells were incubated in 5 μg/ml CM-DiI in GRM medium for 20 min in the incubator. Cells were then washed three times (3×5 min) in D-PBS (Invitrogen, 14190-144). The viability of cells before transplantation was determined by Trypan blue exclusion dye assay to be greater than 95%.

Surgical procedure and cell transplantation. The animals were anesthetized with intraperitoneal (i.p.) injections of 50 mg/kg ketamine and 5 mg/kg xylazine and placed in a stereotaxic instrument. A 30-gauge stainless steel needle was used to inject lysolecithin into the chiasm (anterior-posterior: 0.1 mm from the bregma, lateral: 0 mm and vertical: 4.5 mm from the dura) [32]. All animals were administered 2 μl of 1% lysolecithin (Sigma-Aldrich, L1381) at day zero.

This treatment leads to demyelination of axons after one week. However, spontaneous remyelination will occur over longer durations due to endogenous OPs recruited from the adjacent tissues [33–35]. Therefore, one week after lysolecithin administration, rats were divided randomly into three groups: the cell-transplanted group (n = 8) received 200,000 hiPSC-derived OPs in 2 μl medium; the vehicle-transplanted group (n = 8) received 2 μl medium; and a control group (n = 8) received no cells and no vehicle. Cells were transplanted into the chiasm using a 25 μl Hamilton syringe connected to a 30 gauge needle. A microinjection system (Stoelting, Illinois, USA) infused the suspension at a rate of 0.5 μl/minute. After grafting, the needle remained in place for 1 minute to minimize cell reflux into the needle track. The animals were then housed in standard rat cages at a temperature of 27°C. The rats were immune-suppressed by addition of 210 mg/l, cyclosporine-A (Sandimmune, Novartis Pharmaceuticals, East Hanover, NJ, USA) to the drinking water two days before cell transplantation [36,37]. The animals then remained on the same immunosuppressant throughout the experiment. Serum levels of cyclosporine were measured in a random sample of animals at termination and the average concentration was 1750±36 ng/ml (n = 2, mean±SEM).

Visual evoked potential (VEP) recording. Functional changes in the optic nerve were electrophysiologically studied using VEP recording before lysolecithin injection and at 1st, 3nd, 5th and 9th weeks post-lesion in all groups. VEP can provide important diagnostic information regarding the functional integrity of the visual system [38]. VEP recording was performed using a previously described technique [35]. Briefly, two stainless steel screws were placed into the skull to serve as electrodes. The dura was kept intact to minimize cortical damage. The "reference" electrode was placed 5 mm anterior to the bregma and 1.5 mm right of midline, and the "record" electrode was placed 7 mm caudal to the bregma and 3 mm right of midline. Light stimulation was delivered by a general evoked response stimulator (WSI, Iran) 300 times at a frequency of 0.5 Hz. Responses were amplified using an amplifier (Iso-80, UK). The amplified waveforms were averaged. In each VEP recording, the latencies between the light flash and the first positive peak were studied.

Histochemical and immunohistofluorescence analyses. To study the extent of demyelination, the animals were sacrificed using a lethal dose of anesthesia one week after lysolecithin injection and five and nine weeks post-lesion in cell transplanted and vehicle treated groups (n = 3 per group). The chiasms were immediately stored and post-fixed in 4% paraformaldehyde for 24 h. Some chiasms were processed and embedded in paraffin. Slices were stained with Luxol fast blue to stain myelin and nuclei were counterstained with cresyl violet. Tumor formation in the transplanted animals was assessed by H&E staining.

To follow-up the fate of DiI-labeled transplanted cells, after fixation in cryoprotected 30% sucrose in PBS at 4°C for 24 h in a cryostat, some chiasms (n = 3 per group) were processed for immunohistofluorescence analysis of the cell implants. Tissue was frozen in Jung tissue freezing medium (Leica Microsystems) at −30°C and sectioned with a cryotome into pieces 8 μm thick (Leica Microsystems, CM 1850). The sections were permeabilized with 0.04% Triton X-100 and blocked with 10% normal goat serum and 0.5% BSA (Sigma-Aldrich, A3311) in PBS for 1 h. Primary antibodies against PLP, MBP, GFAP, MAP2 (Table S3) were applied overnight at room temperature. Sections were washed, and the appropriate secondary antibodies, which were conjugated with fluorescent dye (Table S3), were applied for 1 h at 37°C. Sections were washed and counterstained with the nuclear dye DAPI. Each protein was evaluated in three chiasms. Images were obtained on an Olympus BX51 fluorescence microscope with a DP72 digital camera and captured by analySIS LS Starter version 3.2.

Statistical analysis

The data are expressed as mean ± SEM. A difference between groups was considered statistically significant if $p < 0.05$. For immunofluorescence staining, an unpaired, two-tailed t-test was used to assess statistically significant differences. For qRT-PCR, randomization tests using REST 2009 V2.0.13 software were applied to indicate statistically significant differences between stage 1 and the remaining stages [39]. All quantitative data and any significant differences in the latency of the VEPs of each group were tested using a mixed-model ANOVA with a repeated factor

(time) and a non-repeated factor (group). One-way ANOVA followed by post-test LSD was performed for each group.

Supporting Information

Figure S1   Relative gene expression using real-time PCR for hiPSC8 oligodendroglial-lineage cell differentiation. Log_2 changes in expression are reported. In real-time PCR, sampling was done in four different stages during the differentiation protocol. The primers of *OCT4* and *SOX2* were used for pluripotency, *TUJ1* for neural lineage, and *PDGFRα* for oligodendrocyte lineage differentiation. Obviously, pluripotent specific genes decreased during the differentiation of hiPSC8 to oligodendrocyte when compared to stage 1. The expression levels of PDGFRα were increased; however its expression deceased in stage 4. b: $p < 0.01$, a: $p < 0.001$; Error bar: SEM.

Figure S2   Immunofluorescence staining of differentiated oligodendrocyte lineage cells from hiPSC8. (A) The representative pictures of SOX10, PDGFRα, NG2, O4, A2B5, GalC, GFAP, and MAP2 expression in hiPSC8-OPs. Oligodendrocyte lineage markers showed high levels of expression in the OP stage whereas, the astrocyte cell protein, GFAP and neuronal protein MAP2 were minimally expressed (A). The downregulation of NG2 ($p < 0.05$) and PDGFRα ($p < 0.05$) and upregulation of GalC ($p < 0.05$) as shown in (B) were observed following removal of EGF. The percentage of positive cells at stage 3 for some markers compared with expression in stage 4 (C). (c) $p < 0.05$. Error bar: SEM. Scale bars in part (A) are 100 μm.

Figure S3   Negative control for DiI labeling. DiI unlabeled transplanted cells were used as negative control, 9 weeks post lesioning.

Table S1   The number of counted cells counterstained with DAPI or PI in different groups.

Table S2   List of primers used for Real-Time PCR analysis.

Table S3   List of antibodies used in this study.

Acknowledgments

We thank Azam Samadian for technical assistance.

Author Contributions

Conceived and designed the experiments: HB MJ. Performed the experiments: AP SK LS. Analyzed the data: AP LS SK MJ HB. Contributed reagents/materials/analysis tools: AP LS SK. Wrote the paper: HB MJ.

References

1. Martino G, Franklin RJ, Van Evercooren AB, Kerr DA (2010) Stem cell transplantation in multiple sclerosis: current status and future prospects. Nat Rev Neurol 6: 247–255.

2. Takahashi K, Yamanaka S (2006) Induction of pluripotent stem cells from mouse embryonic and adult fibroblast cultures by defined factors. Cell 126: 663–676.

3. Stadtfeld M, Hochedlinger K (2010) Induced pluripotency: history, mechanisms, and applications. Genes Dev 24: 2239–2263.

4. Gonzalez F, Boue S, Belmonte JC (2011) Methods for making induced pluripotent stem cells: reprogramming a la carte. Nat Rev Genet 12: 231–242.

5. Plath K, Lowry WE (2011) Progress in understanding reprogramming to the induced pluripotent state. Nat Rev Genet 12: 253–265.

6. Lister R, Pelizzola M, Kida YS, Hawkins RD, Nery JR, et al. (2011) Hotspots of aberrant epigenomic reprogramming in human induced pluripotent stem cells. Nature 471: 68–73.

7. Zhu H, Lensch MW, Cahan P, Daley GQ (2011) Investigating monogenic and complex diseases with pluripotent stem cells. Nat Rev Genet 12: 266–275.

8. Chambers SM, Fasano CA, Papapetrou EP, Tomishima M, Sadelain M, et al. (2009) Highly efficient neural conversion of human ES and iPS cells by dual inhibition of SMAD signaling. Nat Biotechnol 27: 275–280.

9. Nemati S, Hatami M, Kiani S, Hemmesi K, Gourabi H, et al. (2010) Long-term Self-Renewable Feeder-Free Human Induced Pluripotent Stem Cell-derived Neural Progenitors. Stem Cells Dev: [Epub ahead of print].

10. Onorati M, Camnasio S, Binetti M, Jung CB, Moretti A, et al. (2010) Neuropotent self-renewing neural stem (NS) cells derived from mouse induced pluripotent stem (iPS) cells. Mol Cell Neurosci 43: 287–295.

11. Tsuji O, Miura K, Okada Y, Fujiyoshi K, Mukaino M, et al. (2010) Therapeutic potential of appropriately evaluated safe-induced pluripotent stem cells for spinal cord injury. Proc Natl Acad Sci U S A 107: 12704–12709.

12. Crocker SJ, Bajpai R, Moore CS, Frausto RF, Brown GD, et al. (2011) Intravenous Administration of Human ES-derived Neural Precursor Cells Attenuates Cuprizone-induced CNS Demyelination. , Neuropathol Appl Neurobiol, [Epub ahead of print].

13. Erceg S, Ronaghi M, Oria M, Rosello MG, Arago MA, et al. (2010) Transplanted oligodendrocytes and motoneuron progenitors generated from human embryonic stem cells promote locomotor recovery after spinal cord transection. Stem Cells 28: 1541–1549.

14. Cloutier F, Siegenthaler MM, Nistor G, Keirstead HS (2006) Transplantation of human embryonic stem cell-derived oligodendrocyte progenitors into rat spinal cord injuries does not cause harm. Regen Med 1: 469–479.

15. Faulkner J, Keirstead HS (2005) Human embryonic stem cell-derived oligodendrocyte progenitors for the treatment of spinal cord injury. Transpl Immunol 15: 131–142.

16. Zhang YW, Denham J, Thies RS (2006) Oligodendrocyte progenitor cells derived from human embryonic stem cells express neurotrophic factors. Stem Cells Dev 15: 943–952.

17. Hu BY, Zhang SC (2009) Differentiation of spinal motor neurons from pluripotent human stem cells. Nat Protoc 4: 1295–1304.

18. Hu BY, Du ZW, Li XJ, Ayala M, Zhang SC (2009) Human oligodendrocytes from embryonic stem cells: conserved SHH signaling networks and divergent FGF effects. Development 136: 1443–1452.

19. Hu Z, Li T, Zhang X, Chen Y (2009) Hepatocyte growth factor enhances the generation of high-purity oligodendrocytes from human embryonic stem cells. Differentiation 78: 177–184.

20. Keirstead HS, Nistor G, Bernal G, Totoiu M, Cloutier F, et al. (2005) Human embryonic stem cell-derived oligodendrocyte progenitor cell transplants remyelinate and restore locomotion after spinal cord injury. J Neurosci 25: 4694–4705.

21. Nistor GI, Totoiu MO, Haque N, Carpenter MK, Keirstead HS (2005) Human embryonic stem cells differentiate into oligodendrocytes in high purity and myelinate after spinal cord transplantation. Glia 49: 385–396.

22. Sharp J, Frame J, Siegenthaler M, Nistor G, Keirstead HS (2010) Human embryonic stem cell-derived oligodendrocyte progenitor cell transplants improve recovery after cervical spinal cord injury. Stem Cells 28: 152–163.

23. Kerr CL, Letzen BS, Hill CM, Agrawal G, Thakor NV, et al. (2010) Efficient differentiation of human embryonic stem cells into oligodendrocyte progenitors for application in a rat contusion model of spinal cord injury. Int J Neurosci 120: 305–313.

24. Hu BY, Du ZW, Zhang SC (2009) Differentiation of human oligodendrocytes from pluripotent stem cells. Nat Protoc 4: 1614–1622.

25. Tokumoto Y, Ogawa S, Nagamune T, Miyake J (2010) Comparison of efficiency of terminal differentiation of oligodendrocytes from induced pluripotent stem cells versus embryonic stem cells in vitro. J Biosci Bioeng 109: 622–628.

26. Czepiel M, Balasubramaniyan V, Schaafsma W, Stancic M, Mikkers H, et al. (2011) Differentiation of induced pluripotent stem cells into functional oligodendrocytes. Glia 59: 882–892.

27. Hatch MN, Nistor G, Keirstead HS (2009) Derivation of high-purity oligodendroglial progenitors. Methods Mol Biol 549: 59–75.

28. Totonchi M, Taei A, Seifinejad A, Tabebordbar M, Rassouli H, et al. (2010) Feeder- and serum-free establishment and expansion of human induced pluripotent stem cells. Int J Dev Biol 54: 877–886.

29. Pakzad M, Totonchi M, Taei A, Seifinejad A, Hassani SN, et al. (2010) Presence of a ROCK inhibitor in extracellular matrix supports more undifferentiated growth of feeder-free human embryonic and induced pluripotent stem cells upon passaging. Stem Cell Rev 6: 96–107.

30. Baharvand H, Ashtiani SK, Taee A, Massumi M, Valojerdi MR, et al. (2006) Generation of new human embryonic stem cell lines with diploid and triploid karyotypes. Dev Growth Differ 48: 117–128.

31. Livak KJ, Schmittgen TD (2001) Analysis of relative gene expression data using real-time quantitative PCR and the 2(-Delta Delta C(T)) Method. Methods 25: 402–408.

32. Paxinos G, Watson C (2007) The rat brain in stereotaxic coordinates. Academic Press/Elsevier 6th ed.

33. Hall SM (1972) The effect of injections of lysophosphatidyl choline into white matter of the adult mouse spinal cord. J Cell Sci 10: 535–546.

34. Woodruff RH, Franklin RJ (1999) The expression of myelin protein mRNAs during remyelination of lysolecithin-induced demyelination. Neuropathol Appl Neurobiol 25: 226–235.

35. Mozafari S, Sherafat MA, Javan M, Mirnajafi-Zadeh J, Tiraihi T (2010) Visual evoked potentials and MBP gene expression imply endogenous myelin repair in adult rat optic nerve and chiasm following local lysolecithin induced demyelination. Brain Res 1351: 50–56.

36. Idelson M, Alper R, Obolensky A, Ben-Shushan E, Hemo I, et al. (2009) Directed differentiation of human embryonic stem cells into functional retinal pigment epithelium cells. Cell Stem Cell 5: 396–408.

37. Vugler A, Carr AJ, Lawrence J, Chen LL, Burrell K, et al. (2008) Elucidating the phenomenon of HESC-derived RPE: anatomy of cell genesis, expansion and retinal transplantation. Exp Neurol 214: 347–361.

38. Hudnell HK, Boyes WK, Otto DA (1990) Rat and human visual-evoked potentials recorded under comparable conditions: a preliminary analysis to address the issue of predicting human neurotoxic effects from rat data. Neurotoxicol Teratol 12: 391–398.

39. Pfaffl MW, Horgan GW, Dempfle L (2002) Relative expression software tool (REST) for group-wise comparison and statistical analysis of relative expression results in real-time PCR. Nucleic Acids Res 30: e36.

40. Zhou Q, Wang S, Anderson DJ (2000) Identification of a novel family of oligodendrocyte lineage-specific basic helix-loop-helix transcription factors. Neuron 25: 331–343.

41. Reubinoff BE, Itsykson P, Turetsky T, Pera MF, Reinhartz E, et al. (2001) Neural progenitors from human embryonic stem cells. Nat Biotechnol 19: 1134–1140.

42. Kuhlbrodt K, Herbarth B, Sock E, Hermans-Borgmeyer I, Wegner M (1998) Sox10, a novel transcriptional modulator in glial cells. J Neurosci 18: 237–250.

43. Takebayashi H, Yoshida S, Sugimori M, Kosako H, Kominami R, et al. (2000) Dynamic expression of basic helix-loop-helix Olig family members: implication of Olig2 in neuron and oligodendrocyte differentiation and identification of a new member, Olig3. Mech Dev 99: 143–148.

44. Zhang SC (2001) Defining glial cells during CNS development. Nat Rev Neurosci 2: 840–843.

45. Zhang SC, Wernig M, Duncan ID, Brustle O, Thomson JA (2001) In vitro differentiation of transplantable neural precursors from human embryonic stem cells. Nat Biotechnol 19: 1129–1133.

46. Cai Z, Pang Y, Xiao F, Rhodes PG (2001) Chronic ischemia preferentially causes white matter injury in the neonatal rat brain. Brain Res 898: 126–135.

47. Durand B, Raff M (2000) A cell-intrinsic timer that operates during oligodendrocyte development. Bioessays 22: 64–71.

48. Brolen G, Sivertsson L, Bjorquist P, Eriksson G, Ek M, et al. (2010) Hepatocyte-like cells derived from human embryonic stem cells specifically via definitive endoderm and a progenitor stage. J Biotechnol 145: 284–294.

49. Espinosa-Jeffrey A, Wakeman DR, Kim SU, Snyder EY, de Vellis J (2009) Culture system for rodent and human oligodendrocyte specification, lineage progression, and maturation. Curr Protoc Stem Cell Biol Chapter 2: Unit 2D 4.

50. Buchet D, Baron-Van Evercooren A (2009) In search of human oligodendroglia for myelin repair. Neurosci Lett 456: 112–119.

51. Allt G, Ghabriel MN, Sikri K (1988) Lysophosphatidyl choline-induced demyelination. A freeze-fracture study. Acta Neuropathol 75: 456–464.

52. Dousset V, Brochet B, Vital A, Gross C, Benazzouz A, et al. (1995) Lysolecithin-induced demyelination in primates: preliminary in vivo study with MR and magnetization transfer. AJNR Am J Neuroradiol 16: 225–231.

53. Bull ND, Irvine KA, Franklin RJ, Martin KR (2009) Transplanted oligodendrocyte precursor cells reduce neurodegeneration in a model of glaucoma. Invest Ophthalmol Vis Sci 50: 4244–4253.

54. Einstein O, Friedman-Levi Y, Grigoriadis N, Ben-Hur T (2009) Transplanted neural precursors enhance host brain-derived myelin regeneration. J Neurosci 29: 15694–15702.

55. Gore A, Li Z, Fung HL, Young JE, Agarwal S, et al. (2011) Somatic coding mutations in human induced pluripotent stem cells. Nature 471: 63–67.

56. Zhao T, Zhang ZN, Rong Z, Xu Y (2011) Immunogenicity of induced pluripotent stem cells. Nature 474: 212–215.

15

Virotherapy using Myxoma Virus Prevents Lethal Graft-versus-Host Disease following Xeno-Transplantation with Primary Human Hematopoietic Stem Cells

Eric Bartee[1], Amy Meacham[2], Elizabeth Wise[2], Christopher R. Cogle[2], Grant McFadden[1]*

1 Department of Molecular Genetics and Microbiology, University of Florida, College of Medicine, Gainesville, Florida, United States of America, 2 Division of Hematology/Oncology, Department of Medicine, University of Florida, College of Medicine, Gainesville, Florida, United States of America

Abstract

Graft-versus-host disease (GVHD) is a potentially lethal clinical complication arising from the transfer of alloreactive T lymphocytes into immunocompromised recipients. Despite conventional methods of T cell depletion, GVHD remains a major challenge in allogeneic hematopoietic cell transplant. Here, we demonstrate a novel method of preventing GVHD by *ex vivo* treatment of primary human hematopoietic cell sources with myxoma virus, a rabbit specific poxvirus currently under development for oncolytic virotherapy. This pretreatment dramatically increases post-transplant survival of immunocompromised mice injected with primary human bone marrow or peripheral blood cells and prevents the expansion of human CD3$^+$ lymphocytes in major recipient organs. Similar viral treatment also prevents human-human mixed alloreactive T lymphocyte reactions *in vitro*. Our data suggest that *ex vivo* virotherapy with myxoma virus can be a simple and effective method for preventing GVHD following infusion of hematopoietic products containing alloreactive T lymphocytes such as: allogeneic hematopoietic stem and progenitor cells, donor leukocyte infusions and blood transfusions.

Editor: Gary P. Kobinger, Public Health Agency of Canada, Canada

Funding: This study was supported by funding to GM from National Institutes of Health R01 CA138541 and R21 CA149869 from National Cancer Institute (www.nih.gov). GM and CRC are supported by the Florida Department of Health Bankhead Coley Research Program Team Science grant 1BT02 (http://floridabiomed.com/funding_bc.html). CRC is supported by a Scholar in Clinical Research Award from the Leukemia & Lymphoma Society (www.lss.org). EB is supported by STOP! Children's Cancer, Inc (http://www.stopchildrenscancer.org/). The funders had no role in study design, data collection and analysis, decision to publish, or preparation of the manuscript.

Competing Interests: GM, EB and CRC hold IP rights for the use of MYXV to prevent GVHD. Title: METHODS FOR TREATING OR PREVENTING GRAFT VERSUS HOST DISEASE.

* E-mail: grantmcf@ufl.edu

Introduction

Graft-versus-host disease (GVHD) affects approximately 25–50% of patients receiving allogeneic hematopoietic cell transplantation (alloHCT), of which 15% will die [1,2]. In addition, GVHD occurs in approximately 1% of patients receiving high-risk blood transfusions where it is often fatal [3]. One major cause of GVHD is the transfer of mature donor CD3$^+$ T lymphocytes into an immunocompromised recipient. Once infused, a subset of alloreactive T lymphocytes recognizes recipient cellular antigens and undergo activation and amplification, resulting in an severe immunoreactive cascade which affects many internal organs, particularly the liver, gastrointestinal tract and skin [4,5].

Current methods to prevent and treat GVHD include: general immune suppression following transplant, reduced intensity conditioning, and depletion or inhibition of alloreactive donor CD3$^+$ lymphocytes prior to transfusion [6,7,8,9,10]. The clinical effectiveness of these methods, however, is limited. For example, general immune suppression leads to an increased risk of viral reactivation and other opportunistic infections, while reduced intensity conditioning regimens are associated with increased relapse [7]. Currently, the most promising prophylactic treatment for GVHD appears to be depletion or inhibition of alloreactive donor T lymphocytes prior to infusion [11,12]. This can be

accomplished through a variety of methods, including lymphoablative cytotoxic agents, specific T lymphocyte inhibitors, and antibody based selections. Unfortunately, while these methods have proven effective at lowering the rates of GVHD; they are also associated with slower reconstitution of the recipient immune system, increased risk for life-threatening infections, and reductions in the beneficial graft-versus-leukemia (GVL) effect [13,14]. There is currently no effective treatment for GVHD resulting from high risk blood transfusions [3]. Due to its frequency and severity, GVHD is currently the major factor limiting the use of alloHCT and therefore represents a significant, unresolved clinical issue for the treatment of a wide variety of diseases, including leukemias, lymphomas, bone marrow failure syndromes, and autoimmune diseases. Novel strategies to mitigate GVHD, particularly strategies that maintain the beneficial GVL effect, are therefore needed to advance transplant and transfusion technology, especially in higher risk transplant regimens such as haploidentical transplant where risks of GVHD are extremely high.

Our lab has recently demonstrated that the rabbit specific poxvirus, myxoma virus (MYXV), can be used as a novel *ex vivo* purging agent to functionally eliminate specific malignant cell populations from human HCT samples [15,16,17,18]. MYXV has several advantages as a virotherapeutic in humans. First, MYXV's natural host range is tightly restricted to rabbits and no instances of MYXV infection have been documented in any non-rabbit species, even following injection of live virus into human subjects or immunocompromised mice [19,20]. Second, MYXV binding is thought to depend on relatively ubiquitous glycosaminoglycans at the cell surface rather than specific protein entry receptors making this virus a good candidate for treating a wide variety of human cancers. In contrast, one notable cell type that myxoma virus cannot either bind or infect is normal human $CD34^+$ hematopoietic stem and progenitor cells (HSPCs), thus MYXV treatment does not alter the efficient engraftment of this cell population into immunodeficient mice [15,16,17]. Finally, the *ex vivo* application of MYXV to hematopoietic products is relatively quick and uncomplicated, making it an attractive adjunct therapy for clinical administration.

During our ongoing studies to optimize the purging of contaminating cancer cells from normal human stem cell samples, we unexpectedly observed that immunodeficient mice transplanted with MYXV-treated human hematopoietic products displayed significantly prolonged survival times compared to mock-treated transplant controls. To better understand this observation, we examined the ability of *ex vivo* MYXV treatment to functionally eliminate GVHD-inducing T lymphocytes from human alloHCT samples. Our data shows that MYXV infects a small subset of primary human $CD3^+$ lymphocytes found in both bone marrow and peripheral blood derived HCT samples. Additionally, *ex vivo* treatment of these HCT samples with MXYV delayed or eliminated development of lethal GVHD in xenotransplanted mice, while fully preserving GVL. Our results indicate that *ex vivo* treatment of HCT samples with MYXV prior to infusion shows promise as a novel method to clinically prevent development of GHVD following alloHCT.

Materials and Methods

Normal Human Cells

Fresh normal human bone marrow aspirate cells and peripheral blood mononuclear cells were obtained commercially from Lonza (Walkersville, Maryland). Bone marrow mononuclear cells (BM-MNCs) were then enriched over a Ficoll gradient using a clinical Sepax device (Biosafe Inc.) as per manufacturer's recommendations.

Myxoma virus and viral Infections

MYXV infections were carried out by incubating primary human cells with vMyx-GFP (a MYXV construct which expresses eGFP at an intergenic location in the viral genome from a synthetic viral early/late promoter [21]). Human BM-MNCs were exposed to virus at a multiplicity of infection (MOI) of 10 for 1 hour in PBS + 10% FBS in a humidified chamber at 37°C and 5% CO_2. Mock treated cells were incubated in PBS plus 10% FBS containing no virus under the same incubation conditions.

Human Stem Cell Xenografts in NSG mice

For GVHD studies, NOD/Scid/IL2Rγ$^{-/-}$ (NSG) mice were sublethally irradiated using 175 cGy total body irradiation from a Cs^{137} source. Within twenty-four hours after irradiation, mice were injected through the tail vein with $1 \times 10^6 - 10 \times 10^6$ primary human BM-MNCs or peripheral blood mononuclear cells (PBMCs) that had been either mock treated or treated with vMyx-GFP. Prophylactic antibiotics were administered in the drinking water for two weeks after transplantation to prevent opportunistic bacterial infection. Mice showing evidence of post-transplant disease were sacrificed if they reached a body condition score of 2 according to [22] in accordance with approved

University of Florida IACUC protocol 201105023. Surviving mice were euthanized six weeks after transplantation and bone marrow was harvested. Human hematopoietic cell engraftment was quantified using flow cytometry (BD FACSCaliber) for human $CD45^+$ and HLA-A, B, C^+ cells. Mice were scored as engrafted if flow cytometry confirmed populations of cells present in bone marrow that were human $CD45^+$/HLA-A, B, C^+ double positive. The number of $CD45^+$/HLA-A, B, C^+ cells in each bone marrow sample is presented as level of engraftment. Lineage analysis of engrafted cells was determined by co-staining extracted murine bone marrow with the following antibodies: HLA-APC, CD3-PE, CD19-FitC, CD15-PerCP.

Immunohistochemistry

Analysis of infiltration of human $CD3^+$ lymphocytes into murine peripheral tissues was accomplished by surgically removing six tissues post mortem: lung, liver, kidney, spleen, skin, and intestine. Tissues were fixed in 10% formalin buffered with PBS for 24 hours and then washed in 70% ethanol for an additional 24 hours. Five-micron sections of formalin-fixed, paraffin-embedded blocks were cut and picked-up onto plus charged slides (Fisher Scientific). Slides were deparaffinized and rehydrated through a series of xylenes and graded alcohols and blocked in 3% peroxide/methanol for 10 minutes at room temperature. Heat mediated antigen retrieval was performed in Citra buffer pH 6.0 for 25 minutes. This was immediately followed by blocking with normal goat serum and avidin/biotin using a commercially available kit (Vector Labs). Rabbit anti-huCD3 was applied to the sections at 1:100 overnight at 4°C. Staining was completed using an ABC-Elite kit (Vector Laboratories). The antigen-antibody complex was observed by reaction with DAB (Vector Labs) and slides were counterstained with hematoxylin prior to coverslipping.

Magnetic bead cell sorting

$CD3^+$ and $CD34^+$ human cells were fractionated from primary human BM-MNCs using the $CD3^+$ (Cat#130-050-101) and $CD34^+$ (Cat#130-046-702) microbead separation kits from Miltenyi Biotec as per manufacturer's recommendations. Cells were then positively selected on an autoMACS pro separator (Miltenyi Biotec) as per manufacturer's recommendations. The relative purity of each fractionated population was confirmed after separation using flow cytometry. The total number of fractionated cells was determined after separation using a hemocytometer.

Human:Human Mixed Lymphocyte Reaction Assays

1×10^6 SEPAX purified human BM cells were plated in triplicate into each well of a 96-well plate. Cells were then irradiated using 1000 cGy from a Cs^{137} source to create replication incompetent feeder cells. BM-MNCs cells from a second HLA-mismatched donor were either mock-treated or treated with MYXV and then 1×10^6 cells were plated in triplicate into empty wells or wells containing irradiated feeder cells. At the indicated time points, the total number of viable cells in each well was determined using a commercial MTT assay (Pierce) as per manufacturer's recommendations.

Graft-versus-Leukemia Studies

To pre-establish cancer niches in the bone marrow of mice prior to transplant of human HCT samples, non-irradiated NSG mice were injected through the tail vein with 1×10^6 human multiple myeloma cells (U266 cell line expressing the HLA-A2.1 haplotype). Two weeks after injection of the myeloma cells, mice were sublethally irradiated and injected with 10×10^6 human BM-MNCs cells that had been either mock treated or treated with vMyx-GFP as described above. Six weeks after transplant of human BM-MNCs, surviving mice were euthanized and bone marrow was harvested. Levels of human hematopoietic cell engraftment and pre-existing U266 myeloma load were distinguished and quantified using flow cytometry (BD FACSCaliber). Cells were distinguished based on expression of HLA-A, B, C, HLA-A2.1 and CD45 (hematopoietic stem cell progeny are HLA-A, B, C^+/HLA-A2.1$^-$/CD45$^+$ while U266 myeloma cells are HLA-A, B, C^+/HLA-A2.1$^+$/CD45$^-$).

Statistical Analysis

Statistical differences between different experimental groups were determined by log-rank and Student's t-test. The reported values represent the mean plus or minus the standard error of the mean. A P value of less than 0.05 was considered statistically significant.

Ethic Statement

All animal work in this study was carried out in strict accordance with the recommendations in the Guide for the Care and Use of Laboratory Animals of the National Institutes of Health. The protocol was approved by the University of Florida Institutional Animal Care and Use Committee (Protocol Number: 201105023).

Results

MYXV binds and infects a subset of CD3$^+$ cells

Chahroudi et al have previously demonstrated that vaccinia virus, a related poxvirus from a distinct genus, infects a subset of CD3$^+$ lymphocytes found in human peripheral blood [23]. To determine whether MYXV might also infect CD3$^+$ lymphocytes found in HCT samples, primary human BM-MNCs (Figure 1A) or primary human PBMCs (Figure 1B) were incubated with vMyx-GFP at MOI = 10. After 24 hours, cells were washed, stained with anti-CD3, anti-CD4 and anti-CD8 antibodies, and analyzed using flow cytometry. Successful infection of lymphocytes was readily detected by expression of GFP encoded by vMyx-GFP. Consistent with previous reports for vaccinia virus [23], MYXV infection was observed in a small subset of CD3$^+$ lymphocytes ranging from 1% to 15%, depending on the patient. No significant preference was observed for infection of CD4$^+$ vs CD8$^+$ lymphocytes in individual patient samples (data not shown).

MYXV treatment prevents lethal GVHD following xenotransplant of human BM-MNCs

A previous report indicated that vaccinia virus preferentially infects mature CD3$^+$ lymphocytes, compared to naïve T cells [23]. Since mature CD3$^+$ T lymphocytes are thought to be a major driver of GVHD, we wanted to examine whether treatment with MYXV could prevent development of GVHD in a murine model of allo-HCT. We therefore injected sublethally irradiated NSG mice with either normal human BM-MNCs or PBMCs, which are known to cause a highly lethal form of xeno-GVHD [24]. In our study, 50–70% of sub-lethally irradiated NSG mice transplanted with healthy human BM-MNCs developed a lethal wasting disease by 4–6 weeks after transplant (Figure 2A and 2B). This disease was not observed in irradiated mock-injected control mice or in irradiated mice injected with established cancer cell lines but was consistently observed following injection of primary BM obtained from three distinct healthy donors (Figures S1 and Table S1). Similar results were observed in mice infused with human PBMCs

from two distinct donors (Figure 3). Consistent with these mice developing GVHD, post-mortem histology of diseased mice revealed significant edema as well as infiltration of human CD3$^+$ T lymphocytes into several organs, including the liver, intestines, skin, lung, kidney and spleen (Figures 2C and S1). In sharp contrast, mice injected with normal human BM or PBMCs which had been pretreated ex vivo with MYXV universally survived without evidence for any obvious disease (Figures 2 and 3). Additional post-mortem histology revealed that mice injected with MYXV-treated BM displayed virtually no infiltration of human CD3$^+$ T lymphocytes into any major internal organ (Figures 2C and S1). These data suggest that ex vivo pretreatment of allo-HCT samples with MYXV prior to transplant might prevent the subsequent development of GVHD.

Xeno-GVHD results from transfusion of human CD3$^+$ lymphocytes

Our in vivo experiments indicate that MYXV can prevent GVHD after xeno-transplant of either human BM-MNCs or PBMCs. While allo-reactive donor CD3$^+$ lymphocytes are the primary cause of human GVHD, other cell types, such as NK cells or CD34$^+$, might play a role in the development of GVHD in the murine xeno-transplant model. We therefore wished to confirm that CD3$^+$ lymphocytes were the population causing disease in our xeno-transplant model. To accomplish this, we used immuno-magnetic enrichment or depletion of CD3$^+$ T lymphocytes or CD34$^+$ HSPC from primary human BM. Consistent with T lymphocyte-mediated acute GVHD, mice xenotransplanted with either positively selected CD3$^+$ lymphocytes or BM depleted of CD34$^+$ cells succumbed to GVHD with kinetics similar to mice transplanted with unfractionationed BM (Table S1). In contrast, mice transplanted with BM depleted of CD3+ lymphocytes or positively selected CD34+ HSPCs failed to develop GVHD (Table S1). In all cohorts, NSG mice transplanted with enriched or depleted human cells pretreated with MYXV universally survived and presented no evidence of GVHD (Table S1).

MYXV prevents in vivo expansion of transfused human CD3$^+$ cells

Consistent with our previous observations [16], pretreatment of human hematopoietic stem cell grafts with MYXV did not significantly alter the proportion of mice achieving human hematopoietic cell engraftment six weeks after transplant (Figure 4A). However, mice transplanted with ex vivo MYXV treated whole BM did display a non-significant trend towards decreased numbers of total human repopulating cells in the BM (Figure 4B). In contrast, while all mice transplanted with CD34$^+$ depleted BM or CD3$^+$ selected cells also showed evidence of engrafted human cells in the bone marrow six weeks after transplant, the levels of these cells was significantly reduced by MYXV treatment (Figure 4C and 4D). Unlike the engraftment pattern of unselected BM or CD34+ selected stem cells, lineage analysis of bone marrow from mice transplanted with CD34-depleted samples revealed significant T lymphocyte skewing (Figure 4F). A similar trend was observed in mice transplanted with normal donor PBMCs, which contain CD3$^+$ lymphocytes but virtually no CD34$^+$ HSPCs (data not shown). In mice transplanted with ex vivo MYXV treated CD34$^+$ HSPCs, on the other hand, we observed no reduction in the percentage of human hematopoietic cells in the bone marrow (Figure 4E) and lineage analysis revealed multi-lineage engraftment with B lymphocyte skewing typically seen xeno-transplanted immunocompromised mice (Figure 4F). These data show that ex vivo MYXV treatment of human HCT

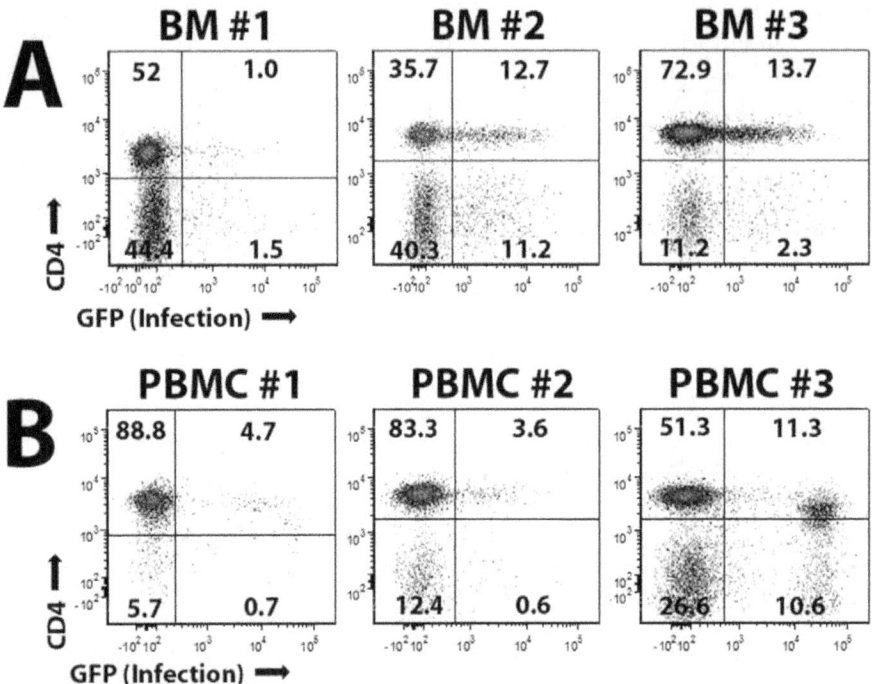

Figure 1. MYXV infects a subset of primary human CD3$^+$ lymphocytes. To determine if MYXV can infect CD3$^+$ lymphocytes found in human HCT samples, 1×10^6 whole BM cells (**A**) or 1×10^6 human PBMCs (**B**) were treated with vMyx-GFP at MOI = 10. Twenty-four hours after MYXV exposure, cells were stained with antibodies against CD3 and CD4 and the levels of GFP$^+$ cells in each population was determined using flow cytometry.

samples does not impair normal human HSPC engraftment in immunocompromised recipients but selectively inhibits expansion of transferred donor CD3$^+$ lymphocytes in the transplant recipient.

MYXV inhibits human:human haplo-mismatched mixed-lymphocyte-reactions

Since our *in vivo* data used a human-mouse xeno-expansion based GVHD model, we next wanted to confirm that MYXV treatment also prevented expansion of reactive cells in human:human allo-mismatched one-way mixed lymphocyte reactions (MLR). BM samples from three different donors were either mock-treated or treated with MYXV and then incubated with lethally irradiated BM feeder cells derived from an independent donor. Expansion of viable allo-reactive cells was measured at the indicated times by measuring total ATP generation using the commercial MTT assay. We found that mock-treated human BM showed a significant increase in viable cells when added to lethally irradiated HLA-mismatched human feeder cells, indicative of a typical alloreactive MLR. In contrast, pre-treatment of BM from all three test donors with MYXV prevented this MLR proliferation (Figure 5) suggesting that MYXV could also prevent expansion of allo-reactive cells from primary human BM samples when stimulated with mismatched human tissue samples.

MYXV treatment does not abrogate beneficial graft-versus-leukemia

Adoptive transfer of mature CD3$^+$ cells contained in alloHCT samples has been shown to improve patient prognosis through the highly beneficial GVL effect where alloreactive donor T cells engage in clearance of minimal residual disease that survived prior conditioning therapy [13,14]. Unfortunately, the most common

method for preventing GVHD, complete elimination of CD3$^+$ lymphocytes, also eliminates the potential for GVL. Since MYXV treatment efficiently prevented GVHD while only directly infecting a small subset of the total CD3$^+$ lymphocytes in the transplant sample, we questioned whether MYXV might selectively prevent GVHD while still permitting GVL. We therefore tested the effectiveness of the MYXV *ex vivo* purging strategy using a transplant model that measures both GVL and GVHD. Initially, non-irradiated NSG mice were injected with human multiple myeloma U266 cells and the myeloma cells were allowed to establish for two weeks. Mice were then sublethally irradiated and infused with human BM-MNCs that had either been mock-treated or treated with MYXV. Mice were observed for evidence of GVHD and mice meeting endpoint criteria were euthanized accordingly. Six weeks after injection of BM, surviving mice that had not succumbed to GVHD were euthanized and their BM analyzed for engraftment of any remaining residual myeloma as well as the expanded progeny of the HSPCs from the donor BM (Figure 6). Consistent with our previous findings, progeny of the donor HSPCs were readily observed in the BM of mice injected with normal human BM and the level of this engraftment was not significantly reduced by pretreatment of the BM with MYXV. Also consistent with our previous findings, 55% (11/20) mice transplanted with untreated human BM died from GVHD while none of the mice (0/20) transplanted with MYXV pretreatment human BM suffered any signs of GVHD. Control mice that had been pre-seeded to carry residual myeloma, sub-lethally irradiated, and then transplanted with saline showed significant remaining residual myeloma load demonstrating that the sublethal irradiation used to permit efficient BM engraftment did not clear the pre-existing myeloma niches in the mouse bone marrow. Injection of free MYXV virions alone caused no significant long term effects on existing myeloma load in the bone marrow, supporting the

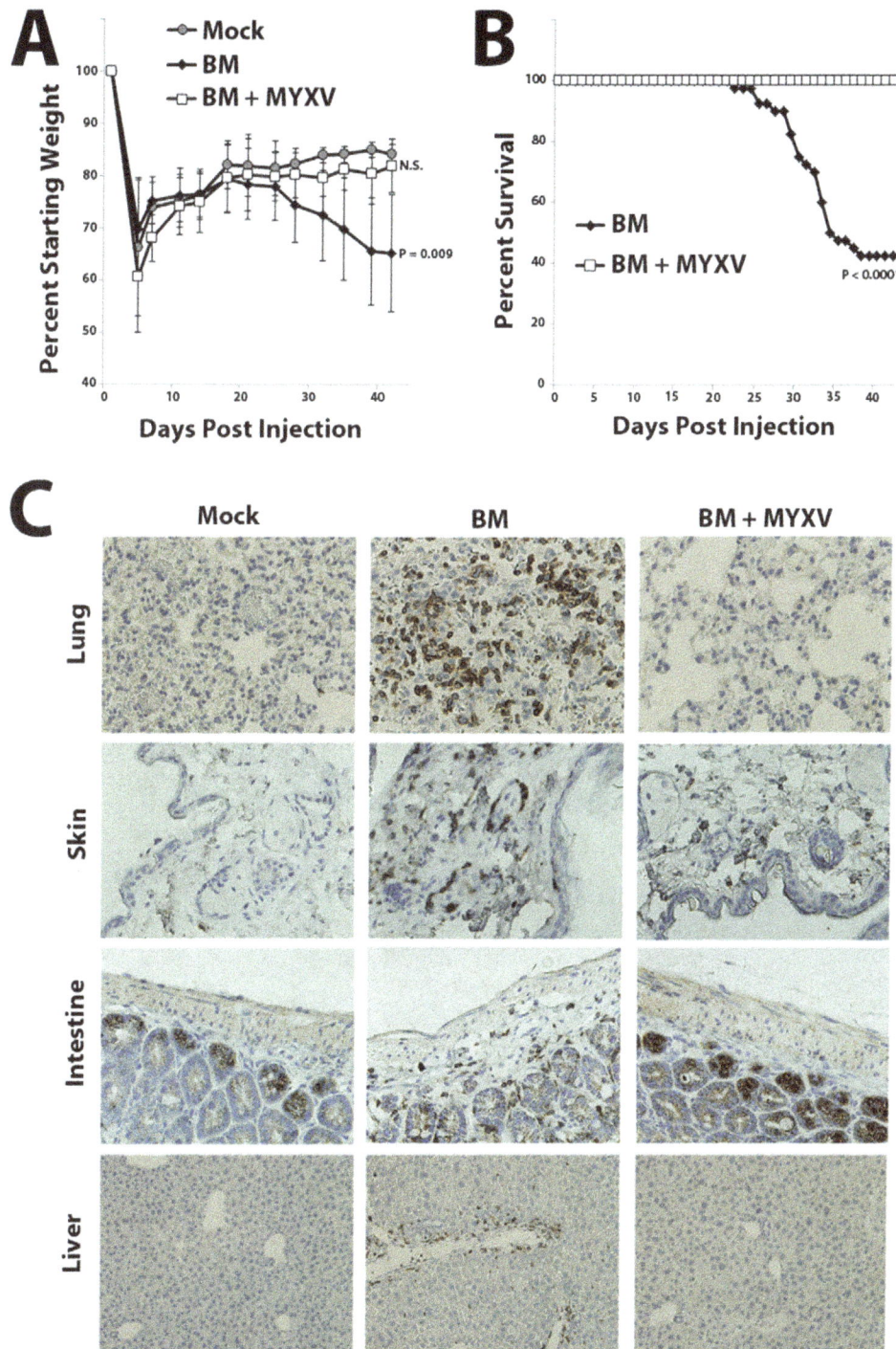

Figure 2. MYXV-treatment prevents lethal GVHD in immunodeficient mice following infusion of primary human BM. NSG mice were sublethally irradiated and then transplanted with either PBS (mock, n = 5), 1×10^7 primary human BM (n = 36) or 1×10^7 primary human BM pre-treated with MYXV (n = 36). Mice were weighed twice per week to monitor body condition (**A**) and sacrificed either six weeks after transplant or when their body condition score measured 2 (**B**). Significant differences in survival were determined using the log-rank test (P<0.05). N.S. = not significant. Post-mortem, organs were extracted, fixed in formalin, sectioned and stained for the presence of infiltrating human CD3+ lymphocytes (**C**). Immunohistochemistry images shown are representative of results observed in five separate mice from the three engrafted cohorts stained for the presence of human CD3+ cells.

expectation that most of the IV-administered virus does not reach the bone marrow. Mice pre-seeded with human multiple myeloma cells, sublethally irradiated, and then transplanted with untreated BM-MNCs showed no signs of remaining cancer six weeks after transplant, indicating that the GVL effect of the donor transplant BM was highly effective at clearing pre-existing myeloma in the bone marrow in this model. Despite this beneficial effect, 50% (10/20) of mice in this cohort died from GVHD. This cohort

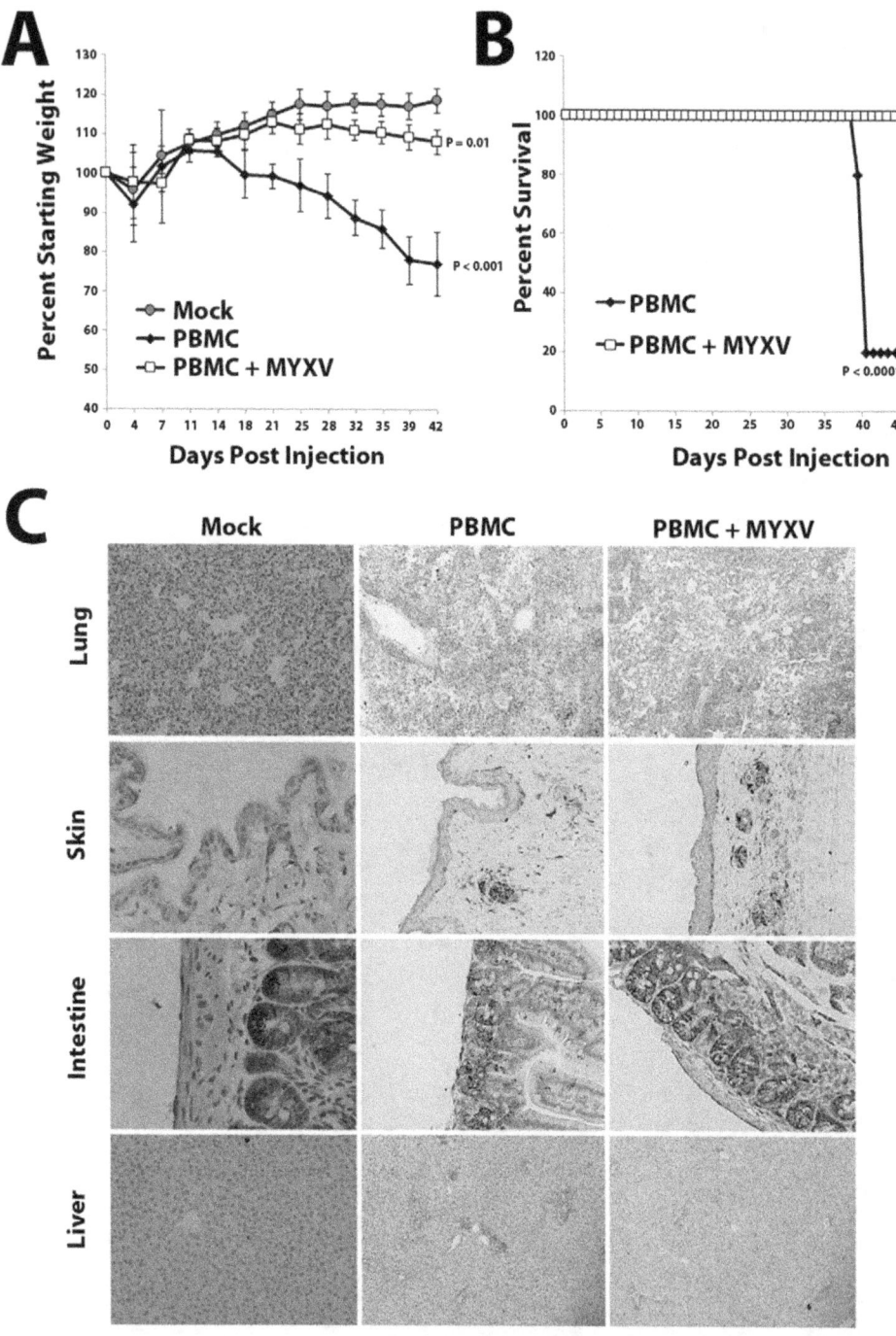

Figure 3. MYXV-treatment prevents lethal GVHD in immunodeficient mice following infusion of primary human PBMCs. NSG mice were sublethally irradiated and then transplanted with either 5×10^6 primary human PBMCs (n = 6) or 5×10^6 primary human PBMCs pre-treated with MYXV (n = 6). Mice were weighed twice per week to monitor body condition (**A**) and sacrificed either seven weeks after transplant or when their body condition score measured 2 (**B**). Significant differences in survival were determined using the log-rank test (P<0.05). N.S. = not significant. Post-mortem, organs were extracted, fixed in formalin, sectioned and stained for the presence of human CD3$^+$ lymphocytes (**C**). Immunohistochemistry images shown are representative of results observed in three separate mice from the three engrafted cohorts stained for the presence of human CD3$^+$ cells.

represents the current clinical scenario of allogeneic transplant for high risk hematological malignancies. Results from this cohort also show that the presence of residual myeloma in the recipient bone marrow does not affect the development of GVHD. In the MYXV treatment cohort, only 1/20 (5%) mice showed evidence of cancer in the mouse bone marrow six weeks after injection, suggesting

that *ex vivo* treatment of the human donor BM with MYXV did not inhibit the ability of this treated BM to elicit a potent GVL effect. Importantly, none of these mice (0/20) showed evidence of GVHD. Together, these results show that *ex vivo* MYXV treatment of human BM effectively prevents GVHD while still preserving beneficial GVL.

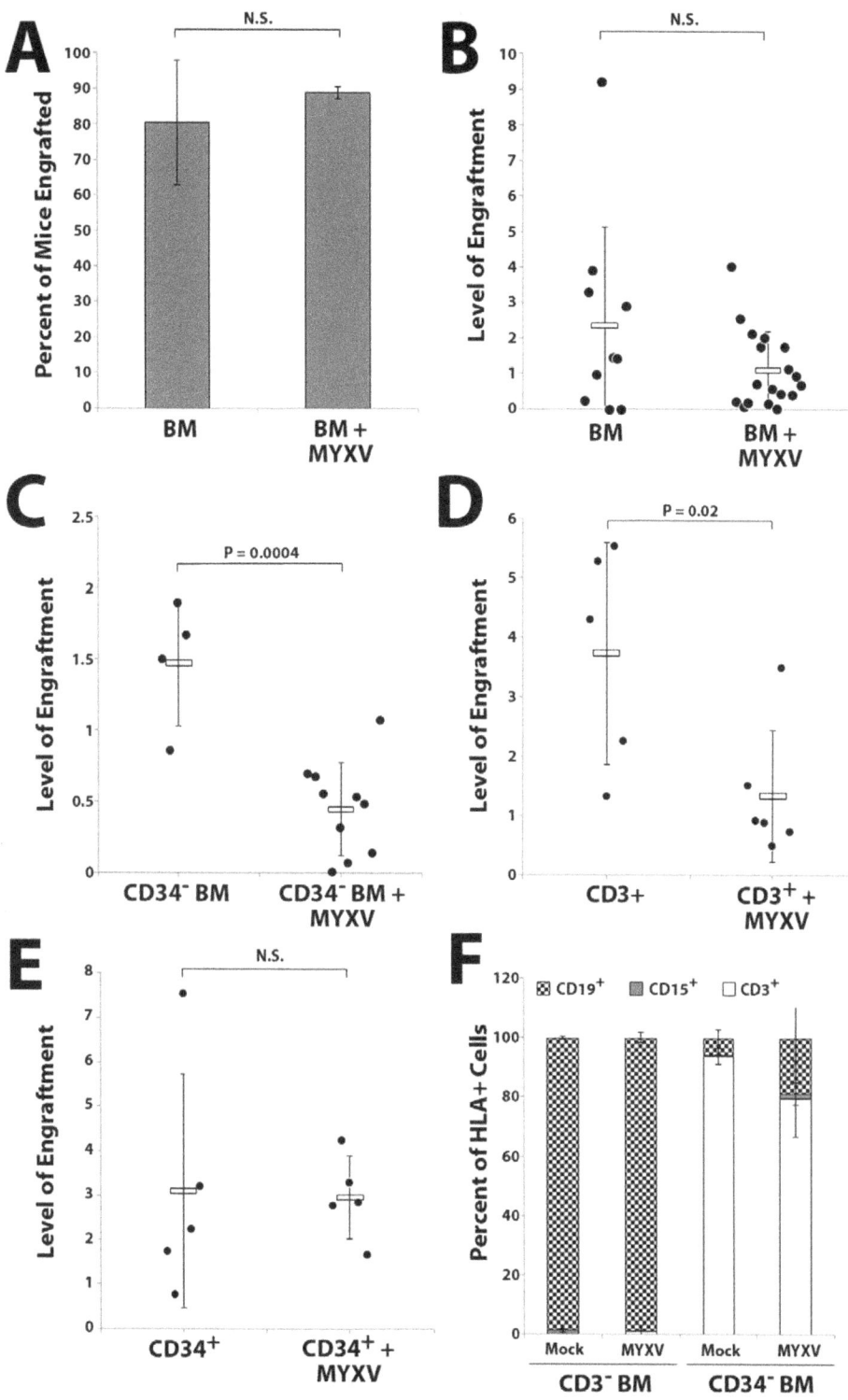

Figure 4. MYXV treatment prevents in vivo expansion of human donor T lymphocytes after transplant into immunodeficient mice while sparing engraftment of normal HSPCs. NSG mice were sublethally irradiated and transplanted with 1×10^7 whole human BM cells. Six weeks after transplant, bone marrow from mice was harvested and analyzed for human hematopoietic engraftment (human CD45+/HLA-A, B, C+ double positive cells) by flow cytometry. Treatment with MYXV did not alter the proportion of animals with successful human hematopoietic engraftment (**A**) but did slightly reduce the total numbers of engrafted human cells in mouse bone marrow, which did not reach statistical significance (**B**). Irradiated mice transplanted with 1×10^7 CD34-depleted BM (**C**) or 1×10^6 human CD3+ cells (**D**) displayed lower overall levels of engraftment and this engraftment was significantly reduced by *ex vivo* MYXV-treatment. Irradiated mice transplanted with 1×10^5 CD34+ selected human cells showed levels of human cell engraftment similar to those observed in mice transplanted with whole human BM. Levels of human cell engraftment were not affected by *ex vivo* MYXV-treatment (**E**). Significance was determined using Student's t-test (P<0.05). N.S = not significant. Lineage of engrafted cells was determined by staining HLA-A, B, C+ cells from murine BM with antibodies against human CD3, CD15, or CD19 (**F**).

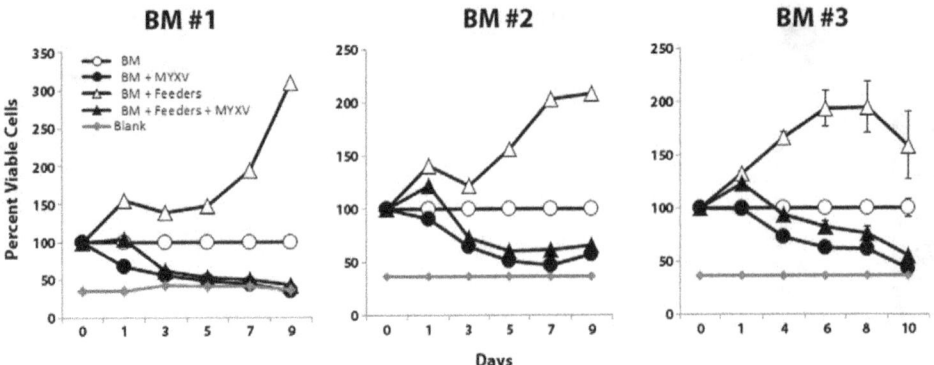

Figure 5. MYXV treatment prevents alloreactive human:human mixed lymphocyte expansion. To determine if MYXV inhibited expansion of allo-reactive human cells in HCT samples following human/human allo-stimulation in a mixed lymphocyte reaction assay, mock-treated or MYXV-treated human BM cells were incubated for 10 days with irradiated HLA-mismatched human feeder cells. Mock-treated BM stimulated with irradiated feeder cells showed significantly increased numbers of viable cells while MYXV-treated BM did not.

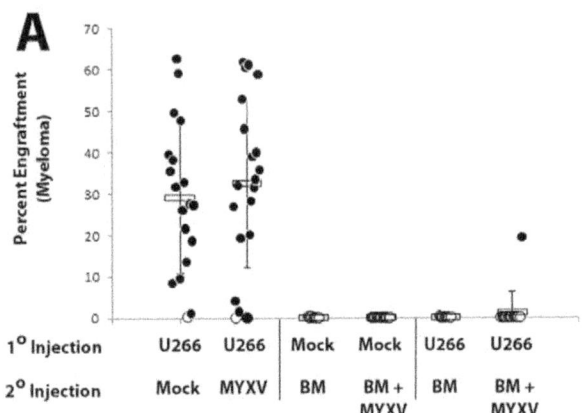

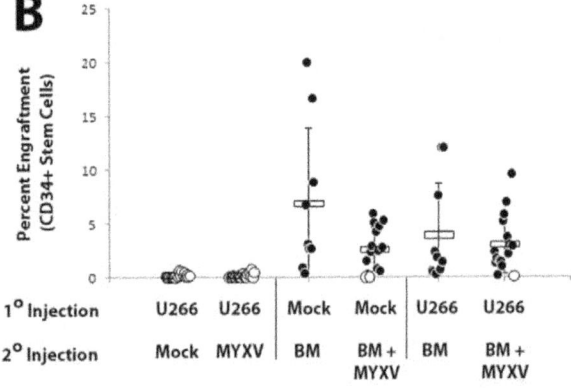

Figure 6. *Ex Vivo* MYXV treatment prevents GVHD while still preserving GVL. NSG mice either naïve or carrying preexisting U266 myeloma were sublethally irradiated and injected with 10×10^6 human donor BM cells that had been either mock treated or treated with vMyx-GFP. Mice were monitored for signs of GVHD for six weeks after which BM was harvested from surviving mice and the levels of both pre-existing U266 myeloma load (**A**) and normal human HSC engraftment (**B**) were quantified using flow cytometry. Cells can be distinguished based on expression of HLA-A, B, C, HLA-A2.1 and CD45 (hematopoietic stem cell progeny are HLA-A, B, C^+/HLA-A2.1$^-$/CD45$^+$ while U266 myeloma cells are HLA-A, B, C^+/HLA-A2.1$^+$/CD45$^-$).

Discussion

Previously, we demonstrated that *ex vivo* MYXV treatment prevents engraftment of primary human acute myeloid leukemia and multiple myeloma cells into NSG mice while sparing the engraftment of normal human HSPCs [16,17]. Based on this evidence, we proposed MYXV as a novel virotherapeutic agent for purging cancer cells that contaminate autologous hematopoietic stem cell grafts [15,25]. The data in this report present an entirely novel application of this *ex vivo* MYXV purging strategy, namely the prevention of GVHD by purging alloreactive T cells from allogeneic transplant samples, which should prove to be applicable for clinical settings such as alloHCT, donor leukocyte infusions and high-risk blood product transfusions. This is the first report of using an intact replicating virus to selectively prevent development of an allo-immune disease.

Various T lymphocyte purging methods, including positive or negative cell separations as well as treatment with specific cytotoxic agents have been previously employed to delete alloreactive T cells in order to improve alloHCT for treatment of hematologic malignancies. These methods, however, carry high risks of life-threatening infections due to delayed immunologic recovery and graft failure [13,14]. In contrast, our data show that MYXV treatment *ex vivo* appears to have no adverse effects on normal human HSPC engraftment, which is related to the inability of this virus to bind or infect normal human CD34$^+$ hematopoietic stem cells [15,17,18]. However, this same *ex vivo* MYXV treatment results in infection of a subset of alloreactive CD3$^+$ T lymphocytes, while still allowing for the adoptive transfer of sufficient functional T lymphocytes into the recipient for beneficial GVL effects. Additionally, the *ex vivo* MYXV treatment strategy requires only a single, brief virus adsorption step prior to donor graft infusion, which could be performed with minimal changes in current good tissue practice clinical conditions (our unpublished observation and [16]). Therefore, translating this new observation into a clinical setting will not require significant deviation from the current standard of care for alloHCT, donor leukocyte infusions and high-risk blood product transfusions.

It should be noted that purging of alloreactive T lymphocytes from alloHCT samples is a fundamentally similar process to purging cancer cells from autologous hematopoietic cell grafts. Both are based on the ability of the purging agent (in this case, a virus that does not infect normal human HSPCs) to distinguish the disease-inducing cells (either contaminating cancer cells in autologous grafts or resident alloreactive donor T lymphocytes in allogeneic grafts) from the normal stem cells whose immune-reconstituting functions must be maintained (in this case CD34$^+$ HSPCs). While the mechanism of MYXV's ability to discriminate alloreactive CD3$^+$ T lymphocytes from HSPCs requires further investigation; our preliminary observations suggests that the safety of MYXV in terms of human hematopoietic engraftment is based on a failure of MYXV to physically bind to normal human CD34$^+$ HSPCs [17,18]. Due to the extremely broad nature of poxvirus binding for most mammalian cells [26] this suggests that MYXV might be an effective purging agent for functionally deleting a wide variety of deleterious non-stem cells from hematopoietic grafts, possibly including various classes of donor B and T lymphocytes as well as contaminating cancer cells from a wide variety of hematopoietic malignancies.

Interestingly *ex vivo* MYXV virus treatment completely abrogated CD3$^+$ lymphocyte driven GVHD in 100% of xeno-transplanted animals and also prevented alloreactive human:human MLR reactions *in vitro* despite the fact that only a small, and highly variable (ranging from 2% to 25%, depending on the donor), subset of human donor CD3$^+$ lymphocytes were detectably infected by MYXV, as measured by the ability to express virus-encoded EGFP. Since GVHD is highly dependent on the infused dose of donor CD3$^+$ lymphocytes [27,28], it initially appears contradictory that MYXV could block development of disease while only infecting as little as 1% of potentially disease-causing T cells. While the molecular mechanism(s) through which MYXV prevents GVHD will require further investigation, we can envision several scenarios whereby infection of only a subset of the total CD3$^+$ lymphocyte population could lead to highly efficient protection from disease. For example, it is possible that MYXV might prevent GVHD by specifically infecting a minor subset of CD3$^+$ lymphocytes essential for development of GVHD, such as those alloreactive T lymphocytes that actually respond to allo-antigens and proliferate in the recipient post-transplant. In a similar fashion, specific CD3$^+$ subsets important for disease development, such as T$_{regs}$, or NKT lymphocytes, could also be preferentially infected. Alternatively, MYXV might bind to a higher fraction of the total T lymphocyte population but only result in measurable GFP$^+$ infection once these cells are activated, which could happen rapidly upon exposure to recipient allo-antigens following infusion. This latter hypothesis is supported by the observation that a related poxvirus, vaccinia virus, infects activated T lymphocytes at a much greater frequency than naïve T lymphocytes [23]. This explanation could also provide a potential mechanism for the ability of MYXV *ex vivo* treatment of the donor graft to prevent GVHD while sparing GVL: for example, transplant cells causing GVHD would be activated (and infected) immediately following infusion whereas cells responsible for GVL would first have to home to the murine BM before activation was initiated. Similar to what we have observed in various human myeloid leukemia cells [18], adsorption of MYXV might also inhibit T lymphocyte expansion even in the absence of fully permissive viral infection (monitored as GFP expression).

The low levels of MYXV infection observed in donor T lymphocytes are consistent with the modest levels of infection observed in several other primary hematopoietic cell types found in human BM or PBMCs, including: CD15$^+$ granulocytes, CD34$^+$ hematopoietic stem and progenitor cells, and platelets (data not shown). In contrast, much higher levels of MYXV infection were observed in professional antigen presenting cells, such as CD19$^+$ B lymphocytes and CD14$^+$ monocytes (data not shown). Therefore, it is formally possible that MYXV inhibits the development of GVHD through blocking or altering the presentation of recipient

tissue antigens. However, the infusion of purified CD3$^+$ lymphocytes fully reconstituted GVHD disease and MYXV treatment of just these cells was fully protective (Table S1), and thus we feel that this model is less likely.

Finally, development of GVHD in this xenograft model requires systemic irradiation prior to infusion of CD3$^+$ lymphocytes (Table S1). This is similar to what is observed in human patients who have undergone myeloablative therapy and suggests that systemic inflammation might promote the development of disease. MYXV encodes several known secreted anti-inflammatory proteins that inhibit myeloid cells, such as the SERP1 glycoprotein that is currently in clinical trial to inhibit systemic inflammation associated with myocardial disease (ADD REF: Tradiff et al, 2011). Therefore, it is also possible that MYXV blocks development of GVHD through a systemic indirect mechanism.

Whether the protective effects of MYXV treatment against GVHD reported in this study are specific to treatment with MYXV, or could be duplicated using other oncolytic viruses, remains unknown. However, any other candidate oncolytic virus would also have to be fully innocuous against CD34$^+$ HSPCs in order to be acceptable as a purging agent. In the case of MYXV, this safety is explained because MYXV neither binds nor infects human CD34$^+$ HSPCs [16,17].

It should also be noted that there are also a variety of autoimmune disorders caused by specific subsets of dysregulated immune cells (such as B cells, NK cells, etc) which could in theory be treated using ablative chemotherapy combined with hematopoietic transplants. However, a treatment regimen involving autologous HSPC transplantation can be complicated by disease-causing immune cells remaining in the patient autograft which can potentially mediate disease relapse. It seems likely that a virus which specifically infects the immune cell type that mediates the disease could also be used as a purging agent to remove potentially allo-reactive/disease-causing immune cells from hematopoietic transplant samples prior to infusion, thus preventing disease relapse. Additional work is obviously needed to address both these issues.

In any event, *ex vivo* MYXV virotherapy prior to infusion of allogeneic hematopoietic cells offers not only the prospect of preventing the onset of GVHD and reducing the risks of severe post-transplant GVHD, but also permits the opportunity for transplant of allogeneic grafts with greater HLA disparity such as that from mismatched unrelated donors and haploidentical donors, thereby potentially opening up alloHCT therapies to a greater number of patients with cancer or autoimmune diseases.

Supporting Information

Figure S1 Development of GVHD is consistently observed between various human bone marrow donors. NSG mice were sublethally irradiated and then transplanted with 1×10^7 human BM cells from three different donors (**A**). Mice were weighed twice per week to monitor body condition and sacrificed either six weeks post-injection or when they reached a body condition score of 2. Significant differences in survival were determined using the log-rank test (P<0.05). Post-mortem, organs were extracted, fixed in formalin, sectioned and stained for the presence of human CD3$^+$ lymphocytes (**B**). Immunohistochemistry images shown are representative of results observed in five separate mice.

Table S1 Development of GVHD in xeno-transplanted mice requires human CD3$^+$ lymphocytes in the donor graft sample. Sublethally irradiated NSG mice were transplanted with various human hematopoietic cell products and each cohort was observed for 6–8 weeks after transplant. Mice were sacrificed when their body condition score measured 2 (reported as death). Significance between survival of mice in the irradiated mock injected cohort and other cohorts was determined using the log-rank test (P<0.05). NS = not significant. N/A = not applicable.

Acknowledgments

We thank Sherin Smallwood for preparing the IACUC protocols, and Dorothy Smith for preparing virus stocks for the study.

Author Contributions

Conceived and designed the experiments: EB GM. Performed the experiments: EB. Analyzed the data: EB GM. Contributed reagents/materials/analysis tools: EB AM EW GM CRC. Wrote the paper: EB CRC GM. Provided access to human specimens: CRC.

References

1. Choi SW, Levine JE, Ferrara JL (2010) Pathogenesis and management of graft-versus-host disease. Immunol Allergy Clin North Am 30: 75–101.
2. Pasquini M, Wang Z (2009) Current use and outcome of hematopoietic stem cell transplantation: CIBMTR Summary Slides, 2010.
3. Anwar M, Bhatti FA (2003) Transfusion associated graft versus host disease. J Ayub Med Coll Abbottabad 15: 56–58.
4. Ferrara JL, Levine JE, Reddy P, Holler E (2009) Graft-versus-host disease. Lancet 373: 1550–1561.
5. Socie G, Blazar BR (2009) Acute graft-versus-host disease: from the bench to the bedside. Blood 114: 4327–4336.
6. Blazar BR, Korngold R, Vallera DA (1997) Recent advances in graft-versus-host disease (GVHD) prevention. Immunol Rev 157: 79–109.
7. Paczesny S, Choi SW, Ferrara JL (2009) Acute graft-versus-host disease: new treatment strategies. Curr Opin Hematol 16: 427–436.
8. Maeda Y, Levy RB, Reddy P, Liu C, Clouthier SG, et al. (2005) Both perforin and Fas ligand are required for the regulation of alloreactive CD8+ T cells during acute graft-versus-host disease. Blood 105: 2023–2027.
9. O'Shaughnessy MJ, Vogtenhuber C, Sun K, Sitcheran R, Baldwin AS, et al. (2009) Ex vivo inhibition of NF-kappaB signaling in alloreactive T-cells prevents graft-versus-host disease. Am J Transplant 9: 452–462.
10. Davies JK, Barbon CM, Voskertchian AR, Nadler LM, Guinan EC (2011) Induction of Alloantigen-specific Anergy in Human Peripheral Blood Mononuclear Cells by Alloantigen Stimulation with Co-stimulatory Signal Blockade. J Vis Exp.
11. Li JM, Giver CR, Lu Y, Hossain MS, Akhtari M, et al. (2009) Separating graft-versus-leukemia from graft-versus-host disease in allogeneic hematopoietic stem cell transplantation. Immunotherapy 1: 599–621.
12. Murphy WJ, Blazar BR (1999) New strategies for preventing graft-versus-host disease. Curr Opin Immunol 11: 509–515.
13. Martin PJ, Hansen JA, Torok-Storb B, Durnam D, Przepiorka D, et al. (1988) Graft failure in patients receiving T cell-depleted HLA-identical allogeneic marrow transplants. Bone Marrow Transplant 3: 445–456.
14. Delain M, Cahn JY, Racadot E, Flesch M, Plouvier E, et al. (1993) Graft failure after T cell depleted HLA identical allogeneic bone marrow transplantation: risk factors in leukemic patients. Leuk Lymphoma 11: 359–368.
15. Rahman MM, Madlambayan GJ, Cogle CR, McFadden G (2010) Oncolytic viral purging of leukemic hematopoietic stem and progenitor cells with Myxoma virus. Cytokine Growth Factor Rev 21: 169–175.
16. Kim M, Madlambayan GJ, Rahman MM, Smallwood SE, Meacham AM, et al. (2009) Myxoma virus targets primary human leukemic stem and progenitor cells while sparing normal hematopoietic stem and progenitor cells. Leukemia 23: 2313–2317.
17. Bartee E, Chan WS, Moreb JS, Cogle CR, McFadden G (2012) Selective purging of human multiple myeloma cells from autologous stem cell transplant grafts using oncolytic myxoma virus. Biol Blood Marrow Transplant.
18. Madlambayan GJ, Bartee E, Kim M, Rahman MM, Meacham A, et al. (2012) Acute myeloid leukemia targeting by myxoma virus in vivo depends on cell binding but not permissiveness to infection in vitro. Leuk Res 36: 619–624.
19. Fenner F, Ratcliffe FN (1965) Myxomatosis. Cambridge, UK: Cambridge University Press.
20. Stanford MM, McFadden G (2007) Myxoma virus and oncolytic virotherapy: a new biologic weapon in the war against cancer. Expert Opin Biol Ther 7: 1415 1425.
21. Johnston JB, Barrett JW, Chang W, Chung CS, Zeng W, et al. (2003) Role of the serine-threonine kinase PAK-1 in myxoma virus replication. J Virol 77: 5877–5888.
22. Ullman-Cullere Foltz (1999) LAboratory Animal Science. 49: 3: 319–323.
23. Chahroudi A, Chavan R, Kozyr N, Waller EK, Silvestri G, et al. (2005) Vaccinia virus tropism for primary hematolymphoid cells is determined by restricted expression of a unique virus receptor. J Virol 79: 10397–10407.
24. Ito R, Katano I, Kawai K, Hirata H, Ogura T, et al. (2009) Highly sensitive model for xenogenic GVHD using severe immunodeficient NOG mice. Transplantation 87: 1654–1658.
25. Bais S, Bartee E, Rahman MM, McFadden G, Cogle CR (2011) Oncolytic virotherapy for hematological malignancies. Adv Virol 2012: 186512.
26. Moss B (2007) Poxviridae: the viruses and their replication (fifth ed.). In: Howley DMKaPM, editor. Fields Virology. New York Lippincott, Williams & Wilkins. p. 2849–2855.
27. Chao N (2012) Control of GVHD: it's in our DNA! Blood 119: 1102–1103.
28. Chao N (2008) Are there effective new strategies for the treatment of acute and chronic GvHD? Best Practice & Research Clinical Haematology 21: 93–98.

16

Genetic or Pharmaceutical Blockade of Phosphoinositide 3-Kinase P110δ Prevents Chronic Rejection of Heart Allografts

Huijun Ying[1♪], **Hongmei Fu**[1♪], **Marlene L. Rose**[2], **Ann M. McCormack**[2], **Padmini Sarathchandra**[2], **Klaus Okkenhaug**[3], **Federica M. Marelli-Berg**[1*¤]

1 Department of Immunology, Division of Medicine, Imperial College London, Hammersmith Campus, London, United Kingdom, **2** National Heart & Lung Institute, Division of Medicine, Imperial College London, Harefield Hospital, London, United Kingdom, **3** Laboratory of Lymphocyte Signalling and Development, Babraham Institute, Cambridge, United Kingdom

Abstract

Chronic rejection is the major cause of long-term heart allograft failure, characterized by tissue infiltration by recipient T cells with indirect allospecificity. Phosphoinositol-3-kinase p110δ is a key mediator of T cell receptor signaling, regulating both T cell activation and migration of primed T cells to non-lymphoid antigen-rich tissue. We investigated the effect of genetic or pharmacologic inactivation of PI3K p110δ on the development of chronic allograft rejection in a murine model in which HY-mismatched male hearts were transplanted into female recipients. We show that suppression of p110δ activity significantly attenuates the development of chronic rejection of heart grafts in the absence of any additional immunosuppressive treatment by impairing the localization of antigen-specific T cells to the grafts, while not inducing specific T cell tolerance. p110δ pharmacologic inactivation is effective when initiated after transplantation. Targeting p110δ activity might be a viable strategy for the treatment of heart chronic rejection in humans.

Editor: Paolo Madeddu, Bristol Heart Institute, University of Bristol, United Kingdom

Funding: This work was entirely funded by the British Heart Foundation (Grants PG/07/090/23697 and RG/09/002). The funders had no role in study design, data collection and analysis, decision to publish, or preparation of the manuscript.

Competing Interests: The authors have declared that no competing interests exist.

* E-mail: f.marelli@imperial.ac.uk

♪ These authors contributed equally to this work.

¤ Current address: William Harvey Research Institute, Heart Centre, Charterhouse Square, London, United Kingdom

Introduction

Chronic rejection is the main cause of late heart allograft failure and the leading cause of death in patients surviving more than 1 year after transplantation [1,2]. Prominent features of chronic heart graft rejection include proximal coronary artery vasculopathy, occlusion, and eventually loss of cardiac function [1–3]. These lesions are associated with substantial parenchymal infiltration by T cells [4]. Host immunity – particularly indirect alloresponses mediated by CD4[+] T cells, as well as antibody-mediated immune responses – to processed fragments of donor major histocompatibility antigens (MHC) and to minor histocompatibility antigens (mHC) have been linked to the development of chronic heart allograft rejection [5–15].

Besides antigen-induced activation, the development of immune responses requires active mechanisms of recruitment of antigen-specific primed T cells into antigenic sites. We and others have shown that T cell receptor (TCR) engagement by antigen-presenting endothelium leads to the migration of antigen-specific memory T cells to non-lymphoid antigen-rich target tissue following priming [16–20]. This effect is required for the development of a number of T cell-mediated diseases in mice [20–22]. The effect of TCR ligation on T lymphocyte motility is likely to engage signaling

pathways linking TCR triggering to the cytoskeleton. Class IA phosphoinositide 3-kinases (PI3Ks) are a family of p85/p110 heterodimeric lipid kinases that generate second messenger signals (e.g., PIP3) downstream of tyrosine kinases, thereby controlling various cell functions, including motility. PI3K p110δ subunit expression is restricted to hematopoietic cells [23]. Following TCR triggering, p110δ is recruited by adaptor proteins [24,25]. Previous studies have shown that mice expressing a catalytically inactive form of p110δ (P110δ[D910A]) display attenuated T cell-mediated immunity, although p110δ[D910A] mice can be primed against nominal antigens [26]. We have recently shown that, while chemotaxis and constitutive trafficking of memory T lymphocytes with impaired p110δ activity are unaffected, these T cells are not susceptible to TCR-mediated T cell recruitment to antigenic sites, which they fail to infiltrate [21].

In this study, we have investigated the effect of PI3K p110δ inactivation on the development of chronic rejection in a murine model of HY-mismatched heart allograft. We show that the establishment of chronic rejection is significantly attenuated in mice lacking p110δ activity in the absence of any additional immunosuppressive treatment. The therapeutic effects of p110δ inhibition correlated with impaired localization of HY-specific memory T cells to the allografts, but did not induce T cell tolerance. Importantly, PI3K p110δ pharmacologic inactivation is effective even when initiated after transplantation. We propose that selective PI3K p110δ inhibitors can be developed into an effective therapeutic tool to control chronic heart allograft rejection.

Results

Genetic abrogation of PI3K p110δ–signaling prevents T-cell-mediated chronic heart allograft rejection

PI3K p110δ has been shown to play a critical and non-redundant role in the activation and differentiation of naive T cells [27]. We therefore sought to investigate the effect of inhibition of PI3K p110δ signaling on the development of immune-mediated mechanisms of chronic heart allograft rejection. A well-established model involving transplantation of HY-mismatched heart allografts, in which grafts develop pathological features of chronic rejection over time [28], was adapted for this study. Development of pathology in this model is strictly T cell-dependent, antibody-independent [29], and occurs without cessation of the heartbeat [28]. For this reason, histopathologic assessments, rather than survival time points, are provided.

Recipient female WT and p110δ^{D910A} mutant mice (bearing an inactive form of p110δ [26]) received either male (antigenic) or female (non-antigenic control) WT hearts. 23 days after transplant, both transplanted and native hearts were harvested and stained with hematoxilin/eosin (HE, representative images in Figure S1), and Miller's elastin combined with SMC alpha actin immuno-staining (Figure 1A). This time point was selected based on previous monitoring of pathology development (data not shown) and license constraints.

As it is shown in Figure 1, heart allografts placed into p110δ^{D910A} female recipients were protected from the development of vasculopathy as assessed by histopathologic criteria. Co-staining of elastine end SMC alpha actin revealed early signs of vasculopathy (narrowing of the lumen and perivascular proliferation of SMC [30]) in female WT recipient of male hearts, which was inhibited in p110δ^{D910A} female recipients (Figure 1A–B). HE staining of the tissues revealed severe inflammatory lesions in WT female recipients of male hearts, which were significantly attenuated in p110δ^{D910A} female recipients (Figure 1C and Figure S1). Female graft and native hearts were free of disease.

Graft infiltration by T cells and macrophages was assessed by immunostaining with FITC-conjugated anti-CD3 and PE-conjugated anti-MAC2 antibodies. As shown in Figure 1D (representative tissue images from each group) and Figure 1E (mean T cell infiltration ± SD), T cell infiltration of male heart grafted into female p110δ^{D910A} mutants was significantly reduced compared with that observed in transplanted male heart grafted into WT female recipients. No difference in T cell infiltration of either female-derived heart grafts or native hearts was observed. Interestingly, no significant difference in the number of infiltrating macrophages was observed in any of the combinations tested. Although p110δ has been shown to affect B cell chemotaxis [31], these data suggest that T cell p110δ activity is selectively targeted in this model, in which the development of chronic rejection is strictly T cell-dependent and B cell-independent [28].

PI3K p110δ inhibition does not induce T cell tolerance

PI3K p110δ has been reported to contribute to T-cell activation and differentiation [23,26]. We therefore sought to investigate whether the lack of PI3K p110δ activity led to loss of responsiveness by HY-specific T cells following transplantation. Splenocytes from female WT and p110δ^{D910A} recipients were harvested 23 days after heart transplantation. T cells were

cultured with increasing concentrations of *Dby* or *Uty* HY epitope peptides for 48 hours, followed by assessment of thymidine incorporation. As shown in Figure 2, both WT and p110δ^{D910A} T cells proliferated in response to HY-derived peptides, suggesting that antigen-specific T cell responsiveness was maintained in mice which did not develop chronic rejection as a result of PI3K p110δ inactivation.

PI3K p110δ is required for male heart graft infiltration by HY-specific T cells

Antigen presentation by graft endothelium has previously been shown to be instrumental to T cell infiltration and rejection of HY-mismatched allografts [21,28].

Given that PI3K P110δ inactivation did not lead to antigen-specific T cell tolerance, we sought to investigate whether the protective effect of abrogation of PI3K p110δ signaling selectively prevented antigen-dependent T cell recruitment to HY-mismatched heart graft. C57BL/6 female mice received a syngeneic male (HY-mismatched) or female (non-antigenic) heart transplant. On day 15 post-heart-grafting (i.e. once a memory T cell response is physiologically established[32]), PKH26-labelled HY-specific H2-A^b-restricted CD4$^+$ WT and CFSE-labeled HY-specific H2-A^b-restricted p110δ^{D910A} CD4$^+$ T cells (10^7/mouse) were injected *i.v.* into female recipients of a WT male heart. The presence of labeled T cells in both transplanted and native hearts was analyzed 24 hours later by wide-field fluorescence microscopy.

As shown in Figure 3, WT T cells promptly infiltrated male (A) but not female-derived (B) heart grafts, while p110δ^{D910A} T cell localization to male transplanted hearts was significantly reduced (A). These results demonstrated that PI3K p110δ activity is required for efficient access of HY-specific T cells to male heart grafts. Interestingly, some T cell infiltration was observed in native hearts of both WT and p110δ^{D910A} recipients of male hearts, possibly driven by non-specific inflammation induced by the allograft, which was nevertheless unable to induce pathology.

PI3K p110δ is not required for constitutive trafficking by memory HY-specific T cells

We have previously suggested that lack of p110δ activity specifically affects antigen-driven migration, but not constitutive memory T cell trafficking [21]. The chronic rejection model allowed us to investigate whether this observation holds true in the presence of inflammation. We therefore assessed the migration of HY-specific T cells in sites of constitutive homing in C57BL/6 female recipients of a syngeneic male heart. On day 15 post-grafting, PKH26-labelled HY-specific H2-A^b-restricted CD4$^+$ WT and CFSE labeled HY-specific H2-A^b-restricted p110δ^{D910A} T cells (10^7/mouse) were injected *i.v.* into female recipients of a WT male heart. T cell localization in the liver, kidney, lymph node, spleen and gut were assessed 24 hours later by wide-field fluorescence microscopy.

As shown in Figure 4, both WT and p110δ^{D910A} T cells re-circulated normally and could be detected in the liver, kidney, lymph node, and spleen of recipient mice in similar numbers. Notably, WT and p110δ^{D910A} T cells displayed similar patterns of distribution within the various organs and localized in the liver and kidney in a scattered pattern, while they clustered in restricted areas in lymph nodes. Some T cell infiltration was observed in native hearts, irrespective of p110δ activity. These observations further confirm that p110δ signaling selectively regulates T cell migration to tissues that do express cognate antigen and it is not required for constitutive trafficking of T cells.

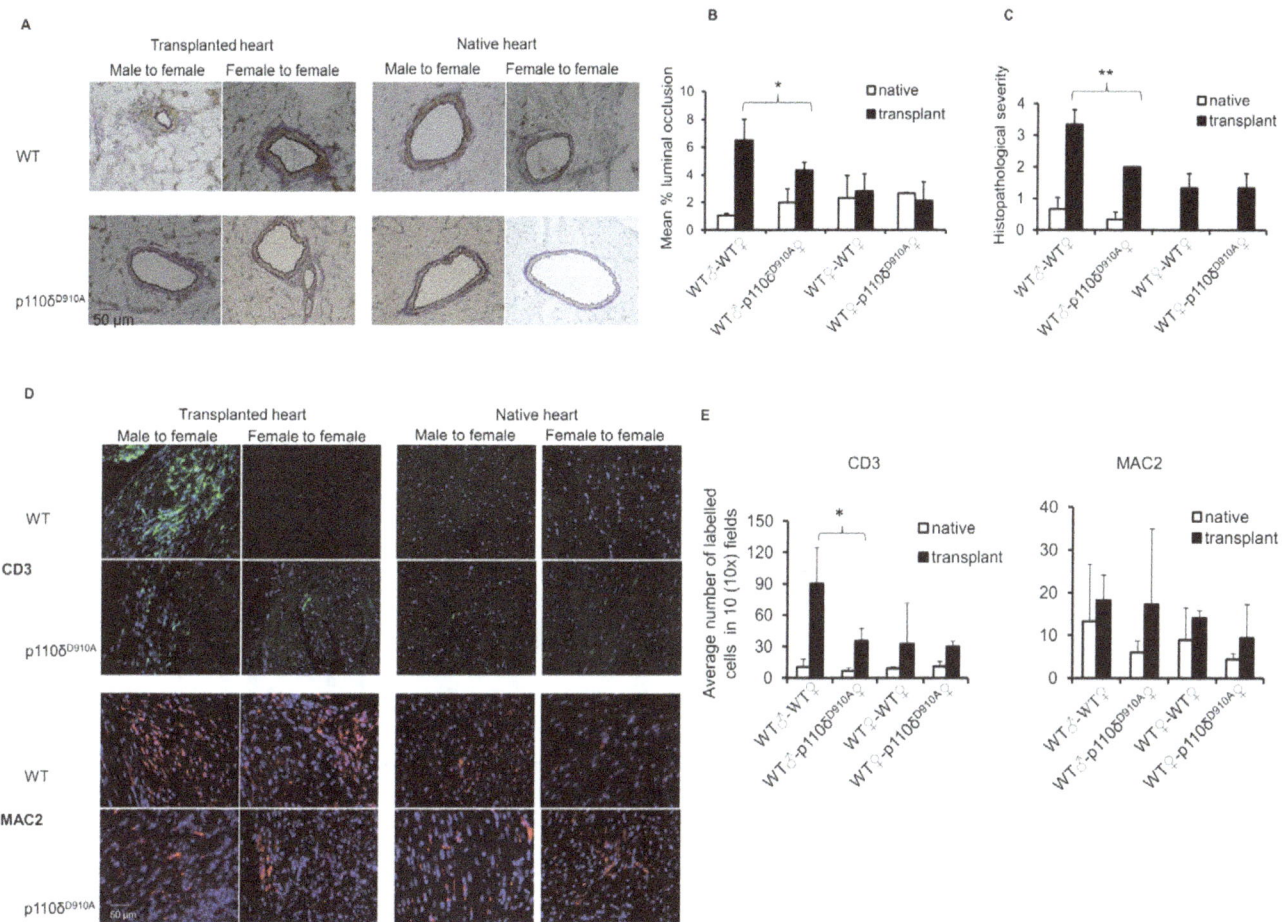

Figure 1. Genetic abrogation of PI3K p110δ signaling prevents T-cell-mediated chronic heart allograft rejection. Recipient female WT and p110δ^D910A mutant mice received either male or female heart. Both transplanted and native hearts were harvested 23 days after transplant. (A) Tissue sections were stained with Miller's elastin followed by immunoperoxidase staining for SMCs using rabbit monoclonal antibody to mouse SMC alpha -actin, then counterstained with hematoxylin. Luminal occlusion was evaluated by tracing the cross-section of each vessel's internal elastic lamina and lumen using software in two transverse sections per graft. Each panel shows a representative tissue image. Magnification: 20x. (B) The mean percentage luminal occlusion ± SD observed in 3 samples obtained from each recipient (at least 3 animals/group) is shown. *p<0.03 (C) The mean histopathological scores ± SD of transplanted hearts stained with HE observed in 3 samples obtained from each recipient (at least 3 animals/group) is shown. 0, no inflammation; 1, light focal lymphohistocytic infiltrate; 2, moderate focal lymphohistocytic infiltrate with myocardial involvement; 3, moderate to severe inflammation with focal vasculopathy and myocyte degeneration; 4, severe inflammation, vasculopathy and myocardial fiber loss. **p<0.01. (D) Tissue sections were stained with FITC-labelled anti-CD3 antibody and PE-labelled anti-MAC2 antibody. Each panel shows a representative tissue image. Magnification: 20x. (E) The mean T cell or macrophage infiltration ± SD observed in 3 samples obtained from each recipients (at least 3 animals/group) is shown. *p<0.05.

Pharmacologic inhibition of PI3K p110δ in HY-mismatched heart allograft recipients inhibits the development of chronic heart allograft rejection

We have previously shown that PI3K p110δ inhibition selectively targets memory T cell trafficking [21]. This opens the possibility that targeting PI3K p110δ might be effective in a therapeutic regime. We therefore investigated whether pharmacologic inactivation of PI3K P110δ delivered after transplantation at a time when the immune response is already established could prevent the development of chronic rejection. Recipient female WT mice received either syngeneic male or female heart grafts. After 7 days, the selective PI3K p110δ inhibitor IC87114 (60mg/kg/day) or vehicle control was administered i.p. daily for 15 days. Mice were sacrificed 24 hours after the last treatment (day 23). Both transplanted and native hearts were harvested for analysis.

As it is shown in figure 5A, histological analysis showed that treatment with PI3K p110δ inhibitor IC87114 prevented the development of pathological signs of chronic rejection (representative images are depicted in Figure S2 panel A). Similarly, T cell infiltration of male heart grafted into WT female mice treated with IC87114 was significantly reduced compared to that observed in transplanted male heart grafted into WT recipient female mice treated with vehicle control (Figure 5B and Figure S2 panel B). No significant differences in T cell infiltrates were observed in either female-to-female transplanted heart grafts or native hearts. Macrophage infiltrates were often observed, but were of similar magnitude in any donor to recipient combination tested, irrespective of the development of pathology.

Similarly to what we observed in p110δ^D910A recipients of male hearts, T cells obtained from WT female recipients treated with or

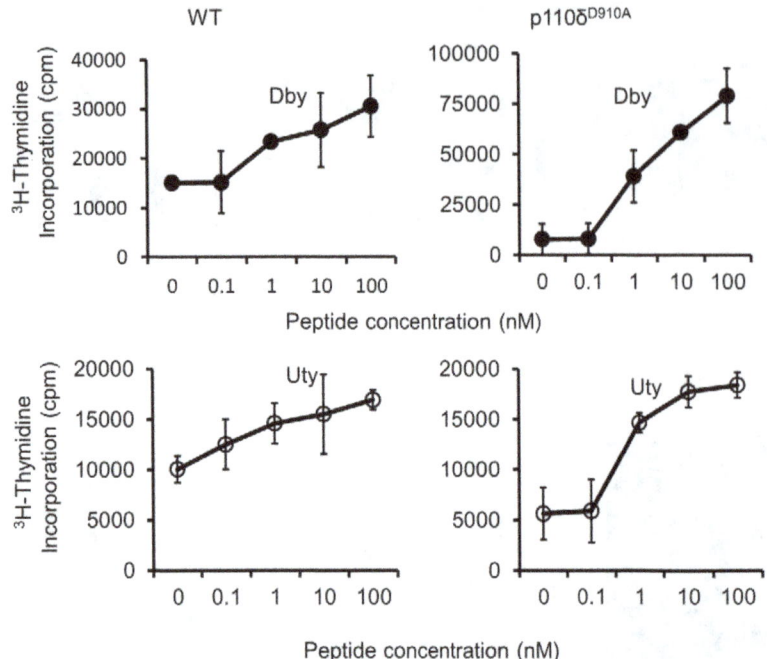

Figure 2. Loss of PI3K p110δ activity does not induce T cell tolerance. Recipient female WT and p110δ[D910A] mutant mice received male WT transplanted heart. 60 days after transplant, splenocytes from either recipient WT or p110δ[D910A] mutant mice were incubated with different concentrations of *Dby* and *Uty* HY peptide epitopes for 48 hours, followed by pulsing with [^{3}H] thymidine to assess T cell proliferation.

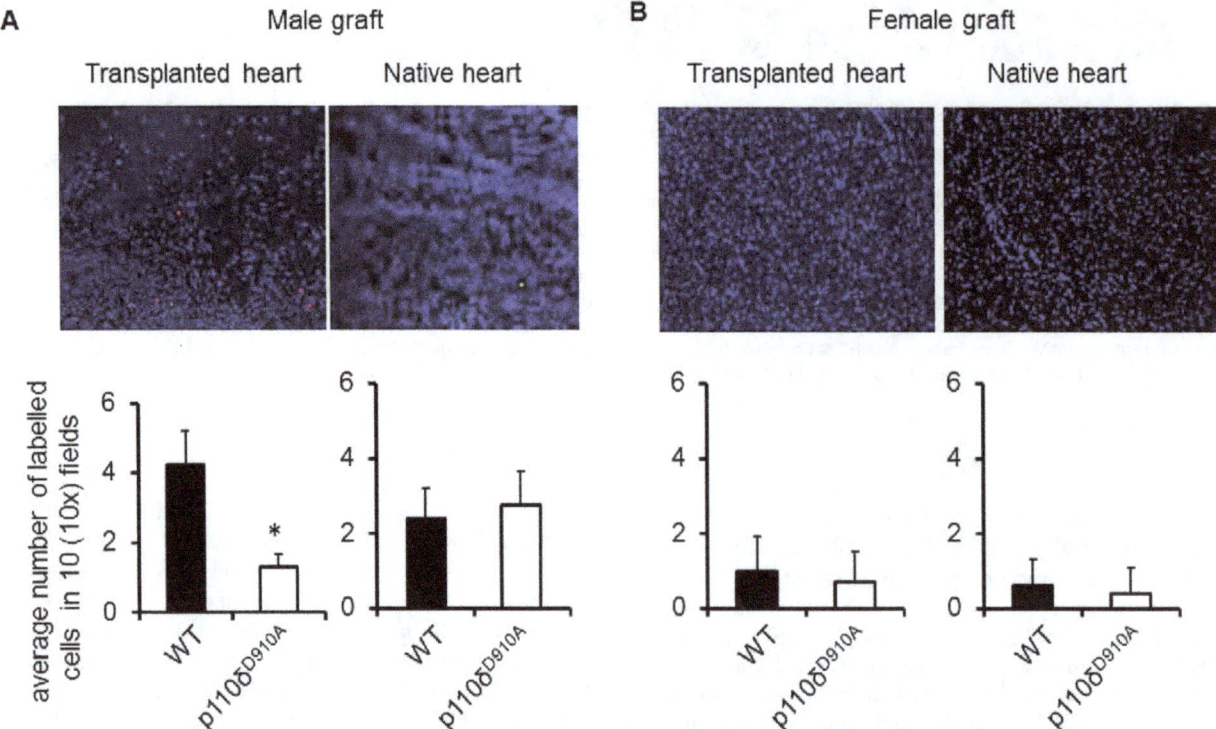

Figure 3. PI3K p110δ is required for heart graft infiltration by antigen-specific T cells. PKH26-labelled HY-specific H2-A^b-restricted CD4$^+$ WT and CFSE labelled HY-specific H2-A^b-restricted p110δ[D910A] T cells were injected *i.v.* into female mice transplanted with either male (A) or female (B) syngeneic heart. T cell localization in the transplanted heart and native heart were assessed 24 hours later by wide-field fluorescence microscopy. Tissue infiltration was quantified by randomly selecting ten ×10-magnified fields from tissue samples obtained from each mouse from all the experimental groups and assessing the number of fluorescent cells in each field. Each panel shows a representative tissue image. The mean T cell infiltration ± SD observed in samples from at least 3 animals is shown. Magnification: 10x. *$p < 0.05$.

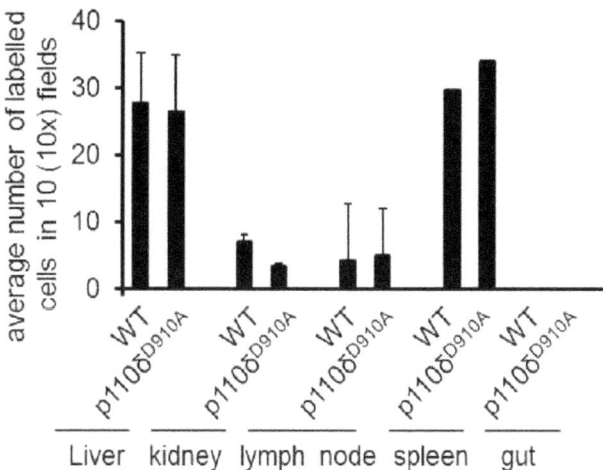

Figure 4. PI3K p110δ is not required for constitutive trafficking by antigen-specific T cells. PKH26-labelled HY-specific H2-A^b-restricted CD4^+ WT and CFSE labelled HY-specific H2-A^b-restricted p110δ^D910A T cells were co-injected *i.v.* into female mice recipient of syngeneic hearts. T cell localization in the liver, kidney, lymph node, spleen, gut and native heart were assessed 24 hours later by wide-field fluorescence microscopy. To minimize the effect of arbitrary choice of field, tissue infiltration was quantified by randomly selecting ten×10-magnified fields from tissue samples from at least 3 animals and assessing the number of fluorescent cells in each field. Each panel shows a representative tissue image. The mean T cell infiltration ± SD observed in samples from at least 3 animals is shown.

without IC87114 responded equally well to HY-derived *Dby* and *Uty* epitopes, suggesting that IC87114 treatment did not affect T cell responsiveness (Figure S3).

Finally, we sought to establish whether, like genetic inactivation, pharmacological inhibition of P110δ selectively affects localization of specific T cells to the heart allograft. Recipient female WT mice received either syngeneic male or female heart grafts. On day 15 post-heart-grafting, PKH26-labelled HY-specific H2-A^b-restricted CD4^+ WT and CD4^+ WT treated with IC87114 (5μM, 1 hour at 37°C) (10^7/mouse) were injected *i.v.* into female mice recipients of syngeneic male or female-derived hearts. The presence of labeled T cells in both transplanted and native hearts were analyzed 24 hours later by wide-field fluorescence microscopy. As shown in Figure 5C, untreated T cells promptly localized to male heart grafts, unlike CD4^+ WT T cells treated with IC87114. No difference in T cell infiltration was observed in female heart grafts or native hearts. These results suggest that pharmacologic PI3K p110δ inactivation is effective at inhibiting access of activated HY-specific T cells to mHC-mismatched heart grafts in a therapeutic regimen.

PI3K p110δ inactivation does not prevent rejection of HY-mismatched skin

Immune-mediated rejection of vascularized (heart) and non-vascularized (skin) allografts relies upon different mechanisms [21,28,33,34]. Having shown that PI3K p110δ inactivation either by genetic mutation or pharmacological inhibition resulted in inhibition of chronic rejection of male heart grafts, we assessed the effect of PI3K p110δ inactivation in a model of HY-mismatched skin transplantation. Recipient female WT or p110δ^D910A mice received WT male skin grafts, and the occurrence of rejection was monitored. Alternatively, WT female recipients of a syngeneic male skin graft were treated daily with PI3K p110δ inhibitor IC87114 at 60mg/kg/day or vehicle control 7 days after

transplantation until rejection. As it is shown in Figure 6A and 6B, neither genetic nor pharmacological inhibition of PI3K p110δ activity led to enhanced skin graft survival. Splenocytes from all groups proliferated equally well to both the HY Dby and Uty epitopes (Figure S4).

We further investigated the ability of HY-specific T cells to infiltrate skin grafts. Both male and female skins were grafted onto female recipient mice. On day 20 post-grafting, PKH26-labelled HY-specific H2-A^b-restricted CD4^+ WT and CFSE labelled HY-specific H2-A^b-restricted p110δ^D910A T cells were injected *i.v.* into recipient mice. In parallel experiment, HY-specific WT T cells were treated with IC87114 (5μM, 1 hour at 37°C) (10^7/mouse) or vehicle (DMSO) before injection. The presence of labelled T cells in skin grafts were analyzed 24 hours later by wide-field fluorescence microscopy.

As shown in Figure 7, inhibition of PI3K p110δ activity either by genetic mutation or pharmacological inhibition prevented HY-specific T cell infiltration to male skin grafts. These results suggest that rejection of non-vascularized skin grafts relies upon inflammatory mechanisms other than graft infiltration by antigen-specific T cells.

Discussion

In this study we have investigated the effect of genetic or pharmacologic inactivation of PI3K p110δ on the development of chronic allograft rejection in a murine model of mHC (HY)-mismatched heart allograft. We show that inhibition of PI3K p110δ activity significantly reduces the development of chronic rejection by inhibiting memory T cell access to the allograft.

Following activation, efficient memory T cell localization to antigen-rich sites requires a sequence of signals, mostly delivered by the endothelium, which include tissue-selective homing interactions such as those mediated by adhesion molecule and chemokine ligand to reach and access target tissue [28,35]. We and others have shown that efficient recruitment of antigen-specific T cells into antigen-rich sites with promiscuous adhesion/chemokine receptor/ligand pairs (such as the heart) is optimized by TCR triggering of specific T cells by antigen-presenting endothelium [19,20,28,36]. Importantly, this effect has been shown to support the localization of effector T cells to mHC-mismatched heart allograft leading to chronic rejection [28]. We have also reported that antigen-dependent recruitment by the endothelium strictly relies upon PI3K p110δ activity, which is initiated upon TCR triggering by MHC:peptide complexes displayed on the endothelial surface[21].

In our study, the prevention of pathological inflammation leading to chronic rejection by PI3K p110δ inhibition correlated with abrogation of antigen-specific T cell access to the transplanted heart. In contrast, loss of PI3K p110δ activity did not affect T cell priming in our system, despite evidence suggesting that this mediator is essential and non-redundant for TCR-induced activation of both naïve and memory T cells [27]. While genetic abrogation of PI3K p110δ activity might have been compensated for by alternative signaling pathways leading to T cell activation and differentiation, pharmacologic inhibition of PI3K p110δ post-priming also appears to selectively affect T cell trafficking to the heart without affecting T cell responsiveness. In the p110δ^D910A mouse, naïve CD4^+ T cell proliferation and cytokine production is particularly impaired under suboptimal stimulation conditions (e.g., in the absence of costimulation)[26]. It is possible that PI3K p110δ signals contributing to T cell activation might be dispensable when antigen is not limiting, such as in transplantation settings.

The role of macrophages in the development of allograft chronic rejection is still controversial [37–39]. In our study,

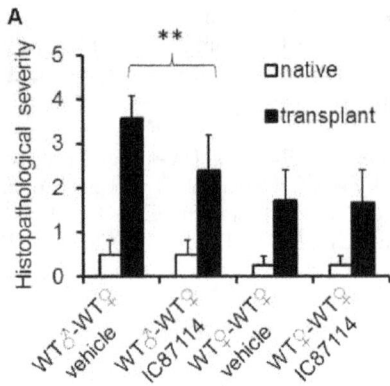

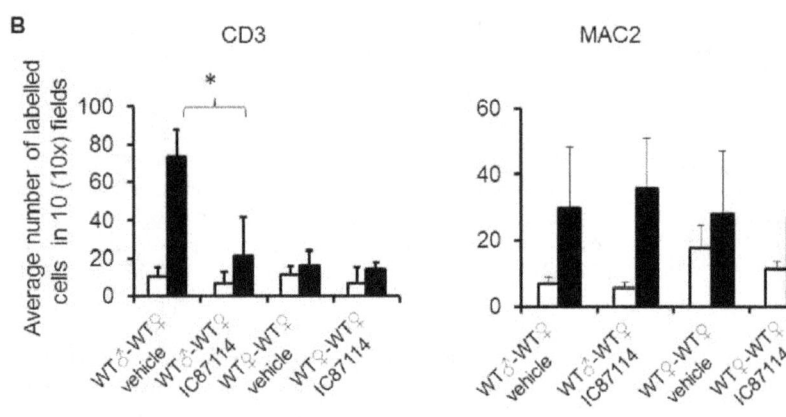

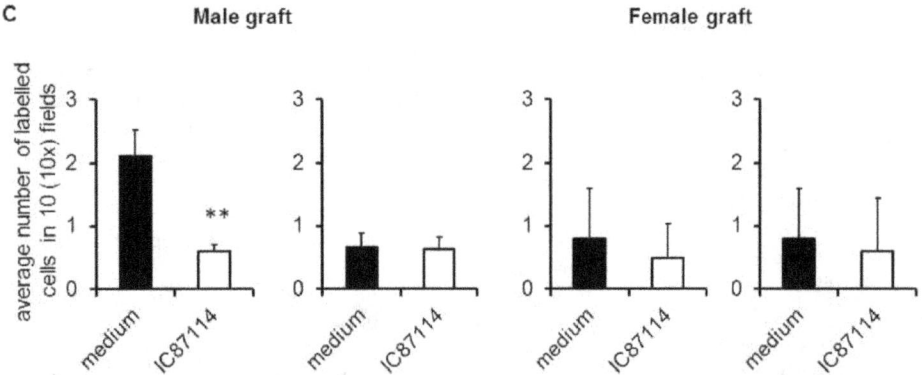

Figure 5. Pharmacologic inhibition of PI3K p110δ inhibits chronic heart rejection by preventing T cell access to the graft. Recipient female WT mice received either syngeneic male or female heart grafts. After 7 days, the selective PI3K p110δ inhibitor IC87114 (60mg/kg/day) or vehicle control were injected i.p daily for 15 days. Mice were sacrificed 24 hours after the last treatment (day 23). (A) The mean histopathological scores ± SD of transplanted hearts stained with HE observed in 3 samples obtained from each recipient (at least 3 animals/group) is shown. 0, no inflammation; 1, light focal lymphohistocytic infiltrate; 2, moderate focal lymphohistocytic infiltrate with myocardial involvement; 3, moderate to severe inflammation with focal vasculopathy and myocyte degeneration; 4, severe inflammation, vasculopathy and myocardial fiber loss. **$p<0.01$ (B) Both transplanted and native hearts were harvested and tissue sections were stained with either FITC-labelled anti-CD3 antibody or PE-labelled anti-MAC2 antibody. The mean T cell infiltration ± SD observed in samples from at least 3 animals is shown. Filled bar: transplanted heart; Non-filled bar: native heart. *$p<0.05$. (C) PKH26-labelled HY-specific H2-A^b-restricted CD4$^+$ WT and CFSE labelled CD4$^+$ WT treated with IC87114 were injected i.v. into female mice with male syngeneic heart transplantation. T cell localization in the transplanted heart and native heart were assessed 24 hours later by wide-field fluorescence microscopy. Tissue infiltration was quantified by randomly selecting ten ×10-magnified fields from tissue samples from at least 3 animals and assessing the number of fluorescent cells in each field. Each panel shows a representative tissue image. The mean T cell infiltration ± SD observed in samples from at least 3 animals is shown. **$p<0.01$.

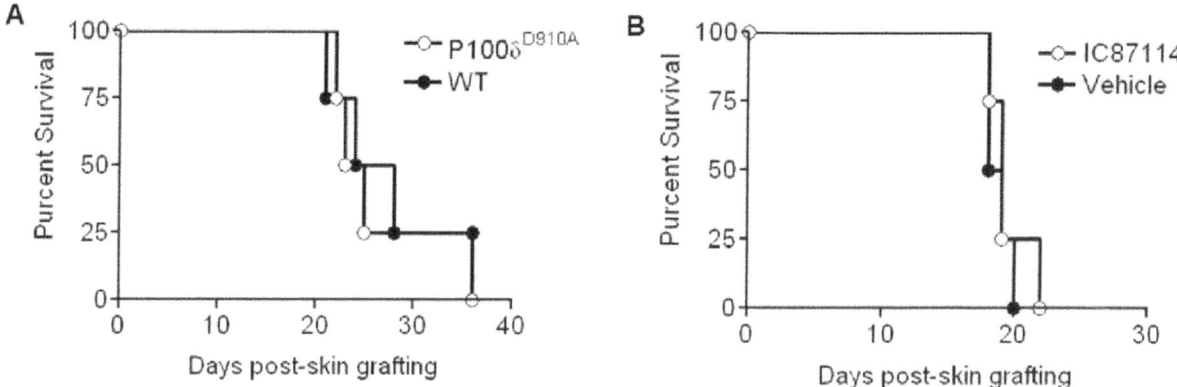

Figure 6. PI3K p110δ inactivation does not prevent rejection of HY-mismatched skin. (A) Recipient female WT or p110δ^{D910A} mice received WT male skin grafts. Graft survival was monitored daily for up to 4 weeks. (B) Recipient female WT mice received male skin grafts. 7 days after transplant, PI3K p110δ inhibitor IC87114 at 60mg/kg/day or vehicle control were injected i.p daily until the grafts were rejected.

macrophage infiltration was increased (while not always significantly) in both female (non-antigenic) and male heart transplants compared to native hearts even in the absence of PI3K p110δ signaling, suggesting that PI3K p110δ activity is not required for monocyte recruitment. However, macrophage infiltration did not affect the clinical outcome, suggesting that either macrophages do not contribute to tissue damage in chronic heart allograft rejection or that a cross talk with infiltrating T cells is necessary for macrophage-mediated pathologic effects.

PI3K p110δ inactivation did not affect HY-mismatched skin rejection, despite inhibiting adoptively transferred HY-specific effector T cell access to the skin graft. The immune responses

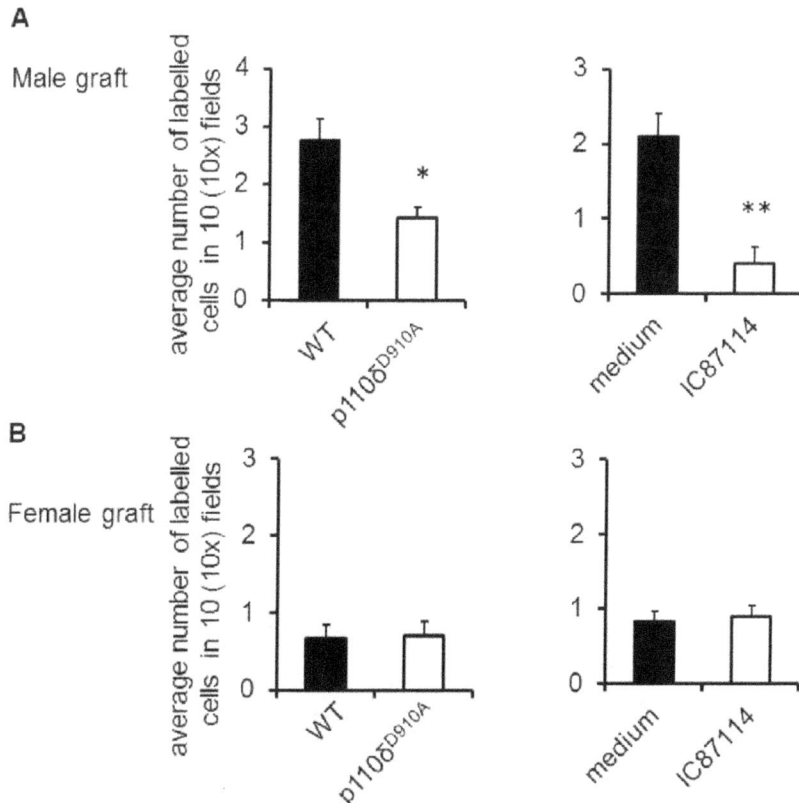

Figure 7. PI3K p110δ inactivation reduces skin graft infiltration by antigen-specific T cells. On day 20 post-skin grafting, PKH26 labelled HY-specific 10x 10^6 WT and CFSE labelled 10^7 P110δ^{D910A} T cells or WT T cells treated with PI3K p110δ inhibitor IC87114 (5µM for 1 hour at 37°C) were injected *i.v.* into recipient mice. T cell localization in male skin (A) and female skin (B) was assessed 24 hours later by wide-field fluorescence microscopy. Tissue infiltration was quantified by randomly selecting ten ×10-magnified fields from at 3 tissue samples from at least 3 animal groups and assessing the number of fluorescent cells in each field. The mean T cell infiltration ± SD observed in samples from at least 3 animals is shown. *p<0.05, **p<0.01.

against mHC antigens of skin and heart grafts have been shown to rely upon different immune mechanisms. First, HY-mismatched heart grafts develop chronic T cell infiltrates and vasculopathy over time but the organ remains viable and the heartbeat is maintained. In contrast, HY-mismatched skin grafts fail on average within 3 weeks of transplantation [28], suggesting that the graft microenvironment (size and antigen presenting cells richness) differently impacts on the strength of the alloresponse. Second, anatomical vascular connection of heart allograft to the host circulation is immediate, while connection of skin graft to the host vascular system occurs within 2–3 weeks post grafting [33,34,40], therefore T cell access to skin grafts is not regulated by endothelial barriers at least in early rejection. Additionally, heart graft endothelium remains of donor origin post grafting [41,42], while skin graft re-vascularization partially relies upon cells of host origin[33,34]. Most importantly, T cell-dependent skin graft rejection can occur acutely in an antigen-independent manner, as H-2b HY-specific, TCR transgenic Mata Hari CD8+ T cells can efficiently reject H-2k skin but not heart allografts [28]. The immune pathway underlying TCR-independent skin rejection has been shown to depend on IFN-γ[28], but its cellular and molecular components have not yet been identified.

Hence, while still inhibiting specific T cell trafficking into the skin, the failure of PI3K p110δ inactivation to improve skin graft survival might be due to inflammation-induced mechanisms leading to by-standing damage, related to the temporary lack of regulating endothelial barrier and possibly triggered by overwhelming host cross-reactive T cell responses against skin-harbored microbial antigens. While the heart is contained within a sterile environment inside the body, the skin is continuously exposed to environmental microorganisms.

In summary, the observations described in this study strongly support the concept that pharmacological inactivation of PI3K p110δ activity is a viable strategy to control heart allograft chronic rejection. Additional advantages of this approach include the possibility of inhibiting T-cell mediated inflammation in the context of an established immune response (i.e. after transplantation, as we have shown in this study), and the maintenance of immune reactivity, which causes severe side-effect associated with conventional immunosuppressive therapies. In this context, a PI3K p110γ?δ dual selective inhibitor has been shown to significantly reduce inflammatory injuries *in vivo* in heart ischemia-reperfusion injury models in rat and pig, while at the same time spare tissue repair processes such as EC mitogenesis [43]. Clearly, the therapeutic application of PI3K p110δ inhibition will require careful planning dictated by the organ-specific immunobiology of graft rejection. We propose that this strategy would be very effective in the context of slow-developing T cell-induced inflammation relying upon antigen-dependent trafficking including chronic rejection of vascularized tissue grafts, such as heart transplants, as well as other chronic, T-cell mediated autoimmune diseases such as type I diabetes and multiple sclerosis.

Materials and Methods

Ethics statement

This study was carried out in strict accordance with the Home Office recommendations and under its authority following approval by the Imperial College London/Central Biomedical Services Ethics Committee (REF. PPL 70/5872 and PPL 80/1842). All surgery was performed under anesthesia and all efforts were made to minimize suffering.

Animals

C57BL/6 mice were purchased from Harlan Olac (Bicester, UK) and used at 7–11 weeks. p110δ^{D910A} mice were generated as previously described [26]. Experimental groups included 3–6 animals per group.

Cell culture

Memory CD4+ T cells specific for the Y-chromosome encoded HY peptide epitope NAGFNSNRANSSRSS and restricted by H2-Ab [44] were obtained from WT and p110δ^{D910A} mice by two fortnightly i.p. immunizations of female mice with male C57BL/6 splenocytes, as previously described [45]. The two T cell populations displayed similar specificity, as assessed by [3H]thymidine incorporation, and phenotype, as established by flow cytometry (Figure S5).

Reagents

The HY peptides encoding the *Dby* and *Uty* epitopes were kindly provided by Dr. Jian Guo Chai (Imperial College, London, UK). The PI3K p110δ inhibitor IC87114 was synthesized as described (D030 from patent WO 01/81346) [27]. IC87114 inhibits p110δ kinase activity in cells with an IC_{50} between 0.1μM and 0.5μM, and only shows cross-reactivity with other PI3K isoforms at concentrations more than 5μM [27,46]. In vivo, IC87114 was administered i.p. at a dose of 60 mg/kg. This dose was chosen based on previous reports of its efficacy in vivo [47]. In our hands, a 30 mg/kg by gavage achieves ~2 μM 90 min post-administration and the drug is cleared from the blood 4–7 hours post admin. IC87114 is selective for p110δ at plasma concentrations of 5 μM [47].

The cell linkers PKH26 and CFSE were purchased from Sigma-Aldrich.

Flow cytometry

For surface staining, cells were labelled with the appropriate concentration of fluorescence-conjugated antibodies or isotype control according to the manufacturer's instructions, and analyzed by a two-laser BD fluorescence activated cell sorter (FACS) Calibur (BD Biosciences, Oxford, UK). Acquired samples were analyzed using Flowjo 7.6 (TreeStar Inc., UK).

T cell proliferation assays

T cells (10^4 /well) isolated from spleen were incubated with irradiated female splenocytes (5×10^5/well) and HY peptides *Dby*, and *Uty* (0–100nM) in 96-well flat-bottomed plates. Plate was pulsed 48 hours later with 1μCi/well [3H] thymidine and incubated overnight, then harvested using the Tomtec harvester 96 and filter and counted using the Wallac Microbeta counter for Windows (all from Wallac/Perkin Elmer, Buckinghamshire, UK).

Heart transplantation

Heterotopic heart transplantation was performed in the pathogen-free facilities at Northwick Park Institute for Medical Research (NPIMR, UK) by placing the donor heart into the recipient (WT and p110δ^{D910A}) sternomastoid cavity, connecting the aortal branch to the carotid artery and the pulmonary vein to the jugular vein. Before surgery, mice were given 0.25ml Saline s.c. to prevent dehydration. Anesthetic agents included Ketamine (80–100mg/kg) and Xylazine 10mg/kg. These were administered s.c. mixed in a syringe at a ratio of 2 (Ketamine):1 (Xylazine) diluted with saline 1:1. For analgesia mice were given Rimadyl (Carprofen 50mg/ml), diluted with saline 1:10 s.c.. at a dose of

5mg/kg s.c.. Analgesics were administered prior to surgery and on day one.

To assess the effect of pharmacological inhibition of PI3K p110δ activity on graft survival, WT recipients received the selective inhibitor IC87114 at 60mg/kg/day or vehicle control i.p. daily starting 7 days after transplantation and for 15 days.

At the indicated time points, all grafts and native hearts were evaluated by histopathologic criteria in a single-blinded manner (G. Stamp, Histopathology, Imperial College London) and scored to grade the degree of inflammation from 0 to 4 [48] (0, no inflammation; 1, light focal lymphohistocytic infiltrate; 2, moderate focal lymphohistocytic infiltrate with myocardial involvement; 3, moderate to severe inflammation with focal vasculopathy and myocyte degeneration; 4, severe inflammation, vasculopathy and myocardial fiber loss).

Histochemistry

Five-micrometer-thick, paraffin-embedded sections were deparaffinized, rehydrated in graded ethanol. For elastin staining, sections were stained with Miller's elastin followed by immunoperoxidase staining for smooth muscle cells (SMCs) using rabbit monoclonal antibody to mouse SMC alpha actin (clone E184, from Epitomics, California), then counterstained with hematoxylin. For the purpose of comparison, tissue sections were taken in corresponding regions of the heart (proximal ventricular areas). Luminal occlusion was evaluated by tracing the cross-section of each vessel's internal elastic lamina and lumen using Lucia NIS elements software (Nikon UK Ltd., United Kingdom) in three transverse sections per graft. All vessels in each section, which demonstrated clear staining of elastin laminar and presence of SMC alpha-actin, were measured in three sections of each heart [48]. For immunohistochemistry, tissue sections were incubated for 1 h at room temperature with either FITC labelled anti-CD3 antibody or PE labelled anti-MAC2 antibody. Nucleus was counterstained with Vectashield mounting medium for fluorescence with DAPI (Vector Laboratories). Cell infiltration was evaluated by wide field microscopy and automated cell counting.

Skin grafting

Skin grafting was conducted by the method of Billingham and Medawar [16] using tail skin from WT donors grafted onto the lateral thorax of either WT or p110δ^{D910A} female mice. Skin graft rejection was assessed as previously described [49]. In the experiments assessing the effect of pharmacological inhibition of p110δ activity on graft survival, WT recipients received the selective inhibitor IC87114 at 60mg/kg/day or vehicle control i.p. daily starting 7 days after transplantation and for 15 days. Prior to surgery, mice received medetomidine (1mg/kg), ketamine (75mg/kg) and atipamezole (2.5mg/kg) s.c..

Recruitment of circulating T cells into tissues

In adoptive transfer experiments HY-specific memory T cells were incubated at 37°C for 10 minutes either with PKH26 (5 μM, red) or CFSE (1 μM, green), washed 3 times with PBS and then co-injected i.v. (10^7/mouse). After 24 hours, mice were sacrificed and tissues were sampled and embedded in optimal cutting temperature compound (CellPath Ltd, Newtown Powys). Tissue infiltration by T cells was assessed by wide-field fluorescence microscopy 24 hours after injection. The following combinations were used: WT (red) and P110δ^{D910A} (green) T cells, WT T cells pre-treated with vehicle (1%DMSO, red) and with PI3K p110δ inhibitor IC87114 (5μM for 1 hour at 37°C, green).

Wide-field fluorescence microscopy and automatic cell counting

Snap-frozen tissue sections were laid onto Polysine Microscope slides (VWR International), and then mounted in Vectashield mounting medium for fluorescence with DAPI (Vector Laboratories), to stain the nuclei. Slides were visualized with a Coolview 12-cooled CCD camera (Photonic Science) mounted over a Zeiss Axiovert S100 microscope equipped with Metamorph software (Zeiss). Tissue infiltration was quantified by randomly selecting ten ×10-magnified fields from tissue samples from at least 3 animals and assessing the number of fluorescent cells in each field. Quantification of T cell infiltrates observed by wide-field fluorescence microscopy was performed using a specifically designed software to run in the LabView (version 7.1; National Instruments) environment. This automatic cell counting algorithm is based on a combination of background subtraction, multiple thresholding, and morphological processing approaches [50], which allow identification of single fluorescent cells within the tissue. The number of infiltrating labelled cells were then averaged and assessed statistically. Infiltration is expressed as the mean of fluorescent cells per ×10 field in a given experimental condition ± SD.

Statistics

Results are given as the mean per group ± SD. The data were analyzed using a two-tailed unpaired Student's t test and Mann-Whitney test. A P value of less than 0.05 was considered significant.

Supporting Information

Figure S1 Histology of transplanted and native hearts. Recipient female WT and p110δ^{D910A} mutant mice received either male or female WT hearts. 23 days after transplant, both transplanted and native hearts were harvested and stained with hematoxilin/eosin. Each panel shows a representative tissue image. Magnification: 20x.

Figure S2 Immunohistochemistry of transplanted and native hearts. Recipient female WT mice received either syngeneic male or female heart grafts. After 7 days, the selective PI3K p110δ inhibitor IC87114 (60mg/kg/day) or vehicle control were injected i.p. daily for 15 days. Mice were sacrificed 24 hours after the last treatment (day 23). (A) Both transplanted and native hearts were harvested and stained with hematoxilin/eosin. Each panel shows a representative tissue image. Magnification: 20x. (B) Both transplanted and native hearts were harvested and tissue sections were stained with either FITC-labelled anti-CD3 antibody or PE-labelled anti-MAC2 antibody. Each panel shows a representative tissue image. Magnification: 20x.

Figure S3 Pharmacologic inactivation of PI3K p110δ does not induce T cell tolerance. Recipient female WT mice received either syngeneic male or female heart grafts. After 7 days, the selective PI3K p110δ inhibitor IC87114 (60mg/kg/day) or vehicle control were injected i.p. daily for 15 days. Mice were sacrificed 24 hours after the last treatment (day 23). Splenocytes obtained from WT female recipients treated with or without IC87114 were incubated with different concentrations of *Dby* and *Uby* HY peptide epitopes for 48 hours, followed by pulsing with [^{3}H] thymidine to assess T cell proliferation.

Figure S4 Genetic or pharmacologic inactivation of PI3K p110δ do not induce T cell tolerance in recipients of skin allografts. (A) Recipient female WT and p110δ^{D910A}

mutant mice received male skin grafts. After skin grafts were rejected, splenocytes from recipient mice were harvested and incubated with different concentrations of *Dby* and *Uty* HY epitopes for 48 hours, followed by pulsing with [^{3}H] thymidine to assess T cell proliferation. (B) Recipient female WT mice received male skin grafts. 7 days after transplant, the PI3K p110δ inhibitor IC87114 at 60mg/kg/day or vehicle control were injected i.p. daily until the grafts were rejected. Splenocytes from recipient mice were harvested and incubated with different concentrations of *Dby* and *Uty* HY epitopes for 48 hours, followed by pulsing with [^{3}H] thymidine to assess T cell proliferation. Filled symbols: *Dby*; Empty symbols: *Uty*.

Figure S5 Characterization of HY-specific WT and p110δ^{D910A} T cells. (A) HY-specific CD4$^+$ WT and p110δ^{D910A} T cells were harvested between days seven and ten post-stimulation with irradiated male splenocytes. T cells were stained with monoclonal antibodies recognizing CD4, CD8, CD62L and CCR7 and appropriate isotype control antibodies and analysed by flow cytometry. Expression of CD4, CD8, CD62L and CCR7 is shown in bold while the dotted line represents the isotype control. (B) WT or p110δ^{D910A} T cells were incubated with 6 x10^6 female irradiated splenocytes and different concentrations of *Dby* (filled symbols) and *Uty* (empty symbols) HY epitopes for 48 hours, followed by pulsing with [^{3}H] thymidine to assess proliferation.

Author Contributions

Conceived and designed the experiments: MR KO FM-B. Performed the experiments: HY HF AMcC PS. Analyzed the data: HY HF AMcC PS. Contributed reagents/materials/analysis tools: KO MR. Wrote the paper: HF FM-B.

References

1. Tanaka M, Fedoseyeva EV, Robbins RC (2005) Graft coronary artery disease in murine cardiac allografts: proposal to meet the need for standardized assessment. JHeart Lung Transplant 24: 316–322.
2. Taylor DO, Edwards LB, Mohacsi PJ, Boucek MM, Trulock EP, et al. (2003) The registry of the International Society for Heart and Lung Transplantation: twentieth official adult heart transplant report--2003. JHeart Lung Transplant 22: 616–624.
3. Taylor DO, Stehlik J, Edwards LB, Aurora P, Christie JD, et al. (2009) Registry of the International Society for Heart and Lung Transplantation: Twenty-sixth Official Adult Heart Transplant Report-2009. J Heart Lung Transplant 28: 1007–1022.
4. van Loosdregt J, van Oosterhout MF, Bruggink AH, van Wichen DF, van Kuik J, et al. (2006) The chemokine and chemokine receptor profile of infiltrating cells in the wall of arteries with cardiac allograft vasculopathy is indicative of a memory T-helper 1 response. Circulation 114: 1599–1607.
5. Lee RS, Yamada K, Houser SL, Womer KL, Maloney ME, et al. (2001) Indirect recognition of allopeptides promotes the development of cardiac allograft vasculopathy. ProcNatlAcadSciUSA 98: 3276–3281.
6. Libby P, Pober JS (2001) Chronic rejection. Immunity 14: 387–397.
7. Liu Z, Colovai AI, Tugulea S, Reed EF, Fisher PE, et al. (1996) Indirect recognition of donor HLA-DR peptides in organ allograft rejection. JClinInvest 98: 1150–1157.
8. Waaga AM, Gasser M, Laskowski I, Tilney NL (2000) Mechanisms of chronic rejection. CurrOpinImmunol 12: 517–521.
9. Chen Y, Demir Y, Valujskikh A, Heeger PS (2003) The male minor transplantation antigen preferentially activates recipient CD4+ T cells through the indirect presentation pathway in vivo. JImmunol 171: 6510–6518.
10. He C, Schenk S, Zhang Q, Valujskikh A, Bayer J, et al. (2004) Effects of T cell frequency and graft size on transplant outcome in mice. JImmunol 172: 240–247.
11. Huddleston SJ, Hays WS, Filatenkov A, Ingulli E, Jenkins MK (2006) CD154+ graft antigen-specific CD4+ T cells are sufficient for chronic rejection of minor antigen incompatible heart grafts. AmJTransplant 6: 1312–1319.
12. Schnickel GT, Whiting D, Hsieh GR, Yun JJ, Fischbein MP, et al. (2004) CD8 lymphocytes are sufficient for the development of chronic rejection. Transplantation 78: 1634–1639.
13. Sun H, Woodward JE, Subbotin VM, Kuddus R, Logar AJ, et al. (2002) Use of recombinase activation gene-2 deficient mice to ascertain the role of cellular and humoral immune responses in the development of chronic rejection. JHeart Lung Transplant 21: 738–750.
14. Szeto WY, Krasinskas AM, Kreisel D, Krupnick AS, Popma SH, et al. (2002) Depletion of recipient CD4+ but not CD8+ T lymphocytes prevents the development of cardiac allograft vasculopathy. Transplantation 73: 1116–1122.
15. Valujskikh A, Zhang Q, Heeger PS (2006) CD8 T cells specific for a donor-derived, self-restricted transplant antigen are nonpathogenic bystanders after vascularized heart transplantation in mice. JImmunol 176: 2190–2196.
16. Billingham RE, Brent L, Medawar PB (1953) Actively acquired tolerance of foreign cells. Nature 172: 603–606.
17. Kawai T, Shimauchi H, Eastcott JW, Smith DJ, Taubman MA (1998) Antigen direction of specific T-cell clones into gingival tissues. Immunology 93: 11–19.
18. Marelli-Berg FM, Frasca L, Weng L, Lombardi G, Lechler RI (1999) Antigen recognition influences transendothelial migration of CD4+ T cells. JImmunol 162: 696–703.
19. Marelli-Berg FM, James MJ, Dangerfield J, Dyson J, Millrain M, et al. (2004) Cognate recognition of the endothelium induces HY-specific CD8+ T-lymphocyte transendothelial migration (diapedesis) in vivo. Blood 103: 3111–3116.
20. Savinov AY, Wong FS, Stonebraker AC, Chervonsky AV (2003) Presentation of antigen by endothelial cells and chemoattraction are required for homing of insulin-specific CD8+ T cells. JExpMed 197: 643–656.
21. Jarmin SJ, David R, Ma L, Chai JG, Dewchand H, et al. (2008) T cell receptor-induced phosphoinositide-3-kinase p110delta activity is required for T cell localization to antigenic tissue in mice. JClinInvest 118: 1154–1164.
22. Sobel RA, Blanchette BW, Bhan AK, Colvin RB (1984) The immunopathology of experimental allergic encephalomyelitis. II. Endothelial cell Ia increases prior to inflammatory cell infiltration. J Immunol 132: 2402–2407.
23. Okkenhaug K, Vanhaesebroeck B (2003) PI3K in lymphocyte development, differentiation and activation. NatRevImmunol 3: 317–330.
24. Wang J, Auger KR, Jarvis L, Shi Y, Roberts TM (1995) Direct association of Grb2 with the p85 subunit of phosphatidylinositol 3-kinase. JBiolChem 270: 12774–12780.
25. Zhang W, Sloan-Lancaster J, Kitchen J, Trible RP, Samelson LE (1998) LAT: the ZAP-70 tyrosine kinase substrate that links T cell receptor to cellular activation. Cell 92: 83–92.
26. Okkenhaug K, Bilancio A, Farjot G, Priddle H, Sancho S, et al. (2002) Impaired B and T cell antigen receptor signaling in p110delta PI 3-kinase mutant mice. Science 297: 1031–1034.
27. Soond DR, Bjorgo E, Moltu K, Dale VQ, Patton DT, et al. (2010) PI3K p110delta regulates T-cell cytokine production during primary and secondary immune responses in mice and humans. Blood 115: 2203–2213.
28. Valujskikh A, Lantz O, Celli S, Matzinger P, Heeger PS (2002) Cross-primed CD8(+) T cells mediate graft rejection via a distinct effector pathway. NatImmunol 3: 844–851.
29. Simpson E, Scott D, Chandler P (1997) The male-specific histocompatibility antigen, H-Y: a history of transplantation, immune response genes, sex determination and expression cloning. Annu Rev Immunol 15: 39–61.
30. Amano J, Ishiyama S, Nishikawa T, Tanaka H, Nagai R, et al. (1997) Proliferation of smooth muscle cells in acute allograft vascular rejection. J Thorac Cardiovasc Surg 113: 19–25.
31. Reif K, Okkenhaug K, Sasaki T, Penninger JM, Vanhaesebroeck B, et al. (2004) Cutting edge: differential roles for phosphoinositide 3-kinases, p110gamma and p110delta, in lymphocyte chemotaxis and homing. J Immunol 173: 2236–2240.
32. Kearney ER, Pape KA, Loh DY, Jenkins MK (1994) Visualization of peptide-specific T cell immunity and peripheral tolerance induction in vivo. Immunity 1: 327–339.
33. de Waal RM, Bogman MJ, Cornelissen IM, Vermeulen AN, Koene RA (1986) Expression of donor class I major histocompatibility antigens on the vascular endothelium of mouse skin allografts. Transplantation 42: 178–183.
34. de Waal RM, Bogman MJ, Maass CN, Cornelissen LM, Tax WJ, et al. (1983) Variable expression of Ia antigens on the vascular endothelium of mouse skin allografts. Nature 303: 426–429.
35. Marelli-Berg FM, Cannella L, Dazzi F, Mirenda V (2008) The highway code of T cell trafficking. JPathol 214: 179–189.
36. Manes TD, Pober JS (2008) Antigen presentation by human microvascular endothelial cells triggers ICAM-1-dependent transendothelial protrusion by, and fractalkine-dependent transendothelial migration of, effector memory CD4+ T cells. JImmunol 180: 8386–8392.
37. Christen T, Nahrendorf M, Wildgruber M, Swirski FK, Aikawa E, et al. (2009) Molecular imaging of innate immune cell function in transplant rejection. Circulation 119: 1925–1932.
38. Murase N, Ichikawa N, Ye Q, Chun HJ, Okuda T, et al. (1999) Dendritic cells/chimerism/alleviation of chronic allograft rejection. JLeukocBiol 66: 297–300.
39. Ozdemir BH, Sezgin A, Haberal M (2009) Apoptosis and proliferation of cardiomyocytes and interstitial mononuclear cells: association with rejection and macrophage infiltration. TransplantProc 41: 2890–2892.

40. Capla JM, Ceradini DJ, Tepper OM, Callaghan MJ, Bhatt KA, et al. (2006) Skin graft vascularization involves precisely regulated regression and replacement of endothelial cells through both angiogenesis and vasculogenesis. PlastReconstrSurg 117: 836–844.

41. Hasegawa S, Becker G, Nagano H, Libby P, Mitchell RN (1998) Pattern of graft- and host-specific MHC class II expression in long-term murine cardiac allografts: origin of inflammatory and vascular wall cells. AmJPathol 153: 69–79.

42. Quaini F, Urbanek K, Beltrami AP, Finato N, Beltrami CA, et al. (2002) Chimerism of the transplanted heart. NEnglJMed 346: 5–15.

43. Doukas J, Wrasidlo W, Noronha G, Dneprovskaia E, Fine R, et al. (2006) Phosphoinositide 3-kinase gamma/delta inhibition limits infarct size after myocardial ischemia/reperfusion injury. ProcNatlAcadSciUSA 103: 19866–19871.

44. Scott D, Addey C, Ellis P, James E, Mitchell MJ, et al. (2000) Dendritic cells permit identification of genes encoding MHC class II-restricted epitopes of transplantation antigens. Immunity 12: 711–720.

45. Millrain M, Chandler P, Dazzi F, Scott D, Simpson E, et al. (2001) Examination of HY response: T cell expansion, immunodominance, and cross-priming revealed by HY tetramer analysis. JImmunol 167: 3756–3764.

46. Knight ZA, Gonzalez B, Feldman ME, Zunder ER, Goldenberg DD, et al. (2006) A pharmacological map of the PI3-K family defines a role for p110alpha in insulin signaling. Cell 125: 733–747.

47. Ali K, Bilancio A, Thomas M, Pearce W, Gilfillan AM, et al. (2004) Essential role for the p110delta phosphoinositide 3-kinase in the allergic response. Nature 431: 1007–1011.

48. Xu Y, Chester AH, Hariri B, McCormack A, Sarathchandra P, et al. (2010) The indirect alloimmune response causes microvascular endothelial dysfunction-a possible role for alloantibody. Transplantation 90: 1157–1164.

49. Schwoebel F, Barsig J, Wendel A, Hamacher J (2005) Quantitative assessment of mouse skin transplant rejection using digital photography. Lab Anim 39: 209–214.

50. Mirenda V, Jarmin SJ, David R, Dyson J, Scott D, et al. (2007) Physiologic and aberrant regulation of memory T-cell trafficking by the costimulatory molecule CD28. Blood 109: 2968–2977.

17

Expression of Calcineurin Activity after Lung Transplantation

Sylvia Sanquer[1]*, Catherine Amrein[2], Dominique Grenet[3], Romain Guillemain[2], Bruno Philippe[3], Veronique Boussaud[2], Laurence Herry[1], Celine Lena[1], Alphonsine Diouf[1], Michelle Paunet[4], Eliane M. Billaud[5], Françoise Loriaux[6], Jean-Philippe Jais[7], Robert Barouki[1], Marc Stern[3]

1 Service de Biochimie Métabolomique et Protéomique, Hôpital Universitaire Necker-Enfants Malades Assistance Publique-Hôpitaux de Paris (AP-HP); INSERM UMR-S 747; and Université Paris Descartes, Centre Universitaire des Saints-Pères, Paris, France, 2 Service de Chirurgie Cardio-Vasculaire, Hôpital Européen Georges Pompidou, AP-HP, Paris, France, 3 Service de Pneumologie, Hôpital Foch, Suresnes, France, 4 Laboratoire de Biologie, Hôpital Foch, Suresnes, France, 5 Service de Pharmacologie, Hôpital Européen Georges Pompidou, AP-HP and Université Paris Descartes, Paris, France, 6 Service de Biochimie, Hôpital Européen Georges Pompidou, AP-HP, Paris, France, 7 Service de Biostatistiques, Hôpital Necker-Enfants Malades, AP-HP, Paris, France; Université Paris Descartes, Paris, France

Abstract

The objective of this pharmacodynamic study was to longitudinally assess the activity of calcineurin during the first 2 years after lung transplantation. From March 2004 to October 2008, 107 patients were prospectively enrolled and their follow-up was performed until 2009. Calcineurin activity was measured in peripheral blood mononuclear cells. We report that calcineurin activity was linked to both acute and chronic rejection. An optimal activity for calcineurin with two thresholds was defined, and we found that the risk of rejection was higher when the enzyme activity was above the upper threshold of 102 pmol/mg/min or below the lower threshold of 12 pmol/mg/min. In addition, we report that the occurrence of malignancies and viral infections was significantly higher in patients displaying very low levels of calcineurin activity. Taken together, these findings suggest that the measurement of calcineurin activity may provide useful information for the management of the prevention therapy of patients receiving lung transplantation.

Editor: Aric Gregson, University of California Los Angeles, United States of America

Funding: Funding for this study was provided by the French association Vaincre la Mucoviscidose. The funders had no role in study design, data collection and analysis, decision to publish, or preparation of the manuscript.

Competing Interests: The authors have declared that no competing interests exist.

* E-mail: sylvia.sanquer@gmail.com

Introduction

Organ transplantation is the last alternative therapeutic option for selected patients with end-stage disease of a given organ. The survival of transplanted organs has markedly improved over the past few decades due to the use of immunosuppressive treatments. However, organ survival remains limited by the onset of chronic rejection and devastating adverse drug events. This is particularly true with lung transplantation. Despite increasing improvement in patient care, lung transplantation has the poorest outcomes mainly because of the development of chronic rejection in response to immunologic, ischemic and infectious injury [1–8]. Chronic rejection, which presents as a bronchiolitis obliterans syndrome (BOS), is defined as a progressive airflow obstruction and a deterioration of graft function. It accounts for more than 30% of all mortality after the third year following lung transplantation [8,9]. Moreover, by promoting factor perivascular and peribronchial infiltration of activated lymphocytes into graft tissue, acute rejection remains an important risk factor for the development of BOS [10].

The standard for rejection prevention in lung transplantation consists of an immunosuppressive regimen which includes a calcineurin (CN) inhibitor (CNI) such as cyclosporine (CsA) and tacrolimus [11]. The CNI prophylactic dose is adjusted according to the whole blood concentration of the drug to avoid the occurrence of dose-dependent toxicities. However, the optimal balance of immunosuppression is difficult to achieve following transplantation. Inadequate immunosuppression may lead to transplant rejection and, on the other hand, excessive immunosuppression facilitates the development of severe complications such as infection or malignancy. To date, there are no robust biomarkers that allow the prediction of the extent of immunosuppression afforded by these treatments. This may be a partial explanation for the frequent failure of the immunosuppressive strategy after lung transplantation as illustrated by the facts that 50 to 60% of the patients develop acute rejection and up to 60% of the recipients who survive 5 years after transplantation are affected by BOS [8,9,12].

Different approaches have aimed at reducing the incidence and severity of acute rejection. As a first attempt, we have developed a pharmacodynamic approach for monitoring the extent of immunosuppression following transplantation. This approach is based on the activity of calcineurin, a calcium-calmodulin-dependent phosphatase. Calcineurin activity reflects the combination of the degree of T lymphocyte activation and the inhibitory effect of CNIs [13–17]. Calcineurin is a key factor involved during the early phase of T lymphocyte activation. When CN is activated, it dephosphorylates the nuclear factor of activated T cells (NFAT) which then allows translocation of NFAT into the nucleus. This leads to the synthesis of cytokines that are involved in T lymphocyte proliferation. It has been demonstrated clearly that T cell activation is dependent upon sustained calcium/CN signaling for maximal proliferation and cytokine production [18,19]. Therefore, the CN activity (CN-a) measured in peripheral blood mononuclear cells (PBMCs) issued from allograft recipients receiving CNIs may be considered to be an index of T cell activation and a marker for graft-versus-host disease [20,21].

In this study, we measured CN-a during the first 24 months after lung transplantation and we correlated the activities with the occurrence of acute rejection, BOS and adverse events which are known to be associated with over-immunosuppression, such as malignancies and infections.

Materials and Methods

Ethics Statement

The CALCILUNG study was a prospective observational study of lung transplant recipients. In accordance with French law, the study protocol was approved by the ethics committee of Paris-Broussais-HEGP. Patients enrolled in this study provided informed written consents.

Patients

The study consisted of measuring CN-a during the first 24 months after lung transplantation. Patients were eligible if they were programmed to receive an immunosuppressive treatment consisting of the association of CsA, azathioprine and steroids. Patients followed a typical care regimen for post-lung transplantation patients, including surveillance fiberoptic bronchoscopy and bronchoalveolar lavage, spirometry, systematic transbronchial biopsies for acute rejection monitoring and blood sampling. The first surveillance biopsy was generally scheduled 7 days after transplantation. Subsequently, transbronchial biopsies were performed during the post-transplantation evaluation tests that were scheduled once a month up to the sixth month after lung transplantation and then every three months up to the 24th month after transplantation. Spirometry, generally, was checked once a week up to the third month after lung transplantation, then once a month up to the first year after transplantation and then every three months. In general, the first CN-a assessment was performed before transplantation during the pre-transplantation evaluation tests. Post-transplantation CN-a measurements were performed at least once a month during the first 6 months after transplantation and then every three months. Sampling for CN-a measurements was concomitant to the other monthly scheduled post-transplantation evaluation tests. The transplantation characteristics of the patients enrolled in this study are listed in **Table 1**.

Drug and Pharmacodynamic Monitoring

CsA and CN-a were both determined before the morning dose of CsA, when it was given orally. The clinical outcome of the patients was unknown to the biologist in charge of CN-a analyses and the results of the analyses were not given to the personnel (physicians and nurses) caring for the lung transplant patients. CsA was routinely measured with a locally available immunoassay. Mononuclear cells were isolated from the samples remaining by a Ficoll gradient method and CN-a measurements were made later. Briefly, 25 μg of proteins from mononuclear cells were incubated at 37°C for 30 min in the presence of phosphorylated RII peptide as a substrate of calcineurin. The dephosphorylation of the substrate was quantified by using high-performance liquid chromatography with ultraviolet detection as previously described [20]. Technical validation of this assay showed a correlation coefficient of the linear regression curves (linearity) greater than

Table 1. Basal characteriwstics of patients.

	Total (n = 107)
Age (yr)	36±12
Sex (M/F)	64(60)/43(40)
Initial disease	
cystic fibrosis	64(60)
emphysema	19(18)
others	24(22)
Type of transplantation (single/bilateral)	16(15)/91(85)
CMV mismatch at transplantaion (D+/R-)	26(24)
EBV mismatch at transplantation (D+/R-)	7(7)
Primary graft dysfunction grade III	15±4
Number of CN-a measurements/24 months	6±3
Time of follow-up (months)	41±16
Patients with acute rejection/6 months	77(72)
Patients with BOS grade ≥ I	40(37)
Patients with malignancies	16(15)
Patients with bacterial infections	
≥1 episode	63(59)
≥2 episodes	31(29)
≥3 episodes	15(14)
Patients with viral infections	
≥1 episode	39(36)
≥2 episodes	20(19)
≥3 episodes	7(6.5)
Patients with fungal infections	
≥1 episode	31(29)
≥2 episodes	9(8.4)
≥3 episodes	2(1.9)

Data are summarized as frequencies and percentage for categorical variables and as mean±SD for continuous variables. A total of 670 peripheral blood samples (mean of 6±3 samples per patient, range: 2–14) were obtained during the first 24 months following transplantation. Yr: year; M: male; F: female; EBV: empstein barr virus; CMV: cytomegalovirus; CN-a: calcineurin activity; BOS: bronchiolitis obliterans syndrome.

0.9971 and a variation coefficient (inter-assay variability) less than 10% [20]. The stability of CN-a under our conditions was previously verified by performing pharmacokinetic and pharmacodynamic measurements over a 10-hr time course in stable renal transplant patients treated with CsA. A peak of inhibition of CN-a occurred at approximately the same time as the peak of CsA in whole blood, and the concentrations of both CN-a and CsA gradually returned to baseline levels [20].

Diagnosis of Acute Rejection

Episodes of acute rejection were diagnosed on the basis of pulmonary function tests and histological evaluation of transbronchial biopsies. Acute rejection was graded according to the ISHLT criteria [22]. During the first six months following transplantation, treatment of acute rejection with steroids was initiated in patients with either an alteration or a 3-month stagnation of their pulmonary function and/or in patients for whom a grade A1 or higher was assessed based on their transbronchial biopies. Very few acute rejections of grade higher than A1 were diagnosed in these patients.

Determination of Pulmonary Function

Pulmonary function was estimated from the spirometric data FEV1, representing the forced expiratory volume in one second. To assess the variation of pulmonary function versus time during the first six months after transplantation, FEV1 ratios were calculated from the ratio of the difference between two spirometric values obtained approximately 1 month apart to the number of days between two spirometric measurements. We expressed these ratios in liters per second per day. Because we considered positive FEV1 ratios as a normal evolution of pulmonary function, only null and negative values of FEV1 ratios, which reveal a negative alteration of pulmonary function were taken into account for the study.

Diagnosis of Chronic Rejection/BOS

BOS was diagnosed and graded according to the ISHLT criteria [23]. BOS was defined as a sustained decrease of at least 20 percent in the FEV1 spirometric data as compared to the patient's maximum values in the absence of other causes [23]. Azithromycin therapy was started in patients displaying a strong reduction in FEF_{25-75}. In this study, we took into account the occurrence of BOS of grade I or higher.

Statistical Analysis

The values are expressed as the means$\pm$SD or the medians and percentiles. For the evaluation of the relationship between CN-a and acute rejection, CN-a values were censored when patients received a first IV bolus of steroids. Kernel smoothing curves were generated and the dispersion of extreme CN-a values was determined. For the evaluation of the relationship between CN-a and pulmonary function, we compared the rates of negative altered FEV1 at different CN-a levels. The survival without BOS, overall survival and the occurrence of adverse events were estimated by the Kaplan-Meier method. Other potentially associated risk factors of BOS occurrence were evaluated by using a stepwise logistic regression model.

Analyses were performed by using SAS 9.2 and Graphpad Prism softwares. Two-tailed P<0.05 were deemed significant. In case of multiple group comparisons, p-values were adjusted by the Bonferroni method.

Results

From March 2004 to October 2008, 107 patients who received lung transplants were examined for CN-a monitoring. The initial clinical-biological characteristics of these patients are shown in **Table 1**. Patients were followed until 2009. A total of 670 blood samples (mean of 6$\pm$3 samples per patient, range: 2–14) were obtained during the first 24 months following transplantation. We compared the levels of CN-a prior to transplantation in patients with or without cystic fibrosis (CF) since this was the main initial end-stage lung disease that led to lung transplantation in this cohort of patients. There was no difference in the average pre-transplantation CN-a between patients with cystic fibrosis and the other patients (**Fig. 1A**).

Calcineurin Activity and Acute Rejection

The relationship between CN-a and acute rejection was assessed during the first six months after transplantation since acute rejection mainly occurred during that period of time. Of the 107 lung-transplant recipients, 30 (28%) were free of any episode of

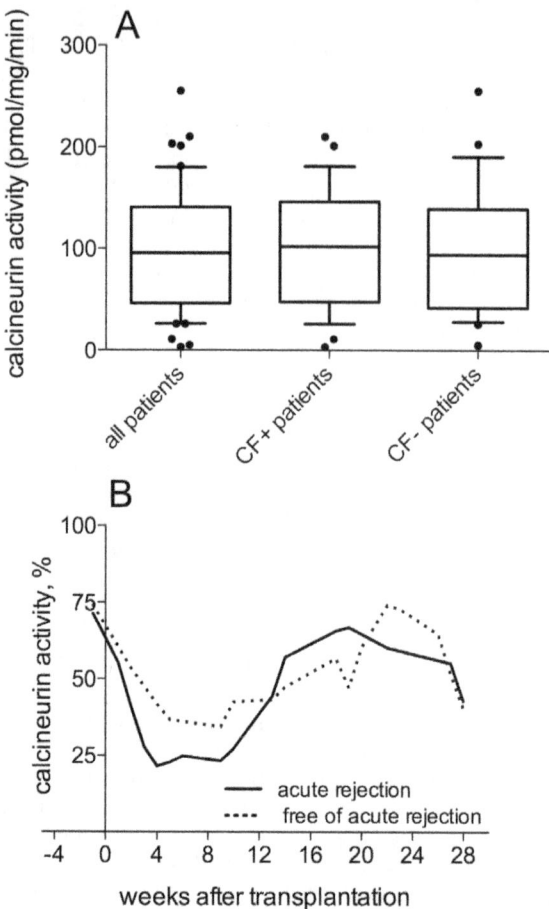

Figure 1. Calcineurin activity and acute rejection. (A) Calcineurin activity (CN-a) was measured before lung transplantation in 52 of the 107 patients enrolled in the participating center. The results are presented as box plots and 10–90 percentile whiskers. We compared CN-a expression prior to transplantation in patients with or without cystic fibrosis (CF) since it is the main initial end-stage lung disease that led to lung transplantation in this cohort of patients and a similar dispersion of the CN-a values was found in CF+ and CF- patients (p = 0.77, Mann-Whitney test). Subsequently, a relationship between extreme values of calcineurin activity and acute rejection was investigated. (B) Comparison across time of the median CN-a levels in patients displaying or not acute rejection: Kernel smoothing curves were generated. The 2 groups of patients displayed similar profiles of CN-a which consist of a phase of enzyme inhibition within the first 10 weeks after transplantation followed by a phase in which enzyme activity is restored. The phase of CN-a inhibition tended to be faster and more marked in patients who had developed acute rejection as compared to patients who were free of acute rejection. Similarly, the increase of enzyme activity to baseline levels tended to be faster and more pronounced in patients who had developed acute rejection.

acute rejection during the first 6 months after transplantation whereas 75 patients (71%) received a first rescue therapy by intravenous bolus (IV) of steroids following a diagnosis of acute rejection based either on their transbronchial biopsies for 68 of them (64%) or on their pulmonary function for 7 of them (7%). Furthermore, 2 patients (2%) were not rescued although an episode of acute rejection was diagnosed. The first episode of acute rejection occurred at a median time of 8 days (extreme values, 5–192 days). A large dispersion of CN-a values was observed, and since no reproducible pattern in CN-a could be discerned, we chose to express the CN-a data using their quartile range. For the

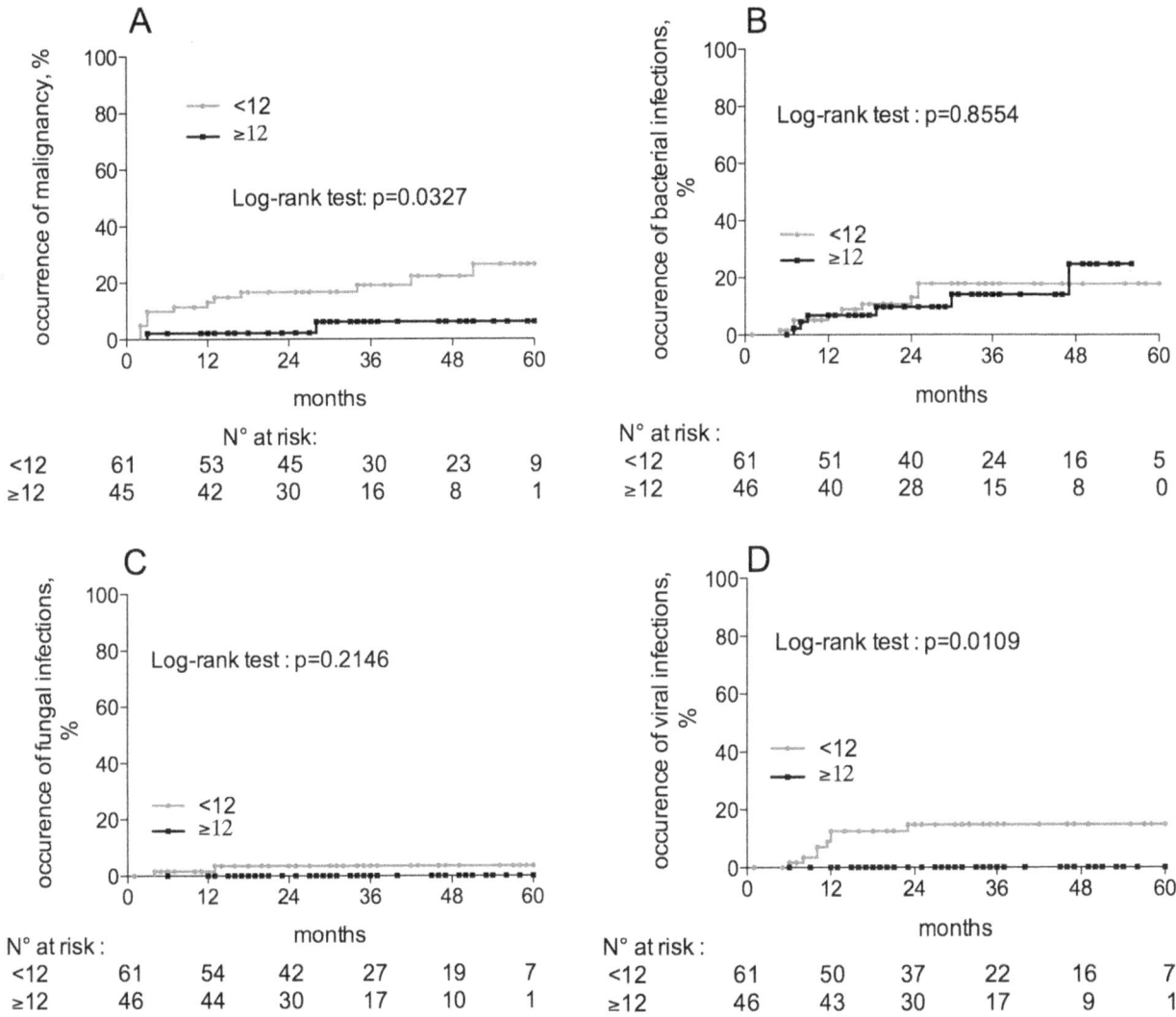

Figure 2. Calcineurin activity and adverse events related to over-immunosuppression. The onset of events known to be related to over-immunosuppression, such as malignancies and infections, was compared between patients displaying or not low CN-a levels by the Kaplan and Meier method. (A) CN-a and malignancies: the occurrence of malignancies was significantly higher in patients displaying at least one CN-a value below 12 pmol/mg/min during the first 24 months after transplantation as compared to patients with higher CN-a values (28% vs 6%, p = 0.0218, Log-rank test). The examination of the relationship between CN-a and infections was performed by separating the infections of bacterial, viral and fungal origin. (B) CN-a and bacterial infections: the occurrence of 3 episodes of bacterial infections was similar in the 2 groups of patients (18% vs 25%, p = 0.85, Log-rank test). (C) CN-a and fungal infections: the occurrence of 3 episodes of fungal infections was similar in the 2 groups of patients (3.5% vs 0%, p = 0.21, Log-rank test). (D) CN-a and viral infections: the occurrence of 3 episodes of viral infections was significantly higher in patients displaying at least one CN-a value below 12 pmol/mg/min during the first 24 months after transplantation compared to patients with higher CN-a values (15% vs 0%, p = 0.01, Log-rank test).

Calcineurin Activity and Overall Survival

Of the 107 patients enrolled in the study, 25 patients (23%) died during follow-up. At this time of the evaluation, no significant difference was found in the overall survival between the 2 groups of patients exhibiting CN-a levels within or outside of the range of 12–102 pmol/mg/min (**Fig. 3D**). This relationship should be re-assessed after a longer period of follow-up.

Calcineurin Activity and Cyclosporine Blood Levels

We next investigated whether CsA blood levels could explain the modification in CN-a that we have observed. However, as shown in **Figure 4**, we did not find any significant correlation between CN-a and CsA blood levels, as also observed in other types of transplantation [20,21,24].

Discussion

The activity of calcineurin measured in the PBMCs of allograft recipients who received inhibitors of calcineurin has been shown to be an index of T cell activation and a marker for graft-versus-host disease [20,21]. It was thought that a high CN-a reflected poor immunosuppression whereas a low CN-a reflected potent immunosuppression. Therefore, our working hypothesis, for the present study, was that the level of CN-a can predict the degree of immunosuppression after lung transplantation, and, thus, be useful for predicting both the occurrence of rejection, related to an inadequate immunosuppression, and the development of severe complications, related to excessively potent immunosuppression. However, we report here that patients who displayed extreme CN-

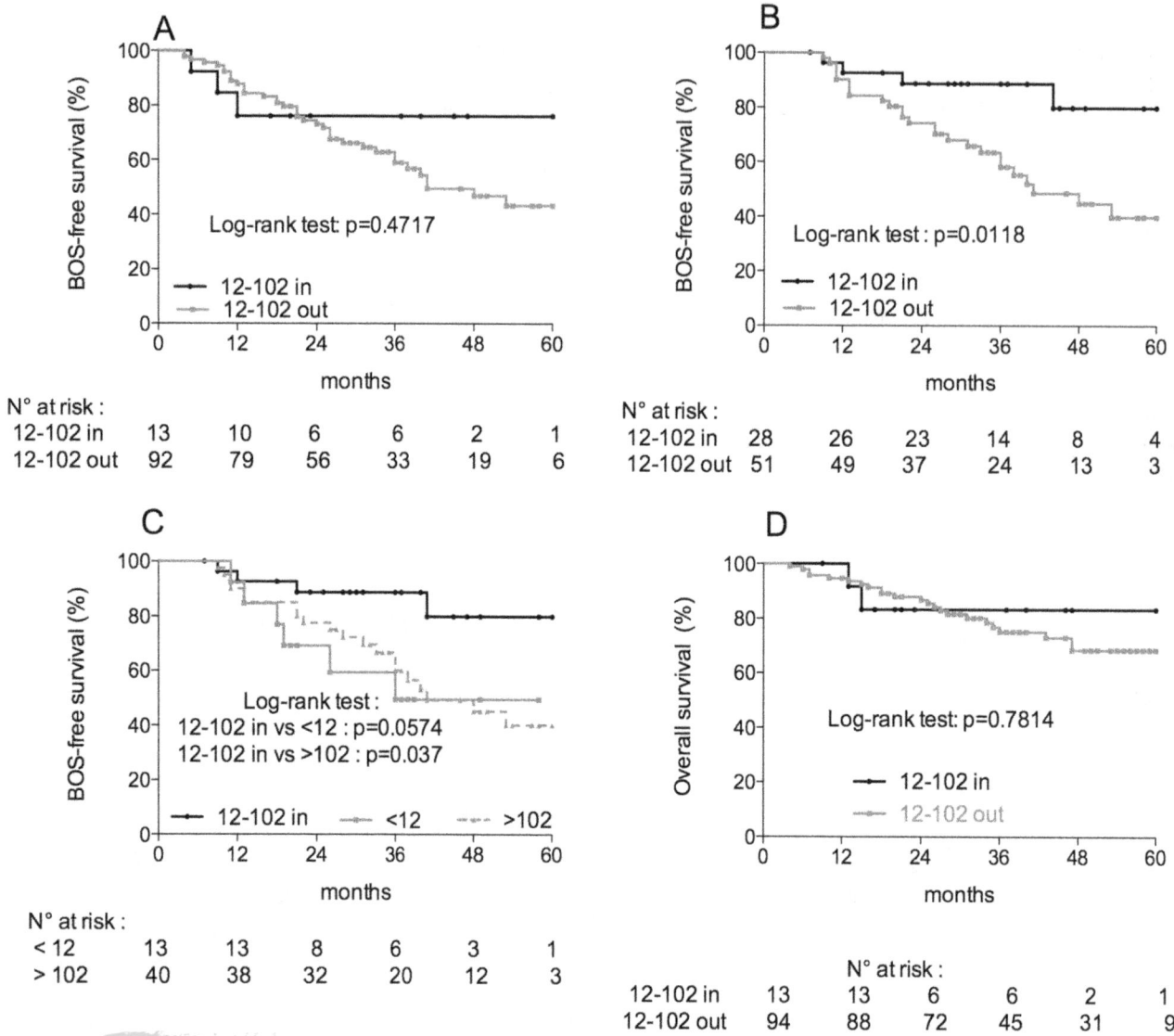

Figure 3. Calcineurin activity, BOS and overall survival. BOS-free survival was estimated at 5 years after transplantation by the Kaplan and Meier method. (A) Calcineurin activity (CN-a) monitoring during the first 24 months after transplantation: although not statistically significant, the survival without BOS was higher in patients who displayed CN-a levels within the range of 12–102 pmol/mg/min as compared to patients who exhibited at least one CN-a value outside this range of 12–102 pmol/mg/min during the first 24 months following transplantation (76% vs 43%, p = 0.4717, Log-rank test). (B) CN-a monitoring from the 6th month to the 24th month after transplantation: the survival without BOS was significantly higher in patients who displayed CN-a levels within the range of 12–102 pmol/mg/min as compared to that of patients who exhibited at least one CN-a value outside this range from the 6th month to the 24th months following transplantation (80% vs 40%, p = 0.0118, Log-rank test). (C) CN-a monitoring from the 6th to the 24th month after transplantation: the threshold values were further separated in 2 groups : <12 pmol/mg/min, >102 pmol/mg/min. The BOS-free survival in patients from each of these groups was compared to that from patients who displayed CN-a levels within the range of 12–102 pmol/mg/min. A significant reduction of the survival without BOS was found in patients who displayed CN-a levels higher than 102 pmol/mg/min (40% vs 80%, p = 0.037, Log-rank test), whereas a reduction in BOS-free survival in the limit of statistical significance was found in patients who displayed CN-a levels lower than 12 pmol/mg/min (49% vs 80%, p = 0.0574, Log-rank test). (D) Calcineurin activity and overall survival: no significant difference was found in the overall survival between the 2 groups of patients exhibiting calcineurin activity levels within or outside of the range of 12–102 pmol/mg/min.

a values, either high or low values, were mainly those patients who developed acute rejection and had an altered pulmonary function. These observations led us to define an optimal activity for CN between two thresholds, 12 and 102 pmol/mg/min. Patients who had CN-a values within this range had a significantly higher survival without BOS. Furthermore, the occurrence of malignancies and viral infections was significantly lower in patients who exhibited CN-a values higher than 12 pmol/mg/min.

With the introduction of more potent immunosuppressive agents and newer combinations during the last ten years, patient and graft survivals have dramatically increased following most types of solid organ transplantation. However the incidence of post-transplantation infections and cancer also has increased. It was thought that potent immunosuppression, as reflected by the occurrence of adverse events, was protective against immunogenic stimulation. However, despite a modern immunosuppressive regimen, lung transplantation is characterized by both poor

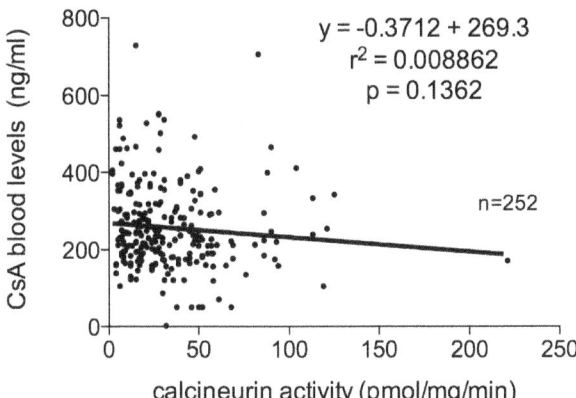

Figure 4. Calcineurin activity and cyclosporine blood levels. The relationship between calcineurin activity (CN-a) and the levels of cyclosporine (CsA) in blood was investigated. No correlation was found between CN-a and the level of CsA in blood.

patient and graft survivals as well as devastating adverse events. The results of the present study may provide a partial explanation for the disappointing long-term outcomes in lung transplant patients. Indeed, we observed extreme CN-a values, below 12 pmol/mg/min or higher than 102 pmol/mg/min, more frequently in the present cohort of lung transplant patients than in other types of transplant patients that we have examined such as hematopoietic stem cell transplant patients [20] or heart transplant patients (unpublished data). In addition, we established a relationship between CN-a and the occurrence of both acute and chronic rejection. This relationship was non-monotonic in that both very low and very high CN-a levels were associated with the onset of acute rejection. As expected, very high CN-a could reflect poor immunosuppression that is not sufficient to counteract the immunogenic activation of T lymphocytes.

On the contrary, the presence of a low threshold was very surprising since very low CN-a levels should have been associated with a strong protection against lymphocyte activation. In fact, the patients with very low CN-a levels were, indeed, strongly immunosuppressed since they developed a higher rate of both malignant diseases and viral infections as compared to patients with higher CN-a levels. Nevertheless, their CN-a levels did not reflect their immunologic potency towards the graft. This finding is consistent with the recently reported activation of a negative feedback loop, via endogeneous CN inhibitors, calcipressins, which down-regulate the CN/NFAT signaling pathway when it is activated [25–28]. Although the calcipressin family has been extensively investigated in brain, heart and endothelial cells, a very limited number of studies has been reported concerning the immune system. Additionally, the impact of calcipressins on the effects of immunosuppressive agents in the context of transplantation has never been assessed. Therefore, we anticipate that low CN-a levels displayed by lung transplant patients developing a rejection are associated first with a lymphocyte activation subsequently followed by a strong endogenous down-regulation of the calcineurin/NFAT signaling pathway.

Taken together, these findings on the relationships between CN-a and acute rejection, pulmonary function and the occurrence of adverse events related to over-immunosuppression led us to define an optimal activity for CN between two thresholds, 12 and 102 pmol/mg/min, and to assess, retrospectively, whether patients who displayed CN-a values between these two thresholds had a significantly higher rate of survival without BOS/chronic

rejection. Lung transplantation is the type of organ transplantation that gives the poorest outcomes, with 45% of the recipients dying within 5 years, mainly due to the development of chronic rejection in response to immunologic, ischemic and infectious injury. Unfortunately, once the clinical signs of BOS/chronic rejection appear, it is usually too late to reverse it. We report here that patients who displayed CN-a values within the range of 12–102 pmol/mg/min had a significantly higher rate of survival without BOS/chronic rejection. In addition, this association of BOS/chronic rejection and CN-a values was not explained by the known risk factors of BOS such as acute rejection, CMV infection, primary graft dysfunction grade III, anti-HLA antibodies or gastro-oesophageal reflux. In a logistic regression model taking into account the other risk factors, the CN-a range was the only variable significantly associated with BOS/chronic rejection. Therefore, CN-a may constitute an additional risk factor of BOS. Currently, overall survival is not significantly associated with CN-a values. However, we have to take into account that, in our study, the median time of occurrence of BOS was 19 months and that it has been shown that the median survival after the onset of BOS is 30 months [29]. Therefore, the overall survival according to CN-a values need to be re-assessed after a longer period of follow-up.

The degree of CN inhibition up to 12 hours after treatment with CsA has been shown to vary directly with the blood levels of CsA [30]. However, this relationship might not persist after several months of treatment with CsA because of the potential contribution of lymphocyte stimulation to the drug effect upon the target. Indeed, we report here that blood levels of CsA and trough levels of CN-a are not correlated. This observation is in agreement with previous findings in hematopoietic stem-cell transplant-, in liver transplant- and in kidney transplant-patients [20,21,24,31,32]. However, the absence of correlation between CN-a levels and CsA whole blood concentrations does not mean that the latter is not a predictor of patient outcome.

There are advantages and limitations to using CN-a as a biomarker. First, interpretation by clinicians of CN-a values, which appear to display a considerable dispersion, may prove to be difficult. Second, other markers, such as the degree of T-cell activation in blood [33], in broncho-alveolar fluid [34,35] or increased T-cell pro-inflammatory cytokine production in the graft [36], have been associated with acute rejection. However, as compared to these studies, the main objective of our study was to identify and characterize a rejection marker that is the most directly related to the degree of immunosuppression produced by an anticalcineurin drug such as CsA. Indeed, only this type of marker aids in determining therapeutic options. Consequently, we believe that our observations can help clinicians in their use of CsA. Our findings suggest that CsA should be administered with much more caution during episodes of acute rejection than might have been thought previously. In particular, monitoring of CN-a sequentially after transplantation might be helpful for facilitating the optimization of multidrug immunosuppressant regimens including those employing CsA. The targeting of CN-a levels between the 25th and 75th percentiles, that is between 17 and 62 pmol/mg/min, can be proposed as a desirable therapeutic range in order to avoid values of CN-a outside the range of 12–102 pmol/mg/min that is associated with poor outcome. Indeed, the dose of CsA should be increased for patients with suspected acute rejection and CN-a levels over 62 pmol/mg/min but not for those patients with CN-a levels below 17 pmol/mg/min. In the latter case, a switch to another class of immunosuppressant can be recommended. Recommendations of this type can be made only when the most specific biomarkers are used and not when general biomarkers, only, are available. However, our data are still preliminary and need to be confirmed through a prospective validation cohort. Further investigation of calcineurin levels need to be carried before considering calcineurin levels as a biomarker.

In summary, we have shown that a relationship exists between CN-a and both acute and chronic rejection in lung transplant patients. Further, we have defined an optimal activity for calcineurin between two thresholds : the risk of rejection was higher when the enzyme activity was above the upper threshold of 102 pmol/mg/min or below the lower threshold of 12 pmol/mg/min. In addition, we report that the occurrence of malignancies

and viral infections was significantly higher in patients displaying CN-a below the lower threshold. Based upon these findings, CN-a appears as a potential predictive biomarker that could lead to new guidelines for the management of lung transplant patients.

Author Contributions

Conceived and designed the experiments: SS RB CA RG MS. Performed the experiments: SS CA DG LH RG BP VB RB MS. Analyzed the data: SS CL CA RB JPJ MS. Contributed reagents/materials/analysis tools: SS CL AD MP EMB FL MS. Wrote the paper: SS RB MS.

References

1. American Thoracic Society (1998) International guidelines for the selection of lung transplant candidates. Am J Respir Crit Care Med 158: 335–339.
2. Lin HM, Kauffman HM, McBride MA, Davies DB, Rosendale JD, et al. (1998) Center-specific graft and patient survival rates: 1997 United Network for Organ Sharing (UNOS) report. JAMA 280: 1153–1160.
3. Bando K, Paradis IL, Similo S, Konishi H, Komatsu K, et al. (1995) Obliterative bronchiolitis after lung and heart-lung transplantation: an analysis of risk factors and management. J Thorac Cardiovasc Surg 110: 4–13.
4. Sharples LD, Tamm M, McNeil K, Higenbottam TW, Stewart S, et al. (1996) Development of bronchiolitis obliterans syndrome in recipients of heart-lung transplantation – early risk factors. Transplantation 61: 560–566.
5. Trulock EP (1993) Management of lung transplant rejection. Chest 103: 1566–1576.
6. Yousem SA (1993) Lymphocytic bronchitis/bronchiolitis in lung allograft recipients. Am J Surg Pathol 17: 491–496.
7. Yousem SA, Duncan SR, Griffith BP (1992) Intersticial and airspace granulation tissue reactions in lung transplant recipients. Am J Surg Pathol 16: 877–884.
8. Estenne M, Hertz MI (2002) Bronchiolitis obliterans after human lung transplantation. Am J Respir Crit Care Med 166: 440–444.
9. Al-Githmi I, Batawil N, Shigemura N, Hsin M, Lee TW, et al. (2006) Bronchiolitis obliterans following lung transplantation. Eur J Cardiothorac Surg 30: 846–851.
10. Sharples LD, McNeil K, Stewart S, Wallork J (2002) Risk factors for bronchiolitis obliterans: a systematic review of recent publications. J Heart Lung Transplant 21: 271–281.
11. Arcasoy SM, Kotloff RM (1999) Lung transplantation. N E J M 340: 1081–1091.
12. Martinu T, Chan DF, Palmer SM (2009) Acute rejection and humoral sensitization in lung transplant recipients. Proc Am Thorac Soc 6: 54–65.
13. Batiuk TD, Kung L, Halloran PF (1997) Evidence that calcineurin is rate-limiting for primary human lymphocyte activation. J Clin Invest 100: 1894–1901.
14. Graef IA, Chen F, Chen L, Kuo A, Crabtree GR (2001) Signal transduced by Ca(2+)/calcineurin and NFATc3/c4 pattern the developing vasculature. Cell 105: 863–875.
15. Beals CR, Sheridan CM, Turck CW, Gardner P, Crabtree GR (1997) Nuclear export of NF-ATc enhanced by glycogen synthase kinase-3. Science 275: 1930–1934.
16. Okamura H, Aramburu J, Garcia-Rodriguez C, Viola JPB, Raghavan A, et al. (2000) Concerted dephosphorylation of the transcription factor NFAT1 induces a conformational switch that regulates transcriptional activity. Mol Cell 6: 539–550.
17. Timmerman LA, Clipstone NA, Ho SN, Northrop JP, Crabtree GR (1996) Rapid shuttling of NF-AT in discrimination of Ca2+ signals and immunosuppression. Nature 383: 837–840.
18. Huppa JB, Gleimer M, Sumen C, Davis MM (2003) Continuous T cell receptor signaling required for synapse maintenance and full effector potential. Nature Immunol 4: 749–755.
19. Feske S, Okamura H, Hogan PG, Rao A (2003) Ca2+/calcineurin signaling in cells of the immune system. Biochem Biophysic Res Com 31: 1117–1132.
20. Sanquer S, Schwarzinger M, Maury S, Yakouben K, Rafi H, et al. (2004) Calcineurin activity as a functional index of immunosuppression after allogeneic stem-cell transplantation. Transplantation 77: 854–858.

21. Fukudo M, Yano I, Masuda S, Fukatsu S, Katsura T, et al. (2005) Pharmacodynamic analysis of tacrolimus and cyclosporine in living-donor liver transplant patients. Clin Pharmacol Therap 78: 168–181.
22. Yousem SA, Berry GJ, Gagle PT, Chamberlain D, Husain AN, et al. (1996) Revision of the 1990 working formulation for the classification of pulmonary allograft rejection: Lung Rejection Study Group. J Heart Lung Transplant 15: 1–15.
23. Estenne M, Maurer JR, Boehler A, Egan JJ, Frost A, et al. (2002) Bronchiolitis obliterans syndrome 2001: An update of the diagnostic criteria. J Heart Lung Transplant 21: 297–310.
24. Caruso R, Perico N, Cattaneo D, Piccinina G, Bonazzola S, et al. (2001) Whole-blood calcineurin activity is not predicted by cyclosporine blood concentration in renal transplant recipients. Clin Chem 47: 1679–1687.
25. Fuentes JJ, Genesca L, Kingsbury TJ, Cunningham KW, Pérez-Riba M, et al. (2000) DSCR1, overexpressed in Down syndrome, is an inhibitor of calcineurin-mediated signaling pathways. Hum Mol Genet 9: 1681–1690.
26. Kingsbury TJ, Cuningham KW (2000) A conserved family of calcineurin regulators. Genes Dev 14: 1595–1604.
27. Gorlach J, Fox DS, Cutler NS, Cox GM, Perfect JR, et al. (2000) Identification and characterization of a highly conserved calcineurin binding protein, CBP1/calcipressin, in Cryptococcus neoformans. EMBO J 19: 3618–3629.
28. Ryeom S, Greenwald R, Sharpe AH, McKeon F (2003) The threshold pattern of calcineurin-dependent gene expression is altered by loss of the endogenous inhibitor calcipressin. Nature Immunol 9: 874–878.
29. Finlen-Copeland CA, Snyder LD, Zaas DW, Turbyfill WJ, Davies WA, et al. (2010) Survival after bronchiolitis obliterans syndrome among bilateral lung transplant patients. Am J Respir Crit Care Med 182: 784–789.
30. Halloran PF, Helms LMH, Kung L, Noujaim J (1999) The temporal profile of calcineurin inhibition by cyclosporine in vivo. Transplantation 68: 1356–1361.
31. Yano I (2008) Pharmacodynamic monitoring of calcineurin phosphatase activity in transplant patients treated with calcineurin inhibitors. Drug Metab Pharmacokinet 23: 150–157.
32. Yano I, Masuda S, Egawa H, Sugimoto M, Fukudo M, et al. (2012) Significance of trough monitoring for tacrolimus blood concentration and calcineurin activity in adult patients undergoing primary living-donor liver transplantation. Eur J Clin Pharmacol 68: 259–266.
33. Schowengerdt KO, Ficker FJ, Bahjat KS, Kuntz ST (2000) Increased expression of the lymphocyte early activation marker CD69 in peripheral blood correlates with histologic evidence of cardiac allograft rejection. Transplantation 69: 2102–2107.
34. Gregson AL, Hoji A, Saggar R, Ross DJ, Kubak BM, et al. (2008) Bronchoalveolar immunologic profile of acute human lung transplant allograft rejection. Transplantation 85: 1056–1059.
35. Crim C, Keller CA, Dunphy CH, Maluf HM, Ohar JA (1996) Flow cytometric analysis of lung lymphocytes in lung transplant recipients. Am J Respir Crit Care med 153: 1041–1046.
36. Hodge G, Hodge S, Chambers DC, Reynolds PN, Holmes M (2012) Increased expression of graft intraepithelial T-cell pro-inflammatory cytokines compared with native lung during episodes of acute rejection. J Heart Lung Transplant 31: 538–544.

18

Disappearance of GFP-Positive Hepatocytes Transplanted into the Liver of Syngeneic Wild-Type Rats Pretreated with Retrorsine

Hiromichi Maeda[1,2,3]*, Masatoshi Shigoka[1], Yongchun Wang[1], Yingxin Fu[1], Russell N. Wesson[1], Qing Lin[1], Robert A. Montgomery[1], Hideaki Enzan[4], Zhaoli Sun[1]*

1 Department of Surgery, Johns Hopkins University School of Medicine, Baltimore, Maryland, United States of America, 2 Department of Surgery, Kochi Medical School, Nankoku, Kochi, Japan, 3 Cancer Treatment Center, Kochi Medical School, Nankoku, Kochi, Japan, 4 Diagnostic Pathology, Chikamori Hospital, Kochi, Kochi, Japan

Abstract

Background and Aim: Green fluorescent protein (GFP) is a widely used molecular tag to trace transplanted cells in rodent liver injury models. The differing results from various previously reported studies using GFP could be attributed to the immunogenicity of GFP.

Methods: Hepatocytes were obtained from GFP-expressing transgenic (Tg) Lewis rats and were transplanted into the livers of wild-type Lewis rats after they had undergone a partial hepatectomy. The proliferation of endogenous hepatocytes in recipient rats was inhibited by pretreatment with retrorsine to enhance the proliferation of the transplanted hepatocytes. Transplantation of wild-type hepatocytes into GFP-Tg rat liver was also performed for comparison.

Results: All biopsy specimens taken seven days after transplantation showed engraftment of transplanted hepatocytes, with the numbers of transplanted hepatocytes increasing until day 14. GFP-positive hepatocytes in wild-type rat livers were decreased by day 28 and could not be detected on day 42, whereas the number of wild-type hepatocytes steadily increased in GFP-Tg rat liver. Histological examination showed degenerative change of GFP-positive hepatocytes and the accumulation of infiltrating cells on day 28. PCR analysis for the GFP transgene suggested that transplanted hepatocytes were eliminated rather than being retained along with the loss of GFP expression. Both modification of the immunological response using tacrolimus and bone marrow transplantation prolonged the survival of GFP-positive hepatocytes. In contrast, host immunization with GFP-positive hepatocytes led to complete loss of GFP-positive hepatocytes by day 14.

Conclusion: GFP-positive hepatocytes isolated from GFP-Tg Lewis rats did not survive long term in the livers of retrorsine-pretreated wild-type Lewis rats. The mechanism underlying this phenomenon most likely involves an immunological reaction against GFP. The influence of GFP immunogenicity on cell transplantation models should be considered in planning in vivo experiments using GFP and in interpreting their results.

Editor: Zhiyuan Gong, National University of Singapore, Singapore

Funding: This study was supported by the Kochi Organization for Medical Reformation and Renewal (http://www.kochi-mrr.or.jp/) to HM. The funders had no role in study design, data collection and analysis, decision to publish, or preparation of the manuscript.

Competing Interests: The authors have declared that no competing interests exist.

* E-mail: hmaeda@kochi-u.ac.jp (HM); zsun2@jhmi.edu (ZS)

Introduction

The accumulation of green fluorescent protein (GFP) in cells is widely used as a molecular tag that can be readily visualized under ultraviolet light illumination. Many different GFP-transgenic (Tg) animals have been generated and utilized for tracking cells in organ and cell transplantation studies. GFP can show weak immunogenicity [1,2] and/or cell toxicity [3,4] that can potentially alter experimental results. Gambotto et al. [1] showed that GFP could generate an antigenic epitope that binds to H2-K^d molecules in BALB/c mice, while Inoue and colleagues [2] generated the GFP-Tg Lewis rat (Major Histocompatibility complex haplotype; RT1^l) and reported that transplanted skin grafts from these rats to wild-type Lewis rats lost viability after about a week, suggesting immunological rejection. Nevertheless,

isolated cells from GFP-Tg rats were observed long after cell transplantation into immune-privileged sites such as the central nervous system and joints [2,5]. In addition, liver harvested from a GFP-Tg Lewis rat survived long term in a wild-type Lewis rat without the use of an immunosuppressant (our unpublished data). These experimental findings imply that GFP is weakly immunogenic, but that organs or cells expressing GFP can survive at sites where there is a weaker immunological reaction.

In general, transplanted allogeneic hepatocytes are eliminated within a few days without the use of an immunosuppressant [6]. Nevertheless, studies with rat models suggest that GFP is minimally immunogenic when GFP-positive hepatocytes or stem/progenitor cells are transplanted into syngeneic liver. Oertel and colleagues [7] transplanted hepatocytes transfected with the

GFP gene into retrorsine-pretreated wild-type syngeneic rat liver. They demonstrated continuous GFP expression, driven by the liver-specific albumin enhancer/promoter, in transplanted hepatocytes up to four months after transplantation. Other studies showed repopulation of injured liver tissue by transplanted syngeneic stem/progenitor cells expressing GFP [8,9]. Therefore, we expected to see long-term survival of GFP-positive hepatocytes after transplantation into a wild-type Lewis rat liver.

In a pilot study, we did not observe proliferation of GFP-positive hepatocytes at six weeks after transplantation of a syngeneic liver specimen. This observation was considered to be important not only for the interpretation of previous data, but also in planning of future experiments using the rat model containing GFP-positive hepatocytes. Therefore, further studies were performed to answer three questions. 1) Did a technical error occur that prevented proliferation of GFP-positive hepatocytes? 2) Was there a loss of GFP-positive hepatocytes or a loss of GFP expression? 3) Was this phenomenon caused by a host immunological response or by GFP toxicity?

Methods

Animals

GFP-Tg Lewis rats, originally generated by Eiji Kobayashi [2], were obtained from the National Institutes of Health (NIH)-funded Rat Resource and Research Center, University of Missouri, Columbia, MO, USA. Male wild-type Lewis rats were purchased from Harlan Sprague-Dawley (Indianapolis, IN, USA) or from Charles-River Laboratories (Wilmington, MA, USA). Animals were maintained in the specific pathogen-free facility of the Johns Hopkins Medical Institutions and were cared for according to NIH guidelines and under a protocol approved by the Johns Hopkins University Animal Care Committee. Rats weighing 150–200 g were used as hepatocyte donors. Recipient rats weighting 180–200 g received an initial treatment of retrorsine as described below. General anesthesia during animal procedures was provided using isoflurane supplied by an isoflurane vaporizer at a concentration of 4% for induction and approximately 2% for maintenance. The muscle tone and respiratory rate of rats were closely monitored to maintain the appropriate depth of anesthesia.

Hepatocyte isolation

Hepatocytes were isolated using a two-step collagenase perfusion procedure [10] with minor modifications. Rats were sacrificed under general anesthesia by exsanguination from the inferior vena cava. The liver was immediately perfused for 10 min with pre-warmed (37°C) first solution, containing 150 mL of HBSS without calcium, 75 mg of EDTA, and 1 mL of 1 M HEPES. At the same time, the portal vein to the left lobe and the left side of the middle lobe of the liver was ligated to reduce the perfusion area. The liver was then perfused for 10 min with pre-warmed (37°C) second solution, containing 90 mL of HBSS with calcium, 10 mL of fetal bovine serum (FBS), 1 mL of 1 M HEPES, and 80 mg of collagenase type IV. The liver was transferred to a dish containing 50 mL of cold HBSS containing 10% FBS. The serous membrane was gently torn with forceps and cells that flowed out were collected. The cells were then transferred to a 50 mL tube after passing through a 70-μm mesh filter without mechanical pressure, and the collected cells were centrifuged at $50 \times g$ for 1 min. The supernatant containing non-parenchymal cells was discarded and the pellet was washed by resuspension in 50 mL of HBSS containing 10% FBS, and then centrifuged. This washing step was repeated. The cell number and viability were calculated and the

cell density was adjusted to 1.5×10^7 cells/mL for cell transplantation and 1×10^8 cells/mL for immunization (Fig. 1). The viability of hepatocytes was maintained at more than 80% throughout the experiments. One donor provided hepatocytes for between four and six recipient rats.

Hepatocyte transplantation

The livers of rats were accessed by laparotomy under general anesthesia. The left lobe and right side of the middle lobe of livers were removed to achieve approximately 40–50% hepatectomy (50% hepatectomy) [11]. A 28 G needle was inserted deep into the right side of the middle lobe and the hepatocytes were injected with the needle slowly being pulled back. This procedure was repeated three times using different puncture sites, allowing the transplanted hepatocytes to distribute throughout the whole right side of the middle lobe. This method prevented embolic injury to the other hepatic lobes and enabled us to safely perform a core needle biopsy one week after cell transplantation. After 1×10^7 cells in total were transplanted, the hemostasis was checked and the wound was closed.

Preparation and administration of retrorsine

Retrorsine treatment was used to inhibit the mitosis of mature hepatocytes and to facilitate the proliferation of transplanted hepatocytes. A 30-mg/kg of retrorsine was administered into the peritoneal cavity of recipient rats twice, two weeks apart, according to the original method [12]. The retrorsine dose was prepared by adding 100 mg of retrorsine into 10 mL of normal saline, whereupon 1 M HCl was added until the solution reached pH 2. Once the retrorsine was completely dissolved, the solution was neutralized with 1 M NaOH. The retrorsine dose was freshly prepared and used immediately for each treatment.

Sample preparation

After laparotomy under general anesthesia, the right edge of the middle liver lobe was cut with a surgical scalpel. Small pieces of tissue were dissected from this site for DNA analysis and the remaining small piece of tissue was fixed in 2% paraformaldehyde for microscopic observation (Fig. 1). After exsanguination, the liver was slowly perfused with 10 mL of cold PBS and then with 30 mL of 2% paraformaldehyde. After excision of the whole liver, the right upper lobe was cut into three pieces and further fixed with 2% paraformaldehyde for 30 min at room temperature in the dark. The liver samples were then immersed in a 30% sucrose solution and stored at 4°C overnight, before embedding in OCT compound (Sakura Finetek USA, Torrance, CA, USA) and storage at −80°C.

Percentage area occupied by transplanted hepatocytes in recipient liver

Sections (6 μm thickness) were prepared from each of four liver tissue samples from each rat. Images of three random fields from each section slide were recorded, providing a total of 12 fields from each rat. The relative area of the transplanted hepatocyte area as a percentage of the total area was calculated by using Photoshop CS3 (Adobe systems, San Jose, CA, USA).

Immunohistochemistry staining

Immunohistochemistry staining was performed to confirm the expression of GFP expression by light microscopy. The tissue sections were incubated with 1% SDS in PBS for 7 min, followed by incubation with 1% H_2O_2 in PBST for 60 min. The presence of endogenous biotin was blocked using an avidin-biotin blocking

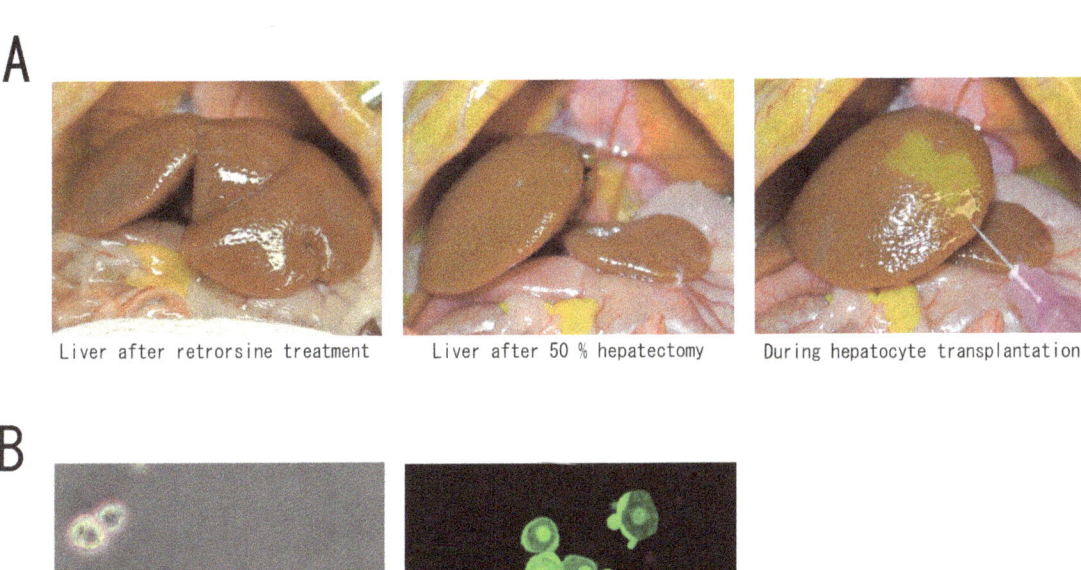

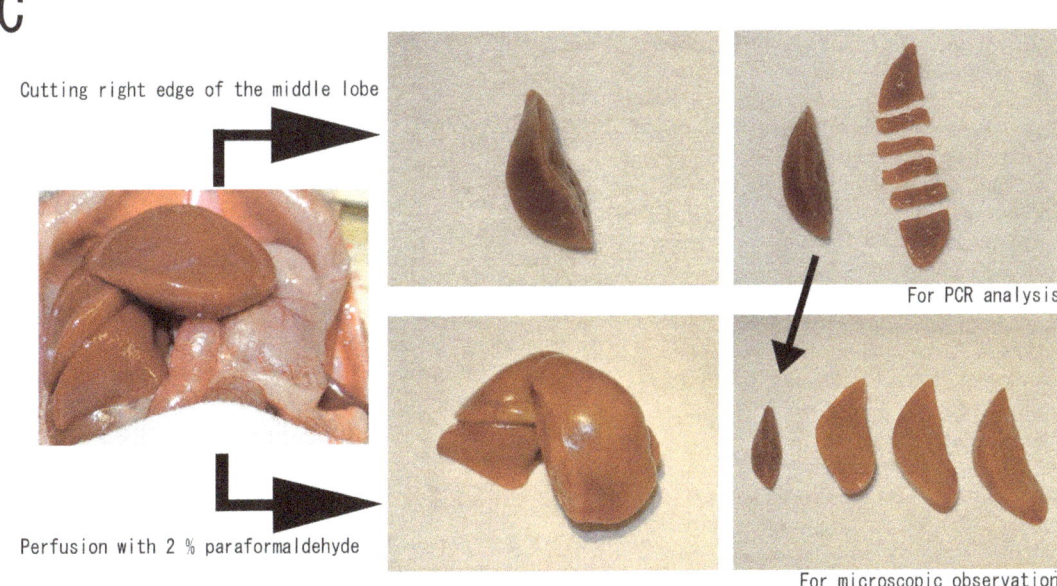

Figure 1. Hepatocyte transplantation and sample preparation. (A) Hepatocyte transplantation. After retrorsine treatment, the parenchyma of the liver became slightly hard and the surface was irregular. After resection of the left lobe and the left side of the middle lobe, hepatocytes were transplanted directly into the liver. The suspended cells spread rapidly according to the blood flow and produced a demarcation line, which disappeared immediately after injection. (B) Isolated hepatocytes. Trypan blue staining identified the viable hepatocytes, which were negative for 7-AAD (red stain) and expressed GFP. GFP-positive hepatocytes lose GFP expression immediately after cell death. The isolated hepatocytes cells were not completely separated. (C) Sample collection. Two weeks after cell transplantation, the remnant liver grew enlarged and swollen. (Upper arm) A small piece of the liver was obtained from the right edge of the middle lobe before perfusion from the portal vein, and then cut into smaller pieces for PCR analysis. The larger part of the liver was fixed with 2% paraformaldehyde for microscopic observation. (Lower arm) The liver was perfused with 2% paraformaldehyde and removed. The right part of the middle lobe was cut into three pieces and further processed for microscopic observation.

reagent (Avidin Blocking System; DAKO, Cambridgeshire, UK), and then sections were incubated with biotin-conjugated anti-GFP antibody (1:200 dilution, Abcam, Cambridge, MA, USA) for 1 h. Tissue sections were then incubated with AB complex (VECTAS-TAIN ABC kit; Vector, Burlingame, CA, USA) for 30 min according to the manufacturer's instructions. The signal was detected with DAB (Liquid DAB+ Substrate Chromogen System; DAKO), and the tissue sections were counterstained with haematoxylin for 20 s.

Immunofluorescent staining

The expression of albumin by the transplanted hepatocytes was detected using immunofluorescent staining. The tissue sections were pre-incubated with 1% SDS in PBS for 12 min, whereupon they were incubated with sheep anti-rat albumin primary antibody (1:800 dilution, Bethyl laboratory Inc, Montgomery, TX, USA) for 30 min. The sections were then washed and incubated with Cy3-conjugated donkey anti-sheep IgG secondary antibody (1:400 dilution, Jackson Immunoresearch Laboratories, West Grove, PA, USA) for 30 min.

The phenotype of infiltrating cells adjacent to GFP-positive transplanted hepatocytes was investigated by assaying the expression of CD4, CD8, and ED-2. The tissue sections were pre-incubated with 1% SDS in PBS for 1–2 min. CD4 was detected using goat anti-CD4 primary antibody (1:100 dilution, Santa Cruz Biotechnology, Dallas, TX, USA) and Cy3-conjugated donkey anti-goat IgG antibody (1:100 dilution, Jackson Immunoresearch Laboratories). CD8 was detected using rabbit anti-CD8 primary antibody (1:100 dilution, Santa Cruz Biotechnology) and Cy3-conjugated donkey anti-rabbit IgG secondary antibody (1:100 dilution, Jackson Immunoresearch Laboratories). ED-2 was detected using mouse anti-ED-2 primary antibody (1:100 dilution, Santa Cruz Biotechnology) and Cy3-conjugated donkey anti-mouse IgG secondary antibody (1:100 dilution, Jackson Immunoresearch Laboratories). In order to characterize GFP-positive non-parenchymal cells, rat endothelial cell antibody (RECA) was detected by using mouse anti-RECA primary antibody ((1:100 dilution, Abcam), and Cy3-conjugated donkey anti-mouse IgG secondary antibody.

Sections were incubated with the primary antibody for 60 min and with the secondary antibody with 30 min. Nuclear staining was performed using DAPI (DAKO) staining when necessary. Serum blocking was performed with 10% donkey serum for 10 min.

Genomic DNA extraction and PCR analysis

Tissue samples were quick-frozen in liquid nitrogen and stored at −80°C until use. Genomic DNA was extracted by first treating the tissue with proteinase K, and then isolating the DNA by phenol-chloroform extraction (Invitrogen, Carlsbad, CA, USA). The presence of the GFP gene in each sample was analyzed using PCR with 1 μg of genomic DNA for each sample, and 0.1 μg of genomic DNA for the positive and negative controls. The PCR comprised 30 cycles of amplification. The DNA content of each sample analyzed for GFP was normalized to that of the *Rattus norvegicus* Sry gene, which is the sex-determining region on Y chromosome. The Sry copy number per haploid genome is similar among all male rat cells. The presence of the Sry gene was analyzed using 0.1 μg of genomic DNA in the samples and controls with 28 amplification cycles.

Bone marrow transplantation

Bone marrow cells were obtained from the bilateral tibia and the femoral bone of male Lewis rats weighing 150–200 g. The bone marrow from one rat provided sufficient donor cells for one recipient rat. Erythroblasts and erythrocytes were removed using red blood cell lysing buffer (Sigma Aldrich, St. Louis, MO, USA). Bone marrow cells were washed and approximately $2–3 \times 10^8$ cells were injected via the tail vein into each recipient rat on the same day that the recipient rat received 11 Gy of whole body irradiation. The relative numbers of GFP-positive leukocytes in peripheral blood was assayed using flow cytometry one day before hepatocyte transplantation at seven weeks after bone marrow transplantation.

Experimental protocol

Experiment 1 - Confirmation of GFP-Tg cell-loss phenomenon (Figs. 2 and 3). A total of 12 wild-type Lewis rats were obtained from Harlan Sprague-Dawley and received hepatocytes from GFP-Tg Lewis rats after retrorsine treatment and 50% hepatectomy. All rats underwent core needle biopsy of the liver seven days after cell transplantation and then were sacrificed on days 14, 28, or 42. For comparison, 12 GFP-Tg Lewis rats received similarly prepared hepatocytes from wild-type Lewis rats. The same studies were performed using the Lewis rats obtained from the Charles River Laboratories and liver samples were collected on days 14 (n = 3) and 42 (n = 3).

Experiment 2 - Effect of an immunosuppressant on GFP-Tg cell loss (Fig. 4). Rats were treated with the immunosuppressive drug, tacrolimus, to investigate if loss of transplanted hepatocytes is related to immunological rejection. Recipient wild-type Lewis rats received 0.3 mg/kg of tacrolimus subcutaneously for five days a week after hepatocyte transplantation, and then were sacrificed on day 42. A control group of rats received the same quantity of normal saline for five days a week.

Experiment 3 - Immunization with GFP-positive hepatocytes (Fig. 4). Wild-type rats received a subcutaneous injection of 1×10^8 isolated hepatocytes from GFP-Tg rats on the same day as retrorsine treatment. A control group of rats received hepatocytes from wild-type Lewis rats. Liver samples were collected two weeks after hepatocyte transplantation (Fig. 4).

Experiment 4 - Modification of the immunological reaction by bone marrow transplantation (Fig. 5). Bone marrow transplantation was performed prior to hepatocyte transplantation to exclude any potential protective effect of tacrolimus on hepatocytes [13] and to confirm the involvement of an immunological reaction. Wild-type Lewis rats received 11 Gy of whole body irradiation and then bone marrow cells from GFP-Tg Lewis rats were transplanted, three weeks prior to retrorsine treatment. Two weeks after the second administration of retrorsine, the rats underwent partial hepatectomy and received hepatocytes from the GFP-Tg Lewis rats (Group 1). Rats in Group 2 received bone marrow transplantation from wild-type Lewis rats. Rats in Group 3 received bone marrow transplantation from GFP-Tg Lewis rats and received HBSS with FBS instead of hepatocyte transplantation. Six weeks after cell transplantation, liver samples were collected.

Results

Mortality and morbidity

One rat from each group in Experiment 1 died of injury to the inferior vena cava or injury to the small intestine during hepatectomy, respectively. No other mortality or late complications, including liver failure and infection, were observed.

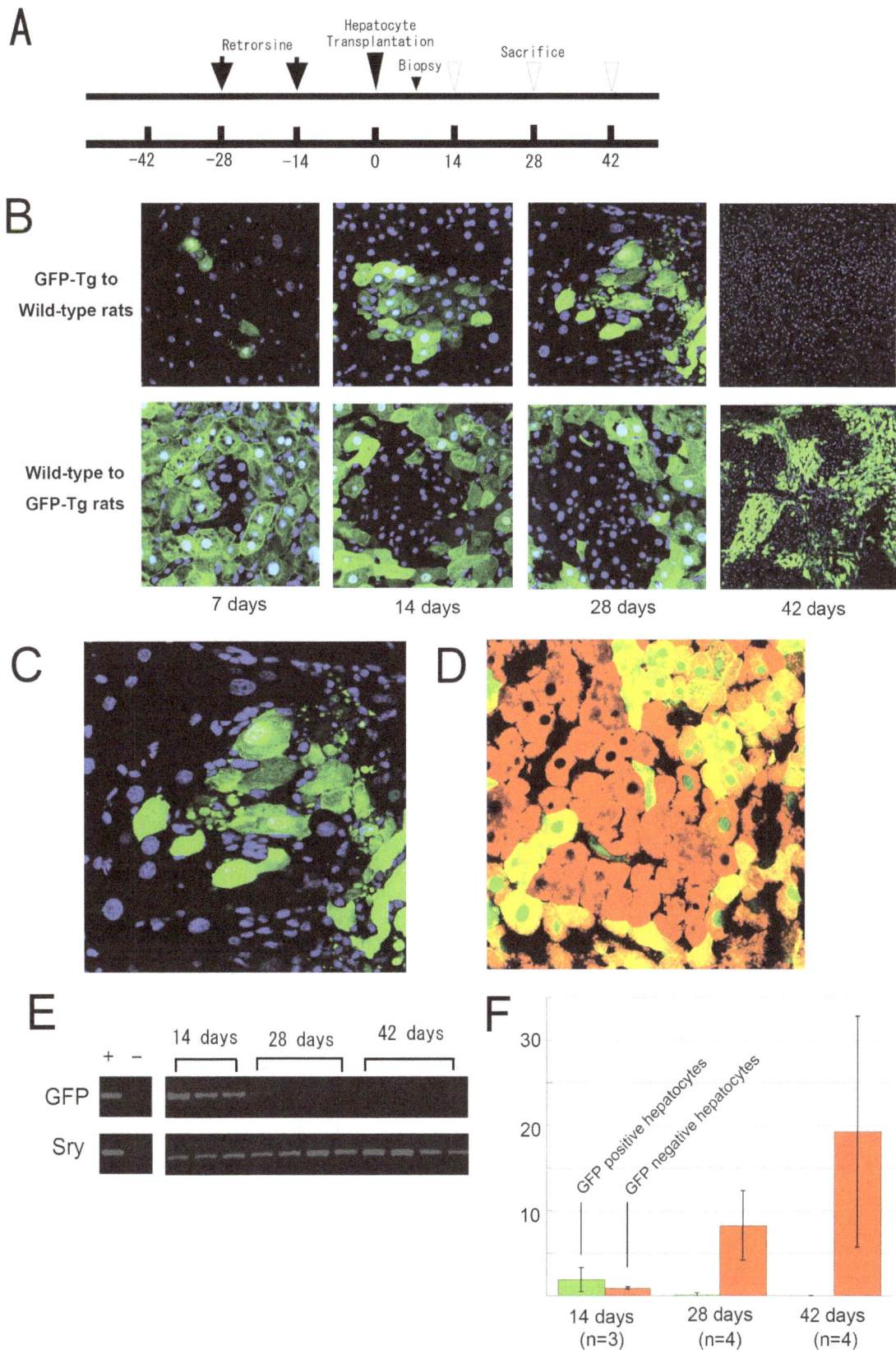

Figure 2. Disappearance of GFP-positive hepatocytes in wild-type syngeneic rat liver. (A) Timeline of Experiment 1. Recipient rats received retrorsine treatment twice (black arrow). One week after hepatocyte transplantation (large black triangle), all rats had a liver biopsy under general anesthesia, and then rats were sacrificed on days 14, 28, or 42 (white triangle). (B) Confocal microscopic observation of GFP fluorescence in hepatocytes after transplantation into wild-type Lewis rats. (Upper lane) The liver biopsy taken at day seven shows engraftment of transplanted hepatocytes in all cases. The nodules of GFP-positive hepatocytes after transplantation were less numerous at day 28 than at day 14. GFP-positive

hepatocytes at 28 days also showed more heterogeneous GFP expression with an irregular cell shape than at day 14, indicating cytoplasmic degenerative changes. The dissociation of GFP-positive hepatocytes was apparent along with nuclear debris (small green dots). The infiltration of GFP-negative cells with a small nucleus (blue stain) was also apparent. (Lower lane) The progressive growth of GFP-negative hepatocytes in GFP-Tg Lewis rat liver resulted in the size of each cluster of transplanted hepatocytes increasing with time. (C) Higher magnification of the liver tissue at 28 days after hepatocyte transplantation from GFP-Tg rats to wild-type rats. (D) Merged image of immunofluorescent staining for albumin (red) and immunohistochemical staining for GFP (green). The transplanted hepatocytes from wild-type rats proliferate and express albumin in GFP-Tg Lewis rat liver. (E)The percentage of transplanted GFP-positive hepatocytes increased by 14 days after cell transplantation, but significantly decreased by 28 days, and no GFP-positive hepatocytes were observed at day 42. In contrast, the percentage of GFP-negative transplanted hepatocytes increased steadily. (F) PCR analysis of the GFP transgene showed a reduction at 28 and 42 days, suggesting elimination of the GFP transgene.

Experiment 1 - Disappearance of GFP-positive hepatocytes

All of the liver biopsies (n = 11) showed engraftment of transplanted hepatocytes from GFP-Tg rats into wild-type rats at seven days after transplantation (Fig. 2). Clusters of GFP-positive hepatocytes were larger and more frequently detected at 14 days after transplantation than at 7 days, suggesting rapid growth of the transplanted hepatocytes. At 28 days after hepatocyte transplan-

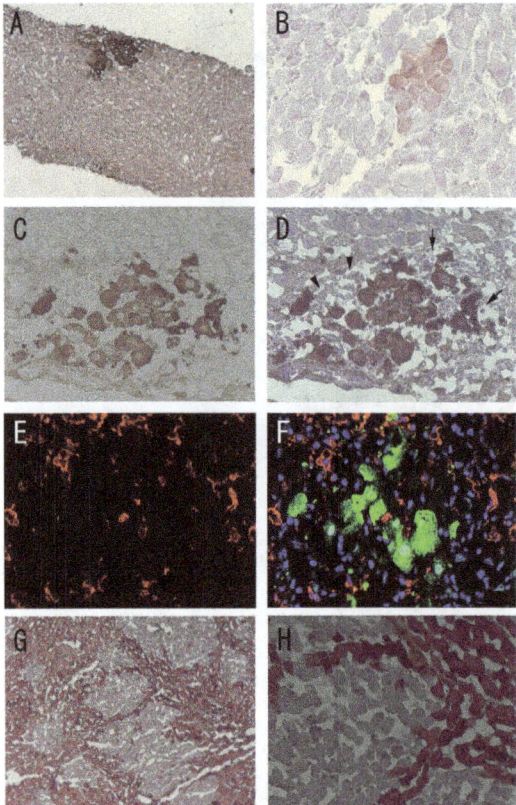

Figure 3. Immunohistochemical staining for GFP and immuno-fluorescent staining for ED-2. (A), (B) The liver specimen showed small clusters of GFP-positive hepatocytes at 7 and 14 days after hepatocyte transplantations into wild-type Lewis rat liver. (C), (D) However, there were fewer GFP-positive hepatocytes apparent at 28 days after hepatocyte transplantation, and dissociated, irregular-shape polygonal cells with debris were observed. Small cells with round nuclei (lymphocytes: arrow) were abundant around the GFP-positive hepatocytes. Cells with a triangular crescent cytoplasmic shape (arrowhead) were reminiscent of Kupffer cells. (E) Some of the infiltrating cells are positive for ED-2 (red). (F) Merged image of GFP (green), ED-2 (red), and DAPI nuclear staining (blue) suggests the accumulation of Kupffer cells adjacent to GFP-positive hepatocytes. (G), (H) The transplanted GFP-positive hepatocytes continued to proliferate at 42 days after hepatocyte transplantation from GFP-negative to GFP-Tg Lewis rats.

tations, the rat livers showed very few clusters of GFP-positive hepatocytes and they exhibited cytoplasmic degenerative changes with nuclear debris (Fig. 2). These cells were surrounded by a large number of GFP-negative, small, round lymphocyte-like cells that were positive for CD4 or CD8 (results not shown). Slightly larger, ED-2-positive, triangular cells that were suggestive of Kupffer cells, were observed in the same region (Fig. 3). A small number of GFP-positive and RECA-positive non-parenchymal cells were also observed. No GFP-positive hepatocytes and only a few GFP-positive non-parenchymal cells were detected at 42 days after transplantation. In contrast, wild-type GFP-negative hepatocytes steadily increased in number after transplantation into GFP-Tg rat liver. At 42 days after transplantation, approximately 19.3% (range; 5.6%–35.2%) of the liver area was occupied by transplanted GFP-negative hepatocytes. The transplanted hepatocytes were largely evenly distributed and each liver specimen from a single rat showed similar features by direct fluorescent microscopy, which is consistent with a previous report [14].

PCR analysis for the GFP transgene in wild-type rat liver showed reduced amounts at four and six weeks after transplantation. This suggests a gradual elimination of GFP-positive cells rather than loss of GFP expression by any remaining viable transplanted cells or their progeny cells. We also examined liver specimens three months after cell transplantation from GFP-Tg Lewis rats to wild-type rats (n = 5), and observed complete loss of GFP-positive hepatocytes and non-parenchymal cells by both fluorescent microscopy and PCR analysis for the GFP transgene (data not shown). This observation was also confirmed using Lewis rats from Charles-River laboratories.

Experiment 2 - Immunosuppressant treatment prolongs survival of transplanted GFP-Tg hepatocytes

The livers of rats treated with the immunosuppressant, tacrolimus, showed abundant GFP-positive hepatocytes and GFP-positive non-parenchymal cells at 42 days after cell transplantation. Control rats that received only saline for 5 days a week showed no GFP-positive hepatocytes at 42 days after cell transplantation (Fig. 4). Non-parenchymal cells were mainly positive for RECA by immunofluorescent staining and few inflammatory cells were found in the vicinity of transplanted hepatocytes.

Experiment 3 - Host pre-immunization with GFP-Tg hepatocytes shortens the survival of transplanted GFP-Tg

The livers of rats treated by pre-immunization with GFP-Tg hepatocytes showed no GFP-positive hepatocytes at 14 days after cell transplantation. Cell-like structures exhibiting green fluorescence were observed in the livers, but no viable cells with GFP expression were identified, nor were GFP-positive hepatocytes detectable at the sites of subcutaneous injection of GFP-Tg hepatocytes. Control rats that were pre-immunized with wild-type hepatocytes showed clusters of GFP-positive hepatocytes at 14 days after cell transplantation.

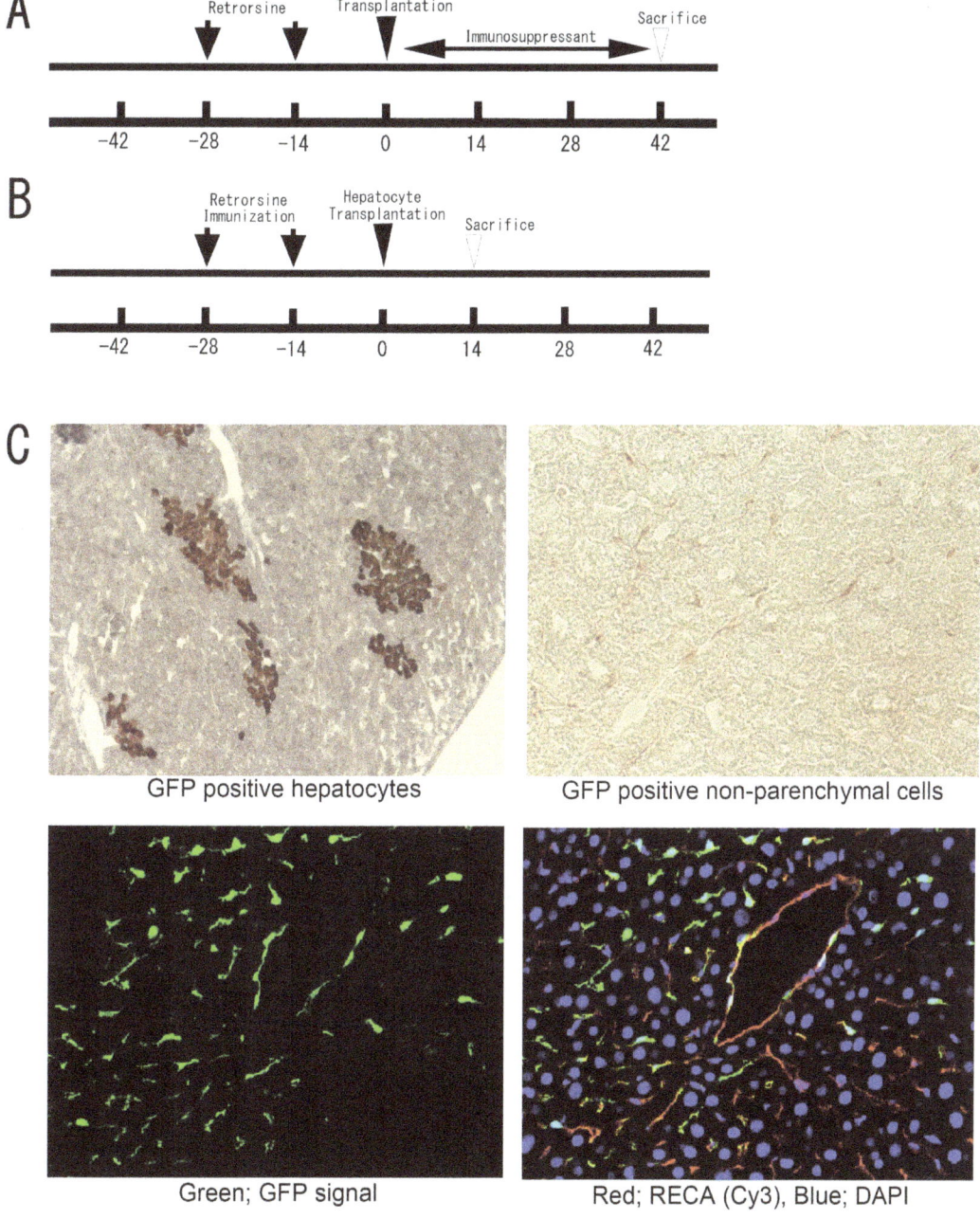

Figure 4. The effect of immunosuppressant or sensitization on GFP-positive hepatocyte survival after transplantation. (A) Timeline of Experiment 2. A dose of 0.3 mg/kg of tacrolimus was administered after hepatocyte transplantation for five days a week, and tissue samples were collected 42 days after transplantation. The control group received normal saline instead of tacrolimus. (B) Timeline of Experiment 3. The recipient rats received a subcutaneous injection of GFP-positive hepatocytes (1×10^8 cells) on the same day as retrorsine treatment. Fourteen days after hepatocyte transplantation into the liver, tissue samples were collected to evaluate the survival of transplanted hepatocytes. (C) After immunosuppressant treatment, the specimen shows GFP-positive hepatocytes and abundant GFP-positive sinusoidal lining cells. These non-parenchymal cells were also positive for the RecA marker of endothelial cells.

Experiment 4 - Modification of the immunological reaction by bone marrow transplantation

More than 90% of leukocytes in the peripheral blood of wild-type rats were positive for GFP expression seven weeks after bone narrow transplantation from GFP-Tg Lewis rats (Fig. 5). In Group 1, GFP-positive hepatocytes continued to survive in wild-type rat liver for at least 42 days after hepatocyte transplantation. In contrast, the rats in Group 2 that received bone marrow of wild-type rats and GFP-Tg

hepatocyte transplantation showed no GFP-positive hepatocytes in the liver except in one rat (n = 4). Abundant GFP-positive non-parenchymal cells were observed, which suggests incomplete reconstruction of their immune system after bone marrow transplantation that resulted in a weaker immunological reaction against transplanted cells. Rats in Group 3 received bone marrow from GFP-Tg Lewis rats and an HBSS injection instead of hepatocyte transplantation. Their livers showed a small number

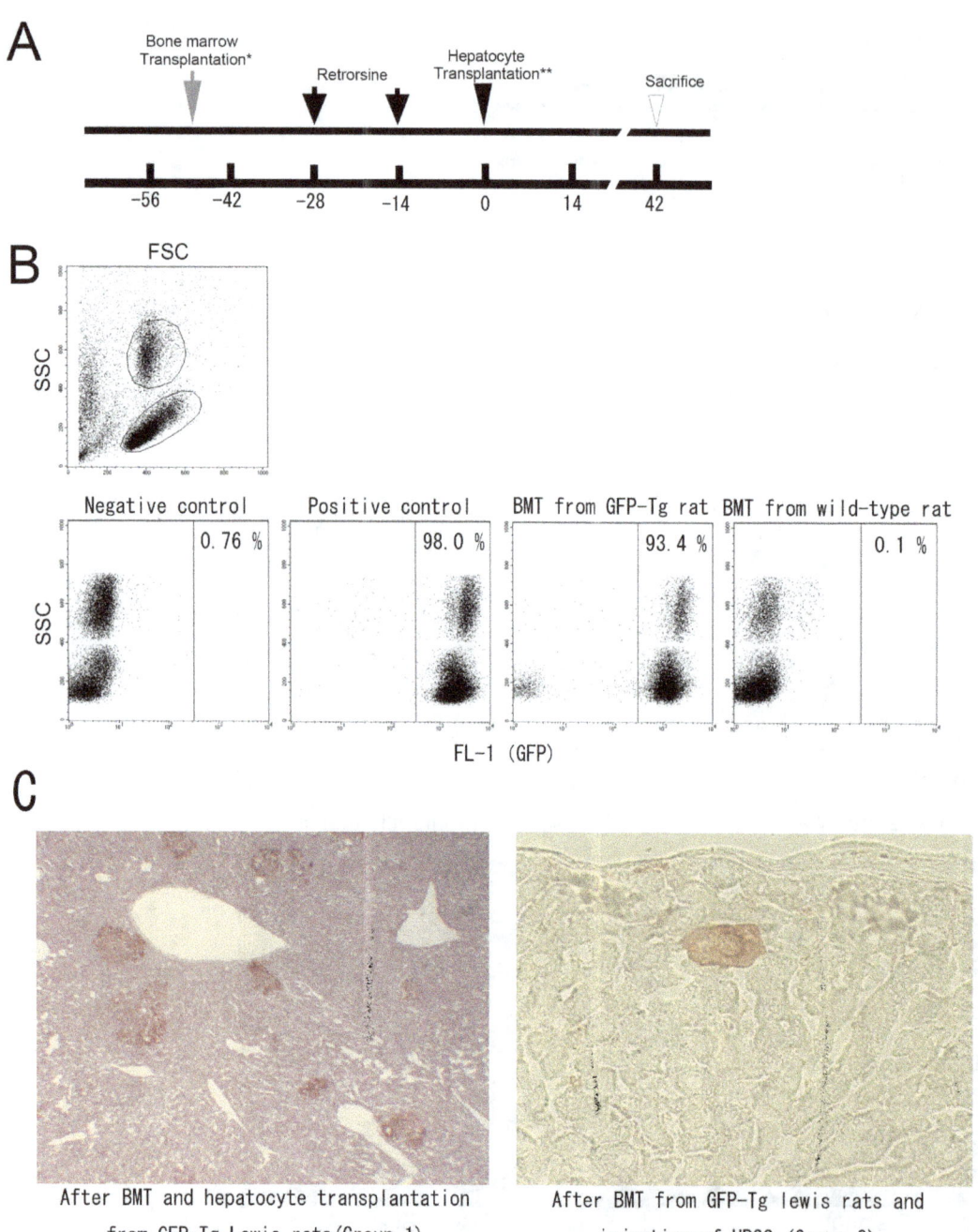

Figure 5. Reconstruction of immune system by bone marrow transplantation and hepatocyte transplantation. (A) Timeline of experiment 5. Wild-type recipient rats received 11Gy of whole body irradiation and bone marrow transplantation (BMT). Rats in Group 1 received bone marrow cells from GFP-Tg Lewis rats and after retrorsine treatment and hepatectomy, GFP-positive hepatocytes were transplanted and the rats were sacrificed on day 42. Rats in Group 2 received bone marrow cells from wild-type Lewis rats and GFP-positive hepatocytes (*). The rats in Group 3 received bone marrow transplantation from GFP-Tg rats and HBSS with 10% FBS instead of hepatocyte transplantation (**). (B) Flow cytometry of peripheral blood 7 weeks after bone marrow transplantation. More than 99% of leukocytes in the blood from GFP-Tg rats were GFP-positive, as compared to more than 90% of leukocytes after transplantation of GFP-positive bone marrow cells. After bone marrow transplantation from wild-type rats to wild-type rats, practically none of the leukocytes were positive for GFP. (C) Livers from Group 1 rats showed clusters of GFP-positive hepatocytes at 42 days after hepatocyte transplantation and from Group 3, a few GFP-positive large polygonal cells were observed residing within hepatic cords. These cells are similar to megalocytic GFP-positive hepatocytes [27]. Clusters of GFP-positive small hepatocyte-like progenitor cells or mature hepatocytes were not detected.

of GFP-positive hepatocyte-like cells that maintained their morphology and were larger than surrounding normal hepatocytes (Fig. 5). Thus, these bone marrow-derived hepatocyte-like cells were distinguishable from transplanted GFP-positive hepatocytes.

Discussion

This study demonstrated that GFP-positive hepatocytes isolated from GFP-Tg rats could engraft in wild-type host rats. Importantly, the transplanted cells did not persist for more than 42 days in a wild-type syngeneic rat liver that was pretreated with retrorsine and by partial hepatectomy. In contrast, hepatocytes transplanted from wild-type rats steadily proliferated in GFP-Tg Lewis rat liver. Immunosuppressant treatment with tacrolimus prolonged the survival of GFP-positive hepatocytes, whereas pre-immunization with GFP-Tg hepatocytes decreased the time to disappearance of transplanted hepatocytes in wild-type rats. Prolonged survival of GFP-positive hepatocytes by bone marrow transplantation eliminated the potential protective effect of tacrolimus on GFP-Tg hepatocytes [13]. These results strongly suggest that the disappearance of transplanted hepatocytes in our model was primarily due to an immunological reaction to the GFP transgene rather than to GFP toxicity.

GFP-Tg Lewis rats were originally generated using Lewis rats obtained from Charles-River Laboratories Japan (Yokohama, Japan), the rats exported from Charles-River Laboratories in the USA in 1981 (personal communication, Charles-River Laboratories, Japan). We initially noticed the disappearance of transplanted hepatocytes by using wild-type Lewis rats from Harlan Sprague-Dawley, and hypothesized that these two rats from two different colonies might express different antigens affecting the immunological reaction. In fact, the phenomenon was reproduced in wild-type Lewis rats from Charles-River Laboratories. Therefore, we consider that the cellular loss after GFP-positive hepatocyte transplantation is due to an immunological reaction against GFP.

Our findings are consistent with the results of a GFP gene transfer study into the liver of immune competent mice [15], although they contradict a transplantation study of hepatocytes expressing GFP [7]. Follenzi et al. [16] used a lentivirus vector to introduce GFP transgenes driven by the cytomegalovirus (CMV) enhancer/promotor into hepatocytes of SCID mice. These authors used fluorescence microscopy to demonstrate the continuous and stable expression of GFP; however, the number of GFP-expressing hepatocytes decreased or disappeared in immune competent mice livers by two weeks after transplantation [15]. Notably, the kinetics of GFP-positive hepatocytes depended on the strain of the mouse, with fewer GFP-positive hepatocytes in C57BL/6 mice, and their disappearance in FVB/N and BALB/c strains within two weeks. That study measured vector DNA content in the liver, and our findings suggested that GFP-positive cells were eliminated from the liver rather than viable cells losing their GFP expression. In contrast, cultured hepatocytes and hepatoblasts with the GFP transgene driven by the albumin promoter showed vigorous proliferation and continuous GFP expression after transplantation into a syngeneic rat liver that did not express dipeptidyl peptidase-4 (DPPIV) in their liver (DPPIV-negative) and had been pretreated with the inhibitor of hepatocyte proliferation, retrorsine. The liver samples from these rats clearly showed groups of GFP-positive hepatocytes which were also positive for DPPIV in DPPIV-negative syngeneic rat liver for at least four months. The reasons for these inconsistent results are not clear as yet, but it is possible that DPPIV-negative animals produce a weak immune response against GFP. DPPIV is also expressed on the surface of T cells [17], where it might play a functional role in regulating the immune system. It is also possible that GFP is minimally antigenic in F344 rats, which were often used in previous studies [7,8,9].

Immunological factors that could affect the outcome of hepatocyte transplantation include conventional immunosuppressants [18], depletion of immune cells [7], and reconstruction of the immune system by bone marrow transplantation. Additional important factors that can affect an immune response include the role of stem/progenitor cells as immune modulators [20], the

amount of antigen, and activation of the immune system by the antigen-presenting cells [15]. Follenzi et al. [15] reported that the absence of GFP expression in antigen-presenting cells results in longer survival of GFP-expressing hepatocytes in a mice model [15]. In our model, cell-to-cell connections were roughly digested and the presence of contaminating non-parenchymal cells in the transplanted hepatocytes was highly likely. This contamination could partially explain the difference between our results and those of Oertel et al. [7]. Severe liver injuries are often utilized to enhance the engraftment and proliferation of transplanted cells. This enhancement occurs by providing both a niche for cell proliferation and a growth stimulus to transplanted cells. In fact, the engraftment of transplanted cells and repopulation of hepatocytes occurs to a lesser extent without liver injury [19]. We also speculate that severe and fulminant liver injury can result in a reduced host capacity for immune response, thereby potentially permitting the survival of transplanted hepatocytes that would be rejected under normal conditions [21].

The characteristics of transplanted cells are important in determining the outcome of their transplantation. A previous study using a retrorsine-treated rat model demonstrated that Thy1-positive hepatocytes grew rapidly in DPPIV-negative rat livers, but disappeared within two months [22]. Under the same conditions mature hepatocytes grew slowly and steadily [22]. Furthermore, mesenchymal stem cells (MSCs) isolated from different species behaved differently. In a liver regeneration model, MSCs isolated from syngeneic rats do not differentiate into hepatocytes [14] whereas transplanted human MSCs could differentiate into functioning hepatocytes in the injured livers of rats or pigs [21,23]. This difference might be attributable to the different properties of human and rat MSCs when human MSCs are xenotransplanted and when rat MSCs undergo syngeneic transplantation [14].

Notably, the liver from GFP-Tg Lewis rats can survive in wild-type syngeneic rats (data not shown) despite vigorous rejection of transplanted hepatocytes in this situation. Typically a liver graft is rejected approximately 10 days after allogeneic transplantation when there is a severe rejection reaction. A shorter treatment with a low dose of tacrolimus resulted in the liver graft surviving in allogeneic recipients despite the MHC barrier [24]. Generally, the same amount of immunosuppressant treatment is insufficient to prevent graft loss of other organs such as heart, kidney, and skin, and the mechanism of liver graft survival after shorter and smaller doses of immunosuppressant includes the release of non-specific immune modulators from the liver graft and the functional role of non-parenchymal cells in the graft [25,26]. In contrast, the majority of the transplanted hepatocytes are eliminated from the host liver within the first few days by a nonspecific immune response [6] that leads to foreign antigen presentation and acceleration of the immune reaction. Identification of the major mechanism determining the tolerance of liver grafts and the rejection of hepatocytes is of major importance. Modulation of the factors involved would be beneficial for the control of immune response after liver and hepatocyte transplantation, as well as other organ transplantation.

Very few large, GFP-positive polygonal cells were residing in the hepatic cords of retrorsine-pretreated livers after bone marrow transplantation but without hepatocyte transplantation, as shown in Experiment 4. Our previous study using transplantation of wild-type retrorsine-pretreated liver into GFP-Tg syngeneic rats identified a similar group of cells that represented less than 0.02% of total hepatocytes at eight weeks after liver transplantation [27]. This population of hepatocytes expressed GFP, albumin, and CYP1A2, suggesting that they were functional hepatocytes.

Majorities of these abnormally large, hepatocyte-like cells resided in hepatic cords solitarily despite the expression of Ki67. We also identified a group of small cells that were capable of vigorous proliferation in the same liver samples. Therefore, it is plausible that the abnormally large GFP-positive polygonal cells are derived from the fusion of endogenous hepatocytes exposed to retrorsine and bone marrow cells, whereas the very small polygonal cells are derived by transdifferentiation of bone marrow cells. Thus, we agree with the model proposed by Masson et al. that cell fusion and cell transdifferentiation depends upon the liver environment [28]. A comprehensive study using sex-mismatched liver or bone marrow transplantation is necessary to clarify this issue.

In this experiment, we have demonstrated that hepatocytes from GFP-Tg Lewis rats are not able to survive long-term in the syngeneic wild-type Lewis rat liver. Liver is not an immune-privileged site for hepatocyte transplantation, and multiple factors determine the death or survival of transplanted hepatocytes. It is

also notable that the progression of the cell loss phenomenon observed in the current study did not alter when more severe treatment such as 2/3 hepatectomy (n = 3) and 80% hepatectomy (n = 1) with retrorsine treatment was employed. This suggests that an immunological reaction against the transplanted GFP-positive hepatocytes is maintained in this strong liver regeneration model. In conclusion, this study demonstrated the need to consider the host immunological reaction in the hepatocyte transplantation model using GFP-Tg Lewis rats as donors.

Author Contributions

Conceived and designed the experiments: HM. Performed the experiments: HM MS YW YF RW QL. Analyzed the data: HM RM ZS HE. Contributed reagents/materials/analysis tools: HM ZS. Wrote the paper: HM ZS.

References

1. Gambotto A, Dworacki G, Cicinnati V, Kenniston T, Steitz J, et al. (2000) Immunogenicity of enhanced green fluorescent protein (EGFP) in BALB/c mice: identification of an H2-Kd-restricted CTL epitope. Gene Ther. 7: 2036–2040.
2. Inoue H, Ohsawa I, Murakami T, Kimura A, Hakamata Y, et al. (2005) Development of new inbred transgenic strains of rats with LacZ or GFP. Biochem Biophys Res Commun. 329: 288–295.
3. Liu HS, Jan MS, Chou CK, Chen PH, Ke NJ (1999) Is green fluorescent protein toxic to the living cells? Biochem Biophys Res Commun. 260: 712–717.
4. Taghizadeh RR, Sherley JL (2008) CFP and YFP, but not GFP, provide stable fluorescent marking of rat hepatic adult stem cells. J Biomed Biotechnol. 2008: 453590.
5. Mizuno K, Muneta T, Morito T, Ichinose S, Koga H, et al. (2008) Exogenous synovial stem cells adhere to defect of meniscus and differentiate into cartilage cells. J Med Dent Sci. 55: 101–111.
6. Han B, Lu Y, Meng B, Qu B (2009) Cellular loss after allogenic hepatocyte transplantation. Transplantation. 87: 1–5.
7. Oertel M, Rosencrantz R, Chen YQ, Thota PN, Sandhu JS, et al. (2003) Repopulation of rat liver by fetal hepatoblasts and adult hepatocytes transduced ex vivo with lentiviral vectors. Hepatology. 37: 994–1005.
8. Watanabe H, Ochiya T, Ueda S, Kominami Y, Gon R, et al. (2007) Differentiation of a hepatic phenotype after heterotropic transplantation of heart, kidney, brain, and skin tissues into liver in F344 rats. Biochem Biophys Res Commun. 354: 841–845.
9. Sgodda M, Aurich H, Kleist S, Aurich I, König S, et al. (2007) Hepatocyte differentiation of mesenchymal stem cells from rat peritoneal adipose tissue in vitro and in vivo. Exp Cell Res. 313: 2875–2686.
10. Seglen PO (1976) Preparation of isolated rat liver cells. Methods Cell Biol. 13: 29–83.
11. Madrahimov N, Dirsch O, Broelsch C, Dahmen U (2006) Marginal hepatectomy in the rat: from anatomy to surgery. Ann Surg. 244: 89–98.
12. Laconi E, Oren R, Mukhopadhyay DK, Hurston E, Laconi S, et al. (1998) Long-term, near-total liver replacement by transplantation of isolated hepatocytes in rats treated with retrorsine. Am J Pathol. 153: 319–329.
13. Sakr MF, Zetti GM, Hassanein TI, Farghali H, Nalesnik MA, et al. (1991) FK 506 ameliorates the hepatic injury associated with ischemia and reperfusion in rats. Hepatology. 13: 947–951.
14. Popp FC, Slowik P, Eggenhofer E, Renner P, Lang SA, et al. (2007) No contribution of multipotent mesenchymal stromal cells to liver regeneration in a rat model of prolonged hepatic injury. Stem Cells. 25: 639–645.
15. Follenzi A, Battaglia M, Lombardo A, Annoni A, Roncarolo MG, et al. (2004) Targeting lentiviral vector expression to hepatocytes limits transgene-specific immune response and establishes long-term expression of human antihemophilic factor IX in mice. Blood. 103: 3700–3709.
16. Follenzi A, Sabatino G, Lombardo A, Boccaccio C, Naldini L (2002) Efficient gene delivery and targeted expression to hepatocytes in vivo by improved lentiviral vectors. Hum Gene Ther. 13: 243–260.
17. Ohnuma K, Takahashi N, Yamochi T, Hosono O, Dang NH, et al. (2008) Role of CD26/dipeptidyl peptidase IV in human T cell activation and function. Front Biosci. 13: 2299–2310.
18. Muraca M, Ferraresso C, Vilei MT, Granato A, Quarta M, et al. (2007) Liver repopulation with bone marrow derived cells improves the metabolic disorder in the Gunn rat. Gut. 56: 1725–1735.
19. Laconi S, Pillai S, Porcu PP, Shafritz DA, Pani P, et al. (2001) Massive liver replacement by transplanted hepatocytes in the absence of exogenous growth stimuli in rats treated with retrorsine. Am J Pathol. 158: 771–777.
20. Avital I, Feraresso C, Aoki T, Hui T, Rozga J, et al. (2002) Bone marrow-derived liver stem cell and mature hepatocyte engraftment in livers undergoing rejection. Surgery. 132: 384–390.
21. Li J, Zhang L, Xin J, Jiang L, Li J, et al. (2012) Immediate intraportal transplantation of human bone marrow mesenchymal stem cells prevents death from fulminant hepatic failure in pigs. Hepatology. 56: 1044–1052.
22. Ichinohe N, Kon J, Sasaki K, Nakamura Y, Ooe H, et al. (2012) Growth ability and repopulation efficiency of transplanted hepatic stem cells, progenitor cells, and mature hepatocytes in retrorsine-treated rat livers. Cell Transplant. 21: 11–22.
23. Sato Y, Araki H, Kato J, Nakamura K, Kawano Y, et al. (2005) Human mesenchymal stem cells xenografted directly to rat liver are differentiated into human hepatocytes without fusion. Blood. 106: 756–763.
24. Cai X, Harnaha J, Rao PN, Flowers J, Venkataramanan R, et al. (1992) Low-dose of FK 506 and associated blood levels in allotransplantation of rat liver, heart, and skin. Transplant Proc. 24: 1403–1405.
25. Kobayashi E, Kamada N, Lord R, Stamatiou S, Goto S, et al. (1994) Mechanisms of tolerance induction by serum from liver-grafted rats: nonspecific immunosuppressive factors induced by liver grafting. Transplant Proc. 26: 1960–1961.
26. Böttcher JP, Knolle PA, Stabenow D (2011) Mechanisms balancing tolerance and immunity in the liver. Dig Dis. 29: 384–390.
27. Maeda H, Ota Y, Wang Y, Ramachandran K, Montgomery RA, Williams GM, Sun Z (2013) Contribution of extrahepatic small cells resembling small hepatocyte-like progenitor cells to liver mass maintenance in transplantation model of retrorsine-pretreated liver. Springerplus. 2: 446.
28. Masson S, Harrison DJ, Plevris JN, Newsome PN (2004) Potential of hematopoietic stem cell therapy in hepatology: a critical review. Stem Cells. 22: 897–907.

19

Interferon-Based Anti-Viral Therapy for Hepatitis C Virus Infection after Renal Transplantation

Fang Wei[1], Junying Liu[2], Fen Liu[1], Huaidong Hu[1], Hong Ren[1], Peng Hu[1]*

1 Department of infectious Disease, Institute for Viral hepatitis, Key Laboratory of Molecular Biology for infectious disease, The second Affiliated Hospital of Chongqing Medical University, Chongqing, PR China, 2 Department of Gastroenterology, The Central hospital of Zhoukou, Henan Province, China

Abstract

Background: Hepatitis C virus (HCV) infection is highly prevalent in renal transplant (RT) recipients. Currently, interferon-based (IFN-based) antiviral therapies are the standard approach to control HCV infection. In a post-transplantation setting, however, IFN-based therapies appear to have limited efficacy and their use remains controversial. The present study aimed to evaluate the efficacy and safety of IFN-based therapies for HCV infection post RT.

Methods: We searched Pubmed, Embase, Web of Knowledge, and The Cochrane Library (1997–2013) for clinical trials in which transplant patients were given Interferon (IFN), pegylated interferon (PEG), interferon plus ribavirin (IFN–RIB), or pegylated interferon plus ribavirin (PEG–RIB). The Sustained Virological Response (SVR) and/or drop-out rates were the primary outcomes. Summary estimates were calculated using the random-effects model of DerSimonian and Laird, with heterogeneity and sensitivity analysis.

Results: We identified 12 clinical trials (140 patients in total). The summary estimate for SVR rate, drop-out rate and graft rejection rate was 26.6% (95%CI, 15.0–38.1%), 21.1% (95% CI, 10.9–31.2%) and 4% (95%CI: 0.8%–7.1%), respectively. The overall SVR rate in PEG-based and standard IFN-based therapy was 40.6% (24/59) and 20.9% (17/81), respectively. The most frequent side-effect requiring discontinuation of treatment was graft dysfunction (14 cases, 45.1%). Meta-regression analysis showed the covariates included contribute to the heterogeneity in the SVR logit rate, but not in the drop-out logit rate. The sensitivity analyses by the random model yielded very similar results to the fixed-effects model.

Conclusions: IFN-based therapy for HCV infection post RT has poor efficacy and limited safety. PEG-based therapy is a more effective approach for treating HCV infection post-RT than standard IFN-based therapy. Future research is required to develop novel strategies to improve therapeutic efficacy and tolerability, and reduce the liver-related morbidity and mortality in this important patient population.

Editor: Wenzhe Ho, Temple University School of Medicine, United States of America

Funding: This research was supported by the National Natural Science Foundation of China (81171560, 30930082, 81171561, 30972584), The National Science and Technology Major Project of China (2008ZX10002-006, 2012ZX1002007001, 2011ZX09302005, 2012ZX09303001-001, 2012ZX10002003), The National High Technology Research and Development Program of China (2011AA020111), the Key Project of Chongqing Science and Technology Commission (cstc2012gg-yyjsB10007), the Chongqing Natural Science Foundation (cstc2011jjA10025), and the Medical Research Fund by Chongqing Municipal Health Bureau (2009-1-71). The funders had no role in study design, data collection and analysis, decision to publish, or preparation of the manuscript.

Competing Interests: The authors have declared that no competing interests exist.

* E-mail: hp_cq@163.com

Introduction

Hepatitis C virus (HCV) infection is a significant public health problem, with an estimated 170 million people infected and three to four million new cases per year [1,2]. HCV infection remains highly prevalent in patients with end-stage renal disease (ESRD) who undergo planned hemodialysis and renal transplantation [3–7]. Renal transplant (RT) recipients have a HCV infection rate of 5–15% in the developed countries, with substantially higher rates reported in the developing world [8,9].

The immunosuppressed state of RT recipients dramatically increases the risk of HCV infection and accelerated disease progression. This condition can lead to severe HCV-related liver damage such as cirrhosis, fibrosing cholestatic hepatitis or liver failure. The risk of liver failure in particular is a major concern, as this condition is the fourth leading cause of mortality (8–28%) in long term survivors after RT [6,10]. Furthermore, HCV also negatively impacts renal graft survival [11,12]. Indeed, current evidence suggests that the long-term graft and patient survival rates of HCV-positive RT recipients were significantly lower than that of HCV-negative patients [13–15]. Thus, prevention and management of HCV infection is a critical factor in RT therapy.

IFN-based therapy is the primary treatment for HCV-related liver disease. However, in the renal transplant setting, the use of IFN therapy has produced unsatisfactory results. Not only are these therapies less effective, but they are also associated with increased risks of acute renal insufficiency and graft rejection

[16,17]. So, physicians managing RT recipients must balance the benefits of reducing HCV infection and subsequent hepatic disease with the complications from antiviral therapy.

The serious complications of HCV infection post-RT have led many researchers around the world to investigate the use of IFN-based antiviral therapy (immunotherapy or combination treatment) to attenuate the aggressive course of HCV infection post-RT. In 2006, a meta-analysis performed by Fabrizi et al [18] had evaluated the efficacy and safety of IFN/IFN-RIB therapy in this patients. However, this study did not include reports of PEG-based (PEG/PEG-RIB) therapies and only used various forms of the conventional IFN doses. Furthermore, Most of the included studies had small sample sizes and the meta-analysis did not include large randomized controlled trials, so the accuracy of these findings remains uncertain.

Currently, most antiviral strategies post-RT employs mono-therapies (i.e. IFN/RIB/Amantadine/PEG) [19–28]. However, there are some case reports that describe successful treatment of chronic HCV infection in RT recipients using combination therapies (i.e. IFN-RIB/PEG-RIB) [29–32]. In particular, PEG-based therapies appear to have fewer side effects, better antiviral efficacy, and more rapidly viral clearance than the standard IFN therapy in most patients [16]. Since earlier meta-analyses did not include PEG-based therapy or combination therapy, an updated meta-analysis is necessary to evaluate IFN-based therapy more appropriately in post-RT patients.

The overall benefits and best strategies for treating HCV infection post-RTwith IFN therapy remain poorly understood. To evaluate the safety and efficacy of IFN-based therapies properly, we carried out a systematic review and an updated meta-analysis of the published clinical trials using of IFN-based monotherapies and combination therapies (IFN or PEG alone or IFN–RIB or PEG–RIB) of HCV infection post-RT. These findings should help determine the optimal treatment strategy for managing HCV in RT recipients.

Materials and Methods

Search strategy

We performed a comprehensive search of the published literature for controlled and observational studies regarding the efficacy of IFN-based therapy (IFN or PEG alone or IFN–RIB or PEG–RIB) for HCV infection post-RT. Studies from January 1997 through April 2013 were pulled from Pubmed, Embase, Web of Knowledge, and the Cochrane Library, using key words "HCV,""interferon," "renal transplant," and their synonyms. The search was restricted using the terms "humans" and "English"; we obtained studies (controlled or non-controlled, randomized or non-randomized) published in full-text or in abstract form for all potentially relevant trials, and the reference list from retrieved documents were also searched to identify additional relevant studies.

Study selection criteria

All retrieved citations were imported into Endnote X4.0.2 reference management software to remove duplicate reports. All potentially eligible full-text articles and abstracts were independently reviewed by two separate reviewers for relevance, inclusion in the meta-analysis, and data extraction using a standardized data collection form. Disagreements between reviewers were resolved with the assistance of an arbiter.

Given the heterogeneity in the published literature, strict inclusion and exclusion criteria were developed to capture all relevant literature, while excluding poorly conducted studies and limiting heterogeneity. If the same patients in different studies were reported two or more studies in controlled and non-controlled form, we included only the studies that reported the complete and adequate data that we needed.

The following inclusion criteria were used to select studies for meta-analysis: i) studies published as peer-reviewed articles; ii) study population must be renal transplant with HCV infection (positive for anti-HCV and/or HCV-RNA and/or biopsy proven) treated with IFN-based scheme (IFN or PEG alone or IFN–RIB or PEG–RIB) and reported the results of the treatment; iii) studies used the sustained virological response (SVR) and/or drop-out rate as a clinical end-point. Review articles, conference abstracts, interim reports of ongoing studies, case reports were excluded from the meta-analysis. In addition, we excluded studies that included patients co-infected with human immunodeficiency virus (HIV) and/or hepatitis B virus (HBV), patients undergoing multiple organ transplantation, clinical trials concerning patients on maintenance dialysis, and studies with inadequate response or treatment data.

Data extraction and outcomes

Intention-to-treat methods were used to extract response rates for all patients in eligible studies. While patients without end-point data were excluded from our analysis. The primary outcome measure in this meta-analysis was SVR rate, a measure of efficacy, which was defined as HCV viraemia (HCV RNA in the blood) undetectable at least six months after cessation of treatment. The secondary outcome measure was Drop-out rate, a measure of tolerability, which was defined as the frequency of patients who stopped treatment due of side-effects.

Additional outcome measures included biochemical response, defined as normalization of serum alanine aminotransferase (ALT) at the end of treatment (ETBR) and at least 6 months of follow-up (EFBR). Virological response at the end of treatment (ETVR) and Rejection rate (the proportion of patients who experienced graft rejection) were also measured. In addition, we measured compliance among treatment groups (completion of full duration at original drug doses defined as A; completion of full duration but at reduced drug doses defined as B; premature termination of treatment defined as C).

Statistical analysis methods

The response rate according to the intention-to-treat method was calculated by the data abstractor. Pooled quantitative summary estimates of the pre-defined outcome rates across individual studies were generated using the random-effects model of DerSimonian and Laird [33]. Unlike a simple arithmetic average, this estimate represents a weighted average of results from individual studies based on study size. The Q-test for heterogeneity was performed for each outcome measurement; a value of <0.10 was considered indicative of statistically significant heterogeneity [34]. The I squared (I^2) value was calculate to assess the consistency of effects across studies [35]. Since the majority of studies in HCV infection post-RT utilized a non-controlled and non-randomized design, we performed the pooled quantitative analysis with consideration for the biases that may result from a lack of randomization [36]. We analyzed five stratifying variables (The SVR and Drop-out rate in Asian countries, in cohort studies, in patients treated with IFN-alone, IFN-RIB, and PEG-RIB).

To explore the potential effect of patients or trial characteristics on the summary estimates, a meta-regression analysis was performed [37]. The dependent variable was the observed logit event rate from each trial for the outcome of interest. Weights were assigned based on the estimated variance of logit event rate.

The residual between-trial variance was estimated by a Restricted Maximum Likelihood Method (REML) using an iterative procedure [37]. The following covariates were included in the meta-regression analysis: Age, male percentage, reference year, rate of cirrhosis, donor source (cadaveric/living), duration of post-RT time before antiviral therapy, duration of antiviral therapy, and IFN dose. A sensitivity analysis using a random-effects model was also performed to assess the consistency of results. Publication bias was assessed by the Begg and Mazumadar adjusted rank-correlation test and by a regression asymmetry test for publication bias [38]. Every estimate was given with its 95% confidence interval (95% CI), with an alpha risk of 0.05. All the statistical analyses were performed using Stata 12.0 (Stata Corporation, College Station, TX, USA).

Results

Search results

According to the search strategy (Figure 1), 789 relevant reports were identified within the searched databases, of which 285 were redundant documents between two or more databases. An additional 391 reports were excluded on the basis of title, resulting in 113 eligible trials. Of these, 39 reports were review articles; eight were case reports [19–23,29,30,39]; one was an interim report [40]; 12 were conference abstracts [24–28,31,32,41–45]; 2 included HCV co-infected with HBV [46,47]; five were combined liver kidney transplantation [48–52] and one included patients on maintenance dialysis [53] at the same time, and seven articles contained confounding factors [54–60]. After these exclusions, 12

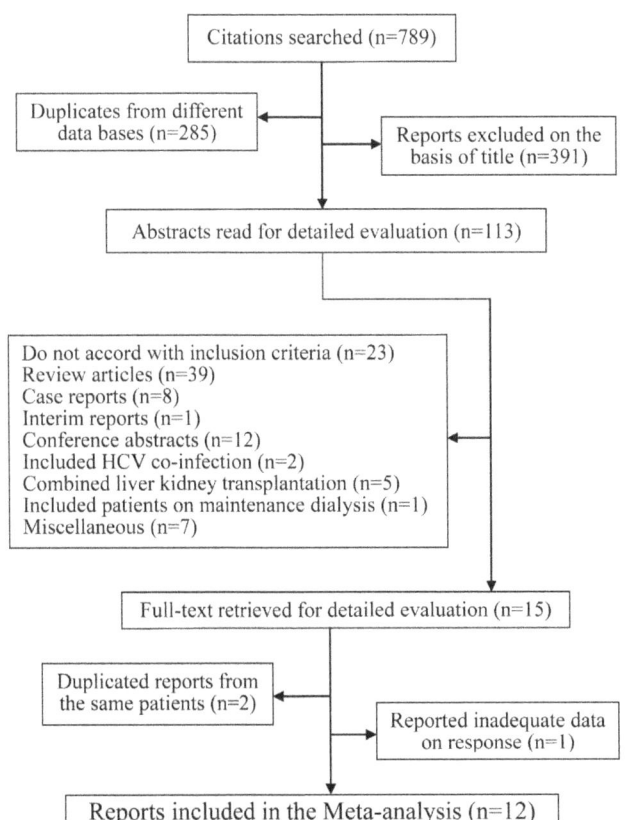

Figure 1. Map of the literature search and selection process.

reports met our eligibility criteria and were included in the meta-analysis [61–72].

Patient characteristics

In Table 1, the lists of studies were analyzed. Seen from the chart, a total of 12 reports, describing a total of 140 patients were included. All of the reports were published in English and conducted between 1997 and 2013. Among them, 11 were conducted as cohort studies, only one used a controlled design approach, although none were randomized, controlled trials (RCTs). Many of the studies were performed in Asian countries (n = 7; 58%). The mean age of the patients ranged from 37 to 52.2 years and the men represented 59.4% to 100% of the study population. The cadaveric source of the donor was recorded in six of the 12 studies (50%). With regard to the viral characteristics, the genotype was reported in eight of the studies indicating that genotype-1 HCV infection predominated in these reports. Also, a liver biopsy was performed in most of the studies (9/12; 75%) suggesting that the frequency of cirrhosis was very low in these patient groups.

In Table 2, the specific treatment schedules are shown, which included the time of IFN-based treatment initiation after renal transplantation, the doses of IFN used, the duration of treatment and follow-up, and the use of immunosuppressant. Five of the studies included patients treated with IFN alone (n = 48), four studies included IFN-RIB therapy (n = 33), and three studies included PEG-RIB therapy (n = 59). Immunosuppressive therapy at the beginning of antiviral therapy included cyclosporine A (CsA), tacrolimus (Tac)/FK506, azathioprine (Aza), corticosteroids (CS), and mycophenolatemophetil (MMF).

In Table 3, the outcomes of IFN-based therapy of each study are shown, recorded as the virological and biochemical responses at the end of treatment and follow up at least six months. The overall SVR rate in PEG-based and standard IFN-based therapy was 40.6% (24/59) and 20.9% (17/81), respectively. Ten patients out of 140 experienced graft rejection and 31 patients out of 140 discontinued treatments because of side-effects such as graft-dysfunction, depression, Flu-like symptoms, anemia, and leucopenia. That is to say, the overall graft rejection rate and drop-out rate was 7% (10/140) and 22% (31/140), respectively.

Data analysis

The quantitative pooled summary estimates for SVR and drop-out rate are shown in Table 4 and Table 5, respectively. The summary estimate for SVR rate and drop-out rate was 26.6% (95% CI: 15.0–38.1%) and 21.1% (95% CI: 10.9–31.2%), respectively. The heterogeneity Q-score was 36.53 and 34.85 for the SVR rate and drop-out rate, respectively. The I^2 value was 69.9% and 68.4% for the SVR rate and drop-out rate respectively. The p-value was >0.10 for our test of study homogeneity, suggesting that the studies included were heterogeneous with respect to the outcome end-points. The summary estimate for ETBR rate, EFBR rate and ETVR rate was 63.6% (95% CI: 44–79.5%), 37.8% (95% CI: 24.9–52.5%) and 42.7% (95% CI: 27.7–57.6%), respectively. The summary estimate of graft rejection rate was 4% (95% CI: 0.8–7.1%). The forest map of SVR rate and drop-out rate are shown in Figure 2 and Figure 3 respectively.

Sensitivity and heterogeneity analysis

The summary estimate for SVR rate in patients treated with IFN alone was 9.6% (95% CI: −0.9–20.2%), 32.8% (95% CI: 17.0–48.7%) in patients treated with IFN-RIB, and 40.6% (95% CI: 28.1–53.1%) in patients receiving PEG-RIB. The summary estimate for SVR rate in studies from Asian countries was 31.7%

Table 1. Characteristics of studies of IFN-based therapy for HCV infection post-RT.

Author	Study Design	Reference Year	Total(n) Male (%)	Age (Year)	Cadaveric donor source	Geno-type 1	Geno-type 2	Cirrhosis %(n/T)
YasumuraT.et al [62]	Co,R	1997	6;100% M	37±5	NA	67.7% (4/6)	33.3%(2/6)	0
Izopet J.et al [61]	Co,P	1997	15;68% M	49 (29–65)	100%	86.7% (13/15)	13.3% (2/15)	13.3% (2/15)
Durlik M.et al [63]	Co,P	1998	11;73% M	38 (20–63)	100%	NA	NA	0
Hanafusa T.et al [64]	Co,P	1998	10; NA M	NA	NA	90%(9/10)	10% (1/10)	0
Tokumoto T.et al [65]	Co,P	1998	6; 83% M	46.8±6.6	67.7%	50%(3/6)	50% (3/6)	0
Baid S.et al [66]	Co,R	2003	12;75% M	48 (30–75)	83.3%	NA	NA	0
Tang S.et al [67]	Co,P	2003	4,100% M	45.8±6.8	100%	50%(2/4)	25% (2/4)	0
Shu K.H.et al [68]	Co,P	2004	11;73% M	42.4±13.1	100%	67.7%(6/9)	33.3% (3/9)	NA
Sharma R.K.et al [69]	CCT	2006	6; NA M	38.7±11.2	NA	NA	NA	NA
Pageaux G.P.et al [70]	Co,R	2009	8;100% M	52.2±5.6	NA	25% (2/8)	50% (4/8)	NA
Aljumah A.A.et al [71]	Co,R	2012	19;68% M	39.9±12.6	NA	NA	NA	0
Sanai F.M.et al [72]	Co,P	2013	32;59% M	46.0±12.4	NA	62.5%(20/32)	0	0

Table 2. Treatment schedules of IFN-based for HCV infection post-RT.

Authors	Interval from RT to treatment (months)	Treatment protocol	Duration of treatment (months)	Duration of follow-up (months)	Immunosuppression (name ; n/T)
Yasumura T et al [62]	97.8±55.4	IFN 6 MU TIW	7.0±0.9	47.2±23.2	CsA 1/6;MZR 1/6;Prelon1/6;
Izopet J et al [61]	51.8±51.4	IFN 3MU TIW	4.7±1.2	12	CsA; Ste; AZ; MP;
Durlik M. et al [63]	60(60–180)	IFN 3MU TIW	6.2±2.2	6.7±1.5	Pred; CsA; AZ; MMF;
Hanafusa T et al [64]	NA	IFN 9MU TIW	6	24	Ste 3/10; OKT3 1/10;
Tokumoto T et al [65]	44.4±23.1	IFN 10MU TIW	6	20.8±3.7	MP; CsA; AZ; OKT3; DSG;
Baid S et al [66]	39.2±40.6	IFN 3MU TIW RIB 200–800 mg/d	18.3±14.8	23.7±18.4	Pred; AZ; CsA; Medrol; Tac; MMF;
Tang S et al [67]	5.3±3.4	IFN 3MU TIW RIB 400–1200 mg/d	6~12	27.3±11.8	CsA;
Shu K.H et al [68]	32.4	IFN 1MU TIW RIB 400–600 mg/d	12	11.1±3.9	CsA; Tac; MMF; Medrol;
Sharma R et al [69]	14.5±7.6	IFN 3MU TIW RIB 600–800 mg/d	12.4±5.5	NA	CsA; Pred;
Pageaux G.P et al [70]	198.9±101.1	PEG 180 ug QW RIB 0–400 mg/d	6~12	36(18–54)	Tac 2/8; MMF 2/8; Aza 3/8; CsA 4/8; Ste 8/8;
Aljumah A.A et al [71]	66.3±45.7	PEG 80–180 µg QW RIB 400–1200 mg/d	12	NA	Pre 19/19; MMF 15/19; CsA 8/19; Tac 9/19;Siro1/19;
Sanai F.M et al [72]	86.4±50.4	PEG 135–180 µg QW RIB 200–1200 mg/d	12	6~12	Tac 65.6%; Cy 28.1%; MMF 87.5%;

AZ: azathioprine; CsA: cyclosporine A; CS: corticosteroids; DSG: deoxyspergualin; IFN: interferon; Medrol: Methylprednisolone; MMF: mycophenolate; MP: methylprednisolone; MZR: mizoribine; MU: million units; Tac: Tacrolimus; Siro: sirolimus; Pred: prednisone; Prelon: Prednisolone; RT: Renal Transplant; Ste: steroid; TIW: three times per week;
In three papers (Yasumura T et al/Hanafusa T et al/Tokumoto T et al) IFN was given on a daily dose for the first two weeks only;
In paper Pageaux G.P et al, PEG was given in three patients at 1.5 ug/kg/week,andone patient at 50 ug QW in paper Sharma R et al;
In two papers (Baid S et al/Tang S et al) the follow-up time calculated from the initiation of antiviral treatment.

Table 3. Outcome of studies of IFN-based therapy for HCV infection post-RT.

Authors	ETBR	ETVR	EFBR	SVR	Rejection rate	Discontinuing	Compliance(A/B/C; n/T)	Side-effect
Yasumura T et al [62]	100%(6/6)	33.3%(2/6)	50%(3/6)	33.3%(2/6)	16.6%(1/6)	0	A(6/6)	Graft dysfunction (n = 1);
Izopet J et al [61]	80%(12/15)	33.3%(5/15)	27%(4/15)	0	0	46.7%(7/15)	A(8/15);C(7/15)	Graft dysfunction (n = 5); backache; fatigue; anorexia; weight loss; alopecia etc;
Durlik M. et al [63]	27.2%(3/11)	0	18.2%(2/11)	0	9.0%(1/11)	0	A(11/11)	Graft dysfunction (n = 2);
Hanafusa T et al [64]	30%(3/10)	20%(2/10)	20%(2/10)	10%(1/10)	40%(4/10)	50%(5/10)	A(5/10);C(5/10)	Graft dysfunction (n = 4);
Tokumoto T et al [65]	100%(6/6)	50%(3/6)	100%(6/6)	50%(3/6)	16.6%%(1/6)	33.3%(2/6)	A(4/6);C(2/6)	Graft dysfunction (n = 2);
Baid S et al [66]	75%(9/12)	33%(4/12)	25%(3/12)	33%(4/12)	16.6%(2/12)	16.6(2/12)	A(4/4);C(6RIB+2/12)	Graft dysfunction (n = 2) thrombocytopenia; Flu-like syndromes; leucopenia; depression;
Tang S et al [67]	75%(3/4)	75%(3/4)	50%(2/4)	50%(2/4)	0	0	A(3/4);B(1RIB/4)	0
Shu K.H et al [68]	91%(10/11)	64%(7/11)	27%(3/11)	27%(3/11)	0	27%(3/11)	A(8/11);C(3/11)	Graft dysfunction(n = 1);Flu-like syndromes; urosepsis;depression;
Sharma R et al [69]	33.3(2/6)	66.7%(4/6)	33.3%(2/6)	33.3%(2/6)	0	33.3%(2/6)	A(4/6);C(2IFN/6)	Graft dysfunction (n = 4); Low platelets; anemia;
Pageaux G.P et al [70]	100%(8/8)	75%(6/8)	100%(4/4)	50%(4/8)	0	62.5% (5/8)	A(2/8);C(5IFN+1RIB/8)	Graft dysfunction (n = 1); depression; anemia; papillary oedema;
Aljumah A.A et al [71]	79%(15/19)	47%(9/19)	79%(15/19)	42%(8/19)	5.3%(1/19)	0	A(19/19)	Graft dysfunction (n = 3)
Sanai F.M et al [72]	NA	47%(9/19)	NA	37.5%(12/32)	0	15.6%(5/32)	A?;B(25RIB+11PEG/32) C(5/32)	Graft dysfunction (n = 2); anemia; Flu-like syndrome; depression etc;

ETBR: end-of-treatment biochemical response; ETVR: end-of-treatment virological response; EFBR: biochemical response of follow-up at least 6 months; SVR: sustained virological response; Compliance (A/B/C): full duration, target dosages/full duration, reduced dosages/premature discontinuation.

(95% CI: 20.5–43%); within the subgroup of cohort trials, the summary estimate for SVR rate was 26.3% (95% CI: 14.2–38.3%).

The summary estimate for drop-out rate in patients treated with IFN alone was 25.4% (95% CI: 5.0–45.7%), 24.4% (95% CI: 8.6–40.2%) in patients treated with IFN-RIB, and 20.1% (95% CI: −1.5–41.6%) in patients receiving PEG-RIB. In Asian countries, the summary estimate for drop-out rate was 16% (95% CI: 4.7–27.4%); within the subgroup of cohort studies, the summary estimate for drop-out rate was 20.5% (95% CI: 10.1–30.9%).

Graft dysfunction occurred in approximately one-fifth of RT recipients (27/140; 19.2%) who received IFN-based therapy for HCV infection. Although 13 patients who reported graft dysfunction were able to complete their treatment. A total of 31 patients discontinued treatment as a result of side-effects, including 14 patients cessation from treatment because of graft dysfunction. Thus, graft dysfunction was the most frequent side-effect of requiring discontinuation from treatment (14/31, 45%).Of the 12 reports included in our meta-analysis, only 3 used PEG-based therapies, and no studies included a control group. Thus, we were unable to conduct a subgroup analysis of IFN and PEG to calculate pooled odds ratios or mean differences in comparison.

As shown in Table S1 and Table S2, meta-regression analysis reported the variance between studies decreased from 0.0241 to 0

Table 4. Summary estimates (with 95%CI) for SVR rate.

Author	SVR rate	[95% Conf. Interval]			Weight (%)
Yasumura T.et al [62]	0.333	−0.044	to	0.71	5.67
Izopet J.et al [61]	0.031	−0.057	to	0.119	13.29
Durik M.et al [63]	0.041	−0.076	to	0.158	12.54
Hanafusa T.et al [64]	0.1	−0.086	to	0.286	10.48
Tokumoto T.et al [65]	0.5	0.1	to	0.9	5.27
Baid S.et al [66]	0.333	0.066	to	0.6	8.14
Tang S.et al [67]	0.5	0.01	to	0.99	4
Shu K.H.et al [68]	0.272	0.009	to	0.535	8.24
Sharma R.K.et al [69]	0.333	−0.044	to	0.71	5.67
Pageaux G.P.et al [70]	0.5	0.154	to	0.846	6.26
Aljumah A.A.et al [71]	0.421	0.199	to	0.643	9.39
Sanai F.M.et al [72]	0.375	0.207	to	0.543	11.04
D+L pooled	0.266	0.15	to	0.381	100
Heterogeneity Q (p value)	36.53(0.000)				

Table 5. Summary estimates (with 95%CI) for Drop-out rate.

Author	Drop-out rate	[95% Conf. Interval]			Weight (%)
Yasumura T.et al [62]	0.07	−0.134	to	0.28	9.22
Izopet J.et al [61]	0.467	0.215	to	0.719	7.73
Durik M.et al [63]	0.041	−0.076	to	0.158	12.41
Hanafusa T.et al [64]	0.5	0.19	to	0.81	6.21
Tokumoto T.et al [65]	0.333	−0.044	to	0.71	4.85
Baid S.et al [66]	0.166	−0.045	to	0.377	9.05
Tang S.et al [67]	0.1	−0.194	to	0.394	6.6
Shu K.H.et al [68]	0.272	0.009	to	0.535	7.42
Sharma R.K.et al [69]	0.333	−0.044	to	0.71	4.85
Pageaux G.P.et al [70]	0.625	0.29	to	0.96	5.65
Aljumah A.A.et al [71]	0.025	−0.045	to	0.095	13.89
Sanai F.M.et al [72]	0.156	0.03	to	0.282	12.1
D+L pooled	0.211	0.109	to	0.312	100
Heterogeneity Q (p value)	34.85(0.000)				

in SVR logit rate, suggesting the covariates included in the studies contribute to heterogeneity of the studies. The variance in drop-out rate logit rate between studies changed from 0.0179 to 0.04422 in meta-regression analysis, suggesting that covariates did not contribute to the heterogeneity. The sensitivity analyses by the random model yielded similar results to the fixed-effects model (Figures S1, S2, S3, S4).

Publication bias

The Egger and Begg tests for publication bias showed that the risk for missing trials was acceptably low. The funnel plots analyzing publication bias for SVR logit rate and Drop-out logit rate are shown in Figure 4 and Figure 5, respectively. The primary publication bias in our study is a preference for small cohort studies, with few large clinical trials.

Discussion

IFN-based combination treatment of HCV infection in the immunocompetent, non-transplant population has been well-studied with large, randomized controlled clinical trials. Meta-analyses of these trials have demonstrated a SVR rate of approximately 41% in IFN-RIB and 55% in PEG-RIB [73,74]. However, in post-RT patients with HCV infection, our present meta-analysis illustrates the limited efficacy, with a SVR rate of 32.8% in IFN-RIB and 40.6% in PEG-RIB, indicating reduced efficacy. Thus, the overall therapeutic advantage of IFN-RIB or PEG-RIB observed in non-transplant chronic HCV infection seemed to be attenuated post RT. Besides, IFN-based combination therapy is more efficient than IFN monotherapy, with at least a two-fold increase in SVR. Moreover, PEG-RIB has a higher SVR than IFN-RIB. The overall SVR in PEG-based therapy is much higher than that of standard IFN-based therapy. This result indicates that PEG-based therapy is a more effective approach for treating HCV infection post-RT than standard IFN-based therapy.

This systematic review showed that the rate of graft rejection was small, with a summary estimate of 4% (0.8–7.1%). At present, the exact mechanism of graft rejection triggered by IFN in RT

recipients is not clear. IFN is a known to be a strong immune modulator, thus, rejection post-RT may involve an immune response. Potential pathways include increased cell surface expression of HLA antigens and induction of cytokines with subsequent stimulation of antibody production by B-cells [75]. It is interesting that the risk of rejection due to IFN is probably lower in liver than in RT recipients, this indicates that the liver being considered as more resistant to rejection than the kidney [76]. In addition, Baid et al noted the risk for acute rejection is higher during the first year after transplantation surgery [66]. Thus, it is strongly recommended to wait at least one year after the surgery to initiate antiviral therapy. Furthermore, antiviral treatment may yield a more effective response if stable renal function and no acute rejection occur during the first year after transplantation [21].

Currently, the limited available data suggests that amantadine monotherapy is safe and tolerated but has limited efficacy in managing HCV infection [77,78]. Analogously, ribavirin mono-therapy appeared to have some biochemical efficacy, but there is no consensus on its affects on liver histology. Furthermore, ribavirin can induce Hemolytic anemia, a serious side effect, though it has been reported to improve the level of proteinuria in HCV-related de novo glomerulopathy. As these data show, the existing alternatives to monotherapies are not clinically effective. Thus it is important to either improve IFN-based therapies or develop novel therapeutic approaches to manage HCV infection post-RT. In recent years, novel protease and polymerase inhibitor agents (e.g. Telaprevir and Boceprevir) were licensed to treat HCV infection. However, they have never been studied in the post-RT population and the newer second generation protease inhibitors as well as the NS5b polymerase inhibitors have likewise not been used, or licensed for use in this important population. These agents may provide additional candidates for combination therapy with PEG-RIB to improve patient outcome.

The ultimate goal of IFN-based treatment of HCV infection post-RT is the eradication of the infection and prevention of HCV-related liver damage. However, as our meta-analysis indicates, IFN therapy has limited efficacy and may induce graft

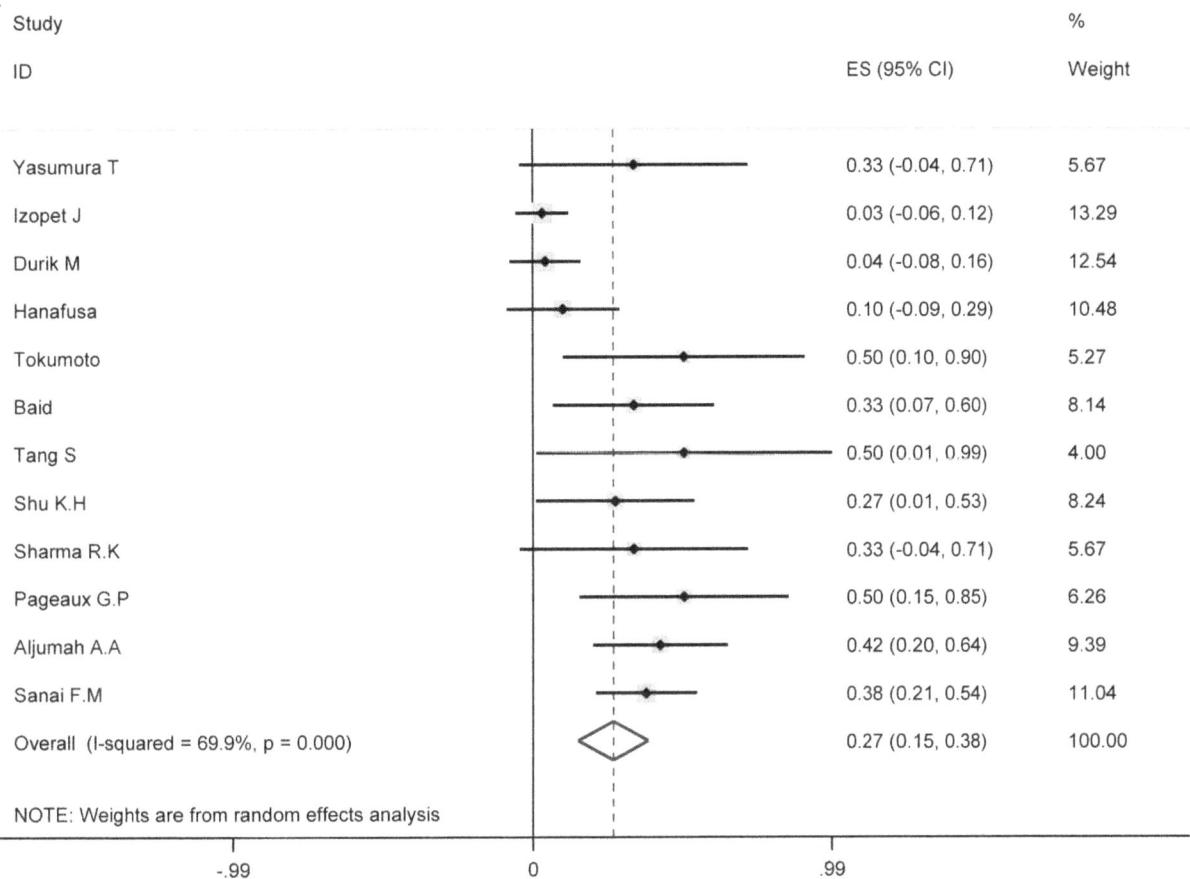

Study ID	ES (95% CI)	% Weight
Yasumura T	0.33 (-0.04, 0.71)	5.67
Izopet J	0.03 (-0.06, 0.12)	13.29
Durik M	0.04 (-0.08, 0.16)	12.54
Hanafusa	0.10 (-0.09, 0.29)	10.48
Tokumoto	0.50 (0.10, 0.90)	5.27
Baid	0.33 (0.07, 0.60)	8.14
Tang S	0.50 (0.01, 0.99)	4.00
Shu K.H	0.27 (0.01, 0.53)	8.24
Sharma R.K	0.33 (-0.04, 0.71)	5.67
Pageaux G.P	0.50 (0.15, 0.85)	6.26
Aljumah A.A	0.42 (0.20, 0.64)	9.39
Sanai F.M	0.38 (0.21, 0.54)	11.04
Overall (I-squared = 69.9%, p = 0.000)	0.27 (0.15, 0.38)	100.00

NOTE: Weights are from random effects analysis

-.99   0   .99

Figure 2. Forest map of summary estimate for SVR rate.

rejection. Therefore, not all RT recipients who are HCV seropositive should receive IFN-based antiviral therapy. The guideline of Kidney Disease Improving Global Outcome (KDIGO) suggests that IFN therapy should limited to cases of recurrent or progressive HCV-related Glomerulopathy in the transplant kidney, and advanced liver diseases such as liver fibrosis or fibrosing cholestatic hepatitis [29,79,80].The strategy of using of IFN therapy to treat HCV infection after RT is based largely on the positive results of this approach in non-transplant settings. However, unlike in non-transplant setting, there are no large, controlled clinical trials to test the efficacy of IFN therapy in post-RT patients. Instead, most of the published reports on IFN therapy post-RT describe small cohort studies. Without detailed clinical trials, it is difficult to predict the efficacy and tolerability of IFN therapy in post-RT patients. The present meta-analysis of 12 clinical trials is the first study, to our knowledge, to pool the results of multiple studies testing the efficacy of IFN-based antiviral therapy for treating HCV infection post-RT.

Compared to the previous meta-analysis of IFN-based therapy post-RT [18], our analysis employed more strict inclusion and exclusion criteria, more accurate data extraction, and incorporated the biochemical response rate and graft rejection rate. Furthermore, earlier studies (included in the prior meta-analysis)

used IFN dosages that are unlikely to produce optimal SVR. In addition, some of these early studies did not describe the method for diagnosing graft rejection, which can potentially cause over-diagnosis of the condition [81]. Due to these factors, the previous meta-analysis may have overestimated the drop-out rate while underestimating the SVR. As a result, our updated meta-analysis may provide a more reliable conclusion regarding the efficacy of IFN therapy in the post-RT setting. Moreover, our meta-analysis included reports of the PEG-based therapies, which have a more beneficial effect on virological and biochemical response than standard IFN-therapies. This finding could have a significant impact on future treatment strategies for HCV patients, as it suggests that PEG-based therapy can be employed to improve the limited efficacy of IFN therapy.

The results of this meta-analysis should facilitate treatment decisions for post-RT patients with HCV infection. Emerging evidence suggests that HCV-related therapy should be performed in patients prior to renal transplantation because when HCV RNA clearance occurred, they experienced no relapse after transplantation despite chronic immunosuppressive treatment [53]. The results of our meta-analysis should be interpreted in the context of the limitations of the included studies. For example, our analysis consisted of eleven small cohort studies and only one controlled

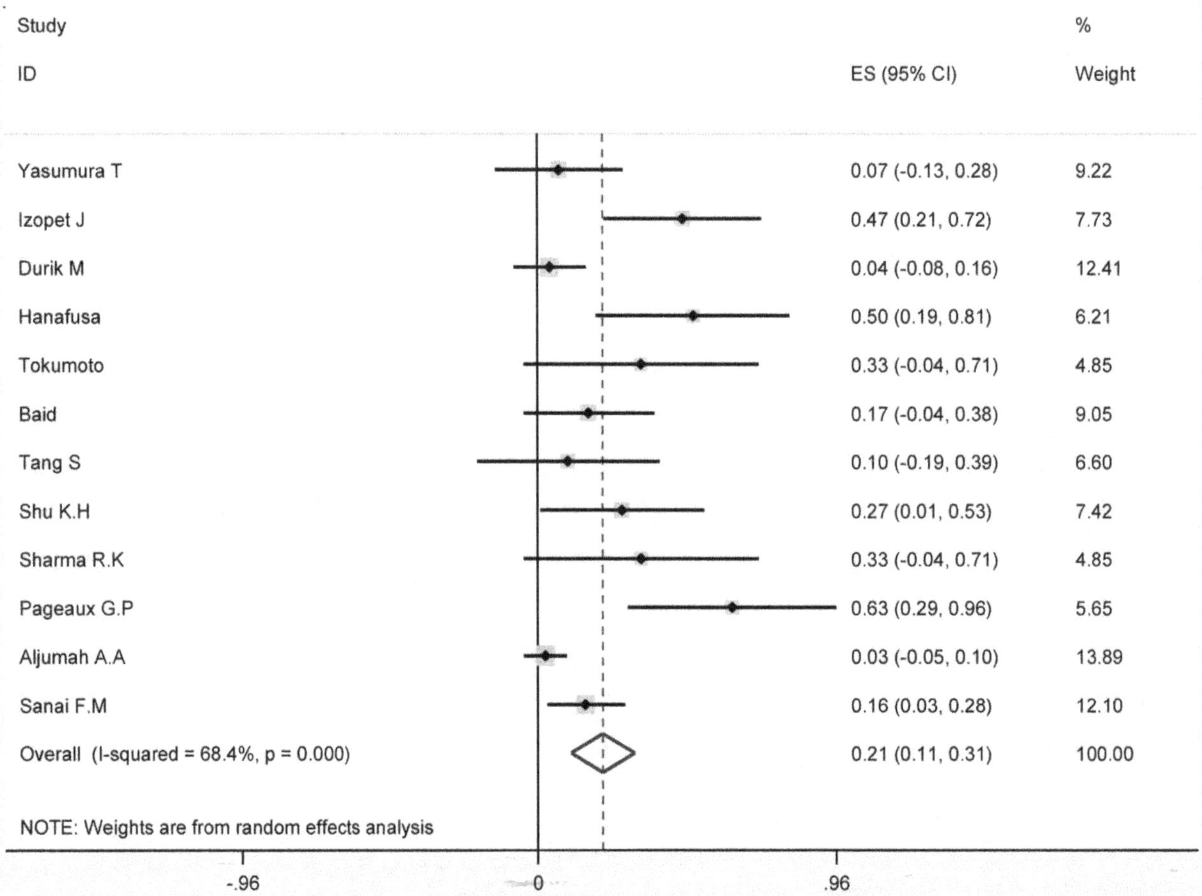

Study
ID
ES (95% CI)
%
Weight
Yasumura T 0.07 (-0.13, 0.28) 9.22
Izopet J 0.47 (0.21, 0.72) 7.73
Durik M 0.04 (-0.08, 0.16) 12.41
Hanafusa 0.50 (0.19, 0.81) 6.21
Tokumoto 0.33 (-0.04, 0.71) 4.85
Baid 0.17 (-0.04, 0.38) 9.05
Tang S 0.10 (-0.19, 0.39) 6.60
Shu K.H 0.27 (0.01, 0.53) 7.42
Sharma R.K 0.33 (-0.04, 0.71) 4.85
Pageaux G.P 0.63 (0.29, 0.96) 5.65
Aljumah A.A 0.03 (-0.05, 0.10) 13.89
Sanai F.M 0.16 (0.03, 0.28) 12.10
Overall (I-squared = 68.4%, p = 0.000) 0.21 (0.11, 0.31) 100.00
NOTE: Weights are from random effects analysis
-.96
0
.96

Figure 3. Forest map of summary estimate for Drop-out rate.

0
-2
-4
logor
0
.2
.4
.6
.8
s.e. of: logor

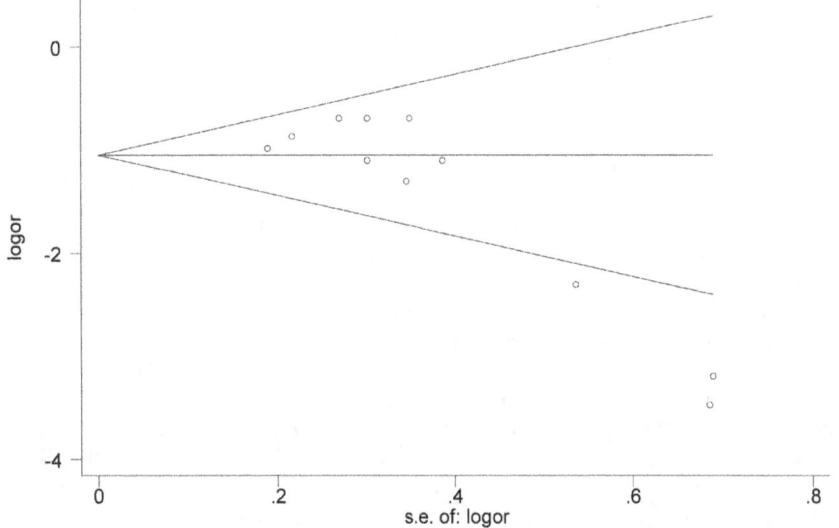

Figure 4. Funnel plot of precision by SVR logit rate.

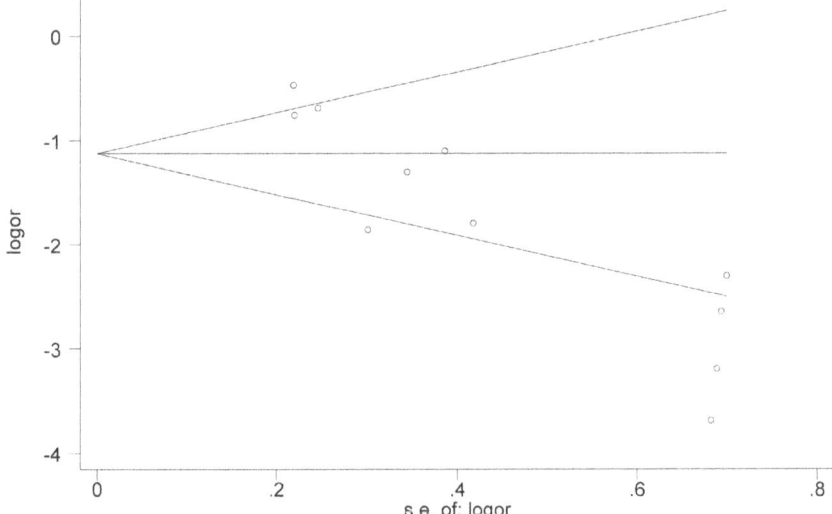

Figure 5. Funnel plot of precision by Drop-out logit rate.

clinical trial, without any large, randomized, controlled clinical trials. Given the stringency of our eligibility criteria, this publication bias likely reflects the need for more comprehensive research on the efficacy of IFN in post-RT patients. Another limitation of the included studies was the lack of a control group (e.g. placebo treated patients). As a result, we were unable to calculate pooled odds ratios or mean differences in comparison to placebo or other therapies. Therefore, it is difficult to provide an accurate estimate of the efficacy and tolerability of IFN treatment in patients with HCV infection post-RT. Additionally, our analysis does not include histological data from the end of treatment, time-points beyond six months of follow up, or patients with end-stage renal disease.

In conclusion, the present review and meta-analysis demonstrates the limited safety and efficacy of IFN-based antiviral therapy for HCV infection post-RT. The therapeutic advantage of IFN-RIB or PEG-RIB therapy observed in non-transplant chronic HCV infection appears to be attenuated post RT.However, PEG-RIB demonstrates greater efficacy on virological and biochemical response compared to IFN-RIB in patients with HCV infection post-RT. We believe this meta-analysis further advances the field of transplant hepatology by clarifying the benefits and risks of IFN-based antiviral therapy post-RT. In particular, our study suggests that the limited benefits of IFN-based therapy post RT need to be weighed against the risk of allograft rejection. Future research is required to develop novel strategies to improve therapeutic efficacy and tolerability, and reduce the liver-related morbidity and mortality in this important patient population.

Supporting Information

Checklist S1   The PRISMA checklist.

Figure S1   Sensitivity analysis by fixed-effects model of SVR logit rate.

Figure S2   Sensitivity analysis by random-effects model of SVR logit rate.

Figure S3   Sensitivity analysis by fixed-effects model of Drop-out logit rate.

Figure S4   Sensitivity analysis by random-effects model of Drop-out logit rate.

Table S1   Meta-regression analysis (dependent variable: SVR logit rate).

Table S2   Meta-regression analysis (dependent variable: Drop-out logit rate).

Author Contributions

Conceived and designed the experiments: FW JL. Performed the experiments: FW JL. Analyzed the data: FW JL FL HH PH. Contributed reagents/materials/analysis tools: HH HR PH. Wrote the paper: FW PH. Proofread the manuscript: PH. Paid for some articles: HR PH.

References

1. World Health Organization (2002) Hepatitis C 2002. In: Resource Centre Communicable Diseases. Available: http://www.who.int/ith/chapter05_m05_hepatitisc.html. Accessed 2005 February 14.
2. Heintges T, Wands JR (1997) Hepatitis C virus: epidemiology and transmission. Hepatology 26: 521–526.
3. Martin P, Fabrizi F (2008) Hepatitis C virus and kidney disease. Journal of Hepatology 49: 613–624.
4. Scott DR, Wong JK, Spicer TS, Dent H, Mensah FK, et al. (2010) Adverse impact of hepatitis C virus infection on renal replacement therapy and renal transplant patients in Australia and New Zealand. Transplantation 90: 1165–1171.
5. Levey AS, de Jong PE, Coresh J, El Nahas M, Astor BC, et al. (2011) The definition, classification, and prognosis of chronic kidney disease: a KDIGO Controversies Conference report. Kidney Int 80: 17–28.
6. Pereira BJ, Levey AS (1997) Hepatitis C virus infection in dialysis and renal transplantation. Kidney Int 51: 981–999.
7. Meyers CM, Seeff LB, Stehman-Breen CO, Hoofnagle JH (2003) Hepatitis C and renal disease: an update. Am J Kidney Dis 42: 631–657.

8. Periera BJ, Wright TL, Schmid CH, Levey AS (1995) The impact of pretransplantation hepatitis C infection on the outcome of renal transplantation. Transplantation 60: 799–805.

9. Mitwalli AH, Alam A, Al-Wakeel J, Al Suwaida K, Tarif N, et al. (2006) Effect of chronic viral hepatitis on graft survival in Saudi renal transplant patients. Nephron Clin Pract 102: c72–80.

10. Rostaing L, Weclawiak H, Izopet J, Kamar N (2012) Treatment of hepatitis C virus infection after kidney transplantation. Contrib Nephrol 176: 87–96.

11. Fabrizi F, Martin P, Ponticelli C (2001) Hepatitis C virus infection and renal transplantation. American Journal of Kidney Diseases 38: 919–934.

12. Morales JM, Campistol JM, Dominguez-Gil B (2002) Hepatitis C virus infection and kidney transplantation. Semin Nephrol 22: 365–374.

13. Morales JM, Dominguez-Gil B, Sanz-Guajardo D, Fernandez J (2004) The influence of hepatitis B and hepatitis C virus infection in the recipient on late renal allograft failure. 19 Suppl 3: iii72–76.

14. Cruzado JM, Carrera M, Torras J, Grinyo JM (2001) Hepatitis C virus infection and de novo glomerular lesions in renal allografts. Am J Transplant 1: 171–178.

15. Seron D, Arias M, Campistol JM, Morales JM (2003) Late renal allograft failure between 1990 and 1998 in Spain: a changing scenario. Transplantation 76: 1588–1594.

16. Kim E, Ko HH, Yoshida EM (2011) Treatment issues surrounding hepatitis C in renal transplantation: A review. Annals of Hepatology 10: 5–14.

17. [No authors listed] (2004) Viral hepatitis guidelines in hemodialysis and transplantation. Am J Transplant 4 Suppl 10: 72–82.

18. Fabrizi F, Lunghi G, Dixit V, Martin P (2006) Meta-analysis: anti-viral therapy of hepatitis C virus-related liver disease in renal transplant patients. Aliment Pharmacol Ther 24: 1413–1422.

19. Ichikawa Y, Kyo M, Hanafusa T, Kohro T, Kishikawa H, et al. (1998) A 20-year case study of a kidney transplant recipient with chronic active hepatitis C - Clinical course and successful treatment for late acute rejection induced by interferon therapy. Transplantation 65: 134–138.

20. Toth CM, Pascual M, Chung RT, Graeme-Cook F, Dienstag JL, et al. (1998) Hepatitis C virus-associated fibrosing cholestatic hepatitis after renal transplantation: response to interferon-alpha therapy. Transplantation 66: 1254–1258.

21. Luciani G, Bossola M, Muscaritoli M, Panocchia N, Ferrante A, et al. (2003) Sustained response with negative serum HCV-mRNA and disappearance of antibodies after interferon-alpha therapy in a kidney transplant recipient with chronic active viral hepatitis C. J Nephrol 16: 417–420.

22. Konishi I, Horiike N, Michitaka K, Ochi N, Furukawa S, et al. (2004) Renal transplant recipient with chronic hepatitis C who obtained sustained viral response after interfon-(beta) therapy. Internal Medicine 43: 931–934.

23. Fraile P, Garcia-Cosmes P, Rosado C, Tabernero JM (2009) Interferon-alpha and its deleterious effects on kidney transplant: regarding one case. Nefrologia 29: 366–367.

24. Tokumoto T, Tanabe K, Oshima T, Ishikawa N, Shinmura H, et al. (1999) Outcome of interferon-alpha (IFN-alpha) treatment in hemodialysis patients and renal transplant recipients with chronic hepatitis C. Transplantation 67: S99–S99.

25. Kim HW, Choi BS, Park JH, Yang CW, Kim YS, et al. (2001) Clinical outcome of Recombinant Interferon-alpha treatment in pre- and post-transplant patients. Journal of the American Society of Nephrology 12: 901A–901A.

26. Sanchez W, Brandhagen DJ, Cosio FG, Poterucha JJ, Gross JB, et al. (2005) Safety and tolerability of interferon for the treatment of chronic HCV in renal transplant recipients. American Journal of Transplantation 5: 301–302.

27. Weclawiak H, Kamar N, Modesto A, Izopet J, Sallusto F, et al. (2007) Acute renal allograft rejection following alpha-interferon therapy for chronic hepatitis C infection in renal transplant patients with failed allografts. Nephrology Dialysis Transplantation 22: 203–203.

28. Kim YK, Yoon HE, Kim SH, Choi BS, Kim Y-s, et al. (2008) Efficacy and safety of interferon alpha treatment in kidney transplant recipients with chronic hepatitis C. American Journal of Transplantation 8: 567–568.

29. Caeiro F, Baptista V, Rodrigues N, Carvalho D, Aires I, et al. (2011) Treatment of hepatitis C virus infection in kidney transplant recipients: Case report. Transplantation Proceedings 43: 259–262.

30. Mukherjee S, Ariyarantha K (2007) Successful Hepatitis C Eradication With Preservation of Renal Function in a Liver/kidney Transplant Recipient Using Pegylated Interferon and Ribavirin. Transplantation 84: 1374–1375.

31. Fujiwara K, Goto N, Tanaka Y, Hayashi K, Yamada T, et al. (2011) Successful treatment of renal transplant recipients infected with chronic hepatitis C genotype 2 with peg-interferon and ribavirin combination therapy. Hepatology 54 SUPPL. 1: 839A.

32. Fujiwara K, Goto N, Hayashi K, Yamada T, Ban T, et al. (2012) Treatment of renal transplant recipients infected with chronic hepatitis C with peg-interferon and ribavirin combination therapy. Hepatology 56 SUPPL. 1: 1047A.

33. Dersimonian R, Laird N (1986) Meta-analysis in clinical trials. control clin Trials 7: 177–178.

34. Petitti DB (2001) Approaches to heterogeneity in meta-analysis. Stat Med 20: 3625–3633.

35. Higgins JP, Thompson SG, Deeks JJ, Altman DG (2003) Measuring inconsistency in meta-analyses. BMJ 327: 557–560.

36. Ozminkowski RJ, Wortman PM, Roloff DW (1988) Inborn/outborn status and neonatal survival: a meta-analysis of non-randomized studies. Stat Med 7: 1207–1221.

37. Thompson SG, Higgins JP (2002) How should meta-regression analyses be undertaken and interpreted? Stat Med 21: 1559–1573.

38. Egger M, Davey Smith G, Schneider M, Minder C (1997) Bias in meta-analysis detected by a simple, graphical test. BMJ 315: 629–634.

39. Siddiqui AR, Abbas Z, Luck NH, Hassan SM, Aziz T, et al. (2012) Experience of fibrosing cholestatic hepatitis with hepatitis C virus in kidney transplant recipients. Transplant Proc 44: 721–724.

40. Sanai FM, Mousa DH, Aleid H, Al Shoail G, Al Mdani AS, et al. (2010) Peginterferon ALFA-2A plus ribavirin combination treatment in chronic hepatitis C postrenal transplant patients: An interim analysis. Hepatology 52 SUPPL. 1: 789A.

41. Kotanko P, Raid H, Skrabal F (2001) Hepatitis C associated cryoglobulinemic vasculitis post-transplant: Efficacy of low-dose interferon alpha and ribavirin therapy. Journal of the American Society of Nephrology 12: 936A–936A.

42. Alfurayh O, Chaaban A, Pall A, Al Mutawa N, Ellis M, et al. (2002) Long-term follow up of haemodialysis (hd) patients with chronic hepatitis (hcv) infection - favorable outcome with a-interferon (ifn) followed by kidney transplantation [abstract no: M221]. Nephrology Dialysis Transplantation. pp. 110.

43. Pageaux G-P, Mourad G, Chermak F, Audin H, Garrigue V, et al. (2006) Late treatment of chronic hepatitis C in renal transplant recipients: An open pilot study. Hepatology 44: 331A–331A.

44. Scott DR, Wong JK, Spicer ST, Dent H, Levy MT (2008) Hepatitis C in Dialysis and Renal Transplant Patients - Analysis of the Australia and New Zealand Dialysis and Transplant Registry Reveals Significant Impact of Hepatitis C Infection after Renal Transplantation. Hepatology 48: 1130A–1130A.

45. Abbas Z, Urrehman A, Hassan Luck N, Hassan SM, Mubarak M, et al. (2012) Fibrosing cholestatic hepatitis C in kidney transplant recipients. Hepatology International 6: 150.

46. Rostaing L, Izopet J, Arnaud C, Cisterne JM, Alric L, et al. (1999) Long-term impact of superinfection by hepatitis G virus in hepatitis C virus-positive renal transplant patients. Transplantation 67: 556–560.

47. Ridruejo E, Diaz C, Davalos Michel M, Soler Pujol G, Martinez A, et al. (2010) Short and long term outcome of kidney transplanted patients with chronic viral hepatitis B and C. Annals of Hepatology 9: 271–277.

48. Schmitz V, Kiessling A, Bahra M, Puhl G, Kahl A, et al. (2007) Peginterferon alfa-2b plus ribavirin for the treatment of hepatitis C recurrence following combined liver and kidney transplantation. Ann Transplant 12: 22–27.

49. Van Wagner LB, Baker T, Ahya SN, Norvell JP, Wang E, et al. (2009) Outcomes of patients with hepatitis C undergoing simultaneous liver-kidney transplantation. Journal of Hepatology 51: 874–880.

50. Molina E, Blum-Guzman JP, Arosemena L, Moon J, Tzakis AG, et al. (2010) Outcomes of Simultaneous Liver and Kidney Transplant Recipients in Hepatitis C Infected Patients. Hepatology 52: 872A–873A.

51. Cimsit B, Schilsky M, Moini M, Cartiera K, Arvelakis A, et al. (2011) Combined liver kidney transplantation: Critical analysis of a single-center experience. Transplantation Proceedings 43: 901–904.

52. Hassan Q, Roche B, Buffet C, Bessede T, Samuel D, et al. (2012) Liver-kidney recipients with chronic viral hepatitis C treated with interferon-alpha. Transplant International 25: 941–947.

53. Kamar N, Toupance O, Buchler M, Sandres-Saune K, Izopet J, et al. (2003) Evidence that clearance of hepatitis C virus RNA after (alpha)-interferon therapy in dialysis patients is sustained after renal transplantation. Journal of the American Society of Nephrology 14: 2092–2098.

54. Voiculescu M, Ionescu C, Ismail G, Mandache E, Hortopan M, et al. (2003) Acute pancreatitis, acute hepatitis and acute renal failure favourably resolved in two renal transplant recipients. Romanian Journal of Gastroenterology 12: 41–46.

55. Carbognin SJ, Solomon NM, Yeo FE, Swanson SJ, Bohen EM, et al. (2006) Acute renal allograft rejection following pegylated IFN-(alpha) treatment for chronic HCV in a repeat allograft recipient on hemodialysis: A case report. American Journal of Transplantation 6: 1746–1751.

56. Fabriz F, Martin P (2006) Management of hepatitis B and C virus infection before and after renal transplantation. Current Opinion in Organ Transplantation 11: 583–588.

57. Montalbano M, Pasulo L, Sonzogni A, Remuzzi G, Colledan M, et al. (2007) Treatment with pegylated interferon and ribavirin for hepatitis C virus-associated severe-cryoglobulinemia in a liver/kidney transplant recipient. Journal of Clinical Gastroenterology 41: 216–220.

58. Sperl J, Petrasek J, Spicak J, Viklicky O (2008) Acute rejection of non-functional allograft in kidney transplant recipients with hepatitis C treated with peginterferon-alpha 2a. J Hepatol 49: 461–462; author reply 462–463.

59. Dale CH, Burns P, McCutcheon M, Hernandez-Alejandro R, Marotta PJ (2009) Spontaneous clearance of hepatitis C after liver and renal transplantation. Canadian Journal of Gastroenterology 23: 265–267.

60. Chang M-L, Lai P-C, Yeh C-T (2011) Sustained eradication of hepatitis C virus by low-dose long-term interferon therapy in a renal transplant recipient with dual infection with hepatitis B and C viruses: a case report. Journal of Medical Case Reports 5: 246–246.

61. Izopet J, Rostaing L, Ton-That H, Dubois M, Cazabat M, et al. (1997) Kinetics of HCV viremia in kidney transplant recipients during and after (alpha)-interferon therapy. American Journal of Nephrology 17: 417–420.

62. Yasumura T, Nakajima H, Hamashima T, Nakai I, Yoshimura N, et al. (1997) Long-term outcome of recombinant INF-alpha treatment of chronic hepatitis C in kidney transplant recipients. Transplant Proc 29: 784–786.

63. Durlik M, Gaciong Z, Rowinska D, Rancewicz Z, Lewandowska D, et al. (1998) Long-term results of treatment of chronic hepatitis B, C and D with interferon-alpha in renal allograft recipients. Transplant international : official journal of the European Society for Organ Transplantation 11 Suppl 1: S135–139.

64. Hanafusa T, Ichikawa Y, Yazawa K, Kishikawa H, Fukunishi T, et al. (1998) Hepatitis C virus infection in kidney transplantation and a pilot study of the effects of interferon-alpha therapy. Transplant Proc 30: 122–124.

65. Tokumoto T, Tanabe K, Ishikawa N, Simizu T, Oshima T, et al. (1998) Effect of interferon-alfa treatment in renal transplant recipients with chronic hepatitis C. Transplant Proc 30: 3270–3272.

66. Baid S, Tolkoff-Rubin N, Saidman S, Chung R, Williams WW, et al. (2003) Acute humoral rejection in hepatitis C-infected renal transplant recipients receiving antiviral therapy. American Journal of Transplantation 3: 74–78.

67. Tang S, Cheng IKP, Leung VKS, Kuok UI, Tang AWC, et al. (2003) Successful treatment of hepatitis C after kidney transplantation with combined interferon alpha-2b and ribavirin. Journal of Hepatology 39: 875–878.

68. Shu KH, Lan JL, Wu MJ, Cheng CH, Chen CH, et al. (2004) Ultra-low dose alpha-interferon plus ribavirin for the treatment of active hepatitis C in renal transplant recipients. American Journal of Transplantation 4: 205–205.

69. Sharma RK, Bansal SB, Gupta A, Gulati S, Kumar A, et al. (2006) Chronic hepatitis C virus infection in renal transplant: Treatment and outcome. Clinical Transplantation 20: 677–683.

70. Pageaux G-P, Hilleret M-N, Garrigues V, Bismuth M, Audin-Mamlouk H, et al. (2009) Pegylated interferon-alpha-based treatment for chronic hepatitis C in renal transplant recipients: an open pilot study. Transplant International 22: 562–567.

71. Aljumah AA, Saeed MA, Al Flaiw AI, Al Traif IH, Al Alwan AM, et al. (2012) Efficacy and safety of treatment of hepatitis C virus infection in renal transplant recipients. World Journal of Gastroenterology 18: 55–63.

72. Sanai FM, Mousa D, Al-Mdani A, Al-Shoail G, Al-Ashgar H, et al. (2013) Safety and efficacy of peginterferon-(alpha)2a plus ribavirin treatment in renal transplant recipients with chronic hepatitis C. Journal of Hepatology.

73. Shepherd J, Brodin H, Cave C, Waugh N, Price A, et al. (2004) Pegylated interferon alpha-2a and -2b in combination with ribavirin in the treatment of chronic hepatitis C: a systematic review and economic evaluation. Health Technol Assess 8: iii-iv, 1–125.

74. Shepherd J, Waugh N, Hewitson P (2000) Combination therapy (interferon alfa and ribavirin) in the treatment of chronic hepatitis C: a rapid and systematic review. Health Technol Assess 4: 1–67.

75. Baid S, Cosimi AB, Tolkoff-Rubin N (2000) Renal disease associated with hepatitis C infection after kidney and liver transplantation. 70: 255–261.

76. Samuel D (2004) Hepatitis C, interferon, and risk of rejection after liver transplantation. Liver Transpl 10: 868–871.

77. Rostaing L (2000) Treatment of hepatitis C virus infection after renal transplantation: new insights. Nephrol Dial Transplant 15 Suppl 8: 74–76.

78. Kamar N, Rostaing L, Sandres-Saune K, Ribes D, Durand D, et al. (2004) Amantadine therapy in renal transplant patients with hepatitis C virus infection. J Clin Virol 30: 110–114.

79. Covic A, Abramowicz D, Bruchfeld A, Leroux-Roels G, Samuel D, et al. (2009) Endorsement of the Kidney Disease Improving Global Outcomes (KDIGO) hepatitis C guidelines: a European Renal Best Practice (ERBP) position statement. Nephrol Dial Transplant 24: 719–727.

80. Ozdemir BH, Ozdemir FN, Sezer S, Colak T, Haberal M (2006) De novo glomerulonephritis in renal allografts with hepatitis C virus infection. Transplant Proc 38: 492–495.

81. Wells JT, Lucey MR, Said A (2006) Hepatitis C in transplant recipients of solid organs, other than liver. Clin Liver Dis 10: 901–917.

20

Alloimmune Activation Promotes Anti-Cancer Cytotoxicity after Rat Liver Transplantation

Stéphanie Lacotte[1]*, Graziano Oldani[1], Florence Slits[1], Lorenzo A. Orci[1], Laura Rubbia-Brandt[2,3], Philippe Morel[1], Gilles Mentha[1,3], Christian Toso[1,3]*

1 Department of Surgery, Geneva University Hospitals, University of Geneva, Geneva, Switzerland, 2 Hepato-pancreato-biliary Centre, Geneva University Hospitals, University of Geneva, Geneva, Switzerland, 3 Department of Pathology, Geneva University Hospitals, University of Geneva, Geneva, Switzerland

Abstract

Liver transplantation for hepatocellular carcinoma (HCC) results in a specific condition where the immune response is potentially directed against both allogeneic and cancer antigens. We have investigated the level of anti-cancer immunity during allogeneic immune response. Dark Agouti-to-Lewis and Lewis-to-Lewis rat liver transplantations were performed and the recipients anti-cancer immunity was analysed at the time of alloimmune activation. The occurrence of rejection in the allogeneic recipients was confirmed by a shorter survival ($p<0.01$), increased liver function tests ($p<0.01$), the presence of signs of rejection on histology, and a donor-specific *ex vivo* mixed lymphocyte reaction. At the time of alloimmune activation, blood mononuclear cells of the allogeneic group demonstrated increased anti-cancer cytotoxicity ($p<0.005$), which was related to an increased natural killer (NK) cell frequency ($p<0.05$) and a higher monocyte/macrophage activation level ($p<0.01$). Similarly, liver NK cell anti-cancer cytotoxicity ($p<0.005$), and liver monocyte/macrophage activation levels ($p<0.01$) were also increased. The alloimmune-associated cytotoxicity was mediated through the NKG2D receptor, whose expression was increased in the rejected graft ($p<0.05$) and on NK cells and monocyte/macrophages. NKG2D ligands were expressed on rat HCC cells, and its inhibition prevented the alloimmune-associated cytotoxicity. Although waiting for *in vivo* validation, alloimmune-associated cytotoxicity after rat liver transplantation appears to be linked to increased frequencies and levels of activation of NK cells and monocyte/macrophages, and is at least in part mediated through the NKG2D receptor.

Editor: Jacques Zimmer, Centre de Recherche Public de la Santé (CRP-Santé), Luxembourg

Funding: This study was supported by grants from the Swiss National Science Foundation (PP00P3_139021), the Artères Foundation, the Astellas European Foundation, and the Boninchi Foundation, the Elsie and Carlos de Reuter, and the Marie-France and Francis Minkoff Foundation. Christian Toso was supported by a Professorship from the Swiss National Science Foundation (PP00P3_139021). The funders had no role in study design, data collection and analysis, decision to publish, or preparation of the manuscript.

Competing Interests: The authors have declared that no competing interests exist.

* E-mail: stephanie.lacotte@unige.ch (SL); christian.toso@hcuge.ch (CT)

Introduction

Liver transplantation is the most effective treatment for patients with early unresectable hepatocellular carcinoma (HCC) [1,2]. However, 15% of recipients experience post-transplant HCC recurrence, which quickly leads to death in almost all patients [3]. Various strategies have been proposed to decrease this risk, including an improved transplant selection criteria, the targeting of circulating HCC cells, the use of adjuvant anti-cancer drugs and a promoted anti-cancer immunity [4].

Transplantation for HCC is a unique condition, with immune activation directed against both allogeneic donor and cancer antigens. This dual activation has rarely been explored. An alloimmune activation may only be directed against specific allogeneic antigens or be linked to a broader activation also promoting a non-specific anti-cancer immune response. The latter hypothesis has been suggested by a number of studies showing a higher risk of post-transplant HCC recurrence in patients with more profound immune inhibition; for example, after the use of anti-lymphocyte antibodies or in case of overexposure to calcineurin inhibitors [5–8]. In addition, a decreased expression of one NKG2D ligand on HCC tumors, low neutrophil-lymphocyte blood ratios and tumor-associated macrophage counts have also been associated with HCC recurrence [9–12].

Ideally, the allogeneic immunity should be prevented and the anti-cancer immunity promoted. A better understanding of the cross-talk between the two is therefore desirable, in order to better define the mediators and the mechanisms involved in each type of immunity. Ultimately, such data will help define the ideal immunosuppression combination after liver transplantation for HCC.

The present study assesses the level of anti-cancer cytotoxicity in the liver, spleen and blood after allogeneic rat liver transplantation. It defines the role of specific immune cell types, including natural killer (NK) cells and monocyte/macrophages, and the action of key NK cell receptors.

Material and Methods

Animals, Liver Transplantation and Ethics Statement

Experiments were performed on male Lewis and Dark Agouti (DA) rats weighing 200–250 g (7 to 8 weeks-old, Janvier). They underwent orthotopic liver transplantation according to a protocol previously described [13]. DA-to-Lewis transplantations (alloge-

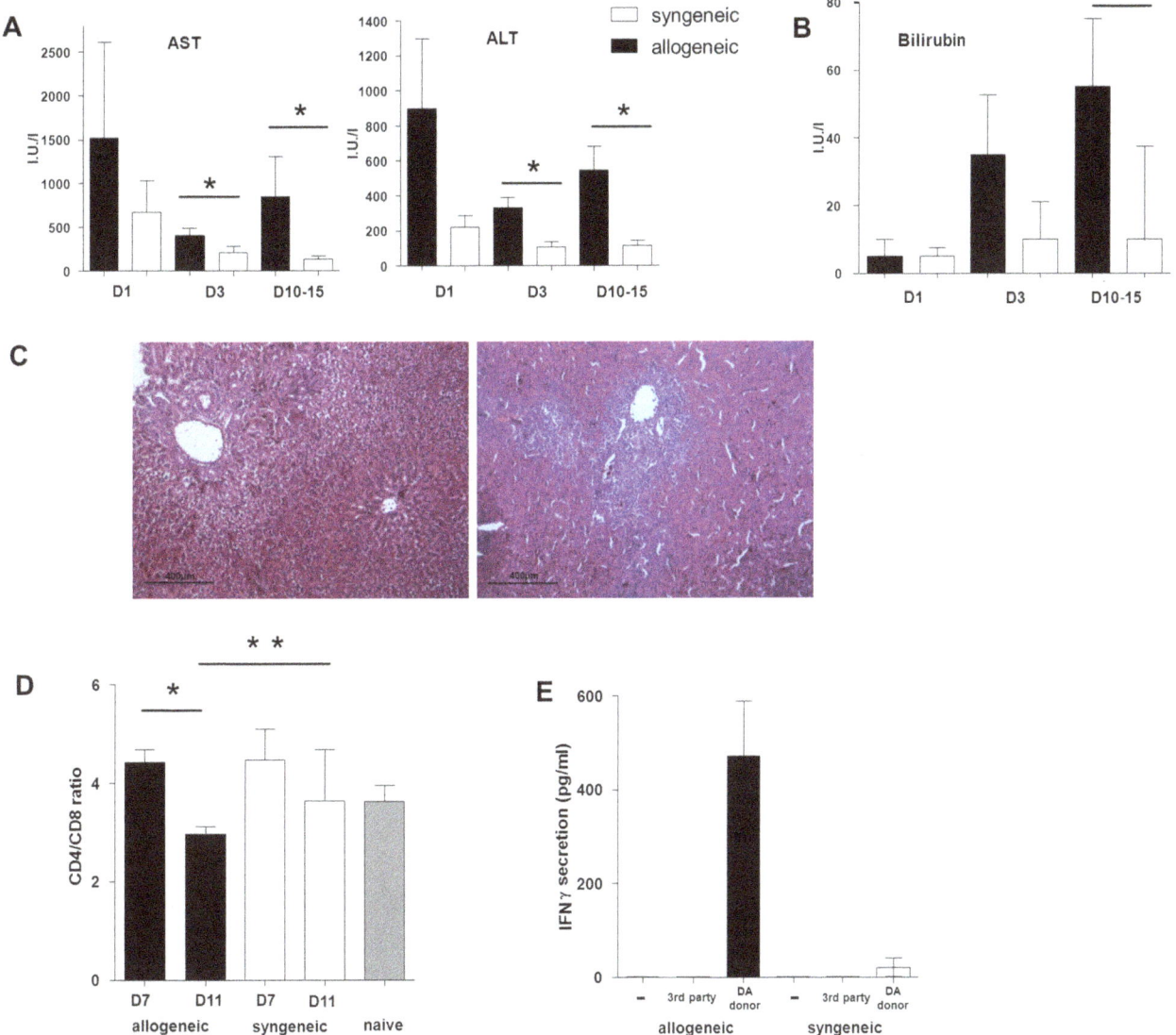

Figure 1. Assessment of alloimmunity and rejection. (A) Serum aspartate aminotransferase (AST) and alanine aminotransferase (ALT) levels after allogeneic Dark Agouti-to-Lewis (black) and syngeneic Lewis-to-Lewis (white) rat liver transplantations. (B) Bilirubine levels after allogeneic (black) and syngeneic (white) transplantation. (C) Representative hematoxilin-eosin stained biopsies on day 10 after allogeneic (right) and syngeneic (left) rat liver transplantation. (D) Post-transplant blood CD4/CD8 ratios on day 7 (D7) and 11 (D11). (E) IFNγ secretion after peripheral blood mononuclear cells (PBMC) mixed lymphocyte reaction on day ten post-transplantation with donor (DA) and third part stimulation. *p<0.05, **<0.01.

neic model) were considered as the study group, and Lewis-to-Lewis transplantations were used as syngeneic controls (six animals in each group for the survival assessment). All animals were cared for according to the international guidelines on Animal Care, and ethical approval was obtained from the ethical committee at the University of Geneva and from the Geneva veterinary authorities (N°1052/3653/3).

Rat HCC cell lines

JM-1 cells were kindly provided by George Michalopoulos (University of Pittsburg) [14]. McA-RH7777 cells were purchased from ATCC (Molsheim, France). Both cell lines were cultured in DMEM medium at high glucose level (Gibco).

Liver Function Test Assessment, Liver Histology and Immunolabelling

To detect signs of liver rejection, serum liver function tests, including aspartate aminotransferase (AST), alanine aminotransferase (ALT) and bilirubin were assessed on day one, three and ten after transplantation. Serum levels were measured in collaboration with the central clinical hospital laboratory (Synchron LX20). Samples from nine animals in each group were analysed.

The presence of rejection was also assessed on histology after hematoxin/eosin staining of liver samples retrieved on day ten after transplantation. The level of rejection was blindly graded by an expert liver pathologist according to the Banff classification [15]. NK cells were labeled on cryosections with anti-NKRP1 (CD161, 10/78, Biolegend) followed by Alexa Fluor®555 donkey anti-mouse IgG (Invitrogen). Macrophages were labeled on

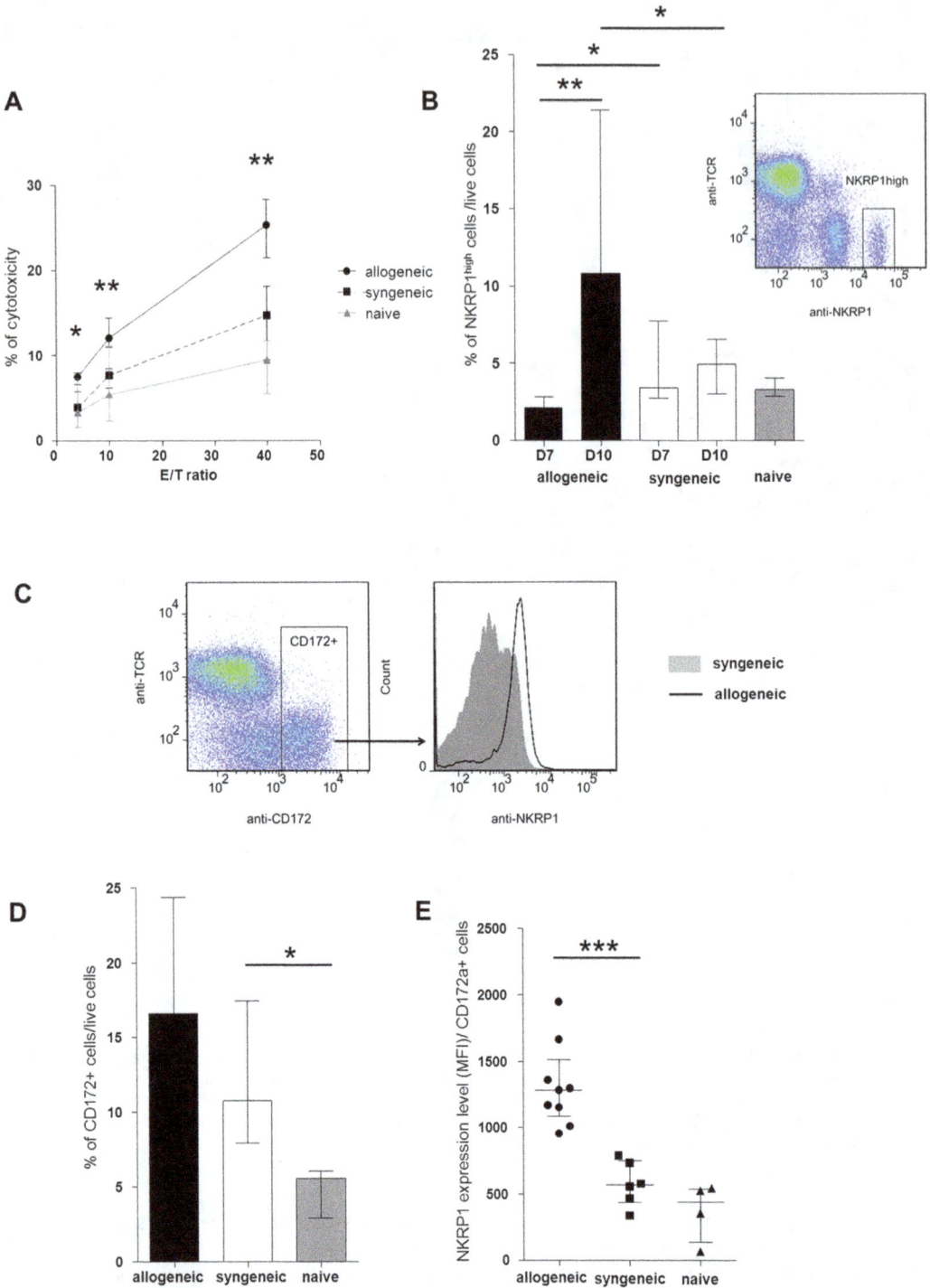

Figure 2. Alloimmunity-associated peripheral cytotoxicity. (A) *Ex vivo* PBMC anti-cancer cytotoxicity on day ten after allogeneic and syngeneic transplantations and in naïve control rats at various effector/target ratio (E/T). (B) Frequency of NKRP1[high] cells (NK cells) among PBMCs on day 7 (D7) and 10 (D10) after transplantation. Flow cytometry dot-plot assessed the gating strategy. (C) Flow cytometry dot-plot and histogram assessing the gating strategy for monocytes/macrophages (CD172+) and NKRP1 expression level on CD172+ cells. (D) Frequency of monocyte/macrophage (CD172+ cells) among PBMCs. (E) Activation level of monocyte/macrophages (NKRP1 expression level (mean fluorescence intensity (MFI)) among CD172a+ cells). *p<0.05, **<0.01.

paraffin-embedded sections with polyclonal rabbit anti-Iba1 (Wako) followed by Alexa Fluor®555 donkey anti-rabbit IgG (Invitrogen).

Peripheral Blood, Spleen and Liver Mononuclear Cell Isolation

Tail vein blood samples (500 μl) were collected in 150 μl of acid citrate dextrose. Liver and spleen were retrieved through a midline

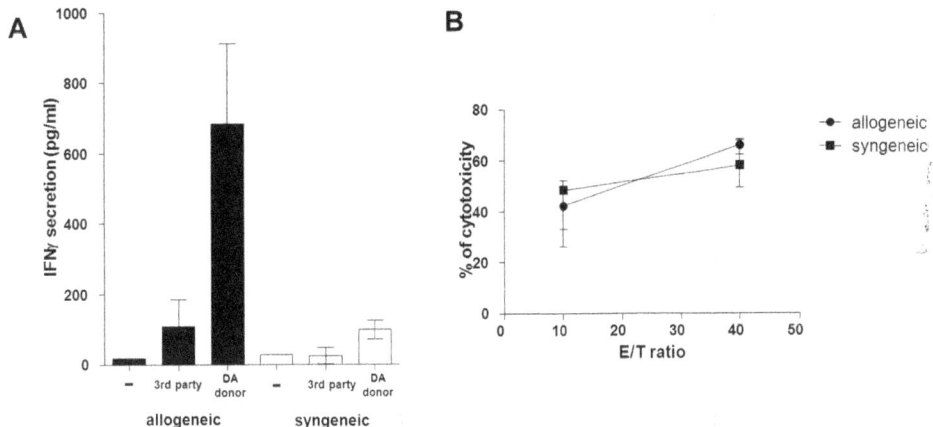

Figure 3. Alloimmunity-associated spleen cytotoxicity on ten days after transplantation. (A) IFNγ secretion after splenocyte mixed lymphocyte reaction on day ten post-transplantation with donor and third part stimulation. (B) *Ex vivo* spleen NK cell anti-cancer cytotoxicity on day ten after allogeneic and syngeneic transplantation.

abdominal incision after 10 U IV heparin injection. The liver was perfused with HBSS containing 0.5 mg/ml of collagenase D (Sigma). It was cut in small pieces, resuspended in HBSS/collagenase solution, digested at 37°C for 20 min. Cell suspension was washed and filtered through a nylon mesh. The spleen was cut in pieces, crushed and filtered through a nylon mesh. Peripheral blood, liver and spleen cells were purified in a Ficoll Paque (GE Healthcare) density gradient. Isolated mononuclear cells were washed and counted.

Mixed Lymphocyte Reaction and ELISA

Peripheral and spleen allogeneic immune activations were tested using mixed lymphocyte reactions. Cell incubations were performed in 96 well-plates in 200 μL RPMI 1640 (Gibco), 10% FCS (Invitrogen), 1 M HEPES (Invitrogen) and 1 U/ml/1 μg/ml Penicillin-Streptomycin and 0.29 mg/ml L-glutamine (Gibco). Responder Lewis cells (2.5×10^5) from four allogeneic and four syngeneic recipients were incubated with 2.5×10^5 irradiated stimulator DA (or third part) splenocytes (5000 rad) at 37°C/5% CO_2 for 24 hours.

The level of interferon gamma (IFNγ) was quantified by ELISA. Polystyrene plates (Costar) were coated overnight at 4°C with purified anti-rat γIFN (1:500, clone DB-1, Biolegend) in carbonate buffer. Plates were washed and saturated for 30 min with supplemented RPMI 1640 medium. Cell culture supernatants were added for two hours, followed by biotin anti-rat IFNγ (1:1000, Poly5109, Biolegend), streptavidin-horseradish peroxidase (1:1000, Biolegend) and the substrate solution (TMB reagent, R&Dsystem). The level of IFNγ was obtained according to a dilution curve.

Flow Cytometry Antibodies and Cytotoxicity Assay

The phenotype of blood, liver and spleen mononuclear immune cells was assessed by flow cytometry. Labeling was performed using antibodies against CD3 (1F4) (BD Pharmingen), CD4 (W3/25) (Biolegend), CD8 (OX-8), CD172a (OX-41) for monocyte/macrophages and NKRP1 (CD161, 10/78) for NK cells. The cell phenotype was assessed in nine animals per group.

NK cell receptors were assessed using anti-NKG2D (11D5F4) (eBiosciences) and anti-NKp30 (sc-33647) (SantaCruz) antibodies. The presence of NKG2D-ligands was tested on JM-1 and McA-RH7777 cell lines after incubation with mouse recombinant NKG2D-Fc chimera (139-NK-050, R&D Systems)(5 μg/well) and anti-human IgG Fc (HP6017, Biolegend).

The level of anti-cancer cell cytotoxicity was assessed with peripheral blood mononuclear cells (PBMC) and NK cells from the liver (six animals per group), the spleen and the blood (seven animals per group). They were incubated with CFSE-labeled Yac-1 target cancer cells (0.5 μM, Invitrogen) at decreasing effector/target ratios ranging from 40/1 to 4/1 for four hours at 37°C. Of note, Yac-1 cells lack the major histocompatibility complex class I and are commonly used for cytotoxic assays. Following labeling with AlexaFluor®647-AnnexinV (1.5 μl, Biolegend) and 7-AAD (1/1000, Invitrogen) in annexin binding buffer, dead cells were assessed using FACS Calibur (BD).

In selected experiments, the inhibition of cytotoxicity was tested upon incubation with anti-NKG2D and anti-NKp30 antibodies (1 μg/well).

NK Cell Magnetic Sorting

In order to specifically look at NK cells, a negative sorting was performed from PBMC and splenocytes. After incubation with mouse anti-CD172a (OX-41, GeneTex), anti-CD45RA (OX-33, Biolegend) and anti-TCR (R73, Biolegend) antibodies, cells were washed with a buffer (PBS 2% BSA 2 mM EDTA), and Dynabeads® coated goat anti-mouse IgG (Invitrogen) were added. After washing, the cell suspension was applied on a magnet in order to remove non-NK cells. The NK cell purity was assessed by flow cytometry (85% in the spleen and 90% in the blood).

Liver NK cells were obtained by a two-step negative/positive selection. Liver mononuclear cells were incubated with biotinylated anti-CD172a and anti-biotin antibodies coupled to microbeads (MiltenyiBiotec). After removal of the CD172a+ cells through a column, the flow-through was incubated with anti-CD161 FITC and anti-FITC microbeads allowing the positive selection of NK cells. The NK cell purity was assessed by flow cytometry (80% in the liver). Sorted cells were immediately used for phenotyping or cytotoxic assay.

Real-Time Polymerase Chain Reaction (qPCR)

Total RNA (cells or liver biopsies) was prepared and purified using the RNeasy Mini Kit (Qiagen, Germantown, MD)

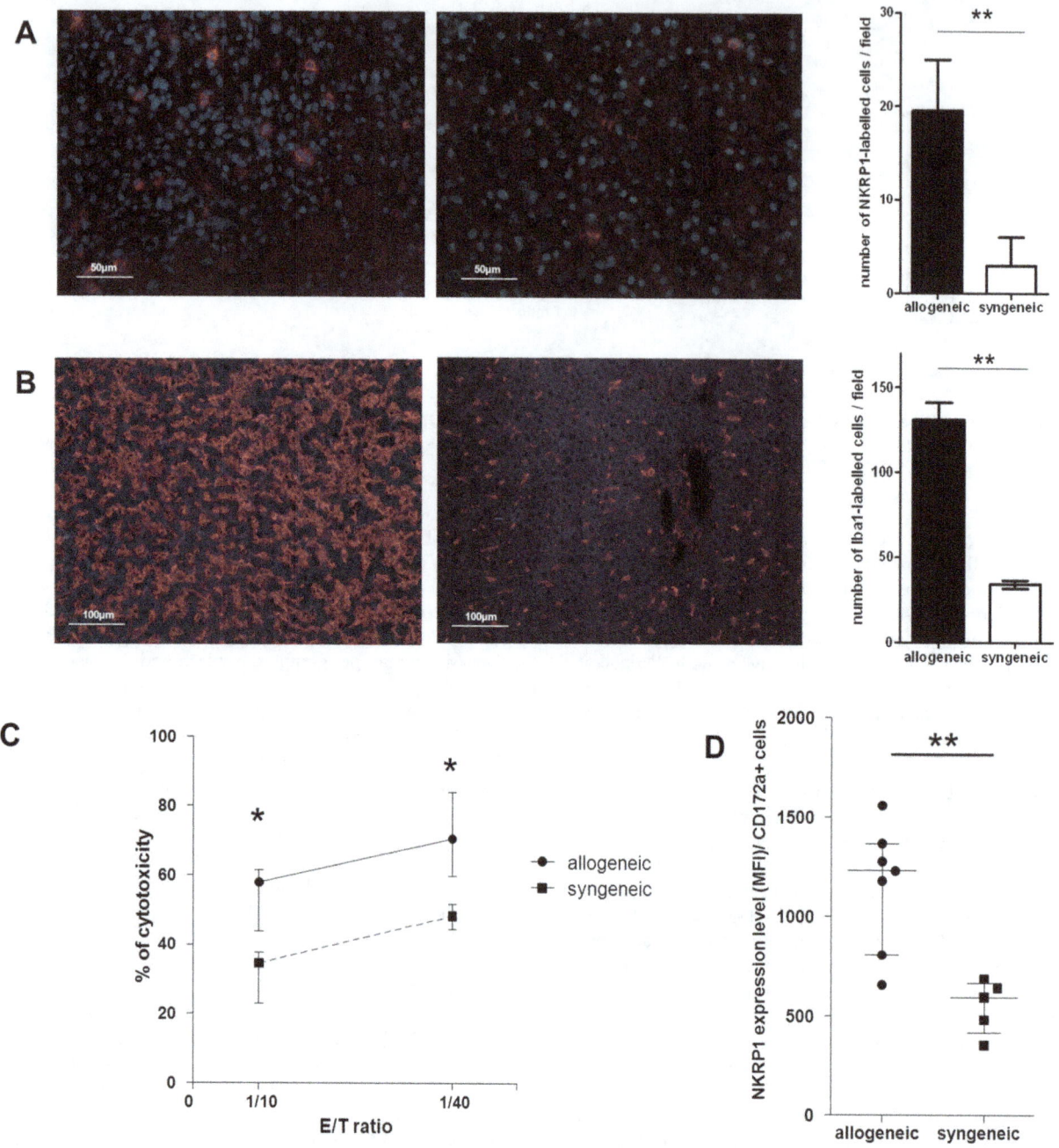

Figure 4. Alloimmunity-associated liver mononuclear cells cytotoxicity on ten days after transplantation. (A) Representative images of sections of allogeneic (left) and syngeneic (right) liver graft labeled with anti-NKRP1 antibodies (red). Nuclei were stained with Hoechst (blue). Number of labeled-NK cells per image counted on multiple liver sections. (B) Representative images of sections of allogeneic (left) and syngeneic (right) liver graft labeled with anti-Iba1 antibodies (red). Number of labeled macrophages per image counted on multiple liver sections. (C) *Ex vivo* liver NK cell anti-cancer cytotoxicity on day ten after allogeneic and syngeneic transplantation. Two effector/target ratio (E/T) were tested. (D) Activation level of liver monocyte/macrophages (NKRP1 expression level (MFI) among CD172a+ cells). *p<0.05, **p<0.01.

according to the manufacturer's instructions. One μg of cDNA was synthesized by extending a mix of random primers with the High Capacity cDNA Reverse Transcription Kit in the presence of RNase Inhibitor (Applied Biosystems). The relative quantity of each transcript was normalized according to the expression of rplp1 (ribosomal protein large P1). Primer sequences for *rplp1, nkg2d, rrlt, rae1l* and *irp94* were designed with AmplifX and Primers3 softwares and are available upon request. Amplification reactions were performed in a total volume of 20 μl using a

Thermocycler sequence detector (BioRad CFX96) with qPCR Core kit for SYBR Green I (Eurogentec).

Statistical analysis

Results were represented as median +/− IQR. Results were statistically compared using Mann-Whitney test. Survivals were plotted on Kaplan-Meier curves and compared with the log-rank test. Statistical significance was set at p<0.05.

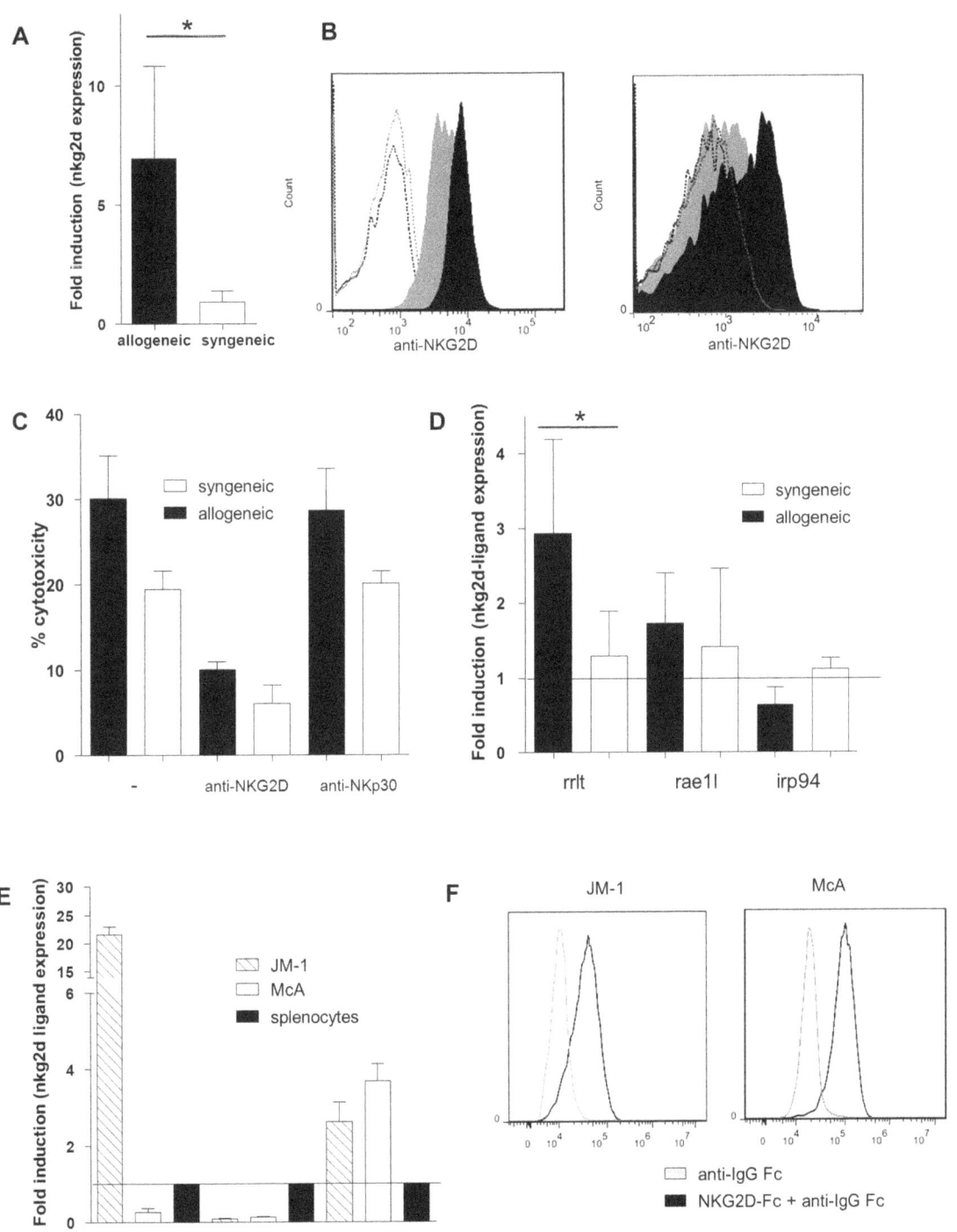

Figure 5. Alloimmunity-associated cytotoxicity is mediated through the NKG2D receptor. (A) Liver expression of *nkg2d* on day ten after liver transplantation. (B) Representative NKG2D expression levels in blood NK cells (left) and monocytes (right) of allogeneic (black) and syngeneic (grey) recipients. Isotype was used as control (dashed lines). (C) Sorted blood NK cell cytotoxicity inhibition with anti-NKG2D antibody or with anti-NKp30 antibody. (D) Levels of NKG2D ligand (*rae1l, rrlt* and *irp94*) expression in the liver on day ten after transplantation. (E) Levels of NKG2D ligand (*rae1l, rrlt* and *irp94*) expression in rat HCC cell lines. (F) Representative level of recombinant NKG2D-Fc binding to rat HCC cells lines. *p<0.05, **<0.01.

Results

Assessment of Alloimmunity and Rejection

The presence of an alloreactivity was specifically looked at because some allogeneic rat-to-rat liver transplantation models induce only low levels of alloimmunity without acute cell rejection [16]. As described in the literature, the studied DA-to-Lewis orthotopic rat liver transplantations were linked to shorter survivals compared to the syngeneic transplantations (median survival: 13 vs. >60 days, p = 0.0037, data not shown). Serum liver function tests (AST and ALT) were increased after day three in the allogeneic recipients (all p<0.01 vs. syngeneic controls, Fig. 1A). Bilirubin level was increased after 10 days in the allogeneic recipients (p = 0.026 vs. syngeneic controls, Fig. 1B).

The presence of cell rejection was confirmed on the day 10 histology and was graded Banff 8 in all studied allogeneic recipients. Syngeneic control recipients were graded Banff 0 (Fig. 1C). In addition, the peripheral CD4/CD8 ratio on day 11 was significantly lower in the allogeneic recipients compared to syngeneic recipients (2.9 vs. 3.6, p = 0.0051, Fig. 1D). Finally, the alloimmunity was specifically directed towards donor antigens as demonstrated by the day 10 mixed lymphocyte reactions against DA splenocytes (supernatant IFNγ concentration: 410 pg/ml vs. undetectable), and the absence of response against third party Fisher rat antigens (Fig. 1E).

Alloimmunity-Associated Peripheral Cytotoxicity

In an effort to assess the impact of rejection on anti-cancer immunity, the cytotoxic activity of peripheral immune cells was tested ex vivo against cancer Yac-1 cells. At the time of alloimmune activation (day 10), the level of peripheral cytotoxicity was increased in the allogeneic recipients compared to the syngeneic controls and naïve rats (effector/target 40/1: 25.2% vs. 14.7% and 9.4% respectively, p = 0.0025, Fig. 2A). This pattern was observed at all tested dilutions (4/1, 10/1, 40/1).

In order to assess whether the altered cytotoxicity was related to a variation in the cell subsets, flow cytometry analyses were conducted on PBMCs. NKRP1 (CD161), a C-type lectin membrane glycoprotein, is highly expressed on NK cells and was used as a marker for rat NK cells [17]. On day seven, the NK cell frequency (CD3$^-$ NKRP1^{high}) was significantly decreased in the allogeneic recipients compared to the syngeneic controls (2.1% vs. 3.4%, p = 0.028, Fig. 2B). This decreased frequency of peripheral NK cells is in line with the previously observed migration of NK cells into the liver early after allogeneic transplantation [18]. On day 10, the observed increased peripheral cytotoxicity was related to an increased blood NK cell frequency (10.79% in allogeneic vs. 4.9% in syngeneic, p = 0.048).

Monocytes/macrophages can also be involved in the cytotoxic events against cancer cells. The day 10 monocyte population (CD172a$^+$) was increased in both allogeneic and syngeneic recipients compared to the naïve non-transplanted controls, likely reflecting some degree of non-specific peri-operative immune activation (16.6% vs. 10.7% vs. 5.58%, respectively; p = 0.1 for allogeneic vs. naïve; p = 0.023 for syngeneic vs. naïve, Fig. 2D). This said, the highest frequency was observed in the allogeneic recipients (yet not reaching statistical significance, p = 0.455 for allogeneic vs. syngeneic). In addition, the frequency of activated monocytes expressing NKRP1 (CD161) was higher in the allogeneic recipients compared to the syngeneic controls and the naïve non-transplanted animals (mean fluorescence intensity 1282 vs. 568 vs. 438, p = 0.0004, Fig. 2E) [19].

Absence of Alloimmunity-Associated Spleen Cytotoxicity

In order to better characterise the observed peripheral cytotoxicity, we assessed the allogeneic and anti-cancer immune events in the spleen. The day 10 splenocytes from allogeneic rats stimulated with donor cells (DA) secreted more IFNγ than the splenocytes from syngeneic rats, confirming the presence of a donor-specific allogeneic response in the spleen (684 vs. 99 pg/ml, p = 0.028, Fig. 3A). Conversely, sorted spleen NK cells demonstrated no difference of cytotoxicity between allogeneic and syngeneic recipients (effector/target ratio 10/1: 42.2 vs. 48.3%,

p = 0.30, Fig. 3B). Similarly, no alteration in the number and the phenotype of spleen cells could be detected (data not shown).

Alloimmunity-Associated Liver Mononuclear Cell Activation

The immune response of liver mononuclear cells was tested on day 10 after transplantation. After isolation, the number of liver mononuclear cells was increased in the allogeneic rats compared to their syngeneic counterparts (16×10^6 vs. 5.35×10^6 cells/liver, p = 0.004).

This rise of the mononuclear cells number was related to an increased number of NK cells in the allogeneic graft (19.5 vs. 3 in the syngeneic graft, p = 0.006, Fig. 4A) and to an increased number of macrophages (131 vs. 34.5 in the syngeneic graft, p = 0.0034, Fig. 4B). These two cells subsets were found both in the hepatic parenchyma and in cell infiltrates of the allogeneic graft. The observed alteration of cell number was associated to an increased activation. Sorted liver NK cells demonstrated an increased anti-cancer cytotoxicity in the allogeneic recipients (effector/target ratio 10/1: 58.8% vs. 32%, p = 0.030, Fig. 4C). Of note, allogeneic rat liver transplant recipients showed a trend towards a higher cytotoxicity in liver-sorted NK compared to spleen-sorted NK cells (effector/target ratio 10/1: 58.8% vs 42.2%, p = 0.101). This higher liver NK cell activity is likely related to the allogeneic rejection primarily located in the liver graft [20].

The level of liver monocyte activation was increased in the allogeneic recipients (MFI: 1232 vs. 590, p = 0.005, Fig. 4D).

Alloimmunity-Associated Cytotoxicity through the NKG2D receptor

In order to define potential receptor/ligand pathways involved in the detected cytotoxicity, qPCR were performed on day nine liver biopsies. Similar to a previous report, the expression of nkg2d, one of the best characterised tumor-related NK receptor, was 6.9 fold higher in the allogeneic liver grafts compared to the syngeneic controls (p = 0.028, Fig. 5A) [21]. As NKG2D receptor is constitutively expressed on NK cells, this result could have been related to the higher number of NK cells in the allogeneic liver. However, the levels of expression of NKG2D in the blood NK cells (median MFI: 7694 vs. 4636, Fig. 5B, left) and monocytes (median MFI: 1180 vs. 666, Fig. 4B, right) were also higher in allogeneic recipients.

The implication of the NKG2D receptor in cytotoxicity was tested with the use of anti-NKG2D antibody. Sorted blood NK cells demonstrated higher cytotoxic levels in the allogeneic animals, and this effect was prevented by the addition of anti-NKG2D antibody (30.1 vs. 10.1, Fig. 5C). This inhibition was receptor-specific as no decrease could be observed with the use of anti-NKp30 antibody.

The expression of NKG2D ligands was further assessed by qPCR on day nine liver biopsies. In rat, three NKG2D ligands were described: Rae1l, Rrlt (retinoic acid early transcript family) and Irp94 (ischemia responsive 94 kDa protein, heat shock protein family) [21,22]. The rrlt gene expression was significantly increased in the allogeneic liver grafts compared to syngeneic liver grafts (2.93 fold increase, p = 0.028, Fig. 5D).

In an effort to determine how the increased NKG2D-mediated cytotoxicity contributed to HCC cell clearance, the expression of NKG2D ligands was also assessed on two rat HCC cell lines, JM-1 and McA. Rrlt was expressed in JM-1 cell line (21.4 fold increase compared to primary splenocytes), but not in McA cells. Rae1l was not expressed in HCC cells and irp94 was expressed at different levels in the two cell lines (JM-1: 2.63, McA: 3.68 fold increase, Fig. 5E). Finally the presence of NKG2D ligands at the surface of HCC cell lines was confirmed with the use of a chimeric recombinant NKG2D-Fc. Both JM-1 and McA expressed high levels of known and potentially still unknown NKG2D ligands (MFI, JM1: $3.53.10^4$ vs. $1.02.10^4$, McA: $9.4.10^4$ vs $1.83.10^4$, Fig. 5F).

Overall, NKG2D-ligands were expressed in all HCC cell lines supporting the idea that activated NKG2D-expressing NK cells and monocytes contribute to HCC cell clearance.

Discussion

This study provides novel insights to the question of the balanced immune activation after allogeneic liver transplantation in the presence of HCC, by demonstrating the presence of an alloimmune-dependent anti-cancer cytotoxic activity after rat liver transplantation. This cytotoxicity is linked to increased frequencies and levels of activation of NK cells and monocyte/macrophages, and is at least in part mediated through the NKG2D receptor.

The studied Dark Agouti-to-Lewis rat liver transplantation model induced a strong alloimmune activation specifically directed against donor antigens [23]. This immune profile was associated with an increased phenotype and level of activation of NK cells and monocytes/macrophages. This is in accordance with previous studies demonstrating the harmful impact of macrophages during a rat kidney allograft rejection and the protective effect of NK cell depletion after allogeneic rat liver transplantation [18,24].

The cross-talk between the allogeneic and anti-cancer immunities has been poorly studied so far, and the present data show an enhanced liver and peripheral (but not spleen) anti-cancer cytotoxicity at the time of liver graft rejection. In human organ transplantation, NK cells were present in endomyocardial cell infiltrates but these cells d, but o not appear as major players in liver graft rejection [25,26]. In fact, an increased alloreactivity of NK cells after liver transplantation has been reported and this activity was not correlated with rejection episodes [26]. However, human liver and secondary lymphoid tissue NK cells have shown strong levels of cytotoxicity after stimulation by IL-2 or in the presence of activated APCs [27,28].

While waiting for in vivo and/or clinical data, the present observation supports the use of milder levels of immunosuppression in patients transplanted for HCC, in order to preserve the anti-cancer cytotoxicity. Of note, many allogeneic rat-to-rat liver transplantation models induce no acute cell rejection, and the perfect model with syngeneic –recipient type- HCC cells and acute allogeneic immunity is currently missing (no Lewis HCC cell line available), thus preventing the in vivo validation of the presented data. Also, the described anti-cancer activity was observed after advanced rejection events, which are seldom seen clinically. However, we hypothesize that milder levels of rejection also promote cancer cell clearance.

Rather than decreasing immunosuppression as a whole, a careful drug selection may also be attempted to spare NK cells and monocyte/macrophages in view of a better HCC cell clearance. The use of depleting anti-lymphocyte antibody has been associated to an increased risk of post-transplant HCC recurrence [8]. Non-depleting anti-IL2-R antibodies may also have an effect, as they alter the phenotype and function of newly produced NK cells [29–31]. Sirolimus and mycophenolate mofetil have been shown to alter the NK cell phenotype and function in vitro, while cyclosporine does not appear to have an effect [32]. In vivo, all maintenance drugs have an impact on various immune cell subsets and the ideal immunosuppression combination remains to be defined in the setting of liver transplantation for HCC [33,34].

The NKG2D receptor/NKG2D ligands pathway appeared as a key player in the alloimmune-associated cytotoxicity. It was already published that NKG2D expression level is raised in liver allogeneic graft [21]. Here, we have demonstrated that the expression of NKG2D is specifically increased in peripheral NK cells and macrophages at the time of rejection, and the ex vivo cytotoxicity of liver NK cells is prevented by blocking the NKG2D receptor (but not the NKp30 receptor). In addition, NKG2D ligands could be found on rat HCC cells, confirming human data with the expression of UL16-binding protein (ULBP) 1, a human NKG2D ligand, on HCC tumors [10]. This pathway has been previously explored in other oncological settings such as colorectal carcinoma, and the level of tumor NKG2D ligand expression has been associated to HCC response and patient survival [10,35]. NKG2D expression on blood NK cells is increased after radiofrequency HCC ablation, and is linked to higher disease-free survival rates [36]. This rise in NKG2D expression is also observed after transarterial chemoembolization and is correlated with a decrease in NKG2D-ligand shedding (soluble MICA) [37]. NKG2D expression after liver transplantation might help in HCC cells clearance. Finally, NKG2D has been recently involved in the macrophage-NK cell cross-talk leading to higher levels of NK cell activation and anti-tumor cell cytotoxicity [38]. The observed increased expression of NKG2D on macrophages at the time of allogeneic liver graft rejection may contribute indirectly to cytotoxicity by promoting NK cell activation and cytotoxicity.

Beyond NKG2D, a wide panel of activating and inhibitory receptors is expressed on NK cells, which pattern of expression can modulate the level of activation of NK cells [39]. To illustrate, inhibitory receptors can recognize class I major histocompatibility complex, and inhibit NK cell cytotoxicity [40]. The receptor profile differs between organ-specific NK cells, as do their function [41], and changes in the balance between activating and inhibitory receptors could explain at least some of the herein described phenotypic and functional NK cell differences between sites in syngeneic and allogeneic recipients. Further exploration is deserved.

The present data demonstrate that the occurrence of a rat liver allograft rejection promotes anti-cancer cytotoxicity through the NKG2D receptor. While waiting for in vivo validation, the observed ex vivo cytotoxicity argue in favor of the use of milder and tailored immunosuppression protocols in patients undergoing liver transplantation for HCC.

Author Contributions

Conceived and designed the experiments: SL LRB PM GM CT. Performed the experiments: SL GO FS LAO CT. Analyzed the data: SL GO LRB CT. Contributed reagents/materials/analysis tools: SL GO FS LAO LRB PM GM CT. Wrote the paper: SL LAO CT.

References

1. Mazzaferro V, Regalia E, Doci R, Andreola S, Pulvirenti A, et al. (1996) Liver transplantation for the treatment of small hepatocellular carcinomas in patients with cirrhosis. N Engl J Med 334: 693–699. doi:10.1056/NEJM199603143341104.

2. Mazzaferro V, Llovet JM, Miceli R, Bhoori S, Schiavo M, et al. (2009) Predicting survival after liver transplantation in patients with hepatocellular carcinoma beyond the Milan criteria: a retrospective, exploratory analysis. Lancet Oncol 10: 35–43. doi:10.1016/S1470-2045(08)70284-5.

3. Sposito C, Mariani L, Germini A, Flores Reyes M, Bongini M, et al. (2013) Comparative efficacy of sorafenib vs. best supportive care in recurrent hepatocellular carcinoma after liver transplantation: A case-control study. J Hepatol 59: 59–66. doi:10.1016/j.jhep.2013.02.026.

4. Toso C, Mentha G, Majno P (2011) Liver transplantation for hepatocellular carcinoma: five steps to prevent recurrence. Am J Transplant 11: 2031–2035. doi:10.1111/j.1600-6143.2011.03689.x.

5. Vivarelli M, Cucchetti A, La Barba G, Ravaioli M, Del Gaudio M, et al. (2008) Liver transplantation for hepatocellular carcinoma under calcineurin inhibitors: reassessment of risk factors for tumor recurrence. Ann Surg 248: 857–862. doi:10.1097/SLA.0b013e3181896278.

6. Vivarelli M, Cucchetti A, Piscaglia F, La Barba G, Bolondi L, et al. (2005) Analysis of risk factors for tumor recurrence after liver transplantation for hepatocellular carcinoma: key role of immunosuppression. Liver Transpl 11: 497–503. doi:10.1002/lt.20391.

7. Cheng J-W, Shi Y-H, Fan J, Huang X-W, Qiu S-J, et al. (2011) An immune function assay predicts post-transplant recurrence in patients with hepatocellular carcinoma. J Cancer Res Clin Oncol 137: 1445–1453. doi:10.1007/s00432-011-1014-0.

8. Decaens T, Roudot-Thoraval F, Bresson-Hadni S, Meyer C, Gugenheim J, et al. (2006) Role of immunosuppression and tumor differentiation in predicting recurrence after liver transplantation for hepatocellular carcinoma: a multicenter study of 412 patients. World J Gastroenterol 12: 7319–7325.

9. Kuang D-M, Zhao Q, Peng C, Xu J, Zhang J-P, et al. (2009) Activated monocytes in peritumoral stroma of hepatocellular carcinoma foster immune privilege and disease progression through PD-L1. J Exp Med 206: 1327–1337. doi:10.1084/jem.20082173.

10. Kamimura H, Yamagiwa S, Tsuchiya A, Takamura M, Matsuda Y, et al. (2012) Reduced NKG2D ligand expression in hepatocellular carcinoma correlates with early recurrence. J Hepatol 56: 381–388. doi:10.1016/j.jhep.2011.06.017.

11. Ding T, Xu J, Wang F, Shi M, Zhang Y, et al. (2009) High tumor-infiltrating macrophage density predicts poor prognosis in patients with primary hepatocellular carcinoma after resection. Hum Pathol 40: 381–389. doi:10.1016/j.humpath.2008.08.011.

12. Motomura T, Shirabe K, Mano Y, Muto J, Toshima T, et al. (2013) Neutrophil-lymphocyte ratio reflects hepatocellular carcinoma recurrence after liver transplantation via inflammatory microenvironment. J Hepatol 58: 58–64. doi:10.1016/j.jhep.2012.08.017.

13. Oldani G, Lacotte S, Morel P, Mentha G, Toso C (2012) Orthotopic liver transplantation in rats. J Vis Exp. doi:10.3791/4143.

14. Novicki DL, Jirtle RL, Michalopoulos G (1983) Establishment of two rat hepatoma cell strains produced by a carcinogen initiation, phenobarbital promotion protocol. In Vitro 19: 191–202.

15. Banff schema for grading liver allograft rejection: an international consensus document (1997). Hepatology 25: 658–663. doi:10.1002/hep.510250328.

16. Zimmermann FA, Davies HS, Knoll PP, Gokel JM, Schmidt T (1984) Orthotopic liver allografts in the rat. The influence of strain combination on the fate of the graft. Transplantation 37: 406–410.

17. Pozo D, Valés-Gómez M, Mavaddat N, Williamson SC, Chisholm SE, et al. (2006) CD161 (human NKR-P1A) signaling in NK cells involves the activation of acid sphingomyelinase. J Immunol 176: 2397–2406.

18. Obara H, Nagasaki K, Hsieh CL, Ogura Y, Esquivel CO, et al. (2005) IFN-gamma, produced by NK cells that infiltrate liver allografts early after transplantation, links the innate and adaptive immune responses. Am J Transplant 5: 2094–2103. doi:10.1111/j.1600-6143.2005.00995.x.

19. Poggi A, Rubartelli A, Moretta L, Zocchi MR (1997) Expression and function of NKRP1A molecule on human monocytes and dendritic cells. Eur J Immunol 27: 2965–2970. doi:10.1002/eji.1830271132.

20. Ishiyama K, Rawson J, Omori K, Mullen Y (2011) Liver natural killer cells play a role in the destruction of islets after intraportal transplantation. Transplantation 91: 952–960. doi:10.1097/TP.0b013e3182139dc1.

21. Zhuo M, Fujiki M, Wang M, Piard-Ruster K, Wai L-E, et al. (2010) Identification of the rat NKG2D ligands, RAE1L and RRLT, and their role in allograft rejection. Eur J Immunol 40: 1748–1757. doi:10.1002/eji.200939779.

22. Srivastava RM, Varalakshmi C, Khar A (2008) The ischemia-responsive protein 94 (Irp94) activates dendritic cells through NK cell receptor protein-2/NK group 2 member D (NKR-P2/NKG2D) leading to their maturation. J Immunol 180: 1117–1130.

23. Hama N, Yanagisawa Y, Dono K, Kobayashi S, Marubashi S, et al. (2009) Gene expression profiling of acute cellular rejection in rat liver transplantation using DNA microarrays. Liver Transpl 15: 509–521. doi:10.1002/lt.21708.

24. Jose MD, Ikezumi Y, van Rooijen N, Atkins RC, Chadban SJ (2003) Macrophages act as effectors of tissue damage in acute renal allograft rejection. Transplantation 76: 1015–1022. doi:10.1097/01.TP.0000083507.67995.13.

25. Sorrentino C, Scarinci A, D'Antuono T, Piccirilli M, Di Nicola M, et al. (2006) Endomyocardial infiltration by B and NK cells foreshadows the recurrence of cardiac allograft rejection. J Pathol 209: 400–410. doi:10.1002/path.1980.

26. Oertel M, Kohlhaw K, Diepolder HM, Schröder S, Schwarz R, et al. (2001) Alloreactivity of natural killer cells in allogeneic liver transplantation. Transplantation 72: 116–122.

27. Ishiyama K, Ohdan H, Ohira M, Mitsuta H, Arihiro K, et al. (2006) Difference in cytotoxicity against hepatocellular carcinoma between liver and periphery natural killer cells in humans. Hepatology 43: 362–372. doi:10.1002/hep.21035.

28. Ferlazzo G, Pack M, Thomas D, Paludan C, Schmid D, et al. (2004) Distinct roles of IL-12 and IL-15 in human natural killer cell activation by dendritic cells from secondary lymphoid organs. Proc Natl Acad Sci USA 101: 16606–16611. doi:10.1073/pnas.0407522101.

29. Chanvillard C, Jacolik RF, Infante-Duarte C, Nayak RC (2013) The role of natural killer cells in multiple sclerosis and their therapeutic implications. Front Immunol 4: 63. doi:10.3389/fimmu.2013.00063.

30. Sageshima J, Ciancio G, Guerra G, Gaynor JJ, Cova D, et al. (2011) Prolonged lymphocyte depletion by single-dose rabbit anti-thymocyte globulin and alemtuzumab in kidney transplantation. Transplant Immunology 25: 104–111. doi:10.1016/j.trim.2011.07.002.

31. Toso C, Edgar R, Pawlick R, Emamaullee J, Merani S, et al. (2009) Effect of different induction strategies on effector, regulatory and memory lymphocyte sub-populations in clinical islet transplantation. Transpl Int 22: 182–191. doi:10.1111/j.1432-2277.2008.00746.x.

32. Eissens DN, Van Der Meer A, Van Cranenbroek B, Preijers FWMB, Joosten I (2010) Rapamycin and MPA, But Not CsA, Impair Human NK Cell Cytotoxicity Due to Differential Effects on NK Cell Phenotype. American Journal of Transplantation 10: 1981–1990. doi:10.1111/j.1600-6143.2010.03242.x.

33. Chen G, Chen H, Wang C, Peng Y, Sun L, et al. (2012) Rapamycin ameliorates kidney fibrosis by inhibiting the activation of mTOR signaling in interstitial macrophages and myofibroblasts. PLoS ONE 7: e33626. doi:10.1371/journal.-pone.0033626.

34. Werner JM, Lang C, Scherer MN, Farkas SA, Geissler EK, et al. (2011) Distribution of intrahepatic T, NK and CD3(+)CD56(+)NKT cells alters after liver transplantation: Shift from innate to adaptive immunity? Transpl Immunol 25: 27–33. doi:10.1016/j.trim.2011.05.006.

35. McGilvray RW, Eagle RA, Watson NFS, Al-Attar A, Ball G, et al. (2009) NKG2D ligand expression in human colorectal cancer reveals associations with prognosis and evidence for immunoediting. Clin Cancer Res 15: 6993–7002. doi:10.1158/1078-0432.CCR-09-0991.

36. Zerbini A, Pilli M, Laccabue D, Pelosi G, Molinari A, et al. (2010) Radiofrequency thermal ablation for hepatocellular carcinoma stimulates autologous NK-cell response. Gastroenterology 138: 1931–1942. doi:10.1053/j.gastro.2009.12.051.

37. Kohga K, Takehara T, Tatsumi T, Ohkawa K, Miyagi T, et al. (2008) Serum levels of soluble major histocompatibility complex (MHC) class I-related chain A in patients with chronic liver diseases and changes during transcatheter arterial embolization for hepatocellular carcinoma. Cancer Sci 99: 1643–1649. doi:10.1111/j.1349-7006.2008.00859.x.

38. Zhou Z, Zhang C, Zhang J, Tian Z (2012) Macrophages help NK cells to attack tumor cells by stimulatory NKG2D ligand but protect themselves from NK killing by inhibitory ligand Qa-1. PLoS ONE 7: e36928. doi:10.1371/journal.pone.0036928.

39. Kveberg L, Jiménez-Royo P, Naper C, Rolstad B, Butcher GW, et al. (2010) Two complementary rat NK cell subsets, Ly49s3+ and NKR-P1B+, differ in phenotypic characteristics and responsiveness to cytokines. J Leukoc Biol 88: 87–93. doi:10.1189/jlb.0110039.

40. Rolstad B, Vaage JT, Naper C, Lambracht D, Wonigeit K, et al. (1997) Positive and negative MHC class I recognition by rat NK cells. Immunol Rev 155: 91–104.

41. Sharma R, Das A (2014) Organ-specific phenotypic and functional features of NK cells in humans. Immunol Res 58: 125–131. doi:10.1007/s12026-013-8477-9.

21

Genetic Polymorphism of Interferon Regulatory Factor 5 (IRF5) Correlates with Allograft Acute Rejection of Liver Transplantation

Xiaobo Yu[1], Bajin Wei[2], Yifan Dai[1], Min Zhang[2], Jian Wu[2], Xiao Xu[2], Guoping Jiang[2], Shusen Zheng[2], Lin Zhou[1]*

1 Key Lab of Combined Multi-Organ Transplantation, Ministry of Public Health, the First Affiliated Hospital, School of Medicine, Zhejiang University, Hangzhou, Zhejiang, China, **2** Division of Hepatobiliary and Pancreatic Surgery, Department of Surgery, the First Affiliated Hospital, School of Medicine, Zhejiang University, Hangzhou, Zhejiang, China

Abstract

Background: Although liver transplantation is one of the most efficient curative therapies of end stage liver diseases, recipients may suffer liver graft loss opst-operation. IRF-5, a member of Interferon Regulatory Factors, functions as a key regulator in TLR4 cascade, and is capable of inducing inflammatory cytokines. Although TLR4 has been proved to contribute to acute allograft rejection, including after liver transplantation, the correlation between IRF5 gene and acute rejection has not been elucidated yet.

Methods: The study enrolled a total of 289 recipients, including 39 females and 250 males, and 39 recipients developed acute allograft rejection within 6 months post-transplantation. The allograft rejections were diagnosed by liver biopsies. Genome DNA of recipients was extracted from pre-operative peripheral blood. Genotyping of IRF-5, including rs3757385, rs752637 and rs11761199, was performed, followed by SNP frequency and Hardy-Weinberg equilibrium analysis.

Results: The genetic polymorphism of rs3757385 was found associated with acute rejection. G/G homozygous individuals were at higher risk of acute rejection, with a P value of 0.042 (OR = 2.34 (1.07–5.10)).

Conclusions: IRF5, which transcriptionally activates inflammatory cytokines, is genetically associated with acute rejection and might function as a risk factor for acute rejection of liver transplantations.

Editor: Song Guo Zheng, Penn State University, United States of America

Funding: This study was supported by grants from Zhejiang Provincial Natural Science Foundation for Young Scholars, Grant number: LQ12H03003; Zhejiang Provincial Education Department Research Foundation, Grant number: Y201120248; National Basic Research Program of China (973 Program), Grant number: 2009CB522400; National S&T Major project, Grant number: 2012ZX10002017 and 2013ZX10002011-006. The funders had no role in study design, data collection and analysis, decision to publish, or preparation of the manuscript.

Competing Interests: The authors have declared that no competing interests exist.

* E-mail: zhoulin99@zju.edu.cn

Introduction

Liver transplantation has been accepted worldwide as an efficient way of treating end stage liver diseases and acute liver failure. Immune system elicits complex and aggressive reaction post-transplantation, which even destroys the graft [1,2]. Although the total incidence of allograft rejection decreases dramatically due to immunosuppressive therapies [3], acute rejection episodes still occur among 15–45% recipients within several months, which leads to higher incidence of chronic organ dysfunction and suboptimal long-term outcomes [3].

For years, acute rejection was considered as response of adaptive immune system. However, it is gradually accepted that, by responding to the released danger signal, innate immune reaction also functions as a pivotal trigger in acute rejection [4]. Toll-like Receptors (TLR), which recognize pathogen-associated molecular patterns (PAMP) on microorganisms in innate immune response, are now proved to initiate inflammation by recognizing

molecules released from damaged cells during organ transplantation [5,6], and prevent graft tolerance in dependence of type I IFNs [7]. Nevertheless, TLRs pathway can also induce immunosuppression [8,9], and we also confirmed the contribution of TLR4 to liver graft rejection [10]. Therefore, regardless of enhanced alloimmune response or immunosuppression, the elucidation of TLR signal pathway in acute rejection, especially TLR4, is urgently needed.

Interferon Regulatory Factors (IRFs), including nine family members, play important roles in TLRs signal cascade [11,12]. Each contains a DNA-binding domain recognizing IFN-Stimulated Response Element (ISRE), which locates upstream of interferon genes [13]. Thus IRFs could involve in regulating the innate immune reaction and immune cell development through transcriptional activation of type I IFNs and other proinflammatory cytokines [14–16]. Studies on gene expression profiling in acute rejection also indicated the association between acute allograft rejection and IRFs, such as IRF9, IRF3 and IRF5 [17–19].

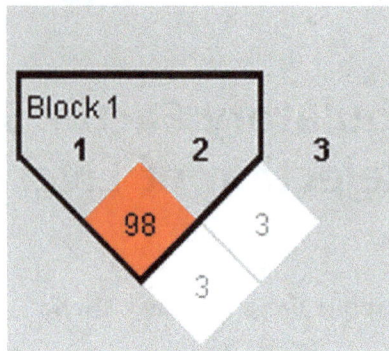

Figure 1. The linkage disequilibrium among 3 SNPs. 1 to 3 represented rs3757385, rs752637 and rs11761199 respectively, and rs3757385 and rs752637 formed a haplotype block by LD analysis.

As a key regulator of TLR4 cascade in innate immune responses, IRF5 can activate the transcription of type I IFNs when it forms homodimers or heterodimers with IRF3, or suppress them via interacting with IRF7 [14,20]. Moreover, IRF5 is also responsible for the production of inflammatory cytokines, such as IL-6 and TNF-α [20,21]. Several studies also associated IRF5 with higher risk of systemic lupus erythematosus (SLE) [22,23], while some other SNPs of IRF5 are proved responsible for a lower risk of its development [24,25]. Researchers further found IRF5 to be critical for IFN-α secretion by dendritic cells in SLE patients [26]. Other genetic studies confirmed its association with rheumatoid arthritis (RA) in different populations [27–29].

Although there has been no direct evidence for the involvement of IRF5 in acute allograft rejection, the fact that IRF5 transcriptionally activates IFNs and other pro-inflammatory genes

in cell apoptosis and T cell activation, and functions as a key factor of TLR4 cascade [26,30], suggests that it is reasonable to perform association studies on acute rejection. Thus understanding of how IRFs participate will help us with the development of treatment of acute rejection. Meanwhile, genetic association studies provide correlation between disease status and genetic variation, such as SNPs and haplotypes that contribute to the disease, and therefore could facilitate identification of new biomarkers for risk prediction and prognosis.

Three SNPs of IRF5 gene were involved in this study, including rs3757385, rs752637 and rs11761199, and among them rs3757385 and/or rs752637 had been found to be associated with SLE and RA [29,31]. Our new findings suggested that rs3757385 might be a genetic marker for acute rejection prognosis, and the biological function of IRF5 as well as other IRFs in acute allograft rejection will be worth studying.

Methods

Population

A total of 289 recipients who received their liver grafts during 2006 to 2011, including 250 males and 39 females, were enrolled in this association study. Those diagnosed with drug-induced hepatitis, autoimmune hepatitis and sclerosing cholangitis were excluded. Moreover, we excluded patients that underwent a second or subsequent liver transplantation or multiple organ transplantation. Data of age, gender and primary diagnoses were collected for population study. All the recipients followed a unique triple combination of immunosuppressive regimen, including tacrolimus, corticosteroid and mycophenolate mofetil. In brief, the minimum level of tacrolimus blood concentration was maintained at 10–12 ng/ml for the first month after transplant, 8–10 ng/ml later in the first year, and 5–8 ng/ml thereafter. Mycophenolate mofetil was administered 1–2 g per day. Cortico-

Table 1. Characteristics and primary diagnosis of 289 liver transplantation recipients assigned to a non-rejection or acute rejection group.

	Non-rejection	Acute Rejection	P value
Age (year)	13–71	31–71	NA
Sex			0.6234
Male	215 (86.0%)	35 (89.7%)	
Female	35 (14.0%)	4 (10.3%)	
MELD Score			0.1945
<10	41 (16.4%)	11 (28.2%)	
10–19	94 (37.6%)	11 (28.2%)	
20–29	77 (30.8%)	9 (23.1%)	
>29	38 (15.2%)	8 (20.5%)	
Primary diagnosis			
HBV infection	148 (59.2%)	30 (76.9%)	0.0351
	102 (40.8%)	9 (23.1%)	
HCC	99 (39.6%)	15 (38.5%)	1.000
	151 (60.4%)	24 (61.5%)	
Fulminant hepatitis	49 (19.6%)	8 (20.5%)	0.8320
	201 (80.4%)	31 (79.5%)	
Decompensated liver cirrhosis	142 (56.8%)	20 (51.3%)	0.6035
	108 (43.2%)	19 (48.7%)	

MELD, model for end-stage liver disease; HCC, hepatocellular carcinoma; NA, not applicable.

Table 2. Association of genetic polymorphism of IRF5 with acute rejection.

SNPs of IRF5	Genetic Model	Non-rejection	Acute Rejection	OR (95% CI)	P value
rs3757385					
T/T	Cod	105 (42.0%)	11 (28.2%)	1.00	0.078
G/T		109 (43.6%)	17 (43.6%)	1.49 (0.67–3.33)	
G/G		36 (14.4%)	11 (28.2%)	2.92 (1.17–7.30)	
T/T	Do	105 (42.0%)	11 (28.2%)	1.00	0.096
G/T+G/G		145 (58.0%)	28 (71.8%)	1.84 (0.88–3.87)	
T/T+G/T	Re	214 (85.6%)	28 (71.8%)	1.00	0.042
G/G		36 (14.4%)	11 (28.2%)	2.34 (1.07–5.10)	
T/T+G/G	Ovd	141 (56.4%)	22 (56.4%)	1.00	1.00
G/T		109 (43.6%)	17 (43.6%)	1.00 (0.51–1.97)	
rs752637					
T/I	Cod	105 (42.0%)	12 (30.8%)	1.00	0.14
C/T		111 (44.4%)	17 (43.6%)	1.34 (0.61–2.94)	
C/C		34 (13.6%)	10 (25.6%)	2.57 (1.02–6.48)	
T/T	Do	105 (42.0%)	12 (30.8%)	1.00	0.18
C/T+C/C		145 (58.0%)	27 (69.2%)	1.63 (0.79–3.36)	
T/T+C/T	Re	216 (86.4%)	29 (74.4%)	1.00	0.067
C/C		34 (13.6%)	10 (25.6%)	2.19 (0.98–4.90)	
T/T+C/C	Ovd	139 (55.6%)	22 (56.4%)	1.00	0.92
C/T		111 (44.4%)	13 (43.6%)	0.97 (0.49–1.91)	
rs11761199					
A/A	Cod	105 (42.0%)	11 (28.2%)	1.00	0.25
A/G		111 (44.4%)	21 (53.9%)	1.81 (0.83–3.93)	
G/G		34 (13.6%)	7 (17.9%)	1.97 (0.71–5.47)	
A/A	Do	105 (42.0%)	11 (28.2%)	1.00	0.096
A/G+G/G		145 (58.0%)	28 (71.8%)	1.84 (0.88–3.87)	
A/A+A/G	Re	216 (86.4%)	32 (82.1%)	1.00	0.48
G/G		34 (13.6%)	7 (17.9%)	1.39 (0.59–3.40)	
A/A+G/G	Ovd	139 (55.6%)	18 (46.1%)	1.00	0.27
A/G		111 (44.4%)	21 (53.9%)	1.46 (0.74–2.34)	

OR, odds ratio; CI, confidence intervals.
Cod, codominant; Do, dominant; Re, recessive; Ovd, overdominant.

steroid treatment was initiated with 1000 mg prednisolone once during the operation, continued with administration of gradually reduced meth-prednisolone starting at 240 mg on day 1 and ending up at 2.5 mg before discontinuation after 2 months [32]. Among the recipients, 39 finally developed acute rejection.

Definition of acute rejection

The diagnoses of acute rejection were confirmed by liver biopsy and graded by Banff schema. Rejection occurred within 6 months was considered as acute rejection [33,34].

Ethics statement

Written informed consents were obtained, and for children, they were obtained from the next of kin. The research procedure was

Table 3. Association of IRF5 Haplotype with acute rejection.

SNPs combination	Non-rejection	Acute Rejection	OR (95% CI)	P value
rs3757385 + rs752637				
T-T	308 (61.6%)	48 (61.5%)	1.00	1.00
G-C	185 (37.0%)	28 (35.9%)	0.97 (0.59–1.60)	

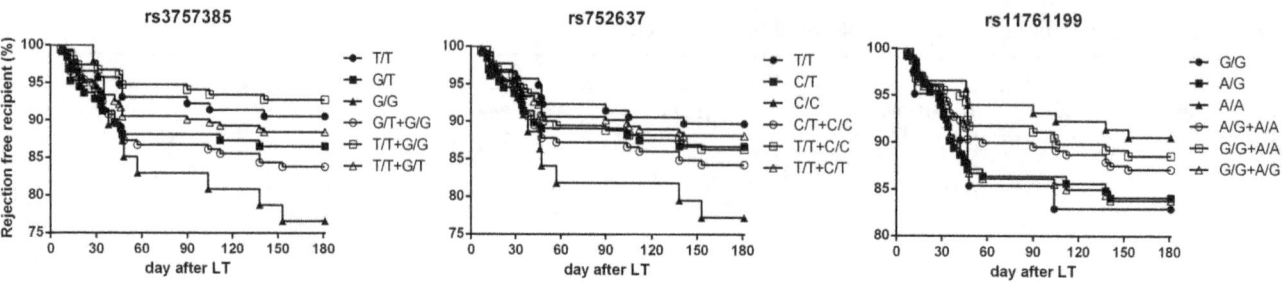

Figure 2. Acute rejection comparisons among SNP groups.

approved and supervised by the Ethical Review Committee of the First Affiliated Hospital, School of Medicine, Zhejiang University, and we followed the World Medical Association's Declaration of Helsinki.

DNA extraction and genotyping

Peripheral blood genomic DNA was extracted for genotyping. Based on the data of Hapmap (http://www.hapmap.org), we selected candidate SNPs of IRF5 in accordance with the rule that minor allele frequency and r^2 should be no less than 20% and 0.8. The genotyping was performed by SNaPshot (Applied Biosystems, CA), followed by data collection and generation from ABI3130xl Genetic Analyzer (Applied Biosystems, CA) and GeneMapper 4.0 (Applied Biosystems, CA), respectively.

Association analysis

Genetic association between SNPs or haplotypes and acute rejection was analyzed by SNPStats (http://bioinfo.iconcologia. net/snpstats) or Haploview (http://www.broad.mit.edu/mpg/haploview).

IRF5 mRNA expression assay

Total RNA was extracted from peripheral blood mononuclear cells of recipients within 6 months post-transplant, and cDNA was synthesized by reverse transcription kit (Bio-Rad, CA). The expression of IRF5 was detected on ABI 7500 Fast Real-Time PCR System (Applied Biosystems, CA) using iTaq Universal SYBR Green Supermix real-time PCR kit (Bio-Rad, CA). The primer pairs of IRF5 and GAPDH for real-time PCR detection were listed as following; IRF5, forward 5'- GACATCCCCAGT-GACAAGCA -3', reverse 5'- AGAACACCTTGCACTGA-CACA -3', and GAPDH, forward 5'-ATGGGGAAGGT-GAAGGTCG-3', reverse 5'-GGGGTCATTGATGGCA-ACAATA-3'. The real-time PCR procedure included a cDNA denaturation at 95°C for 20 sec, and then 40 cycles of amplification with 10 sec at 95°C and 30 sec at 58°C, following with a melt-curve analysis. The relative expression of IRF5 mRNA was calculated by $\Delta\Delta$CT method.

Statistic analysis

For clinical relevance of primary diagnoses and acute rejection, Fisher's exact test was performed with Graphpad Prism 6.0 (Graphpad Software, CA). For survival analysis, cumulative graft rejection rate was estimated using the Kaplan-Meier method. The relationship between risk of acute rejection and genotypes was examined using the log-rank test with Graphpad Prism. For analysis of IRF5 mRNA expression, unpaired t-test or one-way ANOVA test was used for comparison of two groups or more than

Table 4. Comparison of survival curves among SNP groups.

SNPs of IRF5	P value	HR (95% CI)
rs3757385		
T/T vs. G/T vs. G/G	0.075	NA
T/T vs. G/T + G/G	0.102	0.56 (0.31–1.11)
G/T vs. T/T + G/G	0.079	1.95 (0.93–4.12)
G/G vs. T/T + G/T	0.038	2.06 (1.05–5.82)
rs752637		
T/T vs. C/T vs. C/C	0.13	NA
T/T vs. C/T + C/C	0.18	0.63 (0.34–1.22)
C/T vs. T/T + C/C	0.97	0.99 (0.53–1.86)
C/C vs. T/T + C/T	0.057	1.98 (0.98–5.72)
rs11761199		
G/G vs. A/G vs. A/A	0.25	NA
G/G vs. A/A + A/G	0.46	1.36 (0.57–3.48)
A/G vs. A/A + G/G	0.26	1.43 (0.77–2.70)
A/A vs. A/G + G/G	0.098	0.56 (0.31–1.10)

HR, hazard ratio.

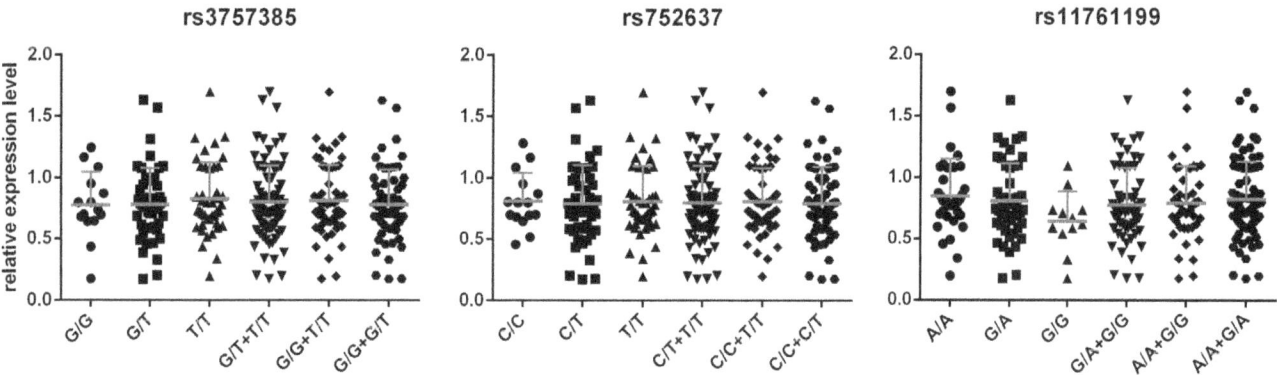

Figure 3. mRNA expression level of IRF5 in PBMC. We performed real-time qPCR to detect the mRNA expression of IRF5 in the PBMC of a total of 104 recipients, of whom the rejection had not been observed within 6 months post-operation.

two groups with Graphpad Prism. A two-tailed P value less than 0.05 was considered statistically significant.

Results

A cohort of 289 recipients was enrolled in the association study. We first analyzed the clinical data from individuals, and no statistical significance was found among age, gender, Model For End-Stage Liver Disease (MELD) score and most of the primary diagnoses, except Hepatitis B Virus (HBV) infection (Table 1). We found HBV infection to be one of the risk factors for acute liver graft rejection, and recipients with HBV infection were at higher risk of rejection. Moreover, our genetic association analysis indicated that the incidence of acute rejection in G/G homozygtes of rs3757385 was relatively higher (Table 2). Linkage disequilibrium analysis showed that haplotypes could be formed by rs3757385 and rs752637 (Figure 1), yet no association was found between haplotype groups and acute rejection (Table 3).

Survival analysis was performed to investigate how genotypes of IRF5 influence the probability of acute rejection. In consistent with the higher risk of rs3757385 G/G homozygous recipients in acute rejection, log-rank test also indicated a predictive value of rs3757385 for rejection, instead of rs752637 and rs11761199 (Figure 2 and Table 4).

Since rs3757385 locates in the promoter region, we assumed that it might cause changes of IRF5 expression level. Meanwhile, IRF5 transcripts could be detected in peripheral blood mononuclear cells (PBMC) [35], which suggest a possibility to evaluate rejection by monitoring IRF5 mRNA in PBMC. Thus we compared IRF5 mRNA expression in PBMC among the different genotype groups of rs3757385, rs752637 and rs11761199 respectively. However, results from real-time PCR exhibited no significant difference among the 3 genotype groups (Figure 3).

Discussion

Although little direct evidence has depicted the involvement of IRF5 in acute rejection, its capability of transcriptionally activating IFNs and pro-inflammatory genes through TLR4 cascade implies potential roles. Moreover, it is genetically associated with autoimmune diseases, such as SLE and RA. Thus genetic polymorphism of IRF5 might function as a marker for risk prediction and prognosis of graft rejection. The rs3757385 SNP, locating in promoter region, participates in regulating IRF5 mRNA expression in atherosclerotic lesions [36], and affects genetic susceptibility to autoimmune diseases [29]. In this article

we proved genetic polymorphism of rs3757385 to be a risk factor for acute rejection for the first time.

Since there have been reports indicating that IRF5 mRNA expression is associated with autoimmune diseases [17,37], in consideration of the detectability of IRF5 mRNA in PBMC [35] and genetic susceptibility of rs3757385 in acute rejection, acute rejection might be predicted by monitoring IRF5 expression. However, in this cohort, IRF5 mRNA expression level was inconsistent with rs3757385 genetic polymorphism, which could be explained from several aspects. IRF5 pre-mRNA generates alternatively spliced transcripts, but little evidence is available on how these transcripts function in physiological regulation. Thus in this study, we used the consensus sequence of IRF5 CDS for real-time analysis of the indistinguishable expression of each isoform, which suggests isoforms specific to acute rejection still need to be identified. The insignificant difference of IRFs expression may also be due to a cell-specific regulation of IRF5 mRNA by rs3757385 in immune cell subpopulations.

According to different cohort studies, MHC mismatch, T cell activity and immunosuppressive regimen, as well as age, gender, pre-LT disease, viral infection and ischemia time were involved in the outcome of graft survival. Based on our study, HBV infection could be a risk factor for acute rejection, while other studies indicated that it would decrease the incidence of acute rejection after liver transplant [38–40]. Therefore, if these inconsistent observations were not due to sampling bias, it might be due to the ways of preventing HBV reinfection that led to such difference. According to some studies [41–43], HBIG administration could benefit the recipients with better immunosuppression, and reduce acute rejection by inhibiting dendritic cells as well as provoking CD4+FoxP3+ T cells. We have developed a substitution therapy combining lamivudine (LAM) and low-dose intramuscular hepatitis B immunoglobulin (HBIG) [44], while many centers adopt a long-term regimen of high-dose administration of HBIG [40]. However, to confirm the survival benefit of HBIG for preventing postoperative HBV reinfection, further examinations and studies will be needed [45].

Genotyping of functional genes has led to improved efficacy of cancer therapy, either providing a targeted course of treatment based on their molecular designation, or avoiding harmful side effects by optimal dosing of drugs [46]. Complex diseases such as autoimmune diseases and transplantation rejections, are caused by the combination of genetic, environmental and some other factors, of which most have not been identified. The elucidation of mechanisms by which they predisposed individuals to graft rejection facilitates the application of genetic polymorphism in the development of new prognosis methods. Scientists can focus on relatively small numbers of genes which are involved in cell differentiation, proliferation and migration, and cytokine signaling, and explore their utility in personalized medicine. In the foreseeable future, personalized medicine associated with genetic information would become embedded in medical units.

In conclusion, for the first time we found the genetic association between IRF5 and liver graft acute rejection. HBV infection of recipients might influence the outcome of liver graft survival, and further studies need to be performed.

Author Contributions

Conceived and designed the experiments: XX GJ SZ LZ. Performed the experiments: XY BW. Analyzed the data: YD. Wrote the paper: XY LZ. Collected the clinical data: BW MZ JW.

References

1. Alex Bishop G, Bertolino PD, Bowen DG, McCaughan GW (2012) Tolerance in liver transplantation. Best Pract Res Clin Gastroenterol 26: 73–84.
2. Rook M, Rand E (2011) Predictors of long-term outcome after liver transplant. Curr Opin Organ Transplant 16: 499–504.
3. Ingulli E (2010) Mechanism of cellular rejection in transplantation. Pediatr Nephrol 25: 61–74.
4. Ponticelli C (2012) The mechanisms of acute transplant rejection revisited. J Nephrol 25: 150–158.
5. Alegre ML, Chong A (2009) Toll-like receptors (TLRs) in transplantation. Front Biosci (Elite Ed) 1: 36–43.
6. Leventhal JS, Schroppel B (2012) Toll-like receptors in transplantation: sensing and reacting to injury. Kidney Int 81: 826–832.
7. Fan H, Cook JA (2004) Molecular mechanisms of endotoxin tolerance. J Endotoxin Res 10: 71–84.
8. Netea MG, Sutmuller R, Hermann C, Van der Graaf CA, Van der Meer JW, et al. (2004) Toll-like receptor 2 suppresses immunity against Candida albicans through induction of IL-10 and regulatory T cells. J Immunol 172: 3712–3718.
9. Peng G, Guo Z, Kiniwa Y, Voo KS, Peng W, et al. (2005) Toll-like receptor 8-mediated reversal of CD4+ regulatory T cell function. Science 309: 1380–1384.
10. Deng JF, Geng L, Qian YG, Li H, Wang Y, et al. (2007) The role of toll-like receptors 2 and 4 in acute allograft rejection after liver transplantation. Transplant Proc 39: 3222–3224.
11. Brown J, Wang H, Hajishengallis GN, Martin M (2011) TLR-signaling networks: an integration of adaptor molecules, kinases, and cross-talk. J Dent Res 90: 417–427.
12. Newton K, Dixit VM (2012) Signaling in innate immunity and inflammation. Cold Spring Harb Perspect Biol 4.
13. Chen W, Royer WE Jr (2010) Structural insights into interferon regulatory factor activation. Cell Signal 22: 883–887.
14. Barnes BJ, Field AE, Pitha-Rowe PM (2003) Virus-induced heterodimer formation between IRF-5 and IRF-7 modulates assembly of the IFNA enhanceosome in vivo and transcriptional activity of IFNA genes. J Biol Chem 278: 16630–16641.
15. Barnes BJ, Richards J, Mancl M, Hanash S, Beretta L, et al. (2004) Global and distinct targets of IRF-5 and IRF-7 during innate response to viral infection. J Biol Chem 279: 45194–45207.
16. Takaoka A, Yanai H, Kondo S, Duncan G, Negishi H, et al. (2005) Integral role of IRF-5 in the gene induction programme activated by Toll-like receptors. Nature 434: 243–249.
17. Morgun A, Shulzhenko N, Perez-Diez A, Diniz RV, Sanson GF, et al. (2006) Molecular profiling improves diagnoses of rejection and infection in transplanted organs. Circ Res 98: e74–83.
18. Spivey TL, Uccellini L, Ascierto ML, Zoppoli G, De Giorgi V, et al. (2011) Gene expression profiling in acute allograft rejection: challenging the immunologic constant of rejection hypothesis. J Transl Med 9: 174.
19. Tannapfel A, Geissler F, Witzigmann H, Hauss J, Wittekind C (2001) Analysis of liver allograft rejection related genes using cDNA-microarrays in liver allograft specimen. Transplant Proc 33: 3283–3284.
20. Honda K, Yanai H, Negishi H, Asagiri M, Sato M, et al. (2005) IRF-7 is the master regulator of type-I interferon-dependent immune responses. Nature 434: 772–777.
21. Barnes BJ, Moore PA, Pitha PM (2001) Virus-specific activation of a novel interferon regulatory factor, IRF-5, results in the induction of distinct interferon alpha genes. J Biol Chem 276: 23382–23390.
22. Cunninghame Graham DS, Manku H, Wagner S, Reid J, Timms K, et al. (2007) Association of IRF5 in UK SLE families identifies a variant involved in polyadenylation. Hum Mol Genet 16: 579–591.
23. Kawasaki A, Kyogoku C, Ohashi J, Miyashita R, Hikami K, et al. (2008) Association of IRF5 polymorphisms with systemic lupus erythematosus in a Japanese population: support for a crucial role of intron 1 polymorphisms. Arthritis Rheum 58: 826–834.
24. Ferreiro-Neira I, Calaza M, Alonso-Perez E, Marchini M, Scorza R, et al. (2007) Opposed independent effects and epistasis in the complex association of IRF5 to SLE. Genes Immun 8: 429–438.
25. Graham RR, Kyogoku C, Sigurdsson S, Vlasova IA, Davies LR, et al. (2007) Three functional variants of IFN regulatory factor 5 (IRF5) define risk and protective haplotypes for human lupus. Proc Natl Acad Sci U S A 104: 6758–6763.
26. Yasuda K, Richez C, Maciaszek JW, Agrawal N, Akira S, et al. (2007) Murine dendritic cell type I IFN production induced by human IgG-RNA immune complexes is IFN regulatory factor (IRF)5 and IRF7 dependent and is required for IL-6 production. J Immunol 178: 6876–6885.
27. Dieguez-Gonzalez R, Calaza M, Perez-Pampin E, de la Serna AR, Fernandez-Gutierrez B, et al. (2008) Association of interferon regulatory factor 5 haplotypes, similar to that found in systemic lupus erythematosus, in a large subgroup of patients with rheumatoid arthritis. Arthritis Rheum 58: 1264–1274.
28. Shimane K, Kochi Y, Yamada R, Okada Y, Suzuki A, et al. (2009) A single nucleotide polymorphism in the IRF5 promoter region is associated with susceptibility to rheumatoid arthritis in the Japanese population. Ann Rheum Dis 68: 377–383.
29. Sigurdsson S, Padyukov L, Kurreeman FA, Liljedahl U, Wiman AC, et al. (2007) Association of a haplotype in the promoter region of the interferon regulatory factor 5 gene with rheumatoid arthritis. Arthritis Rheum 56: 2202–2210.
30. Tailor P, Tamura T, Ozato K (2006) IRF family proteins and type I interferon induction in dendritic cells. Cell Res 16: 134–140.
31. Couzinet A, Tamura K, Chen HM, Nishimura K, Wang Z, et al. (2008) A cell-type-specific requirement for IFN regulatory factor 5 (IRF5) in Fas-induced apoptosis. Proc Natl Acad Sci U S A 105: 2556–2561.
32. Yu X, Xie H, Wei B, Zhang M, Wang W, et al. (2011) Association of MDR1 gene SNPs and haplotypes with the tacrolimus dose requirements in Han Chinese liver transplant recipients. PLoS One 6: e25933.
33. Adeyi O, Fischer SE, Guindi M (2010) Liver allograft pathology: approach to interpretation of needle biopsies with clinicopathological correlation. J Clin Pathol 63: 47–74.
34. Yao J, Feng XW, Yu XB, Xie HY, Zhu LX, et al. (2013) Recipient IL-6-572C/G genotype is associated with reduced incidence of acute rejection following liver transplantation. J Int Med Res.
35. Mancl ME, Hu G, Sangster-Guity N, Olshalsky SL, Hoops K, et al. (2005) Two discrete promoters regulate the alternatively spliced human interferon regulatory factor-5 isoforms. Multiple isoforms with distinct cell type-specific expression, localization, regulation, and function. J Biol Chem 280: 21078–21090.
36. Malarstig A, Sigurdsson S, Eriksson P, Paulsson-Berne G, Hedin U, et al. (2008) Variants of the interferon regulatory factor 5 gene regulate expression of IRF5 mRNA in atherosclerotic tissue but are not associated with myocardial infarction. Arterioscler Thromb Vasc Biol 28: 975–982.
37. Feng D, Stone RC, Eloranta ML, Sangster-Guity N, Nordmark G, et al. (2010) Genetic variants and disease-associated factors contribute to enhanced interferon regulatory factor 5 expression in blood cells of patients with systemic lupus erythematosus. Arthritis Rheum 62: 562–573.
38. Crespo G, Marino Z, Navasa M, Forns X (2012) Viral hepatitis in liver transplantation. Gastroenterology 142: 1373–1383 e1371.
39. Neuberger J (1999) Incidence, timing, and risk factors for acute and chronic rejection. Liver Transpl Surg 5: S30–36.
40. Samuel D, Kimmoun E (2003) Immunosuppression in hepatitis B virus and hepatitis C virus transplants: special considerations. Clin Liver Dis 7: 667–681.
41. Bucuvalas JC, Anand R, Studies of Pediatric Liver Transplantation Research G (2009) Treatment with immunoglobulin improves outcome for pediatric liver transplant recipients. Liver Transpl 15: 1564–1569.
42. Kwekkeboom J, Tha-In T, Tra WM, Hop W, Boor PP, et al. (2005) Hepatitis B immunoglobulins inhibit dendritic cells and T cells and protect against acute rejection after liver transplantation. Am J Transplant 5: 2393–2402.
43. Tha-In T, Metselaar HJ, Bushell AR, Kwekkeboom J, Wood KJ (2010) Intravenous immunoglobulins promote skin allograft acceptance by triggering functional activation of CD4+Foxp3+ T cells. Transplantation 89: 1446–1455.
44. Zheng S, Chen Y, Liang T, Lu A, Wang W, et al. (2006) Prevention of hepatitis B recurrence after liver transplantation using lamivudine or lamivudine combined with hepatitis B Immunoglobulin prophylaxis. Liver Transpl 12: 253–258.
45. Ni YH, Chang MH (2006) The ways paved for prophylaxis against de novo hepatitis B virus infection after liver transplantation: still many stones left unturned. Pediatr Transplant 10: 405–407.
46. PMC (2012) The case of personalized medicine. 3rd ed.

22

Prevention of Allogeneic Cardiac Graft Rejection by Transfer of *Ex Vivo* Expanded Antigen-Specific Regulatory T-Cells

Fumika Takasato[1,2,5], **Rimpei Morita**[1,5], **Takashi Schichita**[1,5], **Takashi Sekiya**[1,5], **Yasuhide Morikawa**[3], **Tatsuo Kuroda**[2], **Masanori Niimi**[4], **Akihiko Yoshimura**[1,5]*

1 Department of Microbiology and Immunology, Keio University School of Medicine, Tokyo, Japan, 2 Department of Pediatric Surgery, Keio University School of Medicine, Tokyo, Japan, 3 Department of Pediatric Surgery, International University Medical Welfare Hospital, Nasushiobara, Tochigi, Japan, 4 Department of Surgery, Teikyo University School of Medicine, Tokyo, Japan, 5 Japan Science and Technology Agency, CREST, Tokyo, Japan

Abstract

The rate of graft survival has dramatically increased using calcineurin inhibitors, however chronic graft rejection and risk of infection are difficult to manage. Induction of allograft-specific regulatory T-cells (Tregs) is considered an ideal way to achieve long-term tolerance for allografts. However, efficient *in vitro* methods for developing allograft-specific Tregs which is applicable to MHC full-mismatched cardiac transplant models have not been established. We compared antigen-nonspecific polyclonal-induced Tregs (iTregs) as well as antigen-specific iTregs and thymus-derived Tregs (nTregs) that were expanded via direct and indirect pathways. We found that iTregs induced via the indirect pathway had the greatest ability to prolong graft survival and suppress angiitis. Antigen-specific iTregs generated *ex vivo* via both direct and indirect pathways using dendritic cells from F1 mice also induced long-term engraftment without using MHC peptides. In antigen-specific Treg transferred models, activation of dendritic cells and allograft-specific CTL generation were suppressed. The present study demonstrated the potential of *ex vivo* antigen-specific Treg expansion for clinical cell-based therapeutic approaches to induce lifelong immunological tolerance for allogeneic cardiac transplants.

Editor: Taishin Akiyama, University of Tokyo, Japan

Funding: This work was supported by special grants-in-aid from the Ministry of Education, Culture, Sports, Science and Technology of Japan, the Japan Society of the Promotion of Science, the Takeda Science Foundation, the Uehara Memorial Foundation, Kanae Foundation for the Promotion of Medical Science, SENSHIN Medical Research Foundation, Astellas Foundation for Research on Metabolic Disorders, and the Mochida Memorial Foundation. The funders had no role in study design, data collection and analysis, decision to publish, or preparation of the manuscript.

Competing Interests: The authors have declared that no competing interests exist.

* E-mail: yoshimura@a6.keio.jp

Introduction

Transplantation is the ultimate treatment for patients with total loss of function of a life-sustaining organ. New immunosuppressive drugs have improved allograft survival rates, but long-term administration of these agents may have serious side-effects, including nephrotoxicity, diabetes, neurotoxicity, and increased risk of infection and cancer [1–3]. These complications could be avoided by establishing a technique for donor-specific unresponsiveness or immunologic tolerance to donor alloantigens in transplant recipients. Active suppression by regulatory T cells (Tregs) is likely ideal for the induction of tolerance to allografts. Several attempts have been made; however, methods for the induction of lifelong tolerance to specific alloantigens have not been established.

We previously reported that systemic injection of an allopeptide, a 15-mer (54–68), corresponding to a hypervariable region of the K^b molecule to CBA ($H2^k$) mice prolonged the survival of a cardiac graft of a C57BL/10 ($H2^b$) but not third party BALB/c ($H2^d$) hearts [4,5]. Adoptive transfer of splenocytes from mice pretreated intratracheally with the K^b peptide to naïve secondary recipients also prolonged the survival of cardiac grafts, suggesting the generation of allograft antigen-specific regulatory cells. Thus, generation of Tregs specific to the K^b peptide ex *vivo* as well as adoptive transfer could achieve successful prevention of cardiac allograft rejection.

Dendritic cells (DCs) are the most potent antigen-presenting cells (APCs), with the unique ability to activate or suppress adaptive immune responses depending on maturation status and cytokine production. "Tolerogenic DCs" or immunoregulatory DCs have been characterized as Treg-inducing cells. These tolerogenic DCs are usually immature, expressing reduced levels of MHC molecules, co-simulators, and inflammatory cytokines but enhanced levels anti-inflammatory cytokines such as IL-10 and TGF-β. It is well established that tolerogenic DCs induce Foxp3+ Tregs through a TGF-β dependent mechanism. Foxp3+ Tregs can be generated from naïve T cells by T cell receptor (TCR) stimulation in the presence of TGF-β and IL-2, so called induced Tregs (iTregs). iTregs have similar suppression activity *in vitro* to thymus-derived naturally occurring Tregs (nTregs). However, Foxp3 expression of iTregs was believed to be unstable *in vivo* under lymphopenic conditions [6–8]. Several methods have been proposed to generate antigen-specific Tregs *in vitro*. All-trance retinoic acids (ATRAs) have been shown to enhance and stabilize Foxp3 expression [9,10]. Experimental generation of tolerogenic

DCs has been accomplished through treatment with maturation-inhibiting agents, blockade of costimulatory molecules, either with antibodies or antisense oligonucleotides, as well as pretreatment with chemical immunosuppressants [11–15].

Cellular therapy with CD4$^+$CD25$^+$ Tregs is limited because of the inability to consistently generate and expand antigen-specific suppressors *in vitro*. Several strategies have been attempted for *ex vivo* propagation of Tregs; however, *in vitro* generated Tregs by tolerogenic DCs could only partially prevented rejection of an allogenic heart graft [16]. Joffre et al have generated *ex vivo*-expanded allograft-specific Tregs by co-culturing with DCs from F1 mice[17]. This method can induce Tregs via both direct and indirect pathways because F1 DCs are expected to express allogenic MHC molecules as well as self-MHCs carrying antigenic MHC peptides. However, this group utilized *in vivo* bone marrow transplantation into irradiated mice to generate Tregs. Therefore, *in vitro* method for the generation of alloantigen-specific Treg is desired to be established. At least two distinct pathways of allorecognition exist: direct and indirect pathways. In the direct pathway, host T cells recognize intact allo-MHC molecules on the donor APCs. In the indirect pathway, T cells recognize processed alloantigen presented as peptides by self-APCs.

In this study, we have tried to establish methods to generate alloantigen specific Tregs to induce long-term tolerance to MHC full-mismatched cardiac grafts. We found that iTregs expanded by peptide-loaded isogenic DCs (indirect pathway) could induce long-term tolerance to MHC full-mismatched cardiac grafts. In contrast, iTregs expanded by allogenic DCs (direct pathway) could prevent acute rejection but not chronic rejection. We also compared nTregs and iTregs expanded by the indirect pathway and found that iTregs were more effective than nTregs in suppressing chronic inflammation. We observed an immunosuppressive feedback loop by DC, Tregs, and CTLA4$^+$CD8$^+$ T cells in the graft. We established a simple and effective protocol to generate alloantigen-specific Tregs that can induce long-term immunological tolerance.

Materials and Methods

Mice

Male C57BL/6 (H-2K^b), CBA/N (H-2K^k), and BALB/c (H-2K^d) mice (6–10 weeks old) were purchased from Sankyo Ltd. (Tokyo, Japan), housed in conventional facilities at the Biomedical Services Unit of Keio University (Tokyo, Japan). Mice were kept in conventional conditions in Keio University (Tokyo, Japan). All experiments using these mice were approved by Institutional Animal Care and Use Committee (IACUC) (approved number 08004) of Keio University and performed according to the guidelines of IACUC. All experiments using these mice were approved by and performed according to the guidelines of the Animal Ethics Committee of Keio University. The donor mouse was anaesthetized with an intraperitoneal injection of pentobarbital sodium 45 mg/kg. The donor mouse was euthanized by cervical dislocation under anesthesia.

Kb Peptide

K^b peptide 54–68 (QEGPEYWERETQKAKG) of class I MHC H2-K^b was used to induce antigen-specific Tregs [4]. The peptide was prepared by chemical synthesis (BEX Corporation Ltd., Tokyo, Japan; SCRUM Corporation Ltd., Tokyo, Japan).

Antibodies

FITC-, PerCP-Cy5.5-, APC-, and PE-conjugated monoclonal antibodies for CD3 (17A2), CD4 (RM4-5), CD25 (PC61.5), CD11c (N418), CD8 (53-6.7), Foxp3 (FJK-16s), CTLA4 (UC10-4B9), CD80 (16-10A1), CD86 (GL-1), CD40 (1C10), CD40L (MR1), CD103 (2E7), I-A/I-E (M5/114.15.2), IFN-γ (XMG1.2), IL-6 (MP5-20F3), Granzyme B (GB11-Biolegend), Perforin (eBioOMK-D), and IL-10 (JES5-16E3) antibodies were purchased from eBioscience. Before IFN-γ, IL-6, and IL-10 intracellular staining, cells were stimulated with 50 nM PMA (Sigma-Aldrich, St. Louis, MO, USA), 1 µg/ml ionomycin (Sigma-Aldrich), and 1 µM Brefeldin A (eBioscience) for 4.5 h. After surface staining for 30 min, the cells were suspended in Fixation Buffer (eBioscience), and intracellular cytokine staining was performed as described [18].

Heart Transplantation

Fully vascularized heterotopic hearts from C57BL/6 donors were transplanted into CBA/N recipients using microsurgical techniques as previously described [19]. In some experiments, CBA mice were used as recipients, and BALB/c or C57BL/6 mice were used as donors of cardiac allografts. Postoperatively, the graft function was assessed daily by palpation for evidence of contraction. Rejection was defined as complete cessation of contraction and confirmed by direct visualization of the graft.

Histologic Studies of Harvested Grafts

Cardiac allografts in untreated mice and mice given Tregs were removed 7, 14–15, 35–40, and 120 days after transplantation and studied histologically. The specimens were fixed with 4% paraformaldehyde phosphate buffer solution and embedded in paraffin using routine procedures. Paraffin sections (4 µm thick) were cut, mounted on saline-coated slides, and stained with hematoxylin-eosin (HE).

Preparation of Naïve CD4$^+$T Cells, nTregs, and Naïve CD8$^+$ T Cells

Spleen and lymph nodes were harvested from CBA mice. Cells were harvested from spleen and lymph nodes and separated using a MACS separator (Miltenyi Biotec, Tokyo, Japan) with both negative selection and positive selection. The purified cells were then used for the experiments, except for nTregs that were separated additionally using fluorescence-activated cell sorting FACSAria (BD Biosciences, Tokyo, Japan) and CD3$^+$CD4$^+$CD25$^+$ cells were collected and used in the experiments as described [20,21]. The purity of the Tregs was determined by the percentage of CD3$^+$CD4$^+$CD25$^+$Foxp3$^+$ cells using anti-Foxp3 antibody staining [22]. For naïve CD8$^+$ T cells, the purified CD8$^+$ T cells were further separated with anti-CD62L MicroBeads (Miltenyi Biotec) and the MACS column. The purity of the naïve CD8$^+$ T cells was >95%.

Preparation of Bone Marrow-Derived Dendritic Cells (BMDCs)

BMDCs were prepared as described previously [23,24]. Briefly, BM cells harvested from the femurs and tibia were cultured in 10 cm dishes (2x10^6/10 ml/dish) in complete medium containing RPMI 1640 supplemented with 10% fetal bovine serum (FBS; Invitrogen, Carlsbad, CA, USA), 1% penicillin/streptomycin, 0.05 mM 2-mercaptoethanol (ME) (Invitrogen), and 10 ng/ml murine GM-CSF (Pepro Tech). At day 4, another 10 ml of complete medium containing 10 ng/ml GM-CSF was added to the plates. At day 6 and day 8, half of the culture supernatant was collected, and the dose of complete medium with 10 ng/ml GM-CSF was added. Days 8–10, non-adherent cells were collected and used for the experiment. The purity of the CD11c$^+$ cells was

>90% based on flow cytometry. For mature DCs, BMDCs were reseeded in 12-well plates (1×10^6/well) on day 8 with complete medium and were stimulated with 10 ng/ml lipopolysaccharide (LPS) (*Escherichia coli* serotype 055:B5, Sigma-Aldrich) for 20–22 h.

Induction of Antigen-Specific iTregs and nTregs

For Tregs expanded via the indirect pathway, purified naïve T cells (5×10^4/well) from CBA mice were cocultured with BMDCs (5×10^4/well). For iTregs, cells were incubated in complete medium with 5 µg/ml anti- IFN-γ Ab (R4-6A2), 5 µg/ml anti-IL-4 Ab, 2 ng/ml human TGF-β (R&D systems), 10 ng/ml IL-2 (PeproTcch), 20 nM all-trans retinoic acid (ATRA; Sigma), and 10 µg/ml K^b peptides using 96-well U-bottom plates. On day 6, half of the medium was changed. Cells harvested on days 8–10 were used for the experiment. For nTregs, CD3$^+$CD4$^+$CD25^{high} cells were incubated in the same medium as the iTregs, except 100 ng/ml IL-2. On day 6, we reseeded them in 4-fold complete medium, with the same cytokines and BMDCs.

For iTreg induction via the direct pathway, purified naïve T cells (5×10^4/well) from CBA mice were cocultured with BMDCs (2.5×10^4/well) from C57BL/6 mice. The cells were incubated in the same medium as the indirect pathway iTregs, except with the addition of 10 µg/ml anti- IFN-γ Ab. On days 5–6, the cells were used for the experiment. For antigen-nonspecific iTreg Induction, naïve CD4$^+$ T-cells were stimulated with anti-mouse CD3 Ab and anti-CD28 Ab in the presence of 10 ng/ml IL-2, 20 nM ATRA, and 2 ng/ml human TGF-β for 3 days as described [25].

Before injection, the cultured cells were labeled with anti-CD3, anti-CD4, and anti-CD25 antibodies, and the CD3$^+$CD4$^+$CD25^{high} cells were then sorted using FACSAria. The Treg purity was >95% judged by anti-Foxp3 antibody staining. Then, 1×10^6 Tregs/mouse were injected intravenously.

Isolation of Cardiac Graft Leucocytes

After perfusion using normal saline, cardiac grafts were excised and washed in ice-cold normal saline. The grafts were minced into 2–3-mm pieces and digested with 1 mg/ml collagenase D (Roche) and 0.25 mg/ml DNaseI in RPMI 1640 with 10% FBS for 30 min at 37°C with constant agitation. The remaining tissues were further minced, and lymphocytes were purified on a 37%/75% Percoll (GE Healthcare) gradient by centrifugation at 2000 rpm for 25 min at 25°C. Infiltrated mononuclear cells were analyzed by FACS as described [26,27].

Statistical analyses

All data are expressed as the mean ± standard error (SE). The data were statistically analyzed using the Log-rank test, Tukey's test, Bonferroni test, and the independent-sample *t*-test. *P*<0.05 was considered statistically significant.

Results

Optimization of Induction of Antigen-Specific Regulatory T Cells

We have tried to establish methods to expand donor-antigen-specific Tregs *in vitro*. We transplanted hearts from donor C57BL/6 mice (H-2K^b) into host CBA (H-2K^k) mice. To induce allospecific T cells via the direct pathway, T cells from CBA mice were stimulated with BMDCs from C57BL/6 mice without any antigens. To induce alloantigen-specific T cells via the indirect pathway, T cells from CBA mice were cultured with BMDCs from CBA mice loaded with the 15-mer (54–68) H-2K^b (K^b) peptide which is located in a hypervariable region of the K^b molecule of the MHC class I of C57BL/6 mice. This peptide was chosen

because we have shown that intratracheal delivery of this peptide induced hyporesponsiveness to allogeneic cardiac grafts and generated regulatory cells [4].

It has been shown that Foxp3$^+$ iTregs can be induced from naïve T cells by co-culture with immature DC in the presence of IL-2 and TGF-β [28–31]. To establish the best conditions for indirect pathway-mediated expansion of alloantigen-specific iTregs, the BMDC/naïve T-cell ratio, peptide concentration, and cytokine combination were examined.

The Treg expansion was assessed with CD25- and Foxp3-positivity using fluorescence-activated cell sorting (FACS). First, naïve CD4$^+$ T cells were cultured with various numbers of BMDCs in the presence of a fixed amount of peptide, IL-2, and TGF-β. The effect of anti- IFN-γ Ab and anti-IL-4 Ab was also examined (**Fig. 1A, B**). Although the number of Foxp3$^+$ Tregs increased as the BMDC number increased, the purity of the Tregs (Foxp3$^+$CD25^{high}/CD4$^+$) decreased. Therefore, we chose a 1:1 ratio (each 5×10^4 cells/well) for optimal iTreg induction. The induction was improved when including anti- IFN-γ and anti-IL-4 antibodies (**Fig. 1A, B**). For the starting cell number, a culture of more than 8×10^4 T cells per well resulted in an increase number of dead cells and a decreased Treg purity. Therefore, we chose a starting cell number of 5×10^4 T cells/well per culture. We also found that 8 days was the best culture period to obtain the highest number of iTregs (**Fig. 1C, D**). Radiation of BMDCs did not affect iTreg induction, while activation of BMDCs with LPS strongly reduced iTreg induction (data not shown). Thus, we used fresh BMDCs for the T cell expansion. We also examined various peptide concentrations and concluded that 10 µg/ml peptide was the most efficient for antigen-specific Treg induction. We also found that 20 nM ATRA increased the Treg purity to 95%. In addition, half of the medium was changed to fresh medium on day 6, and the cells were further cultured to days 8–10 (**Fig. 1C, D**). After co-culture with BMDCs, the CD3$^+$CD4$^+$CD25^{high} fraction was sorted with FACS (**Fig. 1E**). Such optimized conditions (DC:T = 1:1, 10 ng/ml IL-2, 2 ng/ml TGF-β, 5 µg/ml anti-IFN-γ and 5 µg/ml anti-IL-4 antibodies, and 20 nM ATRA) enabled us to obtain more than 1×10^6 iTregs with >95% purity, which is necessary for the transfer to one mouse (**Fig. 1E**). These cells were designated indirect-iTregs.

To induce allogenic iTregs by the direct pathway, BMDCs from C57BL/6 mice and naïve T cells from CBA mice were co-cultured. The best condition was 1:2 DC/naïve T-cell ratio, culture in the presence of IL-2, TGF-β, and ATRA, together with anti- IFN-γ and anti-IL-4 antibodies. Then, the CD3$^+$CD4$^+$CD25^{high} fraction was sorted with FACS (Foxp3 positivity >95%), and these cells were designated direct-iTregs (**Fig. 1E**). CTLA4$^+$ and GITR$^+$ expression in direct-iTregs was slightly higher than that of indirect-iTregs, although two types of Tregs showed similar CD62L^{low} activated phenotypes.

iTregs Induced by the Indirect Pathway but Not by the Direct Pathway Efficiently Prevented Chronic Cardiac Graft Rejection

First, we examined which type of iTreg, direct-iTreg, or indirect-iTreg effectively prevented cardiac graft rejection. As shown in **Fig. 2A**, naïve CBA mice rejected C57BL/6 cardiac grafts acutely (median survival time [MST] = 7 days). Indirect-iTregs extensively prolonged the graft survival, >100 days, while direct-iTregs showed a partial effect (MST = 37 days). Thus, iTregs expanded by a specific MHC class I peptide presented on self-DCs were more effective than those induced by heterogeneous alloantigens on allogeneic DCs. Moreover, third-party BALB/c cardiac grafts were rejected in recipients pretreated with indirect-iTregs induced by the

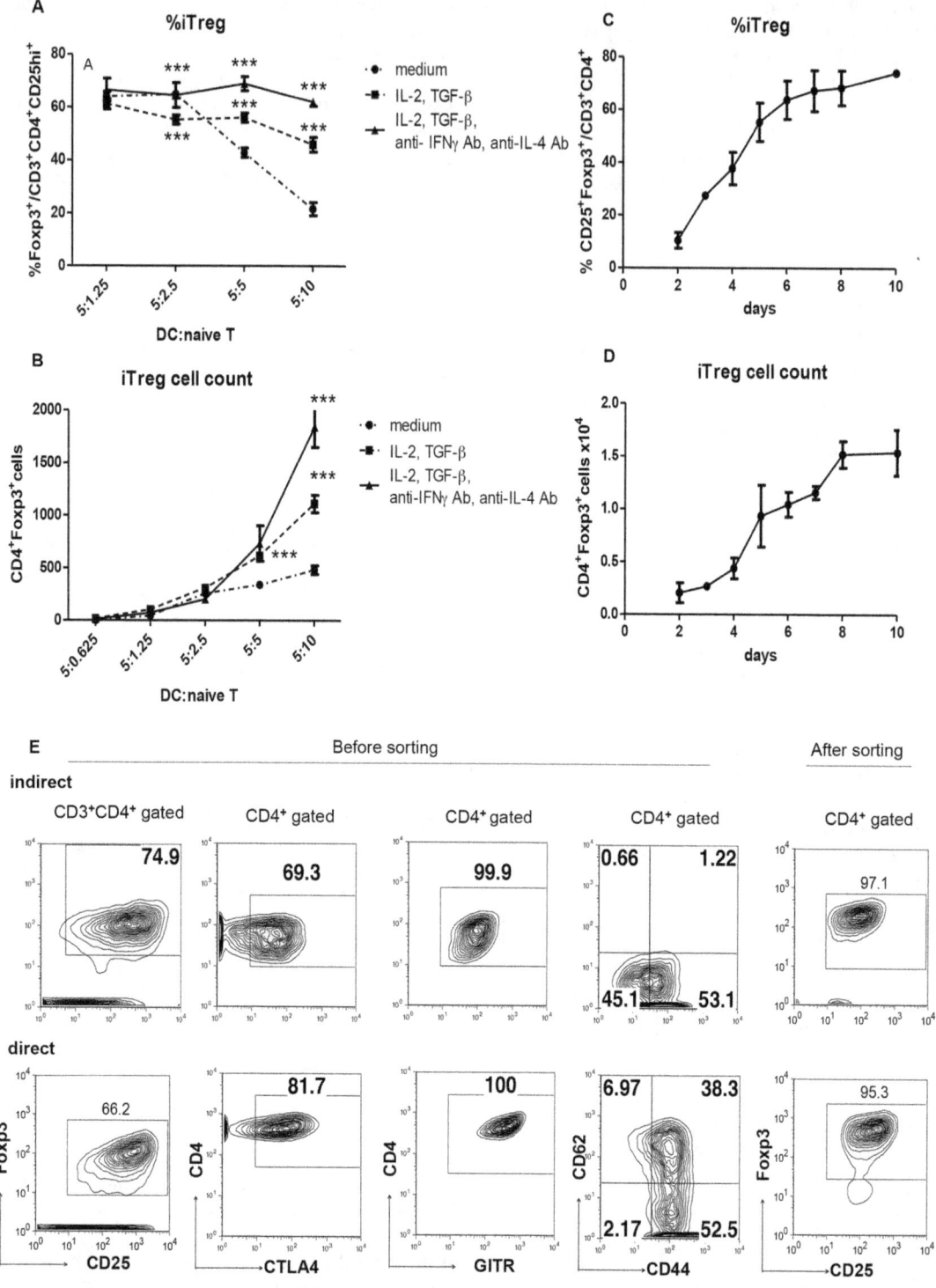

Figure 1. Expansion of Tregs by BMDCs *in vitro.* **A, B,** *In vitro* antigen-specific expansion of iTregs via the indirect pathway. Naïve CD4$^+$ T cells from CBA mice were cultured with BMDCs (CBA) in the presence of the K^b peptide for 7 days at the indicated conditions. The Treg fraction was determined as CD3$^+$CD4$^+$ CD25$^+$Foxp3$^+$ (***P<0.001, Bonferroni test) **C, D,** The-time course of Treg fraction (C) and number (D) in the *in vitro* culture with BMDCs in the presence of 10 μg/ml K^b peptide, 10 ng/ml IL-2, 2 ng/ml TGF-β, 5 μg/ml anti- IFN-γ and anti-IL-4 antibodies, and 20 nM ATRA. **E,** The cell surface marker and purity of the Tregs before and after cell sorting, on day 8 after culture via the indirect and direct pathway. Tregs induced via the direct pathway were cultured with C57BL/6 BMDCs and 10 ng/ml IL-2, 2 ng/ml TGF-β, 10 μg/ml anti- IFN-γ and 5 μg/ml anti-IL-4 antibodies, and 20 nM ATRA. The cells were stained with the indicated antibodies and analyzed with FACS.

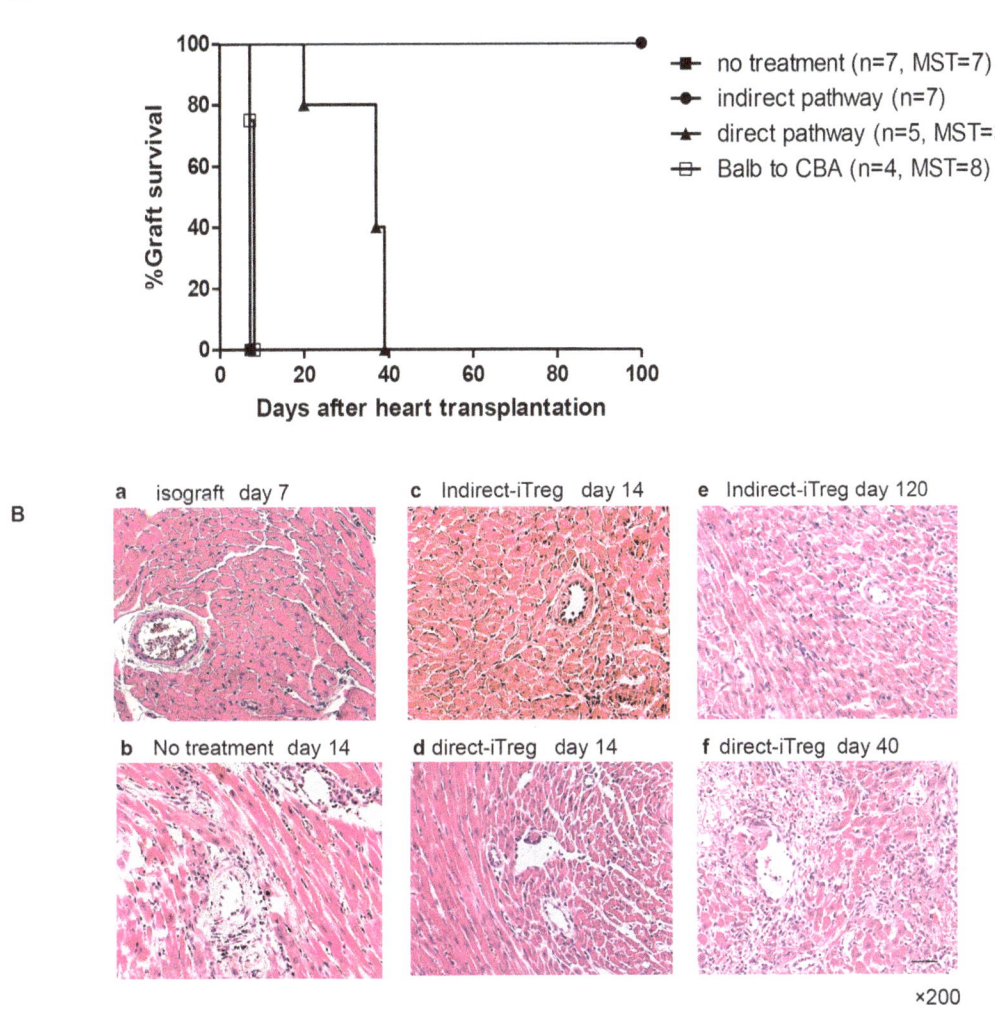

Figure 2. Prevention of graft rejection by Tregs. A, Cardiac graft survival in mice treated with antigen-specific iTregs (CBA background) induced by the indirect pathway and direct pathway. Tregs (1×10^6 cells) were injected intravenously one day before transplantation of the C57BL/6 heart into CBA recipients. BALB/c to CBA cardiac transplantation was performed after injection of indirect-iTregs (CBA) against the K^b peptide. (The Log-rank test was used; P values are compared between the indirect pathway and other pathways; no treatment, $P<0.001$; anti-CD3 Ab/anti-CD28 Ab, $P<0.001$; BALB/c vs. CBA, $P=0.0013$; direct pathway, $P<0.001$. Direct-iTreg treatment vs. no treatment, $P<0.001$) **B,** HE staining of harvest cardiac grafts indicated days after transplantation. The bar of the right lower panels was 10 μm. Magnification; 200×.

K^b peptide (MST = 8 days) (**Fig. 2A**), indicating that the tolerance induced by indirect-iTregs was antigen specific and that the possibility of non-specific immunosuppression by a bystander effect of Tregs could be eliminated.

Histological examination showed all typical signs of chronic cardiac allograft rejection, including diffuse cell filtration and destruction of cardiac myocytes, which were observed in non-treated grafts on day 14 after transplantation (**Fig. 2Bb**). In contrast, little or no obvious signs of cardiac myocyte destruction were observed in grafts administered indirect-iTregs on day 14 (**Fig. 2Bc**). Direct-iTreg treatment also suppressed cardiac myocyte destruction; however, infiltration of mononuclear cells was apparently observed on day 14 (**Fig. 2Bd**). No obvious myocyte destruction, except for a mild angiitis, was observed in grafts in mice treated with indirect-iTregs, even 120 days after transplantation (**Fig. 2Be**). However, the grafts in mice treated with direct-iTregs showed partial fibrosis, destruction of myocytes, and bleeding on day 40 after transplantation, confirming that

direct-iTregs could not suppress chronic rejection. Thus, direct-iTregs had much weaker potential of tolerance induction than indirect-iTregs (**Fig. 2Bf**).

Comparison of iTregs and nTregs Expanded by the Indirect Pathway

Next, we compared the effects of iTregs and nTregs on tolerance induction for cardiac allografts. CD4$^+$CD25^{high} T cells were isolated from CBA mice and co-cultured with auto-BMDCs in the presence the K^b peptide, with the same procedure for iTregs. Because proliferation of nTregs required a higher concentration of IL-2, 100 ng/ml IL-2, instead of 10 ng/ml, was used for nTreg stimulation. Half of the medium was changed on day 6, and the cells were harvested on days 10–12. The CD3$^+$CD4$^+$CD25^{high} fraction of indirect-nTregs was >95% before sorting (**Fig. 3B**); thus, the purity of Tregs in the indirect-nTreg fraction was higher than that of indirect-iTregs after culture with BMDCs. The expression levels of CTLA4 and

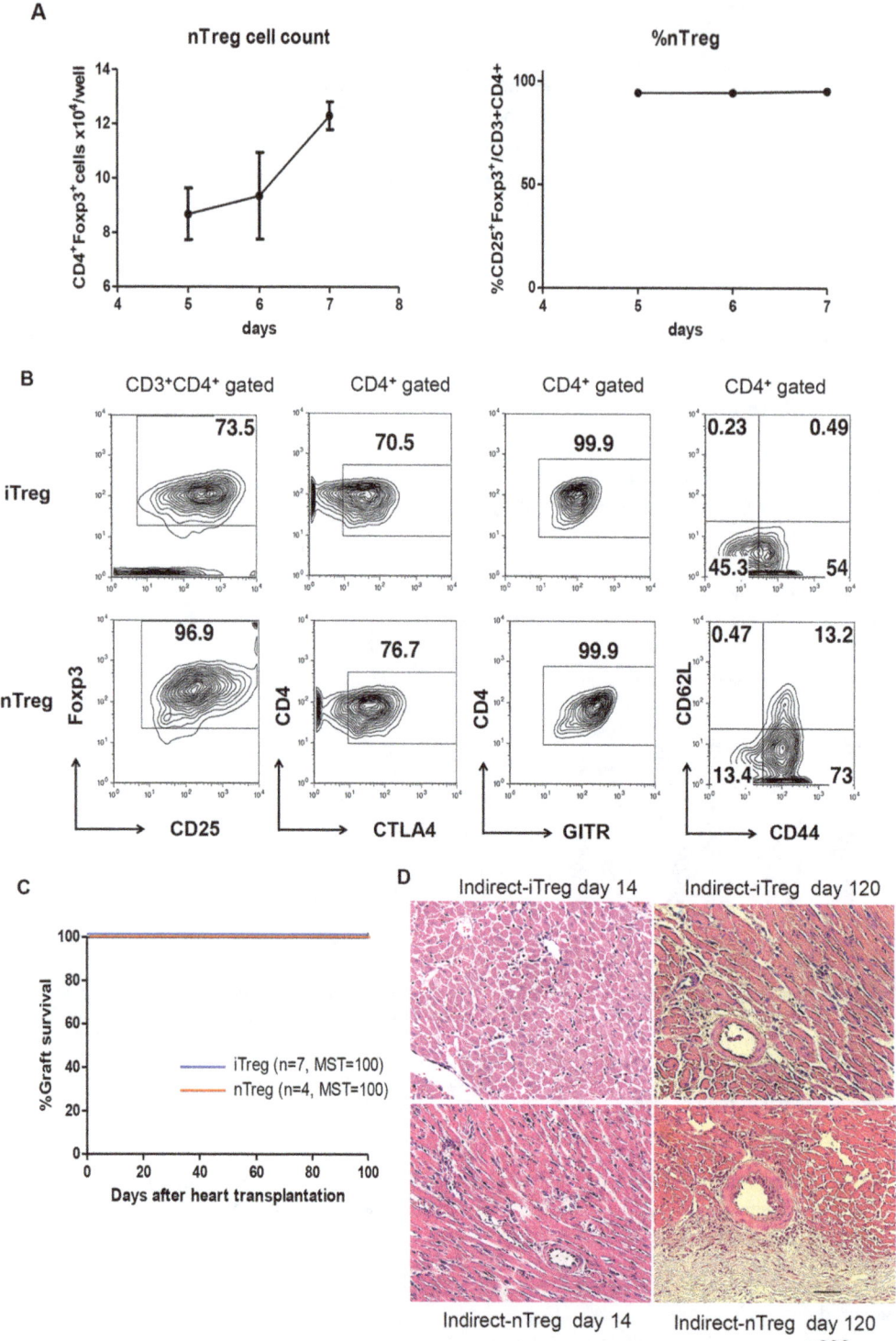

Figure 3. The effect of nTregs expanded by the indirect pathways. A, Expansion of alloantigen-specific nTregs *in vitro*. nTregs (5×10^4) from CBA were cultured with 5×10^4 allo-BMDCs in the presence of 10 μg/ml K^b peptide, 100 ng/ml IL-2, 2 ng/ml TGF-β, 5 μg/ml anti- IFN-γ and anti-IL-4 antibodies, and 20 nM ATRA, and the number (left) and fraction (right) of Tregs were estimated. **B,** Comparison of cell surface markers of iTregs and nTregs expanded by the indirect pathway for 8 days before cell sorting. **C,** Effect of iTregs and nTregs on graft survival in cardiac transplantation models. **D,** HE staining of harvested cardiac grafts.

GITR were similar between iTregs and nTregs, although the CD44^{high}CD62L^{low} fraction of indirect-nTregs was higher (**Fig. 3B**). After sorting, the Foxp3$^+$ fraction was >95% in both the indirect-iTregs and indirect-nTregs (data not shown).

The nTregs and iTregs were then adoptively transferred to CBA mice, and cardiac transplantation was performed 24 h after transfer. As shown in **Fig. 3C**, both the nTregs and iTregs induced strong tolerance to allogenic cardiac grafts, and all grafts survived more than 100 days. However, a small area of destroyed cardiac myocytes associated with infiltration of mononuclear cells around the small blood vessels was frequently found in grafts of mice administered with indirect-nTregs on day 14 (**Fig. 3D**). While more severe vascular hypertrophy was observed in the grafts administered indirect-nTregs than in those with indirect-iTregs on day 120 after transplantation (**Fig. 3D**). These data indicate that indirect-nTregs had weaker potential for the induction of tolerance than indirect-iTregs, although the grafts survived >100 days after transplantation, as judged by heart beating.

Characterization of Tregs infiltrated into Cardiac Grafts

To investigate the mechanism of prevention of allograft rejection by Treg adoptive transfer, we compared the infiltrated Tregs cells on day 7 in the cardiac grafts with the Treg-treated recipient mice. Mononuclear cells were isolated from collagenase-treated grafts by Percoll gradient centrifugation and analyzed with FACS. As shown in **Fig. 4A**, the number of Foxp3$^+$CD4$^+$ Tregs in

the graft on day 7 increased in Treg-treated mice compared with untreated mice. Notably, not only the number but also the fraction of Tregs drastically increased in mice treated with direct-iTregs compared with indirect-iTregs or nTregs. This is consistent with the previous notion that acute organ graft rejection has been attributed mainly to direct antigen presentation [32].

We compared the expression levels of effector molecules of Tregs (**Fig. 4B**). Most CD4$^+$ T cells in the grafts of the mice treated with all types of Tregs expressed high levels of CTLA4. IL-10-positive cells were also increased in graft-associated CD4$^+$ T cells in all Treg-treated mice, although the IL-10$^+$ fraction was lower in direct-iTreg-treated mice than in indirect-Treg-treated mice. Associated with the increase in IL-10-producing Tregs, the number of IFN-γ^+ T cells, which play important roles in chronic rejection, decreased by Treg administration (**Fig. 4C**). However, IL-6 expression did not correlate with the severity of the rejection (**Fig. 4C**).

Induction of immature DCs and CTLA4$^+$CD8$^+$ Tregs in the Grafts with Treg Therapy

As shown in **Fig. 5A**, infiltration of Gr1$^+$ granulocytes was strongly reduced by indirect-iTreg treatment. Direct-iTreg and indirect-nTreg treatments also reduced granulocyte infiltration but were less effective than indirect-iTreg treatment. There is no strong correlation between F4/80-positive macrophage/monocyte infiltration among the Treg treatments (data not shown); however,

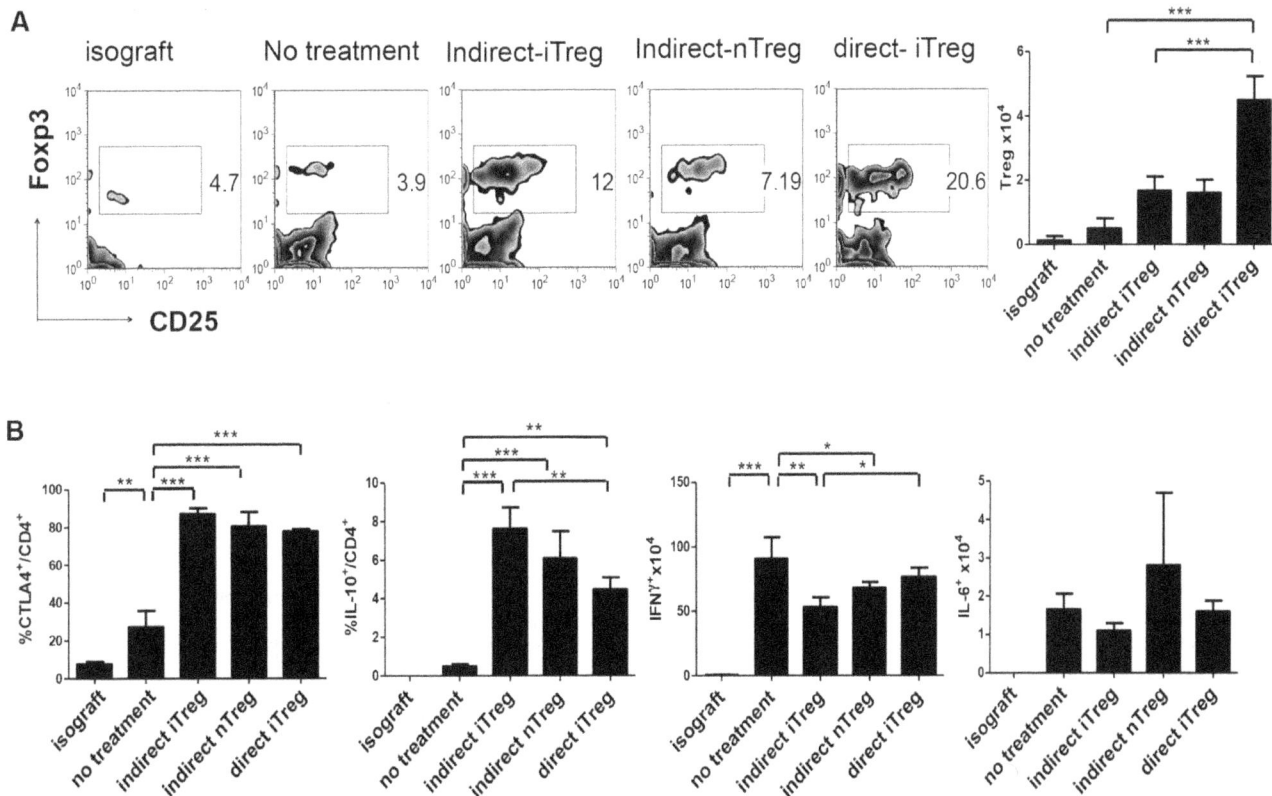

Figure 4. Tregs features in the cardiac grafts on day 7 after transplantation(n = 3–5). A, Proportion and cell number of Tregs in each graft. Mononuclear cells were separated from the graft by collagenase treatment and Percoll gradient centrifugation. After staining with CD3, CD4, CD25 and Foxp3 antibodies, cells were analyzed with FACS. In the lower panel, the number of infiltrated Tregs per graft is shown (n = 5). **B,** Mononuclear cells in the grafts were stained with anti-CTLA4 (left) and anti-IL-10 (left) antibodies after PMA, ionomycin, and brefeldin treatment, and analyzed with FACS (n = 3–5). The proportion of CTLA4- and IL-10-producing cells in the CD4$^+$ T cell population in the grafts is shown. **C,** The cell number of IFN-γ and IL-6-producing cells. The mononuclear cells infiltrated into the grafts were stained with anti- IFN-γ and anti-IL-6 antibodies and analyzed with FACS (n = 3–5). (*** $P<0.01$, ** $P<0.03$, * $P<0.05$, Tukey's Multiple Comparison Test).

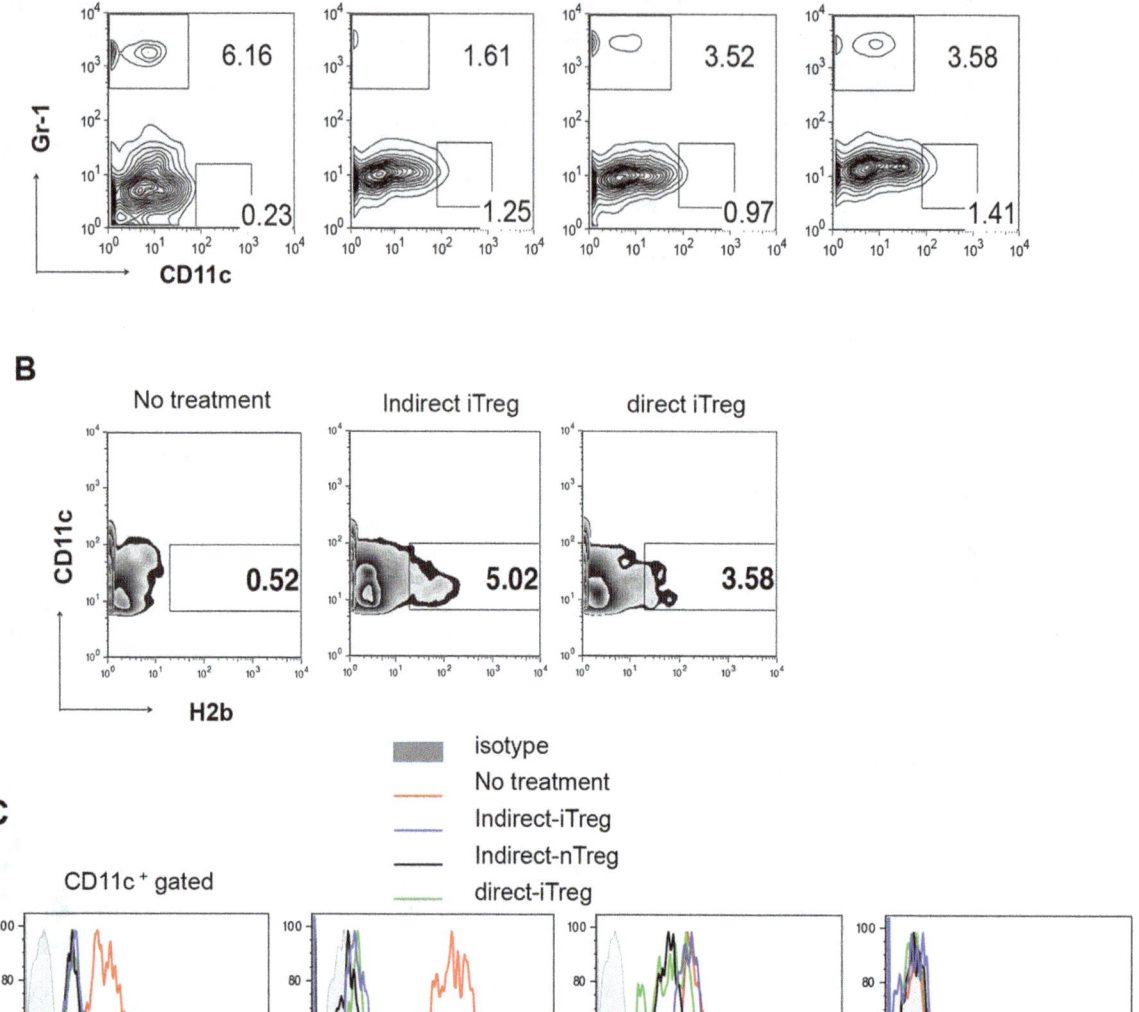

Figure 5. Analysis of DCs in the grafts. A, Gr-1 and CD11c staining in cells filtrated in cardiac grafts 7 days after transplantation in mice with the indicated treatment. **B,** Population of CD11c⁺H2b⁺ cells in the filtrated cardiac graft cells. The graft undergoing no treatment was harvested 14 days after transplantation, and other 2 grafts were harvested 35–40 days after transplantation. **C,** Cell-surface marker expression of CD11c⁺ cells filtrated in the cardiac grafts 14 or 15 days after transplantation in mice tread with the indicated Tregs.

CD11⁺ DCs were increased by the Treg treatment. Thus, we compared the nature of the DCs in the grafts of the mice treated with or without Tregs. Interestingly, as shown in **Fig. 5B**, donor-derived H2b⁺CD11c⁺ cells were present in the grafts in mice treated with iTregs, suggesting that Treg treatment increased the survival of graft DCs. While CD80 and CD86 co-stimulator and CD40 expression levels were lower in Treg-treated graft DCs than in non-treated graft DCs (**Fig. 5C**). There was no upregulation of CD103. These data suggest that transferred Tregs accumulated in the graft, thereby suppressing DC activation.

Not only CD4⁺CTLA4⁺ cells (**Fig. 4B**) but also CD4⁻CTLA4⁺ cells (**Fig. 6A left**) drastically increased via the 3 types of Treg treatments. The CD4⁻CTLA4⁺ cells were maintained in the day 35 grafts in the mice treated with indirect-iTregs and indirect-nTregs; however, the this fraction decreased in grafts of mice treated with direct-iTregs (**Fig. 6A right**), suggesting that the CTLA4 levels correlated with the prevention of chronic rejection. As show in **Fig. 6A lower panels**, these were CD8⁺ T-cells. CD8⁺ T-cells in the graft treated with Tregs showed reduced expression of Granzyme B and perforin molecules compared with

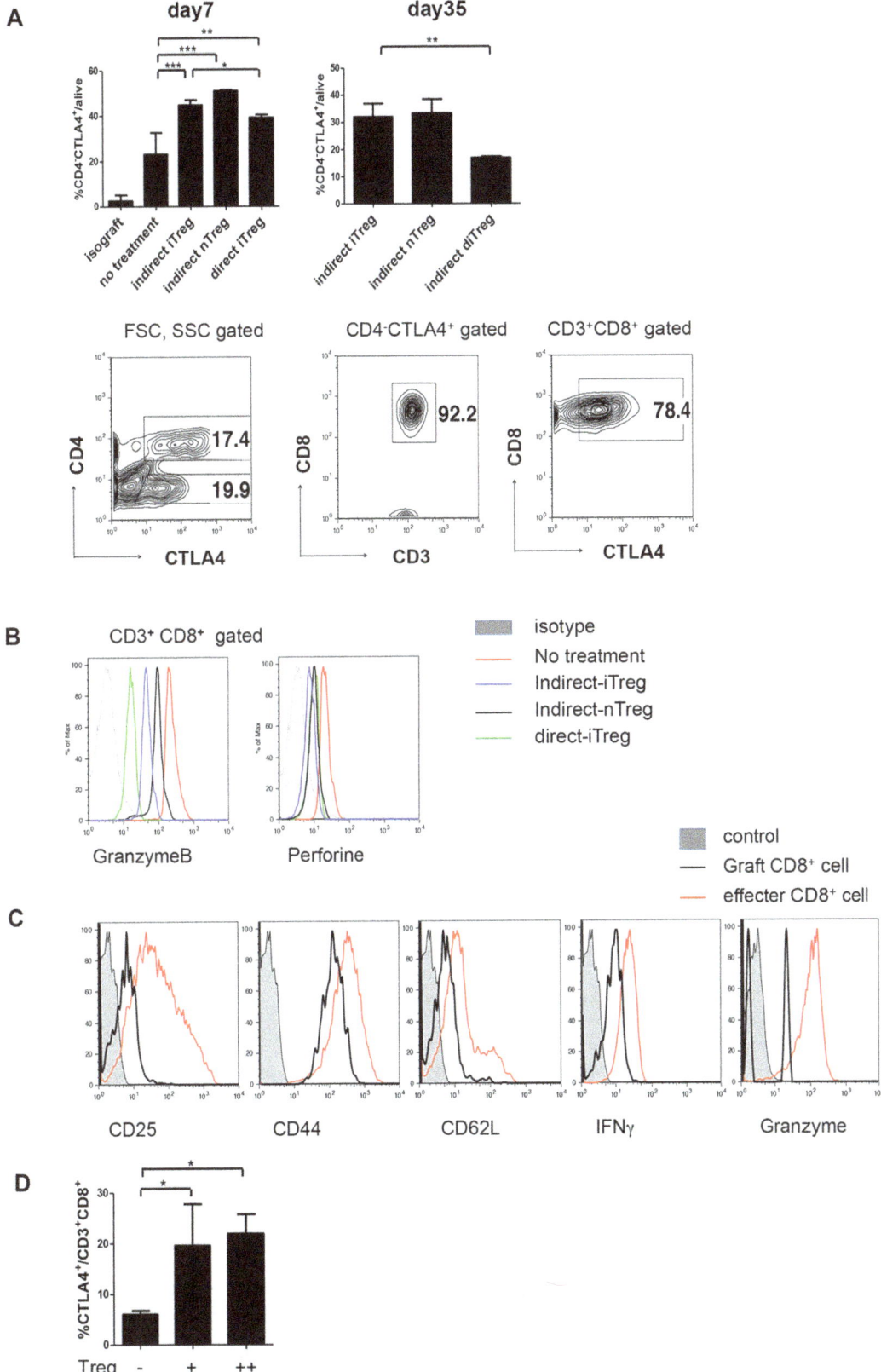

Figure 6. CTLA4+CD8+ cells in filtrated cardiac grafts. A, (upper panels) Fraction of CD4−CTLA4+ cells in mononuclear CD3+ cells in the grafts on day 7 and days 35–40 after transplantation (n = 3–5). *** $P<0.01$ ** $P<0.03$ (lower panels) FACS analysis of CTLA4+ cells in the graft of indirect-iTreg-treated mice on day 35 after transplantation. **B,** Histograms of CD3+CD8+ cells harvested from cardiac grafts 14 or 15 days after transplantation in mice treated with the indicated Tregs. **C,** Comparison of the expression of cell surface marker and cytokines between infiltrated CD8+ cells in indirect-iTreg-treated grafts on day 35, and effector CD8+ cells induced *in vitro*. Effector CD8+ cells were induced from naïve CD8+ T cells from CBA

cultured with BMDCs from C57BL/6 mice (MLR). **D.** Induction of CD8$^+$CTLA4$^+$ cells. Using 96-well U-bottom plates, naïve CD8$^+$ T-cells (2×10^4/well, CBA) were cultured with 15 Gy-irradiated BMDCs (2×10^4/well, C57BL/6) in either the presence or absence of direct-iTregs induced *in vitro* (4×10^4/well (+) or 8×10^4/well (++), CBA), as described above. After 5 days, the cells were analyzed using a FACSCanto. (* $P<0.05$, Bonferroni's Multiple Comparison Test).

those from untreated grafts (**Fig. 6B**). Moreover, in the grafts treated with indirect-iTregs, CD25$^+$, IFNγ and Granzyme B in CD8$^+$ T-cells were reduced compared with activated CD8$^+$ T-cells obtained by allogeneic mixed lymphocyte reaction (MLR) (**Fig. 6C**). To address whether Tregs have potential to induce CTLA4 in CD8$^+$ T cells, naïve CD8$^+$ T-cells were co-cultured with allogeneic BMDCs in the presence or absence of direct-iTregs *in vitro*. As shown in **new Fig. 6D**, direct-iTregs enhanced the CTLA4$^+$ expression in CD8$^+$ T-cells. These data suggest that CTLA4$^+$ tolerogenic CD8$^+$ T-cells were developed by the treatment with Tregs in the cardiac grafts.

Discussion

Tregs are thought to be ideal to prevent allograft rejection during organ transplantation, including heart transplantation, because antigen-specific Tregs are believed to induce antigen-specific tolerance but not systemic immunosuppression. None of the studies has succeeded in generating Tregs specific to a defined peptide ligand that can induce lifelong immunological tolerance. It has been shown that iTregs generated by the direct pathway can prevent the acute phase of cardiac rejection but not chronic phase rejection [32]. Tregs from TCR transgenic mice expanded by auto-antigen-pulsed DCs have been show to reverse hyperglycemia in an animal model of diabetes [33]. This study generated antigen-specific Tregs from TCR transgenic mice; however, this is not applicable to humans. Our method, combining BMDC, TGF-β and an antigen peptide derived from the MHC molecule, is simple and effective for graft-specific Treg generation.

As shown by Joffre et al. [17], we found that direct-iTregs were more efficient than indirect-iTregs for acute phase reaction. The number and purity of Tregs was higher using a direct-Treg injected model, and DC inactivation was also stronger than in indirect-iTreg-injected models at 7 days after transplantation. This was thought to be a result of the difference in infiltration time between indirect-Tregs and direct-Tregs [34].

We found that iTregs induce stronger tolerance than nTregs induced by indirect pathways, although both kept cardiac grafts alive for more than 100 days (**Fig. 3**). This is preferable for clinical application because naïve T cells can be obtained in greater numbers than nTregs. However, this is rather surprising because it has been believed that nTregs are more stable than iTregs. *In vitro*, as well as under lymphopenic conditions, iTregs lost the expression of Foxp3 rapidly and became memory or activated T cells. In contrast to nTregs, adoptively transferred iTregs entirely failed to prevent lethal graft versus host disease (GVHD) [6]. We do not have clear answer yet; however, the expansion rate of the Tregs may be related. We observed that the growth of nTregs was slower than iTregs in the co-culture with the BMDCs, and required higher levels of IL-2. Thus, the survival and/or expansion of iTregs in the graft may be more efficient than those of the nTregs. In addition, TGF-β may exist in high levels in the cardiac graft, which may support iTreg survival. Such environmental factors may contribute to the induction of tolerance by iTregs.

Various mechanisms of prevention of allograft rejection or induction of tolerance by Tregs have been proposed [35–39]. *In vivo* control of DC maturation by Tregs is one of the most likely mechanisms. In this theory, Tregs educate DCs to become

tolerogenic DCs; then, such tolerogenic DCs generate Tregs from naïve T cells. This positive cycle (so called infectious tolerance [40,41]) or "immune regulatory feedback loop" can explain the establishment of long-term tolerance, although early exogenous Tregs die at the early stage of transplantation. This idea is supported by the fact that co-transfer of Tregs and tolerogenic DCs induced stronger tolerance to cardiac grafts than individual transfer events [42]. This mechanism is supported by our observation (**Fig5**) that suppression of DC maturation by Treg therapy. We also observed induction of CD8$^+$CTLA4$^+$ T cells, which has been shown to be related to tolerance to transplants [43,44]. A number of reports have already demonstrated that killing activity of CTLs is indeed suppressed by Tregs [45–47].

To address the question whether recipient Tregs were really induced by transferred iTregs, we performed preliminary experiments by establishing a model to trance Tregs after transfer. We generated allo-specific Tregs by co-culturing recipient naïve T cells from C57BL6, Ly5.1 mice with BMDCs from donor/recipient F1 BMDC in the presence of TGF-β according to the method reported previously [17]. These Tregs were transferred into Ly5.2 C57BL6 mice transplanted with Balb/c heart. F1 mice were obtained by crossing Balb/c, H-2K^d and C57BL6, H-2K^b. By this method, Tregs were induced by both direct and indirect pathway because F1 BMDCs express both allogenic MHC (H-2K^d) as well as recipient syngeneic MHC (H-2K^b). We can distinguish transferred iTregs (Ly5.1) and recipient-derived Tregs (Ly5.2) by flow cytometer. By this method, we have succeeded in counting transferred Tregs and recipient Tregs by FACS on day 7 after cardiac transplantation. In Treg-treated mice, In one cardiac graft, only about 250 Foxp3$^+$Ly5.1$^+$ Tregs were remained. On the other hand, about 8000 Foxp3$^+$Ly5.2$^+$ Tregs were present in the graft. In the absence of Treg transfer, less than 1200 Foxp3$^+$Ly5.2$^+$ Tregs were present in the transplanted heart. Thus, these preliminary data suggests that transferred Tregs cannot survive long in the graft, however, newly generated recipient Tregs are migrated into the graft. Our observations were consistent with the idea of "infectious tolerance".

Our data suggest that indirect-iTregs induced *in vitro* by a specific antigene are the best Tregs to prevent graft rejection and prolong graft survival. even if antigens of grafts are not known, both direct and indirect pathways can mediate generation of Tregs using F1-DCs [17]. If F1-DCs are not available, cell fusion between donor DCs and recipient DCs may also be applicable. Co-culture of recipient DCs with donor cells may also be applicable, however, the efficiency of presentation of allo-antigens by recipient DCs must be high enough to induce antigen-specific Tregs.

We showed here that iTregs induced *in vitro* can be collected with high purity (>95%) using only surface markers. Moreover, iTregs generated from naïve T-cells were easier to harvest and expand than nTregs. We propose that this model might be useful for clinical Treg cellular therapy in the organ transplantation field.

Author Contributions

Conceived and designed the experiments: AY. Performed the experiments: FT RM. Analyzed the data: FT AY. Contributed reagents/materials/analysis tools: T. Shichita T. Sekiya YM TK MN. Wrote the paper: FT AY.

References

1. Cervera C, Fernandez-Ruiz M, Valledor A, Linares L, Anton A, et al. (2011) Epidemiology and risk factors for late infection in solid organ transplant recipients. Transpl Infect Dis 13: 598–607.
2. Sampaio MS, Cho YW, Qazi Y, Bunnapradist S, Hutchinson IV, et al. (2012) Posttransplant malignancies in solid organ adult recipients: an analysis of the u.s. National transplant database. Transplantation 94: 990–998.
3. Zuppan CW, Wells LM, Kerstetter JC, Johnston JK, Bailey LL, et al. (2009) Cause of death in pediatric and infant heart transplant recipients: review of a 20-year, single-institution cohort. J Heart Lung Transplant 28: 579–584.
4. Akiyama Y, Shirasugi N, Aramaki O, Matsumoto K, Shimazu M, et al. (2002) Intratracheal delivery of a single major histocompatibility complex class I peptide induced prolonged survival of fully allogeneic cardiac grafts and generated regulatory cells. Hum Immunol 63: 888–892.
5. Aramaki O, Shirasugi N, Akiyama Y, Takayama T, Shimazu M, et al. (2003) Induction of operational tolerance and generation of regulatory cells after intratracheal delivery of alloantigen combined with nondepleting anti-CD4 monoclonal antibody. Transplantation 76: 1305–1314.
6. Koenecke C, Czeloth N, Bubke A, Schmitz S, Kissenpfennig A, et al. (2009) Alloantigen-specific de novo-induced Foxp3+ Treg revert in vivo and do not protect from experimental GVHD. Eur J Immunol 39: 3091–3096.
7. Floess S, Freyer J, Siewert C, Baron U, Olek S, et al. (2007) Epigenetic control of the foxp3 locus in regulatory T cells. PLoS Biol 5: e38.
8. Sakaguchi S, Yamaguchi T, Nomura T, Ono M (2008) Regulatory T cells and immune tolerance. Cell 133: 775–787.
9. Zhou X, Kong N, Wang J, Fan H, Zou H, et al. (2010) Cutting edge: all-trans retinoic acid sustains the stability and function of natural regulatory T cells in an inflammatory milieu. J Immunol 185: 2675–2679.
10. Lu L, Ma J, Li Z, Lan Q, Chen M, et al. (2011) All-trans retinoic acid promotes TGF-beta-induced Tregs via histone modification but not DNA demethylation on Foxp3 gene locus. PLoS One 6: e24590.
11. van Kooten C, Lombardi G, Gelderman KA, Sagoo P, Buckland M, et al. (2011) Dendritic cells as a tool to induce transplantation tolerance: obstacles and opportunities. Transplantation 91: 2–7.
12. Morelli AE, Thomson AW (2007) Tolerogenic dendritic cells and the quest for transplant tolerance. Nat Rev Immunol 7: 610–621.
13. Woltman AM, van der Kooij SW, de Fijter JW, van Kooten C (2006) Maturation-resistant dendritic cells induce hyporesponsiveness in alloreactive CD45RA+ and CD45RO+ T-cell populations. Am J Transplant 6: 2580–2591.
14. Taner T, Hackstein H, Wang Z, Morelli AE, Thomson AW (2005) Rapamycin-treated, alloantigen-pulsed host dendritic cells induce ag-specific T cell regulation and prolong graft survival. Am J Transplant 5: 228–236.
15. Latek R, Fleener C, Lamian V, Kulbokas E, 3rd, Davis PM, et al. (2009) Assessment of belatacept-mediated costimulation blockade through evaluation of CD80/86-receptor saturation. Transplantation 87: 926–933.
16. Zhang X, Li M, Lian D, Zheng X, Zhang ZX, et al. (2008) Generation of therapeutic dendritic cells and regulatory T cells for preventing allogeneic cardiac graft rejection. Clin Immunol 127: 313–321.
17. Joffre O, Santolaria T, Calise D, Al Saati T, Hudrisier D, et al. (2008) Prevention of acute and chronic allograft rejection with CD4+CD25+Foxp3+ regulatory T lymphocytes. Nat Med 14: 88–92.
18. Ichiyama K, Sekiya T, Inoue N, Tamiya T, Kashiwagi I, et al. (2011) Transcription factor Smad-independent T helper 17 cell induction by transforming-growth factor-beta is mediated by suppression of eomesodermin. Immunity 34: 741–754.
19. Niimi M (2001) The technique for heterotopic cardiac transplantation in mice: experience of 3000 operations by one surgeon. J Heart Lung Transplant 20: 1123–1128.
20. Sekiya T, Kashiwagi I, Yoshida R, Fukaya T, Morita R, et al. (2013) Nr4a receptors are essential for thymic regulatory T cell development and immune homeostasis. Nature immunology 14: 230–237.
21. Tamiya T, Ichiyama K, Kotani H, Fukaya T, Sekiya T, et al. (2013) Smad2/3 and IRF4 play a cooperative role in IL-9-producing T cell induction. Journal of immunology 191: 2360–2371.
22. Takahashi R, Nishimoto S, Muto G, Sekiya T, Tamiya T, et al. (2011) SOCS1 is essential for regulatory T cell functions by preventing loss of Foxp3 expression as well as IFN-{gamma} and IL-17A production. J Exp Med 208: 2055–2067.
23. Lutz MB, Kukutsch N, Ogilvie AL, Rossner S, Koch F, et al. (1999) An advanced culture method for generating large quantities of highly pure dendritic cells from mouse bone marrow. J Immunol Methods 223: 77–92.
24. Koga K, Takaesu G, Yoshida R, Nakaya M, Kobayashi T, et al. (2009) Cyclic adenosine monophosphate suppresses the transcription of proinflammatory cytokines via the phosphorylated c-Fos protein. Immunity 30: 372–383.
25. Takimoto T, Wakabayashi Y, Sekiya T, Inoue N, Morita R, et al. (2010) Smad2 and Smad3 are redundantly essential for the TGF-beta-mediated regulation of regulatory T plasticity and Th1 development. Journal of immunology 185: 842–855.
26. Shichita T, Hasegawa E, Kimura A, Morita R, Sakaguchi R, et al. (2012) Peroxiredoxin family proteins are key initiators of post-ischemic inflammation in the brain. Nature medicine 18: 911–917.
27. Hasegawa E, Sonoda KH, Shichita T, Morita R, Sekiya T, et al. (2013) IL-23-independent induction of IL-17 from gammadeltaT cells and innate lymphoid cells promotes experimental intraocular neovascularization. Journal of immunology 190: 1778–1787.
28. Zheng SG, Wang J, Wang P, Gray JD, Horwitz DA (2007) IL-2 is essential for TGF-beta to convert naive CD4+CD25- cells to CD25+Foxp3+ regulatory T cells and for expansion of these cells. J Immunol 178: 2018–2027.
29. Shevach EM, Davidson TS, Huter EN, Dipaolo RA, Andersson J (2008) Role of TGF-Beta in the induction of Foxp3 expression and T regulatory cell function. J Clin Immunol 28: 640–646.
30. Chai JG, Coe D, Chen D, Simpson E, Dyson J, et al. (2008) In vitro expansion improves in vivo regulation by CD4+CD25+ regulatory T cells. J Immunol 180: 858–869.
31. Sela U, Olds P, Park A, Schlesinger SJ, Steinman RM (2011) Dendritic cells induce antigen-specific regulatory T cells that prevent graft versus host disease and persist in mice. J Exp Med 208: 2489–2496.
32. Brennan TV, Jaigirdar A, Hoang V, Hayden T, Liu FC, et al. (2009) Preferential priming of alloreactive T cells with indirect reactivity. Am J Transplant 9: 709–718.
33. Tarbell KV, Petit L, Zuo X, Toy P, Luo X, et al. (2007) Dendritic cell-expanded, islet-specific CD4+ CD25+ CD62L+ regulatory T cells restore normoglycemia in diabetic NOD mice. J Exp Med 204: 191–201.
34. Gupta S, Balasubramanian S, Thornley TB, Strom TB, Kenny JJ (2011) Direct pathway T-cell alloactivation is more rapid than indirect pathway alloactivation. Transplantation 91: e65–67.
35. Burrell BE, Nakayama Y, Xu J, Brinkman CC, Bromberg JS (2012) Regulatory T cell induction, migration, and function in transplantation. J Immunol 189: 4705–4711.
36. Wood KJ (2011) Regulatory T cells in transplantation. Transplant Proc 43: 2135–2136.
37. Tang Q, Bluestone JA (2008) The Foxp3+ regulatory T cell: a jack of all trades, master of regulation. Nat Immunol 9: 239–244.
38. Kang SM, Tang Q, Bluestone JA (2007) CD4+CD25+ regulatory T cells in transplantation: progress, challenges and prospects. Am J Transplant 7: 1457–1463.
39. Wood KJ, Sakaguchi S (2003) Regulatory T cells in transplantation tolerance. Nat Rev Immunol 3: 199–210.
40. Waldmann H (2008) Tolerance can be infectious. Nat Immunol 9: 1001–1003.
41. Jonuleit H, Schmitt E, Kakirman H, Stassen M, Knop J, et al. (2002) Infectious tolerance: human CD25(+) regulatory T cells convey suppressor activity to conventional CD4(+) T helper cells. J Exp Med 196: 255–260.
42. Li M, Zhang X, Zheng X, Lian D, Zhang ZX, et al. (2008) Tolerogenic dendritic cells transferring hyporesponsiveness and synergizing T regulatory cells in transplant tolerance. Int Immunol 20: 285–293.
43. van Maurik A, Herber M, Wood KJ, Jones ND (2002) Cutting edge: CD4+ CD25+ alloantigen-specific immunoregulatory cells that can prevent CD8+ T cell-mediated graft rejection: implications for anti-CD154 immunotherapy. J Immunol 169: 5401–5404.
44. Jones ND, Brook MO, Carvalho-Gaspar M, Luo S, Wood KJ (2010) Regulatory T cells can prevent memory CD8+ T-cell-mediated rejection following polymorphonuclear cell depletion. Eur J Immunol 40: 3107–3116.
45. Sutmuller RP, van Duivenvoorde LM, van Elsas A, Schumacher TN, Wildenberg ME, et al. (2001) Synergism of cytotoxic T lymphocyte-associated antigen 4 blockade and depletion of CD25(+) regulatory T cells in antitumor therapy reveals alternative pathways for suppression of autoreactive cytotoxic T lymphocyte responses. The Journal of experimental medicine 194: 823–832.
46. Kinter A, McNally J, Riggin L, Jackson R, Roby E, et al. (2007) Suppression of HIV-specific T cell activity by lymph node CD25+ regulatory T cells from HIV-infected individuals. Proceedings of the National Academy of Sciences of the United States of America 104: 3390–3395.
47. Fernandez MA, Puttur FK, Wang YM, Howden W, Alexander SI, et al. (2008) T regulatory cells contribute to the attenuated primary CD8+ and CD4+ T cell responses to herpes simplex virus type 2 in neonatal mice. Journal of immunology 180: 1556–1564.

23

Association of Soluble HLA-G with Acute Rejection Episodes and Early Development of Bronchiolitis Obliterans in Lung Transplantation

Steven R. White[1]*, Timothy Floreth[1], Chuanhong Liao[1], Sangeeta M. Bhorade[2]

1 Departments of Medicine and Health Studies, University of Chicago, Chicago, Illinois, United States of America, **2** Department of Medicine, Northwestern University, Chicago, Illinois, United States of America

Abstract

Lung transplantation has evolved into a life-saving therapy for select patients with end-stage lung diseases. However, long-term survival remains limited because of bronchiolitis obliterans syndrome (BOS). Soluble HLA-G, a mediator of adaptive immunity that modulates regulatory T cells and certain classes of effector T cells, may be a useful marker of survival free of BOS. We conducted a retrospective, single-center, pilot review of 38 lung transplant recipients who underwent collection of serum and bronchoalveolar lavage fluid 3, 6 and 12 months after transplantation, and compared soluble HLA-G concentrations in each to the presence of type A rejection and lymphocytic bronchiolitis in the first 12 months and to the presence of BOS at 24 months after transplantation. Lung soluble HLA-G concentrations were directly related to the presence of type A rejection but not to lymphocytic bronchiolitis. Our data demonstrate that soluble HLA-G concentrations in bronchoalveolar lavage but not in serum correlates with the number of acute rejection episodes in the first 12 months after lung transplantation, and thus may be a reactive marker of rejection.

Editor: Peter Chen, Cedars-Sinai Medical Center, United States of America

Funding: Supported by HL-083527 by NHLBI (National Heart, Lung and Blood Institute) and AI-095230 by NIAID (National Institute of Allergy and Infectious Diseases). The funders had no role in study design, data collection and analysis, decision to publish, or preparation of the manuscript.

Competing Interests: The authors have declared that no competing interests exist.

* Email: swhite@medicine.bsd.uchicago.edu

Introduction

Lung transplantation (LT) remains the best hope for selected patients with end-stage lung diseases. Chronic allograft rejection, clinically manifested as bronchiolitis obliterans syndrome (BOS), remains a major limitation to long-term survival: BOS occurs in 40–60% of lung transplant recipients within 4 years and is the leading cause of death after the first year, despite advances in the use of immunosuppressive therapy [1]. Although several alloimmune-dependent and independent events have been considered as risk factors for BOS, the most common and consistently identified factor associated with the development of BOS is acute lung allograft rejection episodes and alloimmune T-cell reactivity [2,3].

HLA-G is a major histocompatibility complex class I antigen encoded by a gene on chromosome 6p21 [4]. Two HLA-G isoforms exist outside the placenta: membrane-bound G1 and soluble G5 (sHLA-G) that due to alternative splicing lacks the transmembrane and intracellular domains of G1 [5]. HLA-G binds the inhibitory receptor Ig-like transcript (ILT)2/LILRB1/CD85j, expressed by human NK cells, monocytes, T cells, B cells and dendritic cells [6], and the myeloid-specific ILT4/LILRB2/CD85d receptor [7]. HLA-G has effects on both CD4+FoxP3+ regulatory T (Treg) cells and on alloreactive recipient alloreactive CD4+ and CD8+ effector T (Teff) cells that may be beneficial in transplantation: it induces expansion of Treg cells [8], inhibits both NK cell- and CD8+ T cell-mediated cytolysis [9], suppresses CD4+ T cell alloproliferative responses [10], and induces apoptosis of CD8+ T cells [11]. Perhaps more important for long-term tolerance, HLA-G-bearing antigen-presenting cells also induce the differentiation of CD4+ T cells into suppressor cells [12,13].

HLA-G has been demonstrated in heart transplant allografts: patients with higher HLA-G expression had fewer acute rejection episodes (AREs) and less evidence for chronic rejection [14,15]. Circulating sHLA-G was seen only in patients with HLA-G expression in the heart allograft, suggesting the allograft as the source [14]. Similar results were seen in patients following liver [16] and renal [17] transplantation. Suppressor T cells were present in increased number in liver and liver-kidney transplant patients who express HLA-G at high levels [18]. In one recent single-center, retrospective study of 64 LT recipients within the first year of transplant, HLA-G expression was seen in both bronchial and alveolar epithelial cells most frequently in stable patients but less so in patients with frequent AREs or in patients with BOS [19]. This study did not evaluate the presence of either circulating or local (lung) sHLA-G, however.

We have previously demonstrated that low numbers of FoxP3+ Treg cells are associated with accelerated rejection and the development of BOS in LT [20]. Other investigators have demonstrated that increasing the number/function of Treg cells is associated with less alloreactivity in GVHD [21]. Given the association between the presence of HLA-G and other solid-organ transplantation and the potential modulatory role of HLA-G on Treg and Teff function, we asked whether there was an association between HLA-G locally in the recipient lung in the first year after LT and subsequent BOS. To answer this question, we examined a respective cohort of LT recipients to compare the presence of sHLA-G in plasma and in bronchoalveolar lavage (BAL) fluid collected in the first year to the number of acute rejection episodes in the first year and the appearance of BOS after transplantation.

Methods

Ethics statement

Approval was obtained from the University of Chicago Institutional Review Board (IRB) for this study, and was continuously updated as required during the study. Informed written consent done on forms approved by the IRB was obtained from all patients included in this analysis prior to their participation.

Patient population

Adult subjects receiving a single or bilateral sequential lung transplant from June, 2006 to September, 2011 at the University of Chicago Hospitals were evaluated. Clinical data, blood samples, and BAL fluid collected by bronchoscopy in the first 12 months after transplantation, and clinical status and pathology samples to determine the presence or absence of acute rejection episodes and BOS in the first 48 months after transplantation, were evaluated. As the point of the study was to evaluate a potential marker for the development of BOS, patients had to survive for 12 months or longer after transplantation to be included in this study.

Immunosuppression

Baseline immunosuppression for all patients included tacrolimus (target trough level: 10 ng/mL), azathioprine (2 mg/kg/day), and prednisone (tapered to 5 mg/day by 3 months post-transplantation). Daclizumab induction therapy was administered to all patients per the manufacturer's instructions. Immunosuppression was changed because of declining pulmonary function per the discretion of the attending transplant physician.

Bronchoscopy samples

We have previously described these methods [20]. Specimens were collected during surveillance bronchoscopies in the first 12 months post-transplantation. For BAL, one 60 mL and one 30 mL aliquot were instilled into the distal airways and aspirated. In general, 40 to 50 mL of BAL fluid was recovered. An aliquot of this recovered fluid was processed by clinical laboratories to assess clinical infection. Fluid to be used for mediator analysis was centrifuged at $300 \times g$ and $4°C$ for 10 min, after which the supernatant was removed, passed through a 1.2-μm filter, and frozen at $-80°C$ until used. Cell pellets were also frozen at $-80°C$ until analyzed. For transbronchial biopsies, samples were collected by standard technique from the recipient lung and processed for evaluation of rejection.

Plasma samples

Blood was collected on the same day as bronchoscopy in heparin-containing tubes and immediately placed on ice. Plasma was separated by centrifugation and stored in aliquots at $-80°C$ until use.

Acute rejection and BOS

Acute rejection was determined by histological analysis of transbronchial biopsies obtained during each surveillance bronchoscopy and clinical bronchoscopies. Acute rejection was graded

in accordance with International Society of Heart and Lung Transplantation (ISHLT) guidelines [22,23]. All analyses included episodes of both grade A rejection (RA) and lymphocytic bronchiolitis (LB). All rejection episodes that met criteria were included in the data analysis. Determination of BOS was done periodically at clinical encounters for each subject using standard spirometry definitions.

Measurement of sHLA-G

sHLA-G was measured in plasma and in BAL fluid using ELISA (Exbio, Inc., Czech Republic). The capture antibody, MEM-G/9, recognizes both shed G1 and soluble G5. The limit of sensitivity is ~1 U/ml. Concentrations in BAL fluid were not normalized for BAL fluid protein content or other markers.

Data analysis

Clinical data are expressed as the mean ± standard deviation or as the median with interquartile ranges. When HLA-G concentrations were below the limit of detection the value was recorded as '0'. Results were compared using the non-parametric Kruskal-Wallis test. The Spearman correlation was used to determine associations between HLA-G concentrations and grade A or B rejection. The associations between HLA-G, RA or LB and mortality or BOS-free survival were analyzed using Kaplan–Meier analysis and Cox regression model. The log-rank test was used to compare differences of groups. The survival time was measured from the beginning of lung transplant to the date of death or to the end of the study (Jan. 25, 2013) and BOS-free survival was calculated from lung transplant date to the first of observation of BOS or death or the end of study, whichever was earlier. A p value less than 0.05 was considered significant. The data was analyzed using the statistic software Stata/SE 13.0 and IBM SPSS Statistics 20.

Results

Demographics and survival

We performed 53 lung transplants in the time period of this study in which patients survived for 1 year or longer; of these 38 subjects were eligible for inclusion (Figure 1). Subjects characteristics are shown in Table 1. Of the 38 subjects, 28 survived the length of time recorded in the study (mean survival 4.12 ± 1.73 years), whereas 10 subjects died after lung transplant (mean survival 2.77 ± 1.81 years). These subjects were included in our data analysis. BOS-free survival was 3.22 ± 1.49 years in the 15 subjects recorded as not having a clinical diagnosis of BOS during the study, and 1.07 ± 1.62 years in the 23 subjects who did develop clinically-diagnosed BOS. There were no differences in overall survival based on gender, but median BOS-free survival was greater in male subjects: 3.84 years (1.94 to 5.75 years by 95% confidence interval) versus 1.73 years (1.03 to 2.43 years by 95% confidence interval) for female subjects. There were no significant differences in survival or BOS-free survival based on race, type of transplant (single versus bilateral sequential) or diagnosis at the time of transplantation.

Rejection

Both RA and LB were noted in a majority of subjects prior to the onset of BOS (Table 2). There was no difference in overall survival time based on either maximum grade RA or LB score in the first year after transplant. As the numbers of subjects with a RA grade of 2 or 3 were small, these were grouped in subsequent analysis. Three patients had a score of ≥2 for both RA and LB; two patients had a score of 1 for both RA and LB. The association

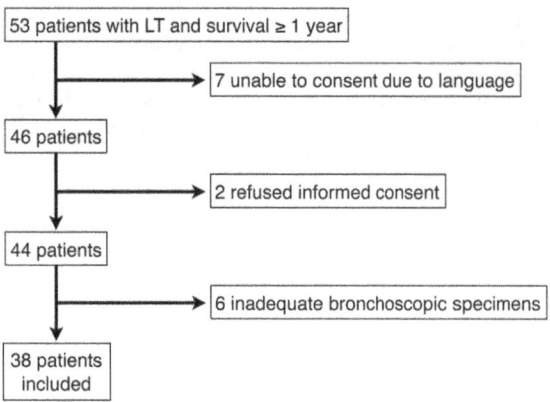

Figure 1. Study enrollment.

between RA and LB was not significant as measured using Kendall's Tau test. There was a significant correlation between BOS-free survival time and maximum RA grade after transplantation (Figure 2) (P = 0.030 for RA by Mantel-Cox log rank test).

sHLA-G concentrations and rejection

A total of 71 plasma and 85 BAL samples were collected in the first year after transplantation in 38 subjects. Plasma sHLA-G concentrations could be measured in every subject at every encounter, whereas 10 BAL samples had an sHLA-G concentration below the limit of sensitivity. Substantial variance was noted in both plasma and BAL maximum concentrations in the first year (Table 2).

There was no relation between either maximum plasma HLA-G concentration recorded in the first year, or in mean plasma HLA-G concentration of all first year samples, and overall survival or BOS-free survival. Likewise, there was no relation between

Table 1. Demographic characteristics of 38 subjects in study.

Age at time of transplantation, years (SD)	
	58.2 (12.3)
Gender, N (%)	
Female	10 (26.3)
Male	28 (73.7)
Type of transplant*, N (%)	
Single lung	24 (64.9)
Bilateral sequential lung	13 (35.1)
Race, N (%)	
European ancestry	24 (63.2)
African ancestry	4 (10.5)
Hispanic ancestry	4 (10.5)
Other	6 (15.7)
Diagnosis at time of transplantation, N (%)	
IPF	20 (52.6)
COPD	12 (31.6)
CF	3 (7.9)
Other	3 (7.9)

*1 missing.

either maximum BAL HLA-G concentration recorded in the first year, or in mean BAL HLA-G concentration of all first year samples, and overall survival. Contrary to our expectations, an increased maximum BAL HLA-G concentration was associated with a higher grade of RA prior to a clinical diagnosis of BOS (P = 0.006 by Kruskal-Wallis test) (Figure 3). In contrast, an increased maximum plasma HLA-G concentration was associated with a lower grade of LB prior to a clinical diagnosis of BOS (P = 0.044 by Kruskal-Wallis test), but not with any grade of RA (Figure 3).

sHLA-G concentrations and infection

Both blood and lung infection, as demonstrated by positive cultures in blood or BAL fluid respectively, were noted in a majority of subjects prior to the onset of BOS (Table 2). There was no significant correlation between the number of infections and either plasma or BAL HLA-G concentrations.

Discussion

Bronchiolitis obliterans syndrome remains the major limitation to long-term survival after lung transplantation despite advances in immunosuppressive therapy, infection control, and management of other complications. The poor prognosis associated with BOS reflects in part an inadequate understanding to date of disease processes which in turn leads either to under-treatment with immunosuppressive medications, and thus BOS progression, or to over-treatment or inappropriate treatment, and thus the increased number of infections and complications seen in this patient population. Our study demonstrates that the local (BAL) presence of HLA-G in the first year after transplantation in the lung correlates with the number of grade A rejection, and that circulating plasma HLA-G in the first year after transplantation correlates inversely with LB. Our study suggests that HLA-G may be a biological marker of rejection in a lung allograft. Such a marker, if confirmed in larger studies, would be useful to segregate those patients with a higher risk of rejection and BOS who require more intense immunosuppressive therapy from those in whom such therapy would entail increased risk without commensurate benefit.

Concentrations of sHLA-G were usually, but not always, detected in BAL fluid collected from LT recipients, and some variance was seen in BAL concentrations. We hypothesized that increased HLA-G levels in the lung would be associated with a lower rejection score as has been seen in patients following other solid-organ transplant [14–17]. Contrary to our hypothesis, however, the highest concentrations in BAL fluid were seen in patients with a RA score ≥2. The reasons for this are not clear: it may suggest that local production of HLA-G (by macrophages or by epithelial cells) is reactive and represent an attempt to induce the presence and generation of regulatory T cells [8]. Alternatively, it may reflect differences in the state of activation of airway macrophages and/or epithelial cells. Further evaluation of this will require studies in which local airway cell production can be ascertained over time.

There was variance also in circulating serum HLA-G concentrations in the first year after transplantation, and these were inversely associated with LB, but not RA, status. Serum HLA-G concentrations in subjects with a score of 1 in LB status was not different than that seen in recipients with a score of 0, while subjects with a score ≥2 had lower HLA-G concentrations. This suggests that mild lymphocytic bronchiolitis demonstrated on transbronchial biopsies may not be associated with changes in immune status sufficient to in turn decrease serum levels. The

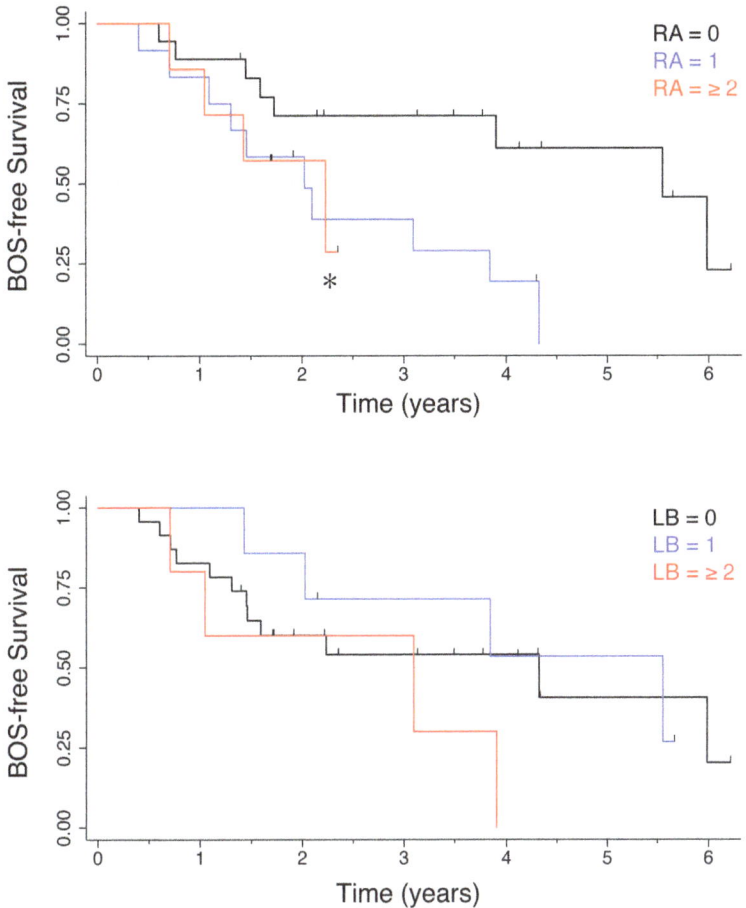

Figure 2. Kaplan-Meier analysis of BOS-free survival in 38 subjects based categorized by grade A rejection status (RA, top panel) or by grade of lymphocytic bronchiolitis (LB, bottom panel). *, P = 0.03 for RA by Mantel-Cox log rank test.

Table 2. Maximum grade A rejection (RA), lymphocytic bronchiolitis (LB), maximum HLA-G concentrations (U/ml), and presence of infection in 38 subjects prior to onset of BOS.

RA*, N (%)	
0	18 (48.6)
1	12 (32.4)
≥2	7 (18.9)
LB**, N (%)	
0	23 (65.7)
1	7 (20.0)
≥2	5 (14.3)
HLA-G, median (interquartile)	
Plasma	41.7 (10.6–74.0)
BAL	26.9 (6.8–49.2)
Number of infections, N (%)	
0	15 (39.5)
1	21 (55.3)
2	2 (5.3)

* 1 missing.
** 3 missing.

downward trend in serum HLA-G concentrations in patients with significant RA noted on transbronchial biopsy is not statistically significant but will need to be examined in the context of a larger study. Serum markers clearly are easier to obtain and, along with other serum markers, provide context for the overall status of the immune system. Correlations with circulating regulatory and effector T cell trafficking to the lung allograft will be needed to understand the potential role of serum sHLA-G in LT recipients.

In one recent single-center, retrospective study of 64 LT recipients within 1 year of transplant, HLA-G protein expression was seen in both bronchial and alveolar epithelial cells most frequently in stable patients but less so in patients with frequent AREs or in patients with BOS [19]. That study however did not evaluate the presence of either circulating sHLA-G in plasma or local sHLA-G in bronchoalveolar lavage. HLA-G also is found in lung macrophages [24], and evaluation of cell pellets by immunofluorescent staining collected from several LT recipients in our study demonstrated significant macrophage expression of sHLA-G (data not shown). Thus, sHLA-G found in bronchoalveolar lavage may represent the combined expression and secretion from both central and alveolar epithelial cells and from macrophages; changes in expression in either cell type might account for changes in the final presence in the lung. Understanding which cells contribute to final expression and presence after lung transplantation, and how that expression is

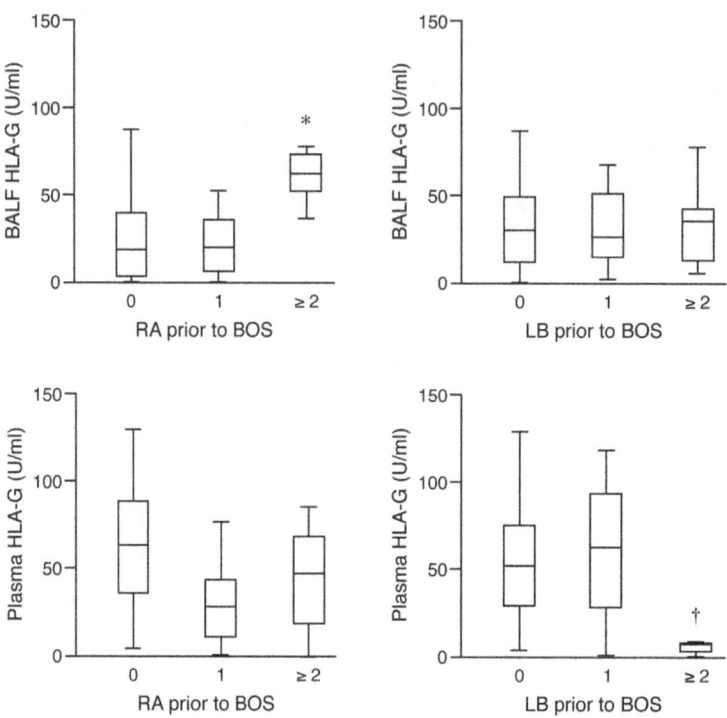

Figure 3. Concentrations of sHLA-G, in maximum U/ml prior to onset of BOS, in bronchoalveolar lavage fluid (BALF) (upper panels) and plasma (lower panels) in 38 subjects based categorized by grade A rejection status (RA, left panels) or by grade of lymphocytic bronchiolitis (LB, right panels). *, P = 0.006 by Kruskal-Wallis test, †, P = 0.044 by Kruskal-Wallis test.

modified by immunosuppressive drug treatment, infection and evolving chronic rejection, will require further study.

HLA-G induces expansion of CD4+FoxP3+ Treg cells [8] which may be important in allograft survival in transplantation. We have previously demonstrated that low numbers of lung FoxP3+ Treg cells are associated with accelerated rejection and the development of BOS in LT recipients [20]. Other investigators have demonstrated similar findings in stem cell [25] and bone marrow [26] transplantation, while increasing their number and function is associated with less alloreactivity in graft versus host disease [21]. Our new data raises the possibility that higher expression of *HLA-G* in the allograft may stimulate the presence and/or survival of lung Treg lymphocytes that then may modulate tolerance; this will need to be confirmed in future studies. In particular, our data do not make clear whether the change in allograft HLA-G expression is reactive, due to some rejection episode or stimulus from cells that ordinarily mediate rejection, or is innate and dependent more on a subject's (or allograft) genotype. HLA-G also inhibits both NK cell- and CD8+ T cell-mediated cytolysis [9], suppresses CD4+ T cell alloproliferative responses [10], and induces apoptosis of CD8+ T cells [11]. Likewise, HLA-G-bearing antigen-presenting cells not only inhibit CD4+ T cell proliferation but also induce the differentiation of CD4+ T cells into suppressor cells [12,13]. Each action may improve allograft outcome, and will require evaluation in the context of LT.

Our study was too small to detect whether either plasma or local lung (BAL) HLA-G concentrations were associated with survival or BOS-free survival. Similarly, given the few time points that were collected for each subject and the missing samples, we were unable to assess changes in sHLA-G concentrations in BAL and serum reliably over time. Both limitations are typical of single-center studies and suggests that a multi-center trial with a

significantly larger number of study subjects will be required to answer this question. Nevertheless our study does suggest that HLA-G is protective against LB; we predict that over a longer period of time and in larger studies that this will translate into improved BOS-free survival.

An additional issue is whether sHLA-G concentrations in BAL fluid reflect the local concentrations of sHLA-G at the tissue level. Previous studies in heart and lung transplant recipients have evaluated sHLA-G presence in endomyocardial and transbron-chial biopsies, respectively [14,19]. In the peripheral lung, sHLA-G presence in BAL fluid may reflect the combined relative contributions of airway epithelial cells [19] and of alveolar macrophages [24]. We did not directly compare the BAL concentrations to tissue presence of sHLA-G in this study, and both the correlation and the assignment of the BAL contribution to epithelial cell and/or macrophage origin will need to be addressed in future studies.

Our study also was too small to examine the potential relation of genotype on lung allograft function and the development of BOS. The influence of *HLA-G* genotype of both the donor graft and recipient has been examined in small studies of other solid organ transplants. While alleles encoding polymorphisms in the coding region apparently have little effect in renal transplantation [27], the 14 bp in/del polymorphism in exon 8 in the 3' un-translated region of *HLA-G* may help predict renal [28] and bone marrow transplant [29] complications. Understanding how both donor and recipient genotypes influence tolerance will have important implications in matching donors to recipients in the future: as one example, if both genotypes predict low HLA-G expression, then clinicians may need to increase immunosuppressive therapy in terms of dosing or combinations of medications; and likewise, if either or both genotypes predict high expression, lower immuno-suppressive therapy may be sufficient. Multi-center studies of

HLA-G and its expression in lung allografts and in recipients will be needed to answer this question.

As may often happen in clinical studies with the collection of biological specimens, data were not available at each pre-specified time point because of the clinical condition (e.g., clinical instability during the bronchoscopy procedure) of the patient or logistics of specimen collection. However, the data remain useful despite these missing samples. In addition, we cannot exclude that different patient phenotypes or the variety of clinical events such as infection may bias our results. The putative use of lung sHLA-G as a biomarker for early allograft rejection clearly will require further study and confirmation in larger cohorts from different transplant centers.

In summary, we demonstrate the presence of sHLA-G in both the lung and serum of LT recipients. There is an association of high BAL sHLA-G presence and the development of grade A rejection within 2 years. While the mechanisms by which lung sHLA-G presence increases are not clear, this adaptive immunity mediator may be a marker of rejection in lung transplantation.

Acknowledgments

We thank Bharathi Laxman, Ph.D., Randi Stern, M.S., and Zhongping Xu, M.S. for assistance in sample analysis.

Author Contributions

Conceived and designed the experiments: SRW SMB. Performed the experiments: SRW SMB TF. Analyzed the data: SRW CL. Contributed reagents/materials/analysis tools: SRW CL. Wrote the paper: SRW CL SMB.

References

1. Christie JD, Edwards LB, Aurora P, Dobbels F, Kirk R, et al. (2008) Registry of the International Society for Heart and Lung Transplantation: twenty-fifth official adult lung and heart/lung transplantation report-2008. J Heart Lung Transplant 27: 957–969.
2. Bando K, Paradis IL, Similo S, Konishi H, Komatsu K, et al. (1995) Obliterative bronchiolitis after lung and heart-lung transplantation. An analysis of risk factors and management. J Thorac Cardiovasc Surg 110: 4–13; discussion 13-14.
3. Todd JL, Palmer SM (2011) Bronchiolitis obliterans syndrome: the final frontier for lung transplantation. Chest 140: 502–508.
4. Nicolae D, Cox NJ, Lester LA, Schneider D, Tan Z, et al. (2005) Fine mapping and positional candidate studies identify HLA-G as an asthma susceptibility gene on chromosome 6p21. Am J Hum Genet 76: 349–357.
5. Ishitani A, Geraghty DE (1992) Alternative splicing of HLA-G transcripts yields proteins with primary structures resembling both class I and class II antigens. Proc Natl Acad Sci U S A 89: 3947–3951.
6. Colonna M, Navarro F, Bellon T, Llano M, Garcia P, et al. (1997) A common inhibitory receptor for major histocompatibility complex class I molecules on human lymphoid and myelomonocytic cells. J Exp Med 186: 1809–1818.
7. Colonna M, Samaridis J, Cella M, Angman L, Allen RL, et al. (1998) Human myelomonocytic cells express an inhibitory receptor for classical and nonclassical MHC class I molecules. J Immunol 160: 3096–3100.
8. Selmani Z, Naji A, Zidi I, Favier B, Gaiffe E, et al. (2008) Human leukocyte antigen-G5 secretion by human mesenchymal stem cells is required to suppress T lymphocyte and natural killer function and to induce CD4+CD25high-FOXP3+ regulatory T cells. Stem Cells 26: 212–222.
9. Riteau B, Rouas-Freiss N, Menier C, Paul P, Dausset J, et al. (2001) HLA-G2, -G3, and -G4 isoforms expressed as nonmature cell surface glycoproteins inhibit NK and antigen-specific CTL cytolysis. J Immunol 166: 5018–5026.
10. Lila N, Rouas-Freiss N, Dausset J, Carpentier A, Carosella ED (2001) Soluble HLA-G protein secreted by allo-specific CD4+ T cells suppresses the allo-proliferative response: a CD4+ T cell regulatory mechanism. Proc Natl Acad Sci U S A 98: 12150–12155.
11. Contini P, Ghio M, Poggi A, Filaci G, Indiveri F, et al. (2003) Soluble HLA-A,-B,-C and -G molecules induce apoptosis in T and NK CD8+ cells and inhibit cytotoxic T cell activity through CD8 ligation. Eur J Immunol 33: 125–134.
12. LeMaoult J, Krawice-Radanne I, Dausset J, Carosella ED (2004) HLA-G1-expressing antigen-presenting cells induce immunosuppressive CD4+ T cells. Proc Natl Acad Sci U S A 101: 7064–7069.
13. Le Rond S, Azema C, Krawice-Radanne I, Durrbach A, Guettier C, et al. (2006) Evidence to support the role of HLA-G5 in allograft acceptance through induction of immunosuppressive/regulatory T cells. J Immunol 176: 3266–3276.
14. Lila N, Amrein C, Guillemain R, Chevalier P, Latremouille C, et al. (2002) Human leukocyte antigen-G expression after heart transplantation is associated with a reduced incidence of rejection. Circulation 105: 1949–1954.
15. Luque J, Torres MI, Aumente MD, Marin J, Garcia-Jurado G, et al. (2006) Soluble HLA-G in heart transplantation: their relationship to rejection episodes and immunosuppressive therapy. Hum Immunol 67: 257–263.
16. Basturk B, Karakayali F, Emiroglu R, Sozer O, Haberal A, et al. (2006) Human leukocyte antigen-G, a new parameter in the follow-up of liver transplantation. Transplant Proc 38: 571–574.
17. Qiu J, Terasaki PI, Miller J, Mizutani K, Cai J, et al. (2006) Soluble HLA-G expression and renal graft acceptance. Am J Transplant 6: 2152–2156.
18. Naji A, Le Rond S, Durrbach A, Krawice-Radanne I, Creput C, et al. (2007) CD3+CD4low and CD3+CD8low are induced by HLA-G: novel human peripheral blood suppressor T-cell subsets involved in transplant acceptance. Blood 110: 3936–3948.
19. Brugiere O, Thabut G, Pretolani M, Krawice-Radanne I, Dill C, et al. (2009) Immunohistochemical study of HLA-G expression in lung transplant recipients. Am J Transplant 9: 1427–1438.
20. Bhorade SM, Chen H, Molinero L, Liao C, Garrity ER, et al. (2010) Decreased percentage of CD4+FoxP3+ cells in bronchoalveolar lavage from lung transplant recipients correlates with development of bronchiolitis obliterans syndrome. Transplantation 90: 540–546.
21. Rezvani K, Mielke S, Ahmadzadeh M, Kilical Y, Savani BN, et al. (2006) High donor FOXP3-positive regulatory T-cell (Treg) content is associated with a low risk of GVHD following HLA-matched allogeneic SCT. Blood 108: 1291–1297.
22. Stewart S, Fishbein MC, Snell GI, Berry GJ, Boehler A, et al. (2007) Revision of the 1996 working formulation for the standardization of nomenclature in the diagnosis of lung rejection. J Heart Lung Transplant 26: 1229–1242.
23. Holtzman MJ, Patel DA, Zhang Y, Patel AC (2011) Host epithelial-viral interactions as cause and cure for asthma. Curr Opin Immunol 23: 487–494.
24. Pangault C, Le Friec G, Caulet-Maugendre S, Lena H, Amiot L, et al. (2002) Lung macrophages and dendritic cells express HLA-G molecules in pulmonary diseases. Hum Immunol 63: 83–90.
25. Hicheri Y, Bouchekioua A, Hamel Y, Henry A, Rouard H, et al. (2008) Donor regulatory T cells identified by FoxP3 expression but also by the membranous CD4+CD127low/neg phenotype influence graft-versus-tumor effect after donor lymphocyte infusion. J Immunother 31: 806–811.
26. Noel G, Bruniquel D, Birebent B, DeGuibert S, Grosset JM, et al. (2008) Patients suffering from acute graft-versus-host disease after bone-marrow transplantation have functional CD4+CD25hiFoxp3+ regulatory T cells. Clin Immunol 129: 241–248.
27. Pirri A, Contieri FC, Benvenutti R, Bicalho Mda G (2009) A study of HLA-G polymorphism and linkage disequilibrium in renal transplant patients and their donors. Transpl Immunol 20: 143–149.
28. Piancatelli D, Maccarone D, Liberatore G, Parzanese I, Clemente K, et al. (2009) HLA-G 14-bp insertion/deletion polymorphism in kidney transplant patients with metabolic complications. Transplant Proc 41: 1187–1188.
29. La Nasa G, Littera R, Locatelli F, Lai S, Alba F, et al. (2007) The human leucocyte antigen-G 14-basepair polymorphism correlates with graft-versus-host disease in unrelated bone marrow transplantation for thalassaemia. Br J Haematol 139: 284–288.

Cytomegalovirus Viral Load Kinetics in Patients with HIV/AIDS Admitted to a Medical Intensive Care Unit: A Case for Pre-Emptive Therapy

Simnikiwe H. Mayaphi[1]*, Marieke Brauer[1], Daniel M. Morobadi[1], Ahmad H. Mazanderani[1], Rendani T. Mafuyeka[1], Steve A. S. Olorunju[2], Gregory R. Tintinger[3], Anton Stoltz[3]

1 Department of Medical Virology, University of Pretoria/National Health Laboratory Service - Tshwane Academic Division (NHLS-TAD), Pretoria, South Africa, **2** Biostatistics unit, Medical Research Council, Pretoria, South Africa, **3** Department of Internal Medicine, University of Pretoria, Pretoria, South Africa

Abstract

Background: Cytomegalovirus (CMV) infection is associated with severe diseases in immunosuppressed patients; however, there is a lack of data for pre-emptive therapy in patients with HIV/AIDS.

Method: This was a retrospective study, which enrolled patients diagnosed with HIV/AIDS (CD4<200 cells/µl), who had detectable CMV viral load (VL) during their stay in an adult medical intensive care unit between 2009–2012.

Results: After screening 82 patients' records, 41 patients met the enrolment criteria. Their median age was 37 (interquartile range [IQR]: 31–46), and median CD4 count was 29 cells/µl (IQR: 5–55). Sixteen patients (39%) had serial measurements of CMV VL before treatment with ganciclovir. Patients whose baseline CMV VL values were between 1,000–3,000 copies/ml had significantly higher values (median of 14,650 copies/ml) on follow-up testing done 4–12 days later. Those with undetectable VLs at baseline testing had detectable VLs (median of 1,590 copies/ml) mostly within 20 days of follow-up testing. Patients who had VLs >1,000 copies/ml at baseline testing had significantly higher mortality compared to those who had <1,000 copies/ml {hazard ratio of 3.46, p = 0.003 [95% confidence interval (CI): 1.55–7.71]}. Analysis of the highest CMV VL per patient showed that patients who had VLs of >5,100 copies/ml and did not receive ganciclovir had 100% mortality compared to 58% mortality in those who received ganciclovir at VLs of >5,100 copies/ml, 50% mortality in those who were not treated and had low VLs of <5,100 copies/ml, and 44% mortality in those who had ganciclovir treatment at VLs of <5,100 copies/ml (p = 0.084, 0.046, 0.037, respectively).

Conclusion: This study showed a significantly increased mortality in patients with HIV/AIDS who had high CMV VLs, and suggests that a threshold value of 1,000 copies/ml may be appropriate for pre-emptive treatment in this group.

Editor: Michael Nevels, University of Regensburg, Germany

Funding: The authors have no support or funding to report.

Competing Interests: The authors have declared that no competing interests exist.

* E-mail: sim.mayaphi@up.ac.za

Introduction

The prevalence of human cytomegalovirus (CMV) in adults is approximately 60% and 95% in developed and developing countries, respectively [1]. CMV is responsible for a variety of clinical diseases in immunosuppressed patients, which include retinitis, pneumonitis, encephalitis, oesophagitis, colitis, hepatitis and others [2]. It is a betaherpesvirus that establishes latency in mature monocyte-derived macrophages and dendritic cells as well as in CD34+ bone marrow progenitor cells, with reactivation only occurring in mature cells [3].

Ganciclovir is the drug of choice for the treatment of CMV, but valganciclovir can be used where oral administration is possible [4]. Common side effects of ganciclovir such as neutropaenia and anaemia can complicate patient management. For this reason, it is very important to properly diagnose or predict CMV disease in order to avoid unnecessary treatment and side effects from these

drugs. The principle of pre-emptive therapy is based on identifying and treating those at high risk of disease in order to avoid CMV-related morbidity and mortality [3].

Diagnosis of CMV disease is complicated by the fact that this virus can reactivate and be shed in various body fluids without causing disease [5]. It is, therefore, always important to differentiate CMV infection from disease or identify those at high risk of disease. Laboratory assays that are commonly used for the diagnosis or prediction of CMV disease are CMV PCR (qualitative/quantitative), pp65 antigen, and histology/cytology (usually from biopsy samples). The latter is regarded as the gold standard for CMV disease as it shows organ invasion by CMV. However, it is not always possible to obtain biopsy samples as this procedure is more invasive [5]. CMV viral load (CMV VL) assays from blood samples are commonly used for prediction of CMV disease as they have high sensitivity, and are simpler to perform and interpret than the other tests [5,6]. Published data from transplant patients show that a CMV VL of 10000 copies/ml or above is associated with high risk of CMV disease in solid organ transplant patients, while a 1000 copies/ml threshold is used for stem cell transplant patients as they are severely immunosuppressed. These values are used for pre-emptive therapy in these groups of patients [4,7]. Some experts have shown a threshold of 2600 copies/ml as appropriate for pre-emptive therapy even in solid organ transplant patients at low risk of CMV reactivation [8].

There is a paucity of data for treatment of CMV infection in patients with HIV/AIDS even though these patients have a similar spectrum of CMV disease manifestations as transplant patients. As a result, extrapolation of transplant data is often used for management of CMV infection in patients with HIV/AIDS. However, it is not known whether patients with HIV/AIDS are as immunosuppressed as solid organ or stem cell transplant patients, thus making the selection of an appropriate CMV VL threshold difficult for this group of patients. Trends observed (unpublished data) in our adult medical intensive care unit (ICU) have shown that the use of a CMV VL threshold of ≥10000 copies/ml for CMV treatment is associated with a high mortality. Consequently, a lower threshold of 1000 copies/ml has been adopted for use in our ICU from around mid-year 2011. The aim of this study was to evaluate the CMV VL kinetics in patients with HIV/AIDS in an ICU environment.

Materials and Methods

This was a retrospective study, which reviewed medical records of patients with CMV VL test results who were admitted in adult medical ICU at Steve Biko Academic hospital between January 2009 to December 2012. The University of Pretoria's Faculty of Health Research Ethics committee granted ethics approval for the study protocol, including approval for authors to access patients' records as almost all patients were no longer hospitalised at the time this study was conducted. Approval for accessing patients' records was also obtained from the superintendent of Steve Biko Academic hospital. Data from the records was anonymized and de-identified prior to analysis in order to ensure patient confidentiality. The study participants were identified through a search in the National Health Laboratory Service (NHLS) database for patients who had a CMV VL test while in ICU. Standard data capturing forms were used to collect patient demographics and clinical data from the records. These forms assessed the following information: dates of admission, discharge or death in ICU; patient diagnosis; ganciclovir use; other drug use (e.g. antibiotics, antivirals, steroids); and timing of antiretroviral initiation (before or after admission). The target group for enrolment were patients with AIDS as defined by CD4 count <200 cells/µl.

Laboratory information was obtained from the NHLS database, and this included CMV VL and serology, HIV tests, CD4 count, *Pneumocystis jirovecii* immunofluorescence, tuberculosis (TB), microbiology culture, and post-mortem results. Confirmed TB infections were based on positive TB culture and/or PCR results. Dates of CMV VL results and the number of these results per patient were documented. CMV VL testing was done on plasma samples using the following assays: Affigene assay (Cepheid, Solna, Sweden) with a limit of detection (LOD) of 235 copies/ml, and R-gene assay (Argene SA, Varilhes, France) with an LOD of 50 copies/ml, and both assays were run on the LightCycler instrument (Roche, Mannheim, Germany). The CMV VL testing was done in three different laboratories, all of which participated in international quality assurance schemes for CMV VL, and two were also approved by the local laboratory accrediting body (South African

National Accreditation System). All the study information was collected by qualified medical doctors.

Intravenous ganciclovir was used at a dose of 5 mg/kg twice a day for 21 days, with dose adjustment for patients with renal dysfunction. All the CMV VL analysis in this study was done before treatment initiation with ganciclovir (i.e. for those who received treatment).

Statistical Analysis

A descriptive analysis was used to present summary statistics (mean, standard deviation, standard error, median and 95% confidence intervals) for the parameters. This was followed by a comparison between the groups using two sample independent t-tests for proportions. Non-parametric survival analysis presenting Kaplan-Meier curve was performed to assess hazard ratios and association of different CMV VL values with mortality. Univariate logistic regression analysis was performed to assess the association of individual variable (age, CD4 count, CMV VL, confirmed TB infections and steroids) with mortality. In addition, multivariable logistic regression was undertaken, adjusting for age, CD4, and ganciclovir use. All the statistics was performed on the STATA version 12.1 software (StataCorp LP, College Station, TX, USA), and survival analysis was also performed on MedCalc version 12.7.0 software (Acacialaan, Ostend, Belgium). A p-value of <0.05 was considered statistically significant.

Results

During the study period, 82 patients were tested for CMV VL while in ICU, and also had HIV and CD4 results available. Of these patients, only 41 met the enrolment criteria for this study, i.e. had a detectable CMV VL and a diagnosis of AIDS as defined by CD4 count <200 cells/µl (Fig. 1). The enrolled participants represented 62% (41/66) of patients with AIDS (Fig. 1). The 25 patients with HIV/AIDS who were excluded did not have detectable CMV VL during their stay in ICU.

The enrolled patients were predominantly black (90%), the remaining 10% were white; and 54% were males. The median age of all patients was 37 (IQR:31–46), and the median CD4 count was 29 cells/µl (IQR:5–55). The majority of patients (65.9%) were diagnosed with pulmonary diseases (mainly community acquired pneumonia) at the time of admission to ICU, followed by renal (14.6%) and central nervous system diseases (12.2%), and septicaemia (7.3%). None of these patients were diagnosed with CMV retinitis. Appropriate antibiotics were used for empiric therapy and later modified based on microbiology cultures. Most patients (78%, n = 32) were not on antiretroviral therapy (ART) at the time of admission to ICU, and 44% (n = 14) of these patients later received ART. The median stay in ICU from admission to discharge or death was 19 days (IQR:12–44).

A large proportion of patients (71%, n = 29) had detectable viral loads at baseline testing with a median CMV VL of 3430 copies/ml (IQR:1380–16450), while others had undetectable viral loads. The latter eventually had detectable viral loads on subsequent testing. Sixteen patients (39%) had serial measurements of CMV VL before treatment with ganciclovir. Patients whose baseline CMV VL values were between 1000–3000 copies/ml had significantly higher values (median of 14650 copies/ml) on follow up testing done 4–12 days later (Table 1). Those with undetectable VLs at baseline testing had detectable VLs (median of 1590 copies/ml) mostly within 20 days of follow up testing (Table 2). Patients (n = 24) who had CMV VLs >1000 copies/ml at baseline testing had significantly higher mortality compared to those (n = 17) who had CMV VLs <1000 copies/ml (hazard ratio of

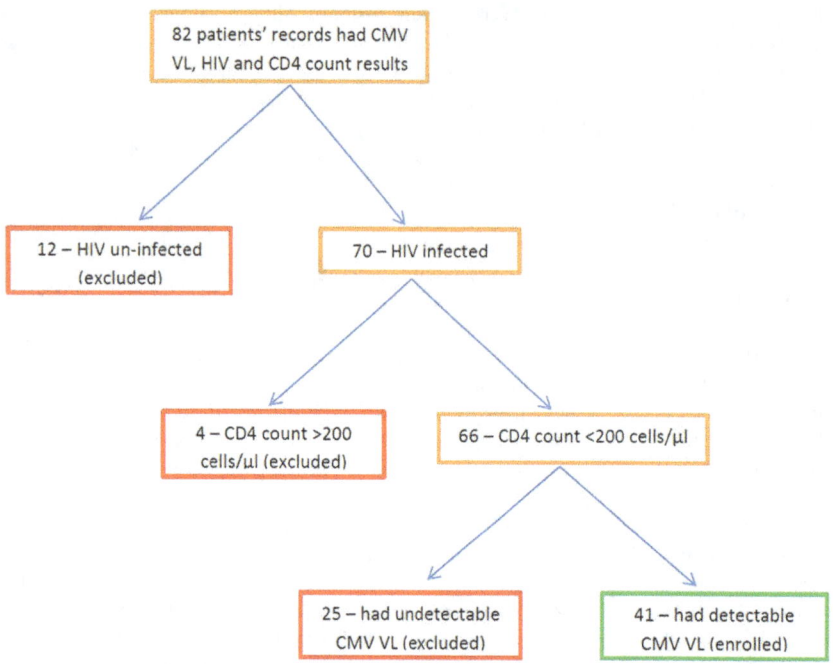

Figure 1. Algorithm showing the selection of study participants. Study participants were selected after a review of records and laboratory results for all the patients who had CMV VL results during ICU stay, within the study period. CMV VL = cytomegalovirus viral load.

3.46, p = 0.003 [95% CI: 1.55–7.71]) (Fig. 2). The trend with higher mortality was also noticed when patients were stratified by a CMV VL of 5000 copies/ml at baseline testing, and no statistical significance noted with a CMV VL of 10000 copies/ml threshold (Fig. 2).

When the highest CMV VLs that patients had during their ICU stay were analysed, it was noticed that patients who were not treated but had high VLs (nt-HVL) of >5100 copies/ml had 100% mortality compared to 58% mortality in those who received ganciclovir at >5100 copies/ml (delayed treatment [DT]), 50% mortality in those who were not treated and had low VLs (nt-LVL) of <5100 copies/ml, and 44% mortality in those who had ganciclovir treatment at <5100 copies/ml (early treatment [ET]) (p = 0.084, 0.046, 0.037, respectively) (Table 3). The reason for non-treatment is that some patients had undetectable or low CMV VL results at baseline testing at the time that we used 10000 copies/ml as a threshold for treatment, and only found to have significantly high CMV VL values on follow-up testing, which was at the time of death for some. Another reason is that some had very high CMV VL results at baseline testing and demised just after testing (more applicable to the nt-HVL group). The majority of patients (53.3%, n = 8) in the nt-LVL group had CMV VLs < 1000 copies/ml. Steroid use was not statistically different amongst all these groups, even though it was slightly lower in the ET group (as compared with DT, nt-LVL and nt-HVL: p = 0.395, 0.476, 0.605, respectively). Confirmed TB infections were higher in the ET group (as compared with DT, nt-LVL and nt-HVL: p = 0.054, 0.627, 0.042, respectively), which had the lowest mortality (Table 3). *Pneumocystis jirovecii* immunofluorescence test was positive in 5 patients; however, most patients were treated or put on prophylaxis for pneumocystis pneumonia despite negative results as there is currently no test that completely excludes this disease [9]. Univariate logistic regression analysis showed that CMV VL was the only variable associated with mortality in this cohort, showing that patients with CMV VL >1000 copies/ml at baseline

had 5 times greater odds (crude odds ratio of 5.5, p = 0.014 [95% CI: 1.4–21.4]) of dying compared to those with CMV VL <1000 copies/ml. Multivariable logistic regression still identified CMV VL as the only factor associated with mortality. The adjusted odds ratios were 5.44 [95% CI: 1.4–21.3], 5.81 [95% CI: 1.5–23.1], and 4.66 [95% CI: 1.1–19.6] after adjusting for age, CD4 count, and ganciclovir use, respectively. The odds ratio was 4.86 [95% CI: 1.1–21.6] after adjusting for all the variables together, and CMV VL association with mortality still remained significant (p = 0.038). Grade 4 neutropaenia was detected in 24% of patients who received ganciclovir.

Only two patients had post-mortem examinations performed, both of whom had CMV inclusion bodies on lung biopsy microscopy. Interestingly, one of these patients belonged to the nt-LVL group with a CMV VL of 880 copies/ml and was therefore not treated (Table 2 - patient 2120). The other patient belonged to the DT group and had a significantly high CMV VL of 21500 copies/ml and did receive ganciclovir treatment (data not shown). The low rate of post-mortem analysis is probably due to general decline in the use of this procedure in modern medicine [10], and failure to obtain consent from the relatives of the deceased.

CMV serology results were available for 7 patients (17%); all had the same profile of negative IgM and positive IgG, 4 of whom had high CMV VLs (median = 32700 copies/ml).

Discussion

This study provides an analysis of the CMV VL kinetics in critically ill patients with HIV/AIDS. It is the first study to report on the CMV VL threshold value that may be appropriate for pre-emptive therapy in patients with AIDS.

The enrolled participants represented 62% (41/66) of the patients with AIDS, showing that CMV reactivation is very common in these patients in the ICU setting. The negative IgM and positive IgG CMV serology profile in all patients who had

Table 1. Clinical characteristics of patients who had low CMV VL at baseline.

Study ID	Age	Sex	CD4 count	CMV VL results and dates (dd/mm/yy)	Ganciclovir initiation date (dd/mm/yy)	Death in ICU and dates (dd/mm/yy)	Group
1707	34	M	35	19100, 26/08/10	29/08/10	Yes, 20/09/10	DT
				2430, 15/08/10			
689	49	F	48	10200, 24/07/10	29/07/10	No	DT
				1150, 20/07/10			
1851	23	F	149	113000, 16/08/10	N/A	Yes, 17/08/10	nt-HVL
				2640, 07/08/10			
8540	67	M	57	5690, 01/02/11	N/A	Yes, 05/02/11	nt-HVL
				1600, 20/01/11			

ID = identity, CMV VL = cytomegalovirus viral load, ICU = intensive care unit, DT = delayed treatment, nt-HVL = non-treatment and high viral load. N/A – ganciclovir was not administered as patients were admitted at a time when a 10000 copies/ml threshold for CMV treatment was used. For consistency, sample collection dates were used for CMV VL results.

serology testing highlights the high prevalence of CMV in an African setting [11], indicating a high likelihood of CMV reactivation in patients with HIV/AIDS or other immunosuppressive conditions. Advanced immunosuppression could account for the negative CMV IgM results despite detectable CMV VLs in some patients [5,12].

The CMV VLs were significantly higher in the group that had 100% mortality (nt-HVL group) compared to other groups (Table 3). This is consistent with data from other immunosuppressed groups of patients, which show that high CMV VLs are associated with CMV disease and high mortality [8,13,14]. In the treated groups, mortality was higher in those where therapy was delayed (DT group, with a median CMV VL of 22150 copies/ml) compared to the early therapy group (ET group, with a median CMV VL of 2690 copies/ml) (Table 3). Even though not statistically significant (p = 0.525), the clinical relevance of this finding cannot be ignored as some published data have shown that treatment started at higher CMV VL (>10000 copies/ml) is associated with delayed response or failure to control viraemia within 4 weeks [1,15].

The significant mortality differences between the nt-HVL group as compared with nt-LVL and ET groups (p-values = 0.046, 0.037, respectively) suggest that pre-emptive therapy for CMV infection in patients with AIDS should be started at low CMV VLs in order to reduce morbidity and mortality. The higher mortality associated with a CMV VL >1000 copies/ml (Fig. 2), and the faster increase of low CMV VL values between 1000–3000 copies/ml to significantly higher values on follow up testing (Table 1) suggest that a CMV VL threshold of 1000 copies/ml may be appropriate to initiate pre-emptive CMV treatment in patients with HIV/AIDS in ICU. This is similar to the threshold VL that is commonly used in stem cell transplant patients at high risk of CMV reactivation [7]. This threshold is supported by the findings of recent studies, which noticed an association between CMV VL and high mortality in ambulatory patients with HIV/AIDS [16–18]. Death hazard ratios of 3.65 and 3.9 were reported by Fielding et al. and Boffi El Amari et al., respectively, when the CMV VL was ≥1000 copies/ml [16,17]; while Durier et al. reported a death hazard ratio of 7.28 when the CMV VL was > 500 copies/ml [18]. A recently published study, which employed a CMV VL threshold of 5000 copies/ml (and 3000 copies/ml for certain patients) showed that pre-emptive therapy prevents CMV end-organ disease by almost 25% in HIV infected patients with advanced immunosuppression [19]. This is; however, lower than 49% CMV disease risk reduction noted by Spector et al. during prophylactic use of oral ganciclovir in patients with AIDS [20]. The difference between the benefits of pre-emptive and prophylactic treatments between these two studies could be explained by a relatively higher CMV VL pre-emptive threshold of 5000 copies/ml, and by undetectable plasma CMV VL in some patients with CMV end-organ disease [21] who would have been missed in the pre-emptive treatment study. Some experts have shown that CMV VL values of <5000 copies/ml are associated with CMV disease. For instance, Rasmussen et al. reported that a CMV VL ≥32 copies/25 µl (i.e. ≥1280 copies/ml) in plasma, particularly when sustained, distinguished patients who developed CMV retinitis from those who did not [22]. The frequency of grade 4 neutropaenia (24%) noticed in this cohort is comparable to a frequency reported by Mizushima et al. for grade 3–4 leukocytopaenia in CMV/HIV co-infected patients receiving ganciclovir [19].

Some published data have shown evidence of CMV disease in autopsy or biopsy samples without detectable viraemia [21,23,24]. Therefore, an undetectable CMV VL in plasma does not exclude

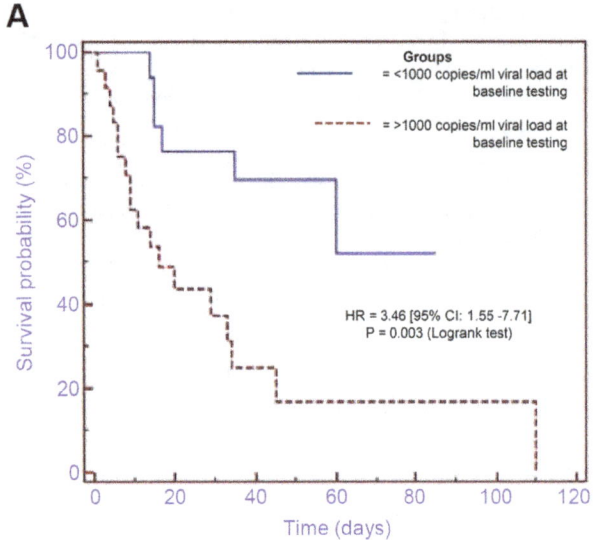

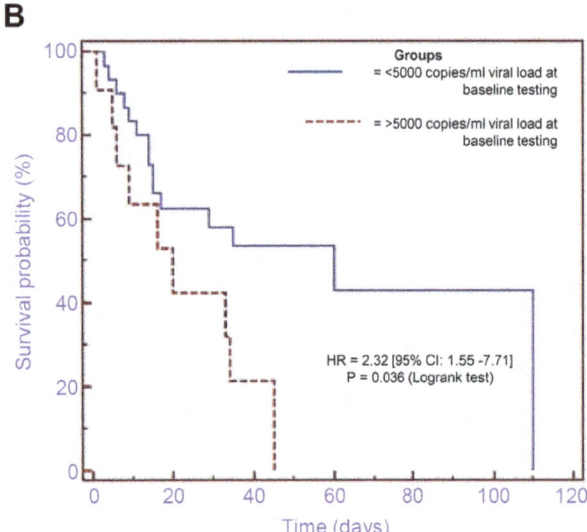

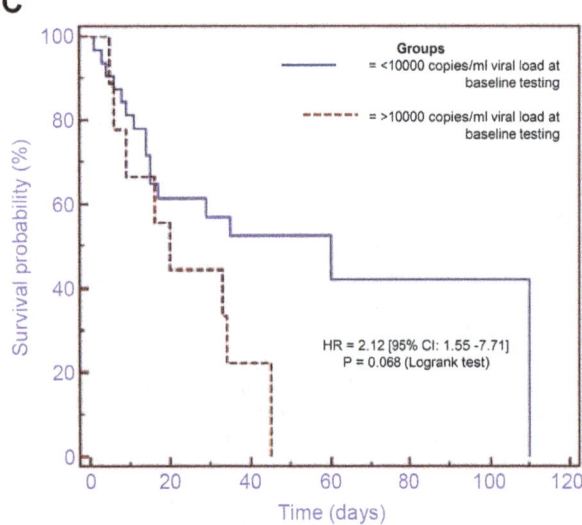

Figure 2. Kaplan-Meier curve analysis showing survival probalities between the groups of patients: (A) who had CMV viral loads <1000 copies/ml compared to those who had viral loads >1000 copies/ml at baseline testing, (B) who had CMV viral loads <5000 copies/ml compared to those who had viral loads >5000 copies/ml at baseline testing, (C) who had CMV viral loads <10000 copies/ml compared to those who had viral loads >10000 copies/ml at baseline testing. HR = hazard ratio, CI = confidence interval.

the presence of CMV disease. In this study patients who initially had undetectable CMV VL later had detectable viral loads in plasma during follow up testing (Table 2). A post-mortem report that showed CMV inclusion bodies on lung microscopy in a patient who had CMV VL results of 880 copies/ml indicates that by the time viraemia is detected in plasma there could already be established end-organ disease in some patients. This highlights the clinical significance of low CMV VL values below 1000 copies/ml in some patients. Where there is uncertainty regarding the relevance of low CMV VL values, follow up testing should be done, particularly if a patient's clinical condition is not improving on appropriate therapy. The detection of CMV VLs during follow up in patients who initially had undetectable viral loads supports the practice of measuring CMV VL in the site of pathology where CMV infection may cause disease before it is detectable in the blood [25–27]. The site to be sampled should be determined by the patient's clinical condition.

The majority of patients presented to ICU with pulmonary disease, mainly community acquired pneumonia. Although CMV can cause pneumonitis in immunosuppressed individuals [2], it is not known if it was the primary cause of pneumonia in this study as CMV disease was not proven by cytology/histology except in two patients who had post-mortem results. Interestingly, confirmed TB infections were higher in the ET group, which had the lowest mortality than the other groups; and the logistic regression analysis identified CMV VL as the only variable associated with mortality. This highlights that CMV infections play a more independent role towards mortality in the setting of high viral loads [13,28,29]. The absence of the CMV retinitis diagnosis in this cohort is surprising; however, this could have been missed as patients' ophthalmology assessment was done without pupil dilatation, and not done by ophthalmologists. Also a recently published South African study showed a low incidence of CMV retinitis in the era of ART [30].

The strengths of this study include the availability of serial CMV VL measurements before treatment initiation in some patients and availability of clinical data (including time to discharge or death). Limitations include the small sample size, inclusion of patients with HIV/AIDS in an ICU setting only, unavailability of CMV VL testing in other samples other than plasma, and that post-mortem data was only available for two patients. The data on the rate of CMV VL increase from lower to higher values should be interpreted with caution as follow up testing was not done at the same regular intervals. Different CMV VL assays used in different laboratories could have influenced results as there was no standardisation of testing. Other opportunistic infectious diseases such as toxoplasmosis were not excluded.

Conclusion

This study has for the first time provided data on CMV VL kinetics in patients with HIV/AIDS admitted to ICU. It showed a significantly increased mortality in patients with HIV/AIDS who had high CMV VLs, and suggests that a threshold value of 1000 copies/ml may be appropriate for pre-emptive treatment in this group of patients. Further studies are needed to confirm the relevance of this threshold.

Table 2. Clinical characteristics of patients who had undetectable CMV VL at baseline.

Study ID	Age	Sex	CD4 count	CMVVLr results and dates (dd/mm/yy)	Ganciclovir initiation date (dd/mm/yy)	Death in ICU and dates (dd/mm/yy)	Group
76	30	M	6	LDL 31/01/11; 2120 01/02/11; 28200 09/02/11	17/02/11	No	DT
8063	40	M	9	LDL 21/05/11; 3820 10/06/11; 4860 17/06/11	17/06/11	No	ET
5558	14	F	5	LDL 27/10/10; 1360 23/11/10; ND	24/11/11	Yes 20/12/10	ET
3938	30	F	8	LDL 02/06/10; LDL 05/06/10; 3000 28/07/10	N/A	No	nt-LVL
7473	49	M	25	LDL 08/09/11; 1590 21/09/11; ND	29/09/11	No	ET
6279	45	M	49	LDL 17/02/10; 4770 02/03/10; ND	N/A	No	nt-LVL
3825	42	M	45	LDL 24/12/09; 14600 09/02/10; ND	15/02/10	No	DT
2120	40	M	54	LDL 17/03/10; 880 26/03/10; ND	N/A	Yes 28/03/10	nt-LVL
3032	47	F	75	LDL 20/10/11; LDL 30/10/11; 4680 23/11/11	N/A	No	nt-LVL
276	49	F	29	LDL 28/06/12; 835 04/07/12; ND	N/A	Yes 06/07/12	nt-LVL
6057	46	F	105	LDL 19/01/12; 44 04/02/12; LDL 04/03/12	N/A	No	nt-LVL
3791	43	F	2	LDL 23/12/09; 29200 30/01/10; ND	08/02/10	No	DT

ID = identity, CMV VL = cytomegalovirus viral load, ICU = intensive care unit, ET = early treatment, DT = delayed treatment, nt-LVL = non-treatment and low viral load, ND = not done, N/A – ganciclovir was not administered as some of these patients were admitted at a time when a 10000 copies/ml threshold for CMV treatment was used, LDL = lower than detectable limit. For consistency, sample collection dates were used for CMV VL results.

Table 3. Characteristics of patients in different groups stratified by CMV VL of 5100 copies/ml and ganciclovir use.

	TREATMENT GROUPS		NON-TREATMENT GROUPS	
	ET	DT	nt-LVL	nt-HVL
	(<5100 copies/ml)	(>5100 copies/ml)	(<5100 copies/ml)	(>5100 copies/ml)
	n = 9	n = 12	n = 15	n = 5
Median age (IQR)	38	34	37	35
	(33–46)	(30–43)	(32–46)	(23–57)
Median CD4 count (IQR)	6	5.5	49	33
	(3–29)	(2–40)	(29–75)	(16–103)
Median CMV VL (IQR)[†]	2690	22150	990	100000
	(1590–4700)	(13000–35900)	(651–3000)	(6655–113000)
Confirmed TB infections	67%	25%	57%	25%
Steroid use	67%	83%	80%	80%
Mortality in ICU	44%	58%	50%	100%

ET = early treatment, DT = delayed treatment, nt-LVL = non-treatment and low viral load, nt-HVL = non-treatment and high viral load, TB = tuberculosis, ICU = intensive care unit.
[†] = highest CMV VL values per patient were used for this analysis.

Acknowledgments

We would like to thank the medical ICU discussion group(s) for their participation in the management of the study participants.

Author Contributions

Conceived and designed the experiments: SHM MB DMM AHM RTM SASO GRT AS. Performed the experiments: SHM MB DMM AHM RTM SASO GRT AS. Analyzed the data: SHM MB DMM AHM RTM SASO GRT AS. Contributed reagents/materials/analysis tools: SHM MB DMM AHM RTM SASO GRT AS. Wrote the paper: SHM MB DMM AHM RTM SASO GRT AS.

References

1. Atkinson C, Emery VC (2011) Cytomegalovirus quantification: Where to next in optimising patient management? J Clin Virol 51: 223–8.
2. Sundar IK (2004) Update: cytomegalovirus infection in HIV-infected patients – a review. Clin Microbiol Newsl 26: 137–44.
3. Mocarski Jr ES, Shenk T, Pass RF (2007) Cytomegaloviruses. In: Knipe DM, Howley PM, Griffin DE, Lamb RA, Martin MA, Roizman B, et al, editors. Fields Virology. 5th ed. Philadelphia: Lippincot Williams & Wilkins, a Wolters Kluwer business. pp. 2701–72.
4. Barron MA, Weinberg A (2005) Common viral infections in transplant recipients, part 1. Herpesviruses. Clin Microbiol Newsl 27: 99–106.
5. De la Hoz RE, Stephens G, Sherlock C (2002) Diagnosis and treatment approaches of CMV infections in adult patients. J Clin Virol 25: 1–12.
6. Li H, Dummer JS, Estes WR, Meng S, Wright PF, et al. (2003) Measurement of Human Cytomegalovirus Loads by Quantitative Real-Time PCR for Monitoring Clinical Intervention in Tranplant Recipients. J Clin Microbiol 41: 187–91.
7. Halfon P, Berger P, Khiri H, Martineau A, Pénaranda G, et al. (2011) Algorithm based on CMV kinetics DNA viral load for preemptive therapy initiation after hematopoietic cell transplantation. J Med Virol 83: 490–5.
8. Martín-Gandul C, Pérez-Romero P, Sánchez M, Bernal G, Suárez G, et al. (2013) Determination, validation and standardization of a CMV DNA cut-off value in plasma for preemptive treatment of CMV infection in solid organ transplant recipients at lower risk for CMV infection. J Clin Virol 56: 13–18.
9. Robberts FJL, Liebowitz LD, Chalkley LJ (2007) Polymerase chain reaction detection of Pneumocystis jiroveci: evaluation of 9 assays. Diagn Microbiol Infect Dis 58: 385–92.
10. Ayoub T, Chow J (2008) The conventional autopsy in modern medicine. J R Soc Med 101: 177–181.
11. Bloch EM, Vermeulen M, Murphy E (2012) Blood Transfusion Safety in Africa: A Literature Review of Infectious Disease and Organizational Challenges. Transfus Med Rev 26: 164–80.
12. Preiser W, Bräuninger S, Schwerdtfeger R, Ayliffe U, Garson JA, et al. (2001) Evaluation of diagnostic methods for the detection of cytomegalovirus in recipients of allogeneic stem cell transplants. J Clin Virol 20: 59–70.
13. De Keyzer K, Van Laecke S, Peeters P, Vanholder R (2011) Human Cytomegalovirus and Kidney Transplantation: A Clinician's Update. Am J Kidney Dis 58: 118–26.
14. Griffiths PD (2012) Burden of disease associated with human cytomegalovirus and prospects for elimination by universal immunisation. Lancet Infect Dis 12: 790–8.
15. Levitsky J, Freifeld AG, Puumala S, Bargenquast K, Hardiman P, et al. (2008) Cytomegalovirus viremia in solid organ transplantation: does the initial viral load correlate with risk factors and outcomes? Clin Transplant 22: 222–8.
16. Fielding K, Koba A, Grant AD, Charalambous S, Day J, et al. (2011) Cytomegalovirus Viremia as a Risk Factor for Mortality Prior to Antiretroviral Therapy among HIV-Infected Gold Miners in South Africa. PLoS One 6: e25571.
17. Boffi El Amari E, Combescure C, Yerly S, Calmy A, Kaiser L, et al. (2011) Clinical relevance of cytomegalovirus viraemia. HIV Med 12: 394–402.
18. Durier N, Ananworanich J, Apornpong T, Ubolyam S, Kerr SJ, et al. (2013) Cytomegalovirus Viremia in Thai HIV-Infected Patients on Antiretroviral Therapy: Prevalence and Associated Mortality. CID 57: 147–55.
19. Mizushima D, Nishijima T, Gatanaga H, Tsukada K, Teruya K, et al. (2013) Preemptive Therapy Prevents Cytomegalovirus End-Organ Disease in Treatment-Naive Patients with Advanced HIV-1 Infection in the HAART Era. PLoS One 8: e65348.
20. Spector SA, McKinley GF, Lalezari JP, Samo T, Andruczk R, et al. (1996) Oral Ganciclovir for the Prevention of Cytomegalovirus Disease in Persons with AIDS. N Engl J Med 334: 1491–7.
21. Ruell J, Barnes C, Mutton K, Foulkes B, Chang J, et al. (2007) Active CMV disease does not always correlate with viral load detection. Bone Marrow Transpl 40: 55–61.
22. Rasmussen L, Zipeto D, Wolitz RA, Dowling A, Efron B, et al. (1997) Risk for Retinitis in Patients with AIDS Can Be Assessed by Quantitation of Threshold Levels of Cytomegalovirus DNA Burden in Blood. JID 176: 1146–55.
23. Metras D, Viard L, Kreitmann B, Riberi A, Pannetier-Mille A, et al. (1999) Lung infections in pediatric lung transplantation: experience in 49 cases. Eur J Cardio-Thorac 15: 490–5.
24. Eid AJ, Arthurs SK, Deziel PJ, Wilhelm MP, Razonable RR (2010) Clinical Predictors of Relapse after Treatment of Primary Gastrointestinal Cytomegalovirus Disease in Solid Organ Transplant Recipients. Am J Transplant 10: 157–61.
25. Chemaly RF, Yen-Lieberman B, Castilla EA, Reilly A, Arrigain S, et al. (2004) Correlation between Viral Loads of Cytomegalovirus in Blood and Bronchoalveolar Lavage Specimens from Lung Transplant Recipients Determined by Histology and Immunohistochemistry. J Clin Microbiol 42: 2168–72.
26. Ganzenmueller T, Henke-Gendo C, Schlué J, Wedemeyer J, Huebner S, et al. (2009) Quantification of cytomegalovirus DNA levels in intestinal biopsies as a diagnostic tool for CMV intestinal disease. J Clin Virol 46: 254–8.

27. Henke-Gendo C, Ganzenmueller T, Kluba J, Harste G, Raggub L, et al. (2012) Improved Quantitative PCR Protocols for Adenovirus and CMV With an Internal Inhibition Control System and Automated Nucleic Acid Isolation. J Med Virol 84: 890–6.

28. Gallant JE, Moore RD, Richman DD, Keruly J, Chaisson RE, et al. (1992) Incidence and Natural History of Cytomegalovirus Disease in Patients with Advanced Human Immunodeficiency Virus Disease Treated with Zidovudine. JID 166; 1223–7.

29. Spector AS, Wong R, Hsia K, Pilcher M, Stempien MJ (1998) Plasma Cytomegalovirus (CMV) DNA Load Predicts CMV Disease and Survival in AIDS Patients. J Clin Invest 101: 497–502.

30. Laher F, Cullen C, Matlala JB (2012) Localised treatment and 6-month outcomes in patients with cytomegalovirus retinitis at a tertiary ophthalmology service in Ga-Rankuwa. S Afr J HIV Med 13: 68–71.

Survival of Skin Graft between Transgenic Cloned Dogs and Non-Transgenic Cloned Dogs

Geon A Kim[1], Hyun Ju Oh[1], Min Jung Kim[1], Young Kwang Jo[1], Jin Choi[1], Jung Eun Park[1], Eun Jung Park[1], Sang Hyun Lim[2], Byung Il Yoon[3], Sung Keun Kang[2], Goo Jang[1], Byeong Chun Lee[1]*

1 Department of Theriogenology & Biotechnology, College of Veterinary Medicine, Seoul National University, Seoul, Republic of Korea, 2 Central Research Institutes, K-stem cell, Seoul, Republic of Korea, 3 Laboratory of Histology and Molecular Pathogenesis, College of Veterinary Medicine, Kangwon National University, Chuncheon, Gangwon-do, Republic of Korea

Abstract

Whereas it has been assumed that genetically modified tissues or cells derived from somatic cell nuclear transfer (SCNT) should be accepted by a host of the same species, their immune compatibility has not been extensively explored. To identify acceptance of SCNT-derived cells or tissues, skin grafts were performed between cloned dogs that were identical except for their mitochondrial DNA (mtDNA) haplotypes and foreign gene. We showed here that differences in mtDNA haplotypes and genetic modification did not elicit immune responses in these dogs: 1) skin tissues from genetically-modified cloned dogs were successfully transplanted into genetically-modified cloned dogs with different mtDNA haplotype under three successive grafts over 63 days; and 2) non-transgenic cloned tissues were accepted into transgenic cloned syngeneic recipients with different mtDNA haplotypes and vice versa under two successive grafts over 63 days. In addition, expression of the inserted gene was maintained, being functional without eliciting graft rejection. In conclusion, these results show that transplanting genetically-modified tissues into normal, syngeneic or genetically-modified recipient dogs with different mtDNA haplotypes do not elicit skin graft rejection or affect expression of the inserted gene. Therefore, therapeutically valuable tissue derived from SCNT with genetic modification might be used safely in clinical applications for patients with diseased tissues.

Editor: Pascale Chavatte-Palmer, INRA, France

Funding: This study was supported by Rural Development Administration (#PJ008975022014), Korea Institute of Planning and Evaluation for Technology (#311062-04-3SB010), NATURE CELL (#2014-0082), Research Institute for Veterinary Science, Nestle Purina PetCare, Natural Balance Korea, and the BK21 plus program. The funders had no role in study design, data collection and analysis, decision to publish, or preparation of the manuscript.

Competing Interests: The authors received funding from NATURE CELL CO., LTD, Nestle Purina PetCare, and Natural Balance Korea. There are no further patents, products in development or marketed products to declare.

* Email: bclee@snu.ac.kr

Introduction

Somatic cell nuclear transfer (SCNT) produces genetically identical cloned animals [1]. Moreover, canine SCNT combined with transgenic technologies can make genetically identical cloned dogs with functional genetic modifications that could be used for gene therapy [2]. For example, transgenic cloned dogs could be used in replacement of diseased (malfunctioning/worn out) organs. However, tissues derived from transgenic cloned dogs, reprogrammed from somatic cells with enucleated oocytes, had not yet investigated whether they are immunologically identical tissues or cell sources of transplantation. Especially, effects of red fluorescent protein (RFP) expression using genetically identical animal models derived from SCNT have not been described and this is a critical subject since RFP has been used as a potential marker for clinical trials of gene therapy [3–5].

In addition, SCNT uses oocytes from animals unrelated to the prospective transplant recipient, oocyte-derived mitochondrial DNA (mtDNA) derived antigen could lead to rejection problems in kidney transplant [6] or not in skin transplant [7,8]. Although tissues derived from SCNT, using the recipient's somatic cells as nuclear donors, provide identical genetics, the absence of immune rejection has not yet been confirmed in cloned dogs.

To our knowledge, no previous report has mentioned *in vivo* skin immune responses against tissue expressing foreign gene or the capable effects of mitochondrial derived minor antigen in cloned animals. Here, we firstly evaluated the anti-foreign gene or minor antigen derived immune responses in cloned dogs with the following design: (1) for investigation of mtDNA derived antigen compatibility, skin graft was performed between transgenic cloned dogs with different mtDNA haplotypes; (2) furthermore, skin graft was also performed between transgenic cloned dogs and non-transgenic cloned dogs for examination of immunogenicity of foreign gene.

Materials and Methods

1. Animals

Two genetically identical cloned female beagles (C1, C2) were generated by SCNT using a beagle fetal fibroblast cell line (BF3) described in a previously study [9]. Transgenic cloned female beagles (R1, R2, R3 and R5) were also produced by SCNT using BF3 transfected with RFP [2].

Non-related controls (Co1, Co2) were healthy age-matched normal female beagles purchased from commercial kennels (Marshall Beijing Biotech Ltd., Beijing, China). All animals used in this study were cared for in accordance with recommendations described in "The Guide for the Care and Use of Laboratory Animals" published by the Institutional Animal Care and Use Committee (IACUC) of Seoul National University (approval number; SNU-110915-2). Dog housing facilities and the procedures performed met or exceeded the standards established by the Committee for Accreditation of Laboratory Animal Care. All surgery was performed under isoflurane anesthesia, and all efforts were made to minimize suffering.

2. DNA extractions and PCR reaction

Blood was collected from two control beagles and six female cloned beagles 4 years of age for DNA extractions, blood typing and blood cross-matching. Approximately 10 ml of blood were collected from the jugular vein into tubes containing EDTA as anticoagulant and used for peripheral blood mononuclear cell isolation and DNA extraction, and 3 ml of blood in plain tubes were collected to provide serum samples for antibody levels. Blood samples were kept at 38°C to maintain cell viability.

Freshly retrieved non-coagulated blood samples were mixed with RBC lysis buffer (Invitrogen, Carlsbad, CA, USA) at room temperature for 15 min. Genomic DNA was isolated according to the manufacturer's protocol. Extracted DNA samples were stored at −30°C. DLA class I (MHC class I) and II (MHC class II) typing analysis was performed by means of PCR and sequencing. The polymorphic exon 2 and exon 3 of the DLA-88 gene was amplified using PCR primers [10]. The polymorphic exon 2 of the DRB1, DQA and DQB genes was also amplified using PCR primers [11]. For PCR, Maxime PCR PreMix kit (iNtRON Biotechnology, Inc., Gyeongi, Korea) was used. In each PCR tube, 1 μl of genomic DNA, 1 μl (10 pM/μl) of forward primer, 1 μl (10 pM/μl) of reverse primer and 17 μl of sterilized distilled water were added according to the manufacturer's instructions. These components were then mixed and centrifuged briefly. PCR was done using a PCR machine (Biometra, Goettingen, Germany). PCR amplification was carried out for 1 cycle with denaturing at 94°C for 5 min, and subsequently for 30 cycles with denaturing at 94°C for 40 sec, annealing at 63°C (DLA-DRB1), 55°C (DLA-DQA1) and 66°C (DLA-DQB1) for 40 sec, extension at 72°C for 40 sec, and a final extension at 72°C for 5 min. Amplified PCR product was run on the gel by gel electrophoresis (Mupid-exu, Submarine electrophoresis system, Advance, Japan) at 100 V for 20 min. A 2% agarose gel was prepared using agarose (Invitrogen) and 1X TAE buffer. The stain (RedSafe, iNtRON Biotechnology Inc.) was used at a concentration of 2.5 μl per 50 ml of gel. After running gels, images were made under ultraviolet light. PCR product was sequenced directly using the Big Dye Terminator kit (Applied Biosystems, Foster City, CA, USA). Sequencing was performed on an automated DNA sequencer model 377 or capillary model 3110 (Applied Biosystems).

3. Sequencing of Mitochondrial DNA haplotype

For mitochondrial DNA analysis, the oligonucleotide primers were synthesized over the hypervariable regions (forward, 5′-CCTAAGACTTCAAGGAAGAAGC-3′; reverse, 5′-TTGACT-GAATAGCACCTTGA-3′) of the complete nucleotide sequence of canine mtDNA (GenBank accession no. U96639). Isolated genomic DNA sample were dissolved in 50 ul TE buffer and used for PCR amplifications. It were performed in a 50 μl volume containing 5 μl of 10× reaction buffer containing 1.5 mM MgCl2, 0.2 mM dNTPs, 0.2 μM each primer, 1.5 U Taq DNA polymerase (Intron, Kyunggi, Korea). Starting denaturing for 1 cycle at 95°C for 3 minutes, subsequently denaturation at 94°C for 30 seconds, annealing at 57°C for 30 seconds, extension at 72°C for

Table 1. Mitochondrial DNA sequences of non-transgenic cloned dog (C2) and four transgenic cloned dogs (R1, R2, R3 and R5).

Sample	Nucleotide positions																					
	15435	15483	15508	15526	15595	15611	15612	15620	15627	15632	15639	15643	15650	15652	15781	15800	15814	15815	15912	15955	16025	16083
Reference[1]	G	C	C	C	C	T	T	T	A	C	T	A	T	G	C	T	C	T	C	C	T	A
C2	G	C	C	C	T	T	T	A	A	C	G	G	T	A	C	T	C	T	C	C	T	A
R1	G	C	C	C	C	C	T	A	A	C	T	A	T	G	C	T	T	T	C	T	T	A
R2	G	C	C	C	C	T	T	A	A	C	A	A	A	G	C	T	T	T	C	C	C	A
R3	G	C	C	C	C	T	T	C	G	C	A	A	A	G	C	T	T	T	C	T	T	A
R5	G	T	C	C	C	T	T	T	G	C	A	A	A	G	C	T	T	T	C	C	T	A

GenBank accession number :U96639 (Kim et al., 1998).

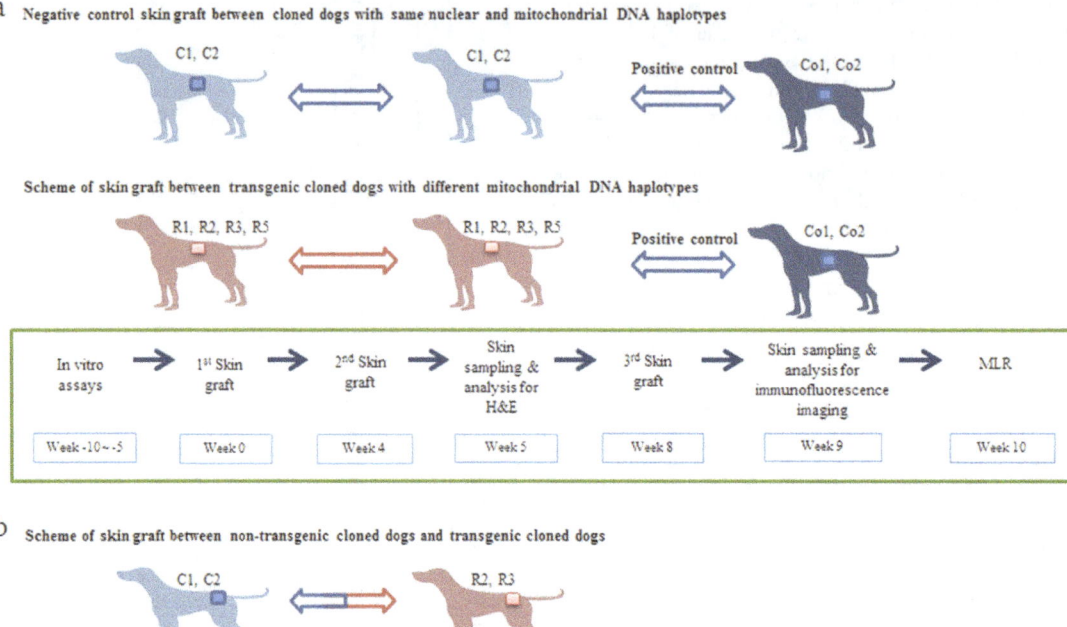

Figure 1. Experimental design and image analysis result between cloned dogs. (a) Experimental design and timeline of skin graft between cloned dogs with different mitochondrial haplotypes. As negative control, auto grafts as well as cloned dogs with same mtDNA haplotype (C1, C2) were used. Before skin graft, all *in vitro* assays were performed. For H&E staining, immunofluorescence imaging, 1st skin graft fragments were analyzed. (b) Experimental design and timeline between transgenic cloned dogs and non-transgenic cloned dogs. Before skin graft, all *in vitro* assays were performed. All dogs were tested twice for each skin graft, then skin samplings were performed. For immunofluorescence imaging, 1st skin graft fragments were analyzed. RFP expression were monitored until 63 days after skin graft.

30 seconds of 35 cycles, and a final extension at 72°C for 3 minutes were carried out. After purification of PCR products using a Gel Extraction Kit (Qiagen, Hilden, Germany), they were sequenced with an ABI3100 instrument (Applied Biosystems). Their identities with mtDNA were confirmed by BLAST search (http://blast.ncbi. nlm.nih.gov/).

4. Blood crossmatching and blood typing

Blood collection was performed from the jugular vein of all cloned dogs (R1, R2, R3, R5, C1 and C2) into an evacuated tube containing EDTA as anticoagulant. Collected samples were submitted to a commercial laboratory kit (Antech Diagnostics, Phoenix, AZ, USA). Blood type was confirmed using the tube agglutination method with antiserum; consisting of 6 types of monoclonal antibodies for canine blood typing [12].

The blood crossmatching test was done on EDTA-treated blood using the tube agglutination method. Isolated RBCs of all dogs were washed 3 times with 0.9% saline, and a 4% RBC suspension was made from the washed cells. RBC suspensions from cloned beagles (C1) were combined with equal volumes of another cloned beagle's serum (C2) and the reverse reaction was also performed. All mixtures were incubated at 37°C for 20 min, centrifuged and then assessed for hemolysis or agglutination. Agglutination was evaluated by comparing the color of supernatant in the test tube with those of the control sample. Each sample was shaken until all red blood cells in the "button" at the bottom of the tube had

become suspended. Again, the degree of RBC clumping of the test sample was compared with that of the auto-mixture of RBC and plasma. When the plasma was clear, no clumping of RBCs was detected at 400× magnification, these results were considered as negative. A positive result showed agglutination resembling stacked coins. Images were obtained using a microscope, the ProgRes Capture camera system, and the ProgRes Capture 2.6 software (JENOPTIK, Jena, Germany).

5. Peripheral blood mononuclear cell isolation and mixed lymphocyte reactions

Blood was collected from two control dogs and six female cloned dogs before and 10 weeks after skin graft. EDTA-treated whole blood was transferred to 50 ml conical centrifuge tubes. An equal volume of phosphate buffered solution (PBS, Gibco, Carlsbad, CA, USA) was mixed with the sample prior to the isolation process. Peripheral blood mononuclear cells (PBMC) were isolated from EDTA-treated blood using lymphocyte separation medium on a Ficoll-paque gradient (Ficoll-Paque Plus, GE Healthcare, Pittsburgh, PA, USA). Mixed lymphocyte reactions were modified from the previous reports [13–15]. Washed cells were diluted in culture medium (RPMI1640, Gibco) supplemented with 10% FBS to 2×10^6 cells/ml. To stimulate proliferation of lymphocytes, PBMCs were preincubated with 2 ug/ml of phytohemagglutin for 24 h before mix reaction. Then 50 ul of this cell suspension was added into each well of a 96-well

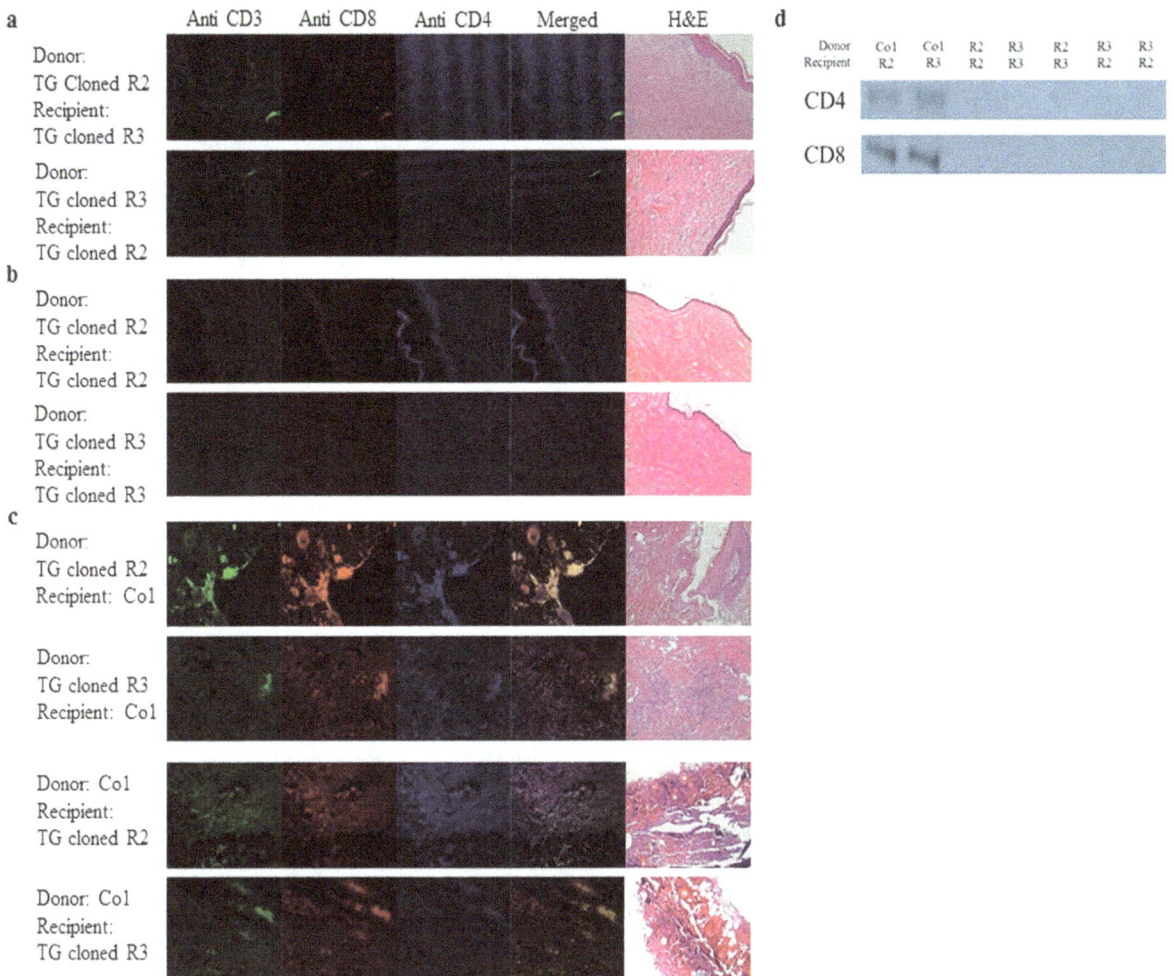

Figure 2. Absence of *in vivo* immunogenicity in skin grafts between cloned dogs with different mitochondrial DNA sequences. No evidence with infiltration of T cell was detected in the skin segments transplanted into the recipient dogs with different mitochondrial haplotypes (a). Sections from skin segments of autografts were used as negative controls (b). Sections from skin segments of cloned dogs transplanted into control dogs were used as positive controls (c). Western blot analysis confirms high protein levels of CD4 and CD8 in the positive controls, whereas CD4 and CD8 expression intensities were significantly lower in allograft of cloned dogs with different mitochondrial haplotypes (d). Upper lane indicates the donor dog and lower lane means recipient dog.

microplate except for the wells required for the blank and cultured at $37.5°C$ in a water-saturated atmosphere containing 5% CO_2. Each cell combination was tested in quadruplicate in a flat-bottomed micro plate containing 0.1 ml of culture medium per well. The mixture was cultured for 5 days and then pyrimidine analogue, bromodeoxyuridine labeling reagent (Cell proliferation ELISA, Roche Applied Science, Indianapolis, IN, USA) was added and re-incubated for 24 h. After removing the labeling medium, results are expressed as absorbance units at 450 nm wavelength read by a micro plate reader, Sunrise (Tecan Sunrise, Hayward, CA, USA). Time-course kinetics was studied by harvesting on day 7 of culture.

6. DNA walking

For confirmation of the transgene (RFP) location, PCR was performed with a DNA Walking SpeedUP Kit (Seegene Inc., Seoul, Korea) and products were gel purified (QIAquick PCR purification kit; QIAGEN, Valencia, CA, USA), and DNA strands were directly sequenced (Macrogen, Seoul, Korea; http://www.

macrogen.com) using a custom-synthesized primer (5′-TCACA-GAAGTATGCCAAGCGA-3′). The sequences, except for known sequences, including primers of each product were aligned by sequence homology analysis using the Basic Local Alignment Search Tool (BLAST) at the National Center for Biotechnology Information (NCBI) GenBank (http://blast.ncbi.nlm.nih.gov/).

7. Skin graft

For skin graft procedures, experimental dogs were anesthetized with ketamine hydrochloride (6 mg/kg) after pretreatment with xylazine (0.05 mg/kg), and were maintained with 2% isoflurane in oxygen. A flank skin segment 1.5 cm×1.5 cm was excised from each donor dog. Simultaneously, the same sized skin piece was excised from recipient dogs, and the excised skin was grafted by suturing into the graft bed of the same region of an anesthetized recipient dog. Bandages were changed every day after surgery and the grafts were observed weekly.

For examination of effects mtDNA haplotypes differences among cloned dogs, skin grafts of three times were performed

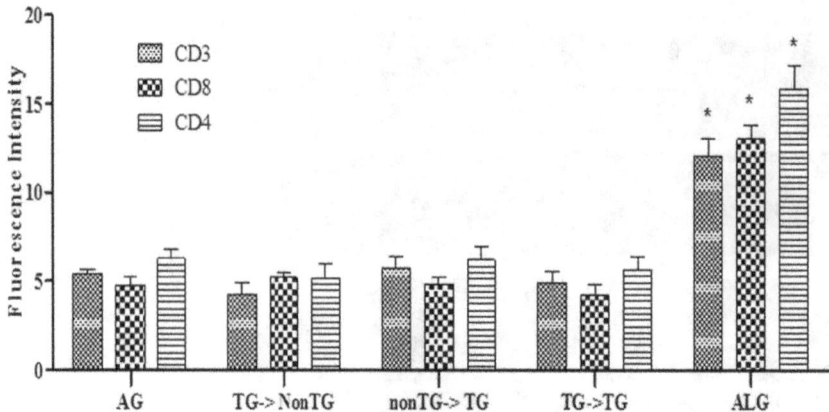

Figure 3. Expression levels of CD3, CD4 and CD8 of skin grafts between cloned dogs using fluorescence image analysis. Immunological response level of CD3, CD4 and CD8 were similar in AG (autograft), TG-> NonTG (donor: transgenic dog, recipient: non-transgenic cloned dogs), NonTG->TG (donor: non-transgenic dog, recipient: transgenic cloned dogs) and TG cloned dogs (donor: transgenic dog, recipient: transgenic cloned dogs). However, Both of ALG (allograft) between TG dogs and non-related control dogs and allograft between non-TG dogs and non-related control dogs shows significantly higher intensity of immunological response (p<0.05). Results are presented as mean ± SEM. Replication number is at least 8 times.

every 4 weeks between non-transgenic cloned dogs with same mtDNA haplotype and between transgenic cloned dogs with disparate mtDNA haplotypes. Accepted tissues were maintained until 9 weeks after skin graft. Biopsies of skin were performed after 63 days after first skin graft. A flank skin segment of 1st graft with size of 0.5 cm×1.5 cm including donor and recipient tissue were excised for H&E staining at 5 weeks of skin graft and remnant tissue were excised for immunofluorescence imaging and western blot at later.

8. Histological and immunofluorescence analysis

Immuno-staining of canine skin immune cells was carried out on formaldehyde-fixed sections using a rabbit monoclonal antibody to CD3 (1:100, ab94756, Abcam, Cambridge, MA, USA), visualized with an anti-rabbit polyclonal DyLight 488 (1:200, ab96895, Abcam) antibody. In these sections, CD4 and CD8 cells were counterstained with a CD4 (1:100, LS c122857, Lifespan Bioscience Inc., Seattle, WA, USA) and CD8 (1:200, ab22505, Abcam) specific antibody detected with a DyLight 405 (1:200, 3069-1, Abcam) and DyLight 649 (1:200, ab98389, Abcam) coupled secondary antibody. Skin sections were also processed for assessing expression of RFP using rabbit polyclonal RFP antibody (1:200, ab62341, Abcam) and visualized with an anti-rabbit polyclonal DyLight 488 (1:200, ab96895, Abcam) antibody. Sections were counterstained with 4′, 6′-diamidino-2-phenylindole (DAPI).

Histology was done by fixing skin fragment in 4% neutral formalin and embedding in paraffin; sections were stained with standard hematoxylin and eosin (H&E) procedures. Fluorescent and bright field images were obtained with a Leica DMI 6000B microscope using a DFC350 camera and LAS software (Leica Microsystems Pty Ltd., North Ryde, Australia) and analyzed by a computer-assisted image analysis system (Metamorph version 6.3r2; Molecular Devices Corporation, PA, USA). To maintain a constant threshold for each image and to compensate for subtle variability of the immune-fluorescent imaging, we only counted cells that were at least 70% lighter than the average level of each positive control image after background subtraction. All image analytical procedures described above were performed blind without knowledge of the experimental scheme.

9. Western blot

Skin fragments of graft was excised and homogenized in PRO-PREP protein extraction solution (iNtRON Biotechnology, Inc.) using a tissue homogenizer. After measuring protein concentration using Nanodrop 2000 (Thermo fischer scientific, Seoul, Korea), equal amounts of proteins were loaded on 10% SDS-PAGE. Proteins were electrophoresed and blotted onto polyvinylidene fluoride membranes. The membranes were blocked with 5% skim milk in TBS with 0.1% Tween-20 and incubated with primary antibodies for 2 hours at room temperature. Monoclonal CD4 and CD8 antibodies were used as markers for immune rejection. Subsequently, membranes were incubated with goat anti-mouse IgG, anti-rat IgG (Pierce, Rockford, IL, USA) with horse radish peroxidase conjugation for 1 h at room temperature. Then, WEST-one™ Western blot detection system (iNtRON Biotechnology, Inc.) was added and visualized after exposing the membrane to X-ray film.

10. Statistical Analysis

The data of mixed lymphocyte reaction, image analysis of immunocytochemistry and western blot were analyzed using one-way ANOVA and a protected least significant different (LSD) test using general linear models to determine differences among experimental groups. Data were analyzed using GraphPad Prism software (GraphPad Software Inc., San Diego, CA, USA). Absorbance mean values were considered significantly different when the P-value was less than 0.05. The observations of mixed lymphocyte reaction among experimental groups were replicated at least 8 times.

Results and Discussions

It has been reported that immune rejection can occur when tissues of genetically identical SCNT cloned animals were transplanted to each other, due to the tissues having different maternally-derived antigens [6,16,17]. Antigens derived from mtDNA in accelerated skin rejection in syngeneic rodent recipients [18,19]. It has also been generally assumed that genetically-engineered tissues with insertion of a foreign gene could invoke immune-rejection by the recipient even in inbred mice [20]. Using embryonic stem cells derived from SCNT, the complete rescues of

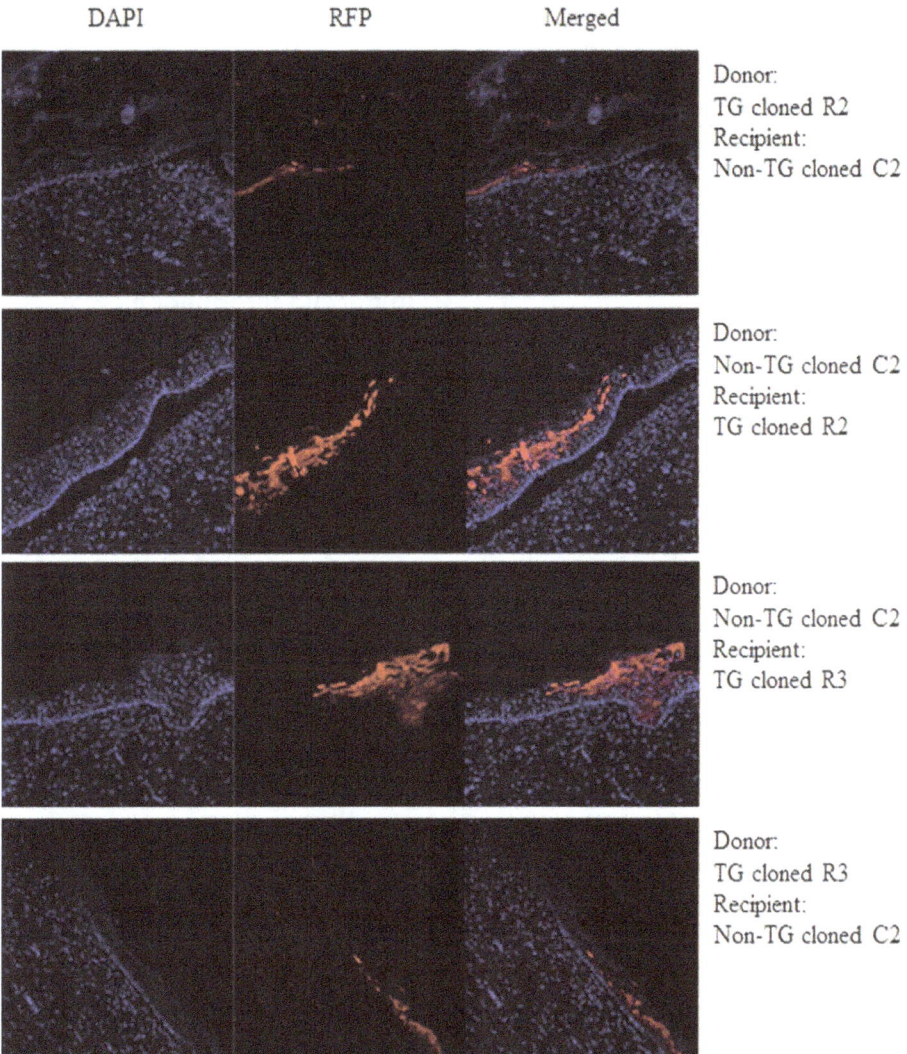

Figure 4. Maintenance of foreign gene expression between transgenic cloned beagle with foreign genes and non-transgenic cloned dogs. No expression of foreign gene in non-transgenic dog (C2) recipient was maintained in skin graft of transgenic cloned dog (R2). The limit between donor and recipient were not changed until 63 days after skin graft.

genetic defect with genetically-engineered cell therapy were not observed [21]. Engraftment of hematopoietic precursor cells differentiated from SCNT or induced pluripotent stem cells (iPSCs) was only successful in the absence of natural killer cells and immunogenicity of iPSCs was reported [21–23].

In the present study, cloned dogs produced by SCNT had different mtDNA haplotypes (Table 1), because canine SCNT used oocytes obtained from several oocyte donor dogs and the oocyte mtDNA was still present after the SCNT procedure. To examine the immunogenicity of skin tissue derived from syngeneic grafts exhibiting different mtDNA haplotypes, we initially performed *in vitro* molecular typing of dog leukocyte antigen (DLA), mixed lymphocyte reaction (MLR) and blood cross-matching using cells derived from cloned dogs with different mtDNA haplotypes (Fig. S1). Despite the different mtDNA haplotypes, they had no effects on *in vitro* immunological compatibility.

To gain insights into the therapeutic applicability of canine skin tissues with different mtDNA haplotypes, skin grafting between cloned dogs was performed to determine immunological compatibility *in vivo* (Fig. 1). Whereas allogeneic Co 1 (non-related control dogs) skin fragments were rapidly rejected in R2 (transgenic cloned dog) and R3 (transgenic cloned dog) recipients with massive infiltration of CD4+, CD8+ T cells, infiltration, edema and perivascular inflammation 7 days after 2nd skin graft, skin tissues of R2 and R3 were accepted in R3 and R2 recipients as well as autografts, without any evidence of immune rejection (Fig. 2). Likewise, skin segments from cloned dogs with different mtDNA sequences did not induce immune rejection in the recipient cloned dogs (Fig. S2). In MLR of 10 weeks after 3rd skin graft, we couldn't detect any sign of mtDNA derived minor antigen immunogenicity with no significant differences compared to those of MLR before skin graft (data not shown).

In mice, mtDNA encoded proteins could elicit rejection by innate immunity in a setting where the genomic DNA matched [24,25]. Furthermore, kidneys transplanted between cloned pigs differing in some mtDNA genes rejected those grafts [6]. Therefore, different antigenicity of grafts from different tissues could be also considered. In our experiment, despite a high level of diversity of mtDNA haplotypes heteroplasmy among domestic dogs [26], skin grafts were successfully accepted in at least 20 donor-recipient combinations. In cattle and pigs, it was shown that SCNT-derived tissues were not rejected by the immune system of the nucleus donor after SCNT in skin graft [7,27,28]. Our findings suggest that differences of canine mtDNA haplotypes could not elicit skin graft rejection among cloned dogs, as previously observed in cattle and pigs.

We also showed genetic identity between tissues of non-transgenic cloned dogs (C1, C2) derived from beagle fibroblasts (BF3) [9] and tissues of transgenic cloned dogs (R1, R2, R3 and R5) derived from BF3 transfected with RFP (Table S1.) [2]. Immunological compatibility between these dogs was completely established through *in vitro* tests such as DLA typing and MLR (Fig. S1). Skin tissues of non-transgenic cloned dogs were transplanted into transgenic cloned dogs and *vice-versa*. Skin tissues derived from cloned dogs were transplanted with no immune rejection, as determined by T cell infiltration of peri-graft skin sections after 7 days of 2nd skin graft. Despite insertion of the foreign gene RFP in transgenic cloned dogs, skin tissue from RFP transgenic cloned dogs was completely accepted in non-transgenic cloned dog recipients (Fig. 3, Fig. S3). These finding indicate that foreign gene insertion in cloned dogs did not induce a T cell-dependent skin graft rejection response in syngeneic recipients. It has been suggested that the nuclear reprogramming process in SCNT could result in surface expression of proteins and molecules unknown to the immune system of the graft recipients. In this regard, in inbred mice, enhanced GFP (eGFP) skin transplantation causes an acute reaction [29]. It was proved that eGFP also induce immune responses that interfere with its applicability in gene insertion of mouse [30]. However, our results suggest that inserted foreign gene, RFP has no immunological effects on the antigens of transgenic cloned dogs against to the non-transgenic cloned dogs. It also suggested that non-transgenic cloned dogs produced by SCNT using transfected cells have no immune regulatory effect on the host immune system and that the canine SCNT process did not result in surface expression of immunogenic molecules. Nonetheless, the possibility of immune rejection of other foreign genes, for example, pathogenically relevant transgene in clinical science remains to be confirmed.

Finally we examined whether functional expression of RFP was maintained in skin tissue grafts. During the course of this experiment, the expression level of RFP positive skin tissues were maintained for at least 63 days after surgery and RFP positive cells were detected in the epidermis, hair follicles and sebaceous glands (Fig. 4 and Table S1). It has been suggested that the co-expression of selection markers can limit or abrogate the persistence of expression of therapeutic genes [31,32]. The potential success of gene therapy or production of transgenic cloned dogs may depend on long-term transgene expression to cure or slow down the progression of disease. In addition, there were no host immune responses to the skin grafts among transgenic dogs and non-transgenic cloned dogs, and it appears that the level and duration of RFP transgene expression was not affected. This also indicates possible successful of therapeutic transplantation of tissues or cells derived from transgenic cloned dogs. In addition, the insertion site of the RFP gene into genomic DNA is not the same in all experimental dogs (Table S2). If the RFP gene insertion site can affect the immune response, it should affect the results of syngeneic skin grafting. However, no immune rejection was apparent in skin grafts with different transgene insertion sites. Our findings indicate that SCNT-derived somatic cells with or without foreign genes can be accepted in syngeneic recipients.

Our study established that tissues derived from canine SCNT can be accepted in syngeneic recipients despite different mtDNA haplotypes. We also provide evidence that skin segments containing a foreign gene are sufficiently acceptable to syngeneic recipients with or without the foreign gene. Taken together, these data indicate that SCNT using transgenic technology can support immunological compatibility between genetically engineered tissues and patients and thereby help to accelerate clinical therapeutic research and its applications.

Supporting Information

Figure S1   Immunological feature of transgenic dogs and non-transgenic dogs. (a) Molecular typing of dog leukocyte antigen, DLA-88 (MHC class I), DRB, DQA1, DQB1(MHC class II) polymorphic region in all cloned dogs (C1, C2, R1, R2, R3, and R5). (b) *In vitro* immunogenicity test using mixed lymphocyte reaction between all experimental dogs before skin graft. (c) Blood typing. (d) Analysis of blood crossmatching in all cloned dogs and control dogs.

Figure S2   Fluorescence image analysis of skin grafts between cloned dogs with different mtDNA haplotypes

Figure S3   Absence of *in vivo* immune rejection between non-transgenic dogs and transgenic dogs. (a) Positive control of skin graft, as donor skin segments were derived from non-related control dogs (Co1, Co2), they were completely rejected in the graft bed in transgenic cloned dogs (R2, R3). (b) However, skin grafts between a transgenic cloned dog, R2 and a non-transgenic cloned dog, C1 showed no apparent immune rejection. Similarly, as shown in (c) R2 - C2, (d) R3-C1, (e) R3-C2, there was no immune rejection in these grafts as well. (f) Western blot analysis of the skin graft between cloned dogs confirmed the expression of CD4 and CD8 protein only in the graft between cloned dogs and non-related control dogs.

Figure S4   Foreign gene expression between skin graft of two transgenic dogs (R2, R3). Red fluorescent protein expression in skin graft was maintained after 63 days skin graft in syngenic graft beds.

Table S1   Genetic background for microsatellite analysis of two non-transgenic cloned dogs and four transgenic cloned dogs.

Table S2   Insertion site of foreign gene, RFP in transgenic cloned dogs.

Acknowledgments

We thank Won Woo Lee for critical reading of the manuscript. We would also like to thank Dr, Barry D. Bavister for his valuable editing of the manuscript.

Author Contributions

Conceived and designed the experiments: GAK HJO MJK SKK GJ BCL. Performed the experiments: GAK YKJ JC JEP EJP SHL. Analyzed the data: GAK HJO BIY BCL. Contributed reagents/materials/analysis tools: JEP BIY BCL. Wrote the paper: GAK HJO SKK BCL.

References

1. Lee BC, Kim MK, Jang G, Oh HJ, Yuda F, et al. (2005) Dogs cloned from adult somatic cells. Nature 436: 641.
2. Hong SG, Kim MK, Jang G, Oh HJ, Park JE, et al. (2009) Generation of red fluorescent protein transgenic dogs. Genesis 47: 314–322.
3. Chang RS, Suh MS, Kim S, Shim G, Lee S, et al. (2011) Cationic drug-derived nanoparticles for multifunctional delivery of anticancer siRNA. Biomaterials 32: 9785–9795.
4. Lee CY, Li JF, Liou JS, Charng YC, Huang YW, et al. (2011) A gene delivery system for human cells mediated by both a cell-penetrating peptide and a piggyBac transposase. Biomaterials 32: 6264–6276.
5. Kinoshita Y, Kamitani H, Mamun MH, Wasita B, Kazuki Y, et al. (2010) A gene delivery system with a human artificial chromosome vector based on migration of mesenchymal stem cells towards human glioblastoma HTB14 cells. Neurol Res 32: 429–437.
6. Kwak HH, Park KM, Teotia PK, Lee GS, Lee ES, et al. (2013) Acute rejection after swine leukocyte antigen-matched kidney allo-transplantation in cloned miniature pigs with different mitochondrial DNA-encoded minor histocompatibility antigen. Transplant Proc 45: 1754–1760.
7. Martin MJ, Yin D, Adams C, Houtz J, Shen J, et al. (2003) Skin graft survival in genetically identical cloned pigs. Cloning Stem Cells 5: 117–121.
8. Theoret CL, Dore M, Mulon PY, Desrochers A, Viramontes F, et al. (2006) Short- and long-term skin graft survival in cattle clones with different mitochondrial haplotypes. Theriogenology 65: 1465–1479.
9. Hong SG, Jang G, Kim MK, Oh HJ, Park JE, et al. (2009) Dogs cloned from fetal fibroblasts by nuclear transfer. Anim Reprod Sci 115: 334–339.
10. Burnett RC, DeRose SA, Wagner JL, Storb R (1997) Molecular analysis of six dog leukocyte antigen class I sequences including three complete genes, two truncated genes and one full-length processed gene. Tissue Antigens 49: 484–495.
11. Kennedy LJ (2007) 14th International HLA and Immunogenetics Workshop: report on joint study on canine DLA diversity. Tissue Antigens 69 Suppl 1: 269–271.
12. Ogawa H, Galili U (2006) Profiling terminal N-acetyllactosamines of glycans on mammalian cells by an immuno-enzymatic assay. Glycoconj J 23: 663–674.
13. Gluckman JC (1980) [Modification of mixed lymphocyte reactivity between DLA-identical dog sibs, after in vivo sensitization]. C R Seances Acad Sci D 290: 105–108.
14. Kolb HJ, Rieder I, Grosse-Wilde H, Scholz S, Kolb H, et al. (1975) Canine marrow grafts in donor-recipient combinations with one-way nonstimulation in mixed lymphocyte culture. Transplant Proc 7: 461–464.
15. Widmer MB, Bach FH (1972) Allogeneic and xenogeneic response in mixed leukocyte cultures. J Exp Med 135: 1204–1208.
16. Do M, Jang WG, Hwang JH, Jang H, Kim EJ, et al. (2012) Inheritance of mitochondrial DNA in serially recloned pigs by somatic cell nuclear transfer (SCNT). Biochem Biophys Res Commun 424: 765–770.
17. Hiendleder S (2007) Mitochondrial DNA inheritance after SCNT. Adv Exp Med Biol 591: 103–116.
18. Chan T, Fischer Lindahl K (1985) Skin graft rejection caused by the maternally transmitted antigen Mta. Transplantation 39: 477–480.
19. Lindahl KF, Burki K (1982) Mta, a maternally inherited cell surface antigen of the mouse, is transmitted in the egg. Proc Natl Acad Sci U S A 79: 5362–5366.
20. Andersson G, Illigens BM, Johnson KW, Calderhead D, LeGuern C, et al. (2003) Nonmyeloablative conditioning is sufficient to allow engraftment of EGFP-expressing bone marrow and subsequent acceptance of EGFP-transgenic skin grafts in mice. Blood 101: 4305–4312.
21. Rideout WM 3rd, Hochedlinger K, Kyba M, Daley GQ, Jaenisch R (2002) Correction of a genetic defect by nuclear transplantation and combined cell and gene therapy. Cell 109: 17–27.
22. Hanna J, Wernig M, Markoulaki S, Sun CW, Meissner A, et al. (2007) Treatment of sickle cell anemia mouse model with iPS cells generated from autologous skin. Science 318: 1920–1923.
23. Zhao T, Zhang ZN, Rong Z, Xu Y (2011) Immunogenicity of induced pluripotent stem cells. Nature 474: 212–215.
24. Ishikawa K, Toyama-Sorimachi N, Nakada K, Morimoto M, Imanishi H, et al. (2010) The innate immune system in host mice targets cells with allogenic mitochondrial DNA. J Exp Med 207: 2297–2305.
25. Loveland B, Wang CR, Yonekawa H, Hermel E, Lindahl KF (1990) Maternally transmitted histocompatibility antigen of mice: a hydrophobic peptide of a mitochondrially encoded protein. Cell 60: 971–980.
26. Webb KM, Allard MW (2009) Mitochondrial genome DNA analysis of the domestic dog: identifying informative SNPs outside of the control region. J Forensic Sci 54: 275–288.
27. Lanza RP, Chung HY, Yoo JJ, Wettstein PJ, Blackwell C, et al. (2002) Generation of histocompatible tissues using nuclear transplantation. Nat Biotechnol 20: 689–696.
28. Oiso N, Fukai K, Kawada A, Suzuki T (2013) Piebaldism. J Dermatol 40: 330–335.
29. Lu F, Gao JH, Mizuro H, Ogawa R, Hyakusoku H (2007) [Experimental study of adipose tissue differentiation using adipose-derived stem cells harvested from GFP transgenic mice]. Zhonghua Zheng Xing Wai Ke Za Zhi 23: 412–416.
30. Stripecke R, Carmen Villacres M, Skelton D, Satake N, Halene S, et al. (1999) Immune response to green fluorescent protein: implications for gene therapy. Gene Ther 6: 1305–1312.
31. Riddell SR, Elliott M, Lewinsohn DA, Gilbert MJ, Wilson L, et al. (1996) T-cell mediated rejection of gene-modified HIV-specific cytotoxic T lymphocytes in HIV-infected patients. Nat Med 2: 216–223.
32. Bonini C, Ferrari G, Verzeletti S, Servida P, Zappone E, et al. (1997) HSV-TK gene transfer into donor lymphocytes for control of allogeneic graft-versus-leukemia. Science 276: 1719–1724.

Permissions

List of Contributors

Patricia Keiko Saito, Roger Haruki Yamakawa and Sueli Donizete Borelli
Department of Basic Health Sciences, Universidade Estadual de Maringá, Maringá, Paraná, Brazil

Erica Pereira Aparecida
Histogene Laboratory of Histocompatibility and Genetics, Maringá, Paraná, Brazil

Waldir Verissimo da Silva Júnior
Department of Statistics, Universidade Estadual de Maringá, Maringá, Paraná, Brazil

Katy Trébern-Launay, Yohann Foucher, Magali Giral, Jean-Paul Soulillou and Jacques Dantal
Institut de Transplantation Urologie Néphrologie (ITUN), Inserm U643, CHU Hôtel Dieu, Nantes, France

Katy Trébern-Launay and Yohann Foucher
Université de Nantes, EA4275 'Biostatistique, Recherche Clinique et Mesures Subjectives en Santé ', Nantes, France

Christophe Legendre and Henri Kreis
Service de Transplantation Rénale et de Soins Intensifs, Hôpital Necker, APHP, Paris, France

Christophe Legendre
Université´s Paris Descartes et Sorbonne Paris Cité, Paris, France

Michè le Kessler and Marc Ladrière
Service de Transplantation Rénale, CHU Brabois, Nancy, France

Nassim Kamar and Lionel Rostaing
Service de Néphrologie, HTA, Dialyse et Transplantation d'Organes, CHU Rangueil, Toulouse, France
Université Paul Sabatier, Toulouse, France

Valérie Garrigue and Georges Mourad
Service de Néphrologie-Transplantation, Hôpital Lapeyronie, Montpellier, France

Emmanuel Morelon
Service de Néphrologie, Transplantation et Immunologie Clinique, Hôpital Edouard Herriot, Lyon, France

Matthias Schaier, Nicole Seissler, Friederike Hug and Martin Zeier
Department of Nephrology, University of Heidelberg, Heidelberg, Germany

Edgar Schmitt
Institute of Immunology, University of Mainz, Mainz, Germany

Stefan Meuer
Institute of Immunology, University of Heidelberg, Heidelberg, Germany

Andrea Steinborn
Department of Obstetrics and Gynecology, University of Heidelberg, Heidelberg, Germany

Ivana R. Ferrer, Maylene E. Wagener, Mingqing Song and Mandy L. Ford
Emory Transplant Center and Department of Surgery, Emory University, Atlanta, Georgia, United States of America

Jenea M. Bin, Soo Yuen Leong, Sarah-Jane Bull, Jack P. Antel and Timothy E. Kennedy
Department of Neurology and Neurosurgery, Montreal Neurological Institute, McGill University, Montreal, Quebec, Canada

Mika Kijima, Noémie Gardiol and Werner Held
Ludwig Center for Cancer Research of the University of Lausanne, Epalinges, Switzerland

Silke Roedder, Szu-Chuan Hsieh and Minnie M. Sarwal
Transplant Research Program Sutter Health Care, California Pacific Medical Center, San Francisco, California, United States of America

Naoyuki Kimura, Homare Okamura and Yongquan Gong
Department of Cardiothoracic Surgery, Stanford University School of Medicine, Stanford, California, United States of America

Beda Muehleisen, Shang Brian Jiang, Julie A. Gladsjo, Monika Gerber, Tissa Hata and Richard L. Gallo
Division of Dermatology, University of California San Diego, La Jolla, California, United States of America

Beda Muehleisen
Department of Dermatology, Zurich University Hospital, Zurich, Switzerland

Richard L. Gallo
Department of Medicine, University of California San Diego, La Jolla, California, United States of America

Richard L. Gallo
Veterans Administration San Diego Healthcare System, San Diego, California, United States of America

Roy Eldor, Roy Abel, Dror Sever, Gad Sadoun and Danielle Melloul
Department of Endocrinology, Hadassah University Hospital, Jerusalem, Israel

Amnon Peled
Goldyne Savad Institute of Gene Therapy, Hadassah University Hospital, Jerusalem, Israel

Ronit Sionov
Department of Biochemistry and Molecular Biology, IMRIC, Hebrew University-Hadassah Medical School, Jerusalem, Israel

Carlos A. Labarrere, Gonzalo L. Campana and Miguel A. Ortiz
Experimental Pathology, Methodist Research Institute, Indiana University Health Methodist Hospital, Indianapolis, Indiana, United States of America

John R. Woods
Outcomes Research, Methodist Research Institute, Indiana University Health Methodist Hospital, Indianapolis, Indiana, United States of America

James W. Hardin
Epidemiology and Biostatistics, University of South Carolina, Columbia, South Carolina, United States of America

Beate R. Jaeger
Dr. Stein und Kollegen, Mönchengladbach, Germany

Lee Ann Baldridge
Department of Pathology and Laboratory Medicine, Indiana University School of Medicine, Indianapolis, Indiana, United States of America

Douglas E. Pitts
St Vincent Medical Group, St Vincent Hospital, Indianapolis, Indiana, United States of America

Philip C. Kirlin
Transplant Center, Indiana University Health Methodist Hospital, Indianapolis, Indiana, United States of America

Benoit Favier, Kiave-Yune HoWangYin, Julien Caumartin, Marina Daouya, Edgardo D. Carosella and Joel LeMaoult
CEA-I2BM-Service de Recherches en Hemato-Immunologie, Paris, France

Institut Universitaire d'Hematologie, Hopital Saint Louis, Paris, France

Kiave-Yune HoWangYins
Biology and Biotechnology Ph.D. Program, University Paris 7, Paris, France

Anatolij Horuzsko
Center for Molecular Chaperone/Radiobiology and Cancer Virology, Georgia Health Science University, Augusta, Georgia, United States of America

Yan Sun, Chong-Chong Xu, Lu Gao, Li-Xiang Ma, Rui-Xi Li and Yu-Wen Peng
Department of Anatomy, Histology and Embryology, Shanghai Medical College, Fudan University, Shanghai, China

Jin Li
Institutes of Biomedical Sciences, Fudan University, Shanghai, China

Xi-Yin Guan and Guo-Pei Zhu
Department of Radiation Oncology, Shanghai Cancer Hospital, Fudan University, Shanghai, China

Qiquan Sun, Song Jiang, Xue Li, Xianghua Huang, Kenan Xie, Dongrui Cheng, Jinsong Chen, Shuming Ji, Jiqiu Wen, Mingchao Zhang, Caihong Zeng and Zhihong Liu
Research Institute of Nephrology, Jinling Hospital, Nanjing University School of Medicine, Nanjing, China

Alireza Pouya, Leila Satarian, Sahar Kiani, Mohammad Javan and Hossein Baharvand
Department of Stem Cells and Developmental Biology, Cell Science Research Center, Royan Institute for Stem Cell Biology and Technology, ACECR, Tehran, Iran

Leila Satarian and Mohammad Javan
Department of Physiology, Faculty of Medical Sciences, Tarbiat Modares University, Tehran, Iran

Hossein Baharvand
Department of Developmental Biology, University of Science and Culture, ACECR, Tehran, Iran

Eric Bartee and Grant McFadden
Department of Molecular Genetics and Microbiology, University of Florida, College of Medicine, Gainesville, Florida, United States of America

Amy Meacham, Elizabeth Wise and Christopher R. Cogle
Division of Hematology/Oncology, Department of Medicine, University of Florida, College of Medicine, Gainesville, Florida, United States of America

Huijun Ying, Hongmei Fu and Federica M. Marelli-Berg
Department of Immunology, Division of Medicine, Imperial College London, Hammersmith Campus, London, United Kingdom

Marlene L. Rose, Ann M. McCormack and Padmini Sarathchandra
National Heart and Lung Institute, Division of Medicine, Imperial College London, Harefield Hospital, London, United Kingdom

Klaus Okkenhaug
Laboratory of Lymphocyte Signalling and Development, Babraham Institute, Cambridge, United Kingdom

Sylvia Sanquer, Laurence Herry, Celine Lena, Alphonsine Diouf and Robert Barouki
Service de Biochimie Métabolomique et Protéomique, Hôpital Universitaire Necker-Enfants Malades Assistance Publique-Hôpitaux de Paris (AP-HP); INSERM UMR-S 747; and Université Paris Descartes, Centre Universitaire des Saints-Pères, Paris, France

Catherine Amrein, Romain Guillemain and Veronique Boussaud
Service de Chirurgie Cardio-Vasculaire, Hô pital Européen Georges Pompidou, AP-HP, Paris, France

Dominique Grenet, Bruno Philippe and Marc Stern
Service de Pneumologie, Hôpital Foch, Suresnes, France

Michelle Paunet
Laboratoire de Biologie, Hôpital Foch, Suresnes, France

Eliane M. Billaud
Service de Pharmacologie, Hôpital Européen Georges Pompidou, AP-HP and Université Paris Descartes, Paris, France

Franc̦oise Loriaux
Service de Biochimie, Hô pital Européen Georges Pompidou, AP-HP, Paris, France

Jean-Philippe Jais
Service de Biostatistiques, Hôpital Necker-Enfants Malades, AP-HP, Paris, France; Université Paris Descartes, Paris, France

Hiromichi Maeda, Masatoshi Shigoka, Yongchun Wang, Yingxin Fu, Russell N. Wesson, Qing Lin, Robert A. Montgomery and Zhaoli Sun
Department of Surgery, Johns Hopkins University School of Medicine, Baltimore, Maryland, United States of America

Hiromichi Maeda
Department of Surgery, Kochi Medical School, Nankoku, Kochi, Japan

Hiromichi Maeda
Cancer Treatment Center, Kochi Medical School, Nankoku, Kochi, Japan

Hideaki Enzan
Diagnostic Pathology, Chikamori Hospital, Kochi, Kochi, Japan

Fang Wei, Fen Liu, Huaidong Hu, Hong Ren and Peng Hu
Department of infectious Disease, Institute for Viral hepatitis, Key Laboratory of Molecular Biology for infectious disease, The second Affiliated Hospital of Chongqing Medical University, Chongqing, PR China

Junying Liu
Department of Gastroenterology, The Central hospital of Zhoukou, Henan Province, China

Stéphanie Lacotte, Graziano Oldani, Florence Slits, Lorenzo A. Orci, Philippe Morel, Gilles Mentha and Christian Tos
Department of Surgery, Geneva University Hospitals, University of Geneva, Geneva, Switzerland

Laura Rubbia-Brandt
Hepato-pancreato-biliary Centre, Geneva University Hospitals, University of Geneva, Geneva, Switzerland

Laura Rubbia-Brandt, Philippe Morel, Gilles Mentha and Christian Tos
Department of Pathology, Geneva University Hospitals, University of Geneva, Geneva, Switzerland

Xiaobo Yu, Lin Zhou and Yifan Dai
Key Lab of Combined Multi-Organ Transplantation, Ministry of Public Health, the First Affiliated Hospital, School of Medicine, Zhejiang University, Hangzhou, Zhejiang, China

Bajin Wei, Min Zhang, Jian Wu, Xiao Xu, Guoping Jiang and Shusen Zheng
Division of Hepatobiliary and Pancreatic Surgery, Department of Surgery, the First Affiliated Hospital, School of Medicine, Zhejiang University, Hangzhou, Zhejiang, China

Fumika Takasato, Rimpei Morita, Takashi Schichita, Takashi Sekiya and Akihiko Yoshimura
Department of Microbiology and Immunology, Keio University School of Medicine, Tokyo, Japan

Fumika Takasato
Department of Pediatric Surgery, Keio University School of Medicine, Tokyo, Japan

Yasuhide Morikawa
Department of Pediatric Surgery, International University Medical Welfare Hospital, Nasushiobara, Tochigi, Japan

Masanori Niimi
Department of Surgery, Teikyo University School of Medicine, Tokyo, Japan

Fumika Takasato, Rimpei Morita, Takashi Schichita, Takashi Sekiya and Akihiko Yoshimuras
Japan Science and Technology Agency, CREST, Tokyo, Japan

Steven R. White, Timothy Floreth and Chuanhong Liao
Departments of Medicine and Health Studies, University of Chicago, Chicago, Illinois, United States of America

Sangeeta M. Bhorade
Department of Medicine, Northwestern University, Chicago, Illinois, United States of America

Simnikiwe H. Mayaphi, Marieke Braue, Daniel M. Morobadi, Ahmad H. Mazanderani and Rendani T. Mafuyeka
Department of Medical Virology, University of Pretoria/National Health Laboratory Service - Tshwane Academic Division (NHLS-TAD), Pretoria, South Africa

Steve A. S. Olorunju
Biostatistics unit, Medical Research Council, Pretoria, South Africa

Gregory R. Tintinger and Anton Stoltz
Department of Internal Medicine, University of Pretoria, Pretoria, South Africa

Geon A Kim, Hyun Ju Oh, Min Jung Kim, Young Kwang Jo, Jin Choi, Jung Eun Park, Eun Jung Park, Goo Jang and Byeong Chun Lee
Department of Theriogenology and Biotechnology, College of Veterinary Medicine, Seoul National University, Seoul, Republic of Korea

Sang Hyun Lim and Sung Keun Kang
Central Research Institutes, Kstem cell, Seoul, Republic of Korea

Byung Il Yoon
Laboratory of Histology and Molecular Pathogenesis, College of Veterinary Medicine, Kangwon National University, Chuncheon, Gangwon-do, Republic of Korea

Index